The object of education is not learning, but discipline
and enlightenment of the mind.

Woodrow Wilson

ACKNOWLEDGMENTS

The writing and editing of a comprehensive text is a complex and tedious process that requires considerable skill and monumental effort. Work on the fifth edition began about two years ago with the assignment of chapters to those physicians listed as "Contributors." Their task was to review the chapters, conduct research into current academic texts and literature and then, make recommendations for changes. Once manuscript is submitted, the editorial work begins. This is an extensive process that involves qualifying, verifying, updating and revising the academic material before "distilling it" into a concise and accurate board-oriented text. Chapters that require further investigation prior to publication are sent to specific physician editors with special expertise in designated areas for final content approval; these physicians are listed as "Associate Editors". The entire manuscript is again re-edited and proofed by the Senior Editor and Editor-in-Chief before being sent to the printer.

Dr. John Howell is the Senior Editor in this edition. His expertise as author and editor is evidenced in his own emergency medicine textbook, Emergency Medicine published in 1998 by W.B. Saunders. I have personally used this as a reference source for three editions of this text. I admire his work and feel very fortunate to have him on board.

Dr. Roger Barkin is a well-known name in pediatric emergency medicine. He has authored several texts in this subspecialty of emergency medicine, all of which I have on my bookshelf. Pediatrics has been one of the weaker areas in EM for those EPs without much exposure to this population of patients. Dr. Barkin was kind enough to review this chapter and provide his expertise.

Without the contributors, I would not have the opportunity to review valuable input from some of the best and brightest emergency physicians it has been my pleasure to know. These EPs research the existing content and submit new/revised content that is state-of-the-art data that I need to consider for inclusion in each new edition. Several new contributors were provided by Dr. Howell and their fresh perspective is greatly appreciated.

Since EMEE is its own publishing company, special services are required to turn the manuscript into a book. All of the services (and service companies) we use are located in Cincinnati. I would like to thank my staff, Susan Cappa, my right hand assistant who organizes and coordinates all aspects of book production. Her skills and dedication are key ingredients to our success. I also am grateful to Bernice Hill for her detailed final proofing of the book . Although not directly involved in book production, a special thanks to Ann Campbell who is responsible for order-taking and processing as well as answering your questions in a kind, caring and considerate manner; she refers to all of you as "my Doctors." The book design and format has been provided by Sue Mitchell, Vice-President, Design Centre of Cincinnati, Inc. Ms. Mitchell designed the book cover and created the original text format with a computer software program. She is also credited with the design and format of our oral board book. Her creative ability and dedication to quality production will always be remembered. Rob Krehbiel, President of Krehbiel Printing Company, is an old friend. He has orchestrated book production for all editions of this text as well as the last seven editions of the oral board book. We keep going back to him because we can depend on books that are professional in appearance, quality bound. . . and delivered on time.

Finally, I would like to thank my associate, mentor and dear friend, June M. Hodge, B.A., M.A. My colleagues call her my "secret ingredient" and, indeed, she is. Thirty years ago, June awakened the "teacher" in me and predicted that I would become a medical educator. A gifted educator herself, she taught me how to teach and encouraged me to write the first book. Today, she manages the business of EMEE and, as vice-president of the company, assures you, our customer, the highest quality in our products and services. Without her, you would not be holding this book in your hands right now.

My sincere thanks to all of you.

Carol S. Rivers, M.D.
Editor-in-Chief
President, EMEE, Inc.

FOREWORD

This book was written and compiled to fill a need — the need for a teaching textbook (not another reference book) aimed directly at the written board examination (not the entire field of emergency medicine) and designed for the busy physician (not the average medical student) who has little time to devote to study and whose study time comes in unequal segments.

I did not understand the need for such a text myself back in 1987 when I began receiving letters and phone calls asking for study material for the written board exam in emergency medicine. Several good emergency medicine textbooks were already in print. Judy Tintinalli's Text: <u>Comprehensive Study Guide in Emergency Medicine</u> and Peter Rosen's <u>Emergency Medicine: Concepts and Clinical Practice</u> were then, and still are, standard reference sources in our specialty. Furthermore, almost every ACEP chapter sponsored a written board course — an intensive five-day review of the body of knowledge in emergency medicine. In addition, there were independent aids (tapes, study programs and review courses) designed to prepare the emergency physician for the written exam. In spite of this, a number of my colleagues continued to express the need for "something else."

The major characteristics of that "something else" finally began to take shape. It had to be something that did not require plowing through from cover to cover, as with the usual textbook. It had to be easy to read and retain important detail. It had to discriminate, to distinguish the material important to the exam from what is not. And, unlike courses — most of which are given a few weeks before the exam, leaving too little time for review — it had to be available any time.

At this point, I plunged into an analysis of available publications and courses. I interviewed physicians who had used more than one review source in their preparation. I discovered that all of the printed sources were of value, some more than others and, if a physician used all the sources, a passing score on the exam was likely — but at a terrible cost in time and energy. It seemed that every text had its own strengths and weaknesses... and none seemed to be succinctly focused on the exam itself.

By the end of 1987, I decided a book was needed that would focus the examinee's attention and time on the material crucial to the exam — and I began to lay the foundation for building the book. I selected 16 board-certified emergency physicians (contributors and editors) who agreed to specialize in specific aspects of the examination. With their assignments in hand, the writers researched their topics, searching for facts and concepts pertinent to the exam. The primary reference sources, Tintinalli's Text and Rosen's Text, were supplemented by notes taken from written board courses and similar programs. The chapters were written, edited, re-written and re-edited — and then re-written and re-edited again — until the editors felt that we had what was needed.

The response to the first edition (published in 1992) was most gratifying. There was, indeed, a need for a board-oriented text. The following year sales doubled which, in my judgment, was sufficient evidence that, those who had used it the previous year, passed the exam. The book also found its way into residency programs where I was delighted to discover an improvement in residency in-service exam scores for those residents who were studying from the text.

In the third edition, we added a new major reference source, the Core Curriculum (published in 1999) since we felt this text covered the new topics contained in the revised Core Content (published in 1997). In the fourth edition, we cross-checked the Core Content with the components of the EM Model (published in 2001) to make sure we included all of the revisions necessary for you to do well on the exam. In this edition, we have incorporated material from ABEM's LLSA-reading lists (2004-2006) we feel is likely to be tested on the ConCert exam. We continue to use more than thirty major text references because they have proven themselves over time...even as the exam changes. We are confident that, with adequate study of this two-volume review text, you will have a solid foundation for your exam preparation.

Carol S. Rivers, M.D.
Editor-in-Chief
President EMEE, Inc.

INTRODUCTION

This book has been written primarily for the emergency physician who is preparing for the written certification exam or the written recertification exam (as well as for residents preparing for in-service exams) in emergency medicine. Its purpose is to provide a concise, focused review of material that usually appears on these exams. Information that may seem "basic" is included because it is essential to your understanding of principles and concepts that are important parts of the exam.

While this book has been used as a reference text, it is primarily a teaching text. The largest division of the book — the academic review section — is essentially a set of notes that contain the knowledge you must have to pass the exam. I suggest you treat them as notes—as your own notes. Read them with a pen, pencil or highlighter in hand. Underline or highlight information you especially want to remember. Use the space provided for writing notes of your own. As you read, you will notice that some material is repeated—on purpose. A teaching text requires some redundancy for emphasis and coherence.

The fifth edition is an expanded and updated revision of the prior editions. A few new topics have been added that are pertinent to both the board exam and the residency in-service exams. Outdated information has been removed and controversial issues have been clarified wherever possible. To enhance clinical acuity for the resident in training, a few bedside diagnostic techniques (in addition to descriptions of selected procedures) are included. The remaining text is essentially unchanged except for those changes required to bring the content in line with the EM Model.

You will be asked to use other materials periodically. Depending on how much time you have to prepare for this exam, (see "Recommended Study Plan"), you may find the following reference and self-assessment books helpful:

1. Tintinalli, et.al., <u>Emergency Medicine: A Comprehensive Study Guide</u>, Sixth ed. (Mosby). Referred to in this text as Tintinalli's Text, Sixth ed.

2. Marx, et. al., <u>Rosen's Emergency Medicine: Concepts and Clinical Practice</u>, Fifth ed., 3 vols. (Mosby). Referred to in this text as Rosen's Text, Fifth ed.

3. Peer VI self-assessment booklet (ACEP).*

4. These and other reference sources you may find useful are listed on our website under "Resources."

*Peer VII is scheduled for publication in mid-2006.

These are complementary texts. If I ask you to review a particular subject — e.g., LeForte facial fractures — you should go to Tintinalli's and/or Rosen's Text and read the appropriate section. If you find something in either of these texts especially important to your understanding, write it in the "Notes" space in this text (which is found at the end of every chapter in the "Condensed Academic Review"). Another text that has become popular with practicing emergency physicians is Ann Harwood's, The Clinical Practice of Emergency Medicine published by Lippincott (Philadelphia). In general, it is easier to read than Tintinalli or Rosen and utilizes a numbered, itemized format similar to that found in this text. There are two additional features that separate Harwood's text from Tintinalli and Rosen: indications for admission as well as "Pearls and Pitfalls."

The Peer VI (and soon-to-be-published Peer VII) self-assessment booklets are valuable in your preparation because they reacquaint you with the process of answering multiple-choice questions and help you define areas of weakness that require further study. I will show you how to use these booklets in the following section entitled, "Recommended Study Plan."

There are several radiologic images on the written exam. Whenever possible, I have noted those that merit review. As you read the "Condensed Academic Review" section of the text, I recommend that you have a pad of note paper and a pen handy. As you come to a paragraph where an x-ray or CT review of a particular entity is recommended, jot it down. When you have completed your list, show it to your favorite radiologist and ask him or her to pull sample films for you to review. I suggest that you set aside a morning or afternoon on one of your "off" days when the radiologist can be available to review these films with you. The best way to conduct this review session is to ask the radiologist to let you read the films. If you miss something, have the radiologist show you what you missed (or misread) and ask that he teach you how to pick it up or interpret it correctly the next time you see it. This is important for you to do because the x-rays, CT and MRI prints on the exam are not usually taken from standard textbooks; they usually come from teaching files. If, after your review session with the radiologist, you are still uncertain about your ability to recognize a specific abnormality (e.g., epiglottitis), ask the radiologist to call you when he comes across one or more of these films during his daily x-ray reading time. If you do this, your ability to read films will improve and you are likely to recognize radiographic abnormalities on prints in the exam booklet. A good text reference is The Radiology of Emergency Medicine by Harris and Harris. You can also view x-rays, CTs and MRIs online on MedPix™, a medical image database supported by the Uniformed Services University Department of Radiology (see link on our website under "resources").

In addition to radiologic images, ECGs and other pictorials are presented on the exam. Again, when I ask you to find sample tracings or prints, I will also tell you (whenever possible) where to look for them or who can help you find and interpret them. Also, you may want to attend a written board course that provides pictorials and a syllabus that contains dozens of ECGs. Several emergency physicians have written or called to ask why ECGs, x-rays, scans and derm photos are not included in this text. You may need to review several examples of a particular entity in order to identify it accurately on the exam. The American College of Cardiology offers a self-assessment course in ECG interpretation — a good course for those who need a solid review. An ECG text that has been recommended is <u>The ECG in Emergency Decision Making</u> by Wellens & Conover (published by Saunders). Board prep courses have <u>hundreds</u> of photos and ECGs that are ideal for many participants. If a course is not feasible, Ohio ACEP has published a book called <u>Photo and X-ray Stimuli for Emergency Medicine</u>. It contains over 200 high-quality photos accompanied by clinical presentations. Answers are provided in separate sections of the book. Another <u>excellent</u> pictorial source is <u>Atlas of Emergency Medicine</u> (Knoop, Stack and Storrow) published by McGraw-Hill. In addition to clinical presentations, each entity includes a differential diagnosis, ED treatment and disposition as well as clinical pearls.

A special feature of this text, found throughout the "Condensed Academic Review," is visual imagery. Clinical presentations of specific diagnoses are presented in a story-telling style called "Clinical Pictures." This concept is based on "the simple chain technique," the object of which is to "chain" or link one item to the next in the order you wish to remember them. Basically, this chain is a story that involves all the items you want to remember in a particular sequence. You will be able to do this by using mental images and tying each item to the next as you move through the story.

How does the chaining technique work? One item acts as a stimulus (or cue) for the next item. It's almost like seeing a slide show or a movie in your mind's eye, where you can automatically anticipate the next scene. You don't have to strain your mental faculty searching for it; it's right there.

Chaining has been tested in scientific studies which have verified its effectiveness as a memory-enhancing tool for simple rote memory tasks. In this respect, imagery is probably the single most important aspect of memory training. In numerous studies, one group of students would be shown pictures of an array of items to remember, and the other group would simply be given a list of words to remember. Both groups would be given the same test to determine what they remembered. The people who had been given images consistently scored higher than those who had been given lists. The important point here is that vivid images of items will improve your memory of those items.

Why should the seemingly insignificant procedure of linking one item to another dramatically improve recall? The answer is found to be in the linking itself. Separate pieces of information become unified when connected to each other. In other words, when 20 pieces of information are presented separately, you have to remember 20 independent segments of information. But when we link the items together, as we do in chaining, the 20 items actually represent only one segment of data.

Now, some areas of this text do contain memory recall facts (i.e., lists) and they are unavoidable. However, these "lists" are easier to remember when they are mixed with imagery. Pure memorizing is a left-brain function. Imagery is a right brain function. When combined, the reader remembers more detail.

Before you begin reading this text, briefly scan each of the sections so that you can get an overview of the information presented. You might want to read the nonclinical/non-academic sections first since other activities are discussed there and you will want to allow time to schedule some or all of them in the time prior to the exam. You have enough information in this text to pass the exam, but other activities can help you as well. So pick and choose those that sound worthwhile and then plan your time to include them in your final preparation for this exam.

TO THE RESIDENT IN TRAINING

When this text was originally written in the late 1980s, it was primarily intended for the practicing emergency physician preparing for the written board exam in emergency medicine. However, I also had the resident in mind because this is what I would want as a resident today. As it was, I had Dr. Judy Tintinalli's "Study Guide" in the early 1970s and it was a godsend. I read it over and over again until I had it inside me. It was my "EM Model" and I carried it with me wherever I went, including Detroit to hear lectures from Dr. Tintinalli herself. Much of this text grew out of those early Tintinalli years in Michigan. Today, of course, her study guide is a major textbook; as the specialty grew, so did her writing. Her work has always been a major reference source for me and thousands of other emergency physicians.

But a "study guide", a primer, is still needed. A resident still needs a basic "nuts and bolts" manual or text from which to learn. The specialty is now almost 40 years old and there are almost as many texts in emergency medicine, most of them comprehensive. In addition, we have had an explosion of technological advances and pharmaceutical agents in the last twenty years. An attempt to learn it all at once would be overwhelming. A primer, on the other hand, provides a foundation from which to begin building an academic database....and the best time to begin using a primer is during training.

Since this text has always been board-oriented, it only made sense that the content would also be aligned with preparation for the inservice exams. Based on feedback we have received, this appears to be the case. Test scores are good and, in some cases, great (10-15% improvement over previous test scores); that can mean a difference of passing or failing or receiving a high score rather than an average one. What's important about this is that many residents are not using any other material to prepare for their exam, which makes the studying process easier.

What this two-volume text is <u>not</u>, is an "all-you-need-to-know-in-emergency-medicine" source. As stated, it is a primer which, by definition, is a place from which to start. When you need more information on a specific topic, it's time to go to reference sources. I recommend Tintinalli and Rosen as first choices. Your faculty physicians will acquaint you with several textbooks as well as other reference material; they can teach you how to become a life-long student.

Take advantage of their knowledge and expertise as academic emergency physicians; ask them how they would reference a topic as a resident in training. Then use this text to add new information; it was designed for that purpose (double spacing, wide margins, blank spaces and pages). In other words, build your own book. This is the best way to really learn, to get it inside of you so that it is with you at the bedside.... where it counts.

Learning is a journey that never ends. Good study habits make the progression easier and more rewarding. Decide now to make this a top priority as you begin your career in emergency medicine. I promise it will serve you well.

Carol S. Rivers, M.D.
Editor-in-Chief
President EMEE, Inc.

RECOMMENDED STUDY PLAN

Engage in regular and consistent study. Learning is acquired by studying over a reasonable period of time. What is learned in a hurry is seldom completely learned and is soon forgotten. Do not "cram" for this exam. Cramming is an attempt to learn in a very short period of time (8 - 10 hours a day in spurts) what should have been learned through regular and consistent study over a period of weeks or months. Cramming seldom pays off in terms of effective learning. It is likely that you will be more confused than prepared on the day of the exam if you have "cram-studied."

Before you start reading this text, an organized approach will be helpful in order to maximize your time and effort. To begin with, you need to be aware that the chapters in the "Condensed Academic Review" appear in a specific order, i.e. the most important chapter is the first one and the least important chapter is the last one: 11% of the questions on the exam cover "Cardiovascular Emergencies" and only 1% of the questions cover "Dermatologic Emergencies." It follows, therefore, that you need to concentrate more on the first ten chapters than the last ten chapters. Take a good look at the following list. You will be referring to it periodically while you are studying.

Written Board Topics Covered By Percentages

1. *Cardiovascular Emergencies* *11%*
2. *ENT, Maxillofacial, Dental Emergencies* *8%*
3. *Pediatric Emergencies* *8%*
4. *Gastrointestinal Emergencies* *7%*
5. *Pulmonary Emergencies* *7%*
6. *Orthopedic Emergencies* *7%*
7. *Major Trauma* *7%*
8. *Urogenital Emergencies* *7%*
9. *EMS and Emergency Dept. Administration* *5%*
10. *Neurologic Emergencies* *5%*
11. *Fluid and Electrolyte Emergencies* *4%*
12. *Toxicologic Emergencies* *4%*
13. *Behavioral Emergencies* *3%*
14. *Eye Emergencies* *3%*
15. *Ethical-Legal Aspects of Emergency Medicine* *3%*
16. *Metabolic and Allergic Emergencies* *3%*
17. *Environmental Emergencies* *3%*
18. *Hematologic/Oncologic Emergencies* *2%*
19. *Physician-Patient Interactive Skills* *2%*
20. *Dermatologic Emergencies* *1%*

Prior to 2002, the "Core Content Categories" served as the basis of the topics covered on ABEM's Written Board Exam. This has been changed to the "Model of the Clinical Practice of Emergency Medicine" (The EM Model) and the categories/topics are listed as "Conditions & Components" below. This is a shorter list than the old Core Content. The reason is that some topics have been incorporated into the remaining topics and others have been given a new name.

Listing of Conditions & Components

1.0	Signs, Symptoms and Presentations	9%
2.0	Abdominal and Gastrointestinal Disorders	9%
3.0	Cardiovascular Disorders	10%
4.0	Cutaneous Disorders	2%
5.0	Endocrine, Metabolic and Nutritional Disorders	3%
6.0	Environmental Disorders	3%
7.0	Head, Ear, Eye, Nose & Throat Disorders	5%
8.0	Hematologic Disorders	2%
9.0	Immune System Disorders	2%
10.0	Systemic Infectious Disorders	5%
11.0	Musculoskeletal Disorders (Non-traumatic)	3%
12.0	Nervous System Disorders	5%
13.0	Obstetrics and Gynecology	4%
14.0	Psycho-behavioral Disorders	3%
15.0	Renal and Urogenital Disorders	3%
16.0	Thoracic-Respiratory Disorders	8%
17.0	Toxicologic Disorders	4%
18.0	Traumatic Disorders	11%
	Appendix I: Procedures & Skills	6%
	Appendix II: Other Components	3%
	Total	100%

Do not be concerned about the differences you see in the two lists. The "EM Model" was designed to facilitate the <u>testing</u> process, and the "Specific Topics" in this book were created to facilitate the <u>learning</u> process. The academic content, however, is the <u>same</u> as that of the "EM Model". It's just packaged differently in this text.

The next point you need to consider is this: How much time do you have left before the exam? Check off the time frame that is most appropriate to your situation:

- Less than one month   _____
- One to two months   _____
- Two to three months   _____
- Three months or more   _____

Now that you know which topics are covered most heavily on the written board exam and how much time you have left to study, a methodical approach is in order. There are four steps in this process:

(1) A self-assessment evaluation to determine strong and weak areas.
(2) A comparison of your self-assessment score with an analysis of your current level of preparedness for the exam.
(3) A study plan that includes the number of hours per day and the number of days per week you need to study.
(4) A method of reading and reviewing that promotes high retention and recall of specific information.

These four points will be described in the paragraphs that follow.

Using the time frame that you previously checked off, select the category that pertains to you and read the program outlined therein. That is your program, your study-approach method. I recommend that you do not allow yourself to be distracted by the content written in other categories. It may confuse you and diffuse your focused approach. Some of you, however, will already have a plan in mind and may decide to incorporate parts of the information from within the different categories... and that's fine. But most of you will not have a plan and will be looking for direction. These categories have been written primarily for those of you who don't have a plan. If you're one of them, stick with me...and I'll get you where you need to go.

CATEGORY I (less than one month)

(1) In front of each academic chapter is a series of multiple choice questions. Go through all of the questions throughout the academic section, recording your answers in the book or on a separate sheet of paper. When you're finished, look at the answers at the end of each series of questions and mark which ones you missed. Use the pre-chapter multiple choice question worksheet (on page xxv) to record and determine the percentage of correct answers for each section. Divide the number of correct answers by the total number of questions to get the percent of correct answers; for example, if the total number of questions for a particular chapter is 14 and you correctly answered 11 of them, the calculation is: $11 \div 14 = .785$ (which is 78.5%).

(2) Compare your scores from each chapter with the specific topics covered by percentages to see where you are in the scheme of things:
  (a) 85% or higher is a good score. Review the questions missed and note the correct answers.
  (b) 75 - 85% is pretty good but further study is needed. For the questions you missed, review those particular subjects within the body of that chapter; the questions are in sequence with the text so the material you need to cover will be easy to find.
  (c) Less than 75% is not a good score. Read the entire chapter and then go through all the questions again. If you have still missed some questions, review those subjects again.
  With this approach in mind, start at the top of the list of specific topics (which are in the same order as the chapters) and work your way down. That way you'll cover the most important topics first.

(3) Plan your study schedule. Since you have less than a month, you'll need to study 4 hours/day, six days a week. I recommend that you study in two 2-hour blocks rather than four straight hours at one time. Your retention will be better and you'll have more stamina.

(4) If you have to read a whole chapter or parts of a chapter, do so with a marker or colored pen in hand, underlining or highlighting (or both) important points. Plan to review this material three times. In addition, allow yourself some additional time to read the two sections after the academic review ("Mechanics of the Written Board Exam" and also "Additional Tips for Good Performance"). If you run out of time and can't finish this program, let it go and don't worry about it. You will have covered the most important material in the time given and your chance of passing will be higher than if you tried to cram-study.

(5) A few days before the exam, review all the pre-chapter questions again. Then go through the Critical Qs&As (in flashcard, palm or pocket PC format) and CME questions (look up the answers if you have to). Do not stay up late the night before the exam. You will have better recall ability during the test if you are not tired.

CATEGORY II (one to two months)

(1) In front of each academic chapter is a series of multiple choice questions. Go through all of the questions throughout the academic section, recording your answers in the book or on a separate sheet of paper. When you're finished, look at the answers at the end of each series of questions and mark which ones you missed. Use the pre-chapter multiple choice question worksheet (on page xxv) to record and determine the percentage of correct answers for each section. Divide the number of correct answers by the total number of questions to get the percent of correct answers; for example, if the total number of questions for a particular chapter is 14 and you correctly answered 11 of them, the calculation is: 11 ÷ 14 = .785 (which is 78.5%).

(2) Compare your scores from each chapter with the specific topics covered by percentages to see where you are in the scheme of things:
  (a) 85% or higher is a good score. Review the questions missed and note the correct answers.
  (b) 75 - 85% is pretty good but further study is needed. For the questions you missed, review those particular subjects within the body of that chapter; the questions are in sequence with the text so the material you need to cover will be easy to find.
  (c) Less than 75% is not a good score. Read the entire chapter and then go through all the questions again. If you have still missed some questions, review those subjects again.
  With this approach in mind, start at the top of the list of specific topics (which are in the same order as the chapters) and work your way down. That way you'll cover the most important topics first.

(3) Plan your study schedule. In this time frame, you will need to study 4 hours/day, five days a week. I recommend that you study in two 2 - hour blocks rather than four hours at one sitting. Your retention will be better and you'll have more stamina.

(4) As you go through the academic chapters (either in whole or in part), read with a marker or colored pen in hand, underlining or high-lighting (or both) important points. Set aside some of your study time to read the two sections that follow the academic review ("Mechanics of the Written Board Exam" and "Additional Tips for Good Performance"). When you have finished, go back and reread the material you covered three more times. Be sure to review the x-rays and other pictorials noted in the text, utilizing the recommended sources. If you still have some time left prior to the exam, go through the rest of the academic chapters that you haven't looked at before and look for "pearls" (info that looks important) and any information that clarifies your understanding of a particular subject; review these points a couple of more times and then stop. You're in pretty good shape. Relax.

(5) A week before the exam, take the CME test and see how you do. Verify your answers in the academic chapters (you won't have time to send the CME test in, get it graded and receive the answers and explanations prior to the exam). If you have them, now is the time to go through the Critical Qs&As (in flashcard, palm or pocket PC format).

CATEGORY III (two to three months)

(1) If you don't already have it, obtain the current PEER self-assessment test booklet* from the ACEP headquarters in Dallas. Go through the entire booklet answering all questions. Determine your score by obtaining the percentage of correct answers; divide the number of correct answers by the total number of questions. For example, if the total number of questions is 350 and you correctly answered 275 of them, the calculation is: $275 \div 350 = .785$ (78.5%).

(2) Compare your score with the following analysis to see where you are in the scheme of things.

    (a) 85% or higher is a good score. Review the questions missed, note the correct answers and read the explanations given in the PEER answer book.

    (b) 75 - 85% is a pretty good score but further study is needed. In addition to reading the explanations to incorrect answers, also read the referenced material in Tintinalli's Text itself.

    (c) Less than 75% is not a good score. More extensive study is necessary, especially if several of the missed questions are found in the first eight topics on the list of specific topics covered by percentages; this amounts to 62% of the material covered on the exam. You should read corresponding chapters in the sixth edition of Tintinalli's Text (as well as in this text). Of the remaining twelve chapters, it will be sufficient to read these in their entirety in this book; no other reference is necessary.

(3) Plan your study schedule. If you have about two months, set aside 3 hours/day, five days a week; I recommend that you do not study more than two hours at one sitting because your ability to retain information is likely to diminish after that time. If you have three months to study, 2 hours/day, five days a week should be sufficient.

(4) As you go through the book, use a pen or marker to underline/highlight key points, i.e. information you didn't know or that seems important. Be sure to review the x-rays and other pictorials noted in the text, utilizing the recommended sources. Divide your material into "Easy Reading" and "Hard Reading" categories. An example might be:

Easy Reading	Hard Reading
(a) Mechanics of the Written Board Exam	(a) PEER VI (or VII) test-taking and review
(b) "Light" academic chapters (Derm, EMS-ED administration, etc.)	(b) The first eight academic chapters (especially "Cardiovascular Emergencies")
(c) Additional Tips for Good Performance	(c) Tintinalli's Text reading

Alternate your study time between the two categories. Do "Hard Reading" during one study session and "Easy Reading" the next. This will maximize your learning time as well as allow you to maintain your

*Peer VII is scheduled for publication in mid-2006.

stamina in the long run. When you have finished, go back and reread the entire book, looking especially for "pearls" (info that looks important) and any information that clarifies your understanding of a particular subject. Be sure to go through the questions in front of each academic chapter and record your scores on p. xxv; it will help focus your attention as you read the academic material. If you have time, reread again but, this time only the material you have underlined, high-lighted or otherwise noted... and then stop.

(5) In the final 7 - 10 days prior to the exam, take the CME test and check your answers within the academic content of the text. Go through the Critical Qs&As (in flashcard, palm or pocket PC format) two or three times and stop studying the day before the exam. You're ready.

CATEGORY IV (three months or more)

(1) If you don't already have it, obtain the PEER VI (or PEER VII if available) self-assessment test booklet from the ACEP headquarters in Dallas. Go through the entire booklet answering all the questions, grading yourself on each topic. Determine your score by obtaining the percentage of correct answers for each topic; divide the number of correct answers by the total number of questions. For example, if the total number of questions is 350 and you correctly answered 275 of them, the calculation is: $275 \div 350 = .785$ (78.5%).

(2) Compare your score with the following analysis to see where you are in the scheme of things.

   (a) 85% or higher is a good score. Review the questions missed, note the correct answers and read the explanations given in the PEER answer book.

   (b) 75 - 85% is a pretty good score but further study is needed. In addition to reading the explanations to incorrect answers, also read the referenced material in Tintinalli's Text itself.

   (c) Less than 75% is not a good score. More extensive study is necessary, especially if several of the missed questions are found in the first eight topics on the list of specific topics covered by percentages; this amounts to 62% of the material covered on the exam. You should read corresponding chapters in the sixth edition of Tintinalli's Text (as well as in this text). Of the remaining twelve chapters, it will be sufficient to read these in their entirety in this book; no other reference is necessary.

(3) Plan your study schedule. If you have three to four months prior to the exam, plan on studying 2 hours/day, five days a week. If you have more than four months, 2 hours/day, four days a week is sufficient. You may also want to attend a written board course. (See the section titled, "Additional Tips for Good Performance" for info on written board courses). You have plenty of time and it might be worth it to you.

(4) As you go through the book, use a pen or marker to underline or highlight key points, i.e. info you didn't know or seems important. Be sure to review x-rays and other pictorials noted in the text, utilizing the recommended sources. Divide your material into "Easy Reading" and "Hard Reading" categories. An example might be as follows:

<u>Easy Reading</u>
(a) Mechanics of the Written Board Exam
(b) "Light" academic chapters (Derm, EMS-ED administration, etc.)
(c) Additional Tips for Good Performance

<u>Hard Reading</u>
(a) PEER VI (or VII) test-taking and review
(b) The first eight academic chapters (especially "Cardio-vascular Emergencies")
(c) Tintinalli's Text reading

Alternate your study time between the two categories. Do "Hard Reading" during one study session and "Easy Reading" the next. This will maximize your learning time as well as allow you to maintain your stamina in the long run. When you have finished, go back and reread the entire book, looking especially for "pearls" (info that looks important) and any information that clarifies your understanding of a particular subject. Be sure to go through the questions in front of each academic chapter and record your scores on the next page; it will help focus your attention as you read the academic material. If you have time, reread again but, this time, only material you have underlined, highlighted or otherwise noted...and then stop.

(5) In the last two weeks before the exam, take the CME test. You should do quite well. Be sure to verify your answers with the material in the text. Then go through the Critical Qs&As (in flashcard, palm or pocket PC format) until you know all the answers...then stop studying. You are well prepared.

An important point for <u>all of you</u> to consider (no matter what "category" you are in) is that test-taking skills and strategies can play a significant role in the bottom line...your exam score. Be sure to read "How to Take a Multiple-Choice Exam" in the section titled, "Mechanics of the Written Board Exam." I recommend that you practice using the techniques described for answering questions you don't know. Start first with the questions in this book. If you have time, do the same with the PEER booklet; use other sources as well (CME booklet and Critical Qs&As that supplement this text); some written board courses have hundreds of questions. Under no circumstances do I recommend that you focus your attention on test-taking techniques at the expense of studying the academics of emergency medicine. If your knowledge-base is lacking, no amount of test-taking skill is going to result in a passing score. In addition, these techniques don't work all the time. But if you're one of those candidates that scores 73 - 74% on exam content, knowing how to use test-taking techniques can raise your score another percent or two... just enough to help you pass.

Pre-Chapter Multiple Choice Question Worksheet

Chapter	topic covered by %	# answered correctly	# of pre chapter questions	percent of correct answers	Missed questions to review
Cardiovascular	11%	_____	/ 41	_____	_____
ENT, Maxillofacial, Dental	8%	_____	/ 26	_____	_____
Pediatric	8%	_____	/ 43	_____	_____
Gastrointestinal	7%	_____	/ 40	_____	_____
Pulmonary	7%	_____	/ 30	_____	_____
Orthopedic	7%	_____	/ 36	_____	_____
Major Trauma	7%	_____	/ 21	_____	_____
Urogenital	7%	_____	/ 31	_____	_____
EMS & EDA	5%	_____	/ 16	_____	_____
Neurologic	5%	_____	/ 24	_____	_____
Fluid and Electrolyte	4%	_____	/ 20	_____	_____
Toxicologic	4%	_____	/ 21	_____	_____
Behavioral	3%	_____	/ 15	_____	_____
Eye	3%	_____	/ 30	_____	_____
Ethical-Legal	3%	_____	/ 16	_____	_____
Metabolic/Allergic	3%	_____	/ 20	_____	_____
Environmental	3%	_____	/ 40	_____	_____
Hematologic/Oncologic	2%	_____	/ 25	_____	_____
Physician-Patient	2%	_____	/ 8	_____	_____
Dermatologic	1%	_____	/ 17	_____	_____
Total			520		

Note:

85% or higher is a good score. Review the questions missed and note the correct answers.

75 - 85% is pretty good but further study is needed. For the questions you missed, review those particular subjects within the body of that chapter; the questions are in sequence with the text, so the material you need to cover will be easy to find.

75% or lower is not a good score. Read the entire chapter and then go through all the questions again. If you have still missed some questions, review those subjects again.

A
CONDENSED
ACADEMIC REVIEW

Volume I

CARDIOVASCULAR EMERGENCIES

📖 **Note: Manual Update**

For New ACLS guidelines published after this printing, refer to Written
Board Manual/Guideline Update link on our website - www.emeeinc.com.

---

1. ECG findings of tall hyperacute T waves, wide QRS complexes, flattened P waves and a prolonged PR interval are most consistent with the presence of:
   (a) Hyperkalemia
   (b) Hypokalemia
   (c) Hypercalcemia
   (d) Hypocalcemia

2. The presence on ECG of sagging ST segments, short QT intervals and flattened or inverted T waves is most accurately described as:
   (a) Digitalis effect
   (b) Hypercalcemia
   (c) Signs of digitalis toxicity
   (d) Hypokalemia

3. The treatment of V-Tach and SVT is:
   (a) Lidocaine
   (b) Adenosine
   (c) Cardioversion
   (d) Dependent upon the hemodynamic stability of the patient

4. All of the following are indications for pacemaker therapy except:
   (a) Hemodynamically unstable bradycardia unresponsive to drug therapy
   (b) Overdrive of tachydysrhythmias refractory to drug therapy or electrical cardioversion
   (c) Asymptomatic bifascicular or trifascicular block
   (d) Mobitz II Second-Degree AV block in the presence of an Acute MI

5. The most common cause of failure to pace is:
   (a) Battery depletion
   (b) Oversensing
   (c) Wire fracture
   (d) Undersensing

6. Which of the following statements regarding the diagnosis of an Acute MI is most accurate?
   (a) One set of normal cardiac enzymes obtained in the ED is sufficient to rule out an MI.
   (b) A positive response to antacids effectively rules out the diagnosis of Acute MI.
   (c) CPK-MB may not reach peak levels for at least 18 hours.
   (d) A normal ECG rules out the presence of an Acute MI.

7. ST segment elevation in Leads I, aVL and V_1-V_6 with reciprocal ST depression in Leads II, III and aVF is characteristic of:

    (a) An acute inferior wall MI
    (b) An acute posterior wall MI
    (c) Myocarditis
    (d) An acute anterior wall MI

8. All of the following drugs may be given through an endotracheal tube except:

    (a) Sodium bicarbonate
    (b) Atropine
    (c) Epinephrine
    (d) Narcan

9. Appropriate first-line therapy for acute pulmonary edema may include all of the following agents except:

    (a) Oxygen
    (b) Digitalis
    (c) Nitroglycerin
    (d) Furosemide

10. What is the earliest radiographic finding of CHF?

    (a) Pulmonary vascular redistribution to the upper lung fields
    (b) Interstitial edema
    (c) Cardiomegaly
    (d) Alveolar edema

11. What is the most effective medical therapy for the treatment of angina pectoris associated with hypertrophic cardiomyopathy?

    (a) Nitroglycerin
    (b) Digitalis
    (c) Beta blockers
    (d) Morphine

12. The diagnostic procedure of choice for detecting a pericardial effusion occurring in association with pericarditis is _____ .

    (a) CXR
    (b) ECG
    (c) Radionuclide scanning
    (d) Echocardiography

13. The differential diagnosis of neck vein distention associated with hypotension includes all of the following except:

    (a) Tension pneumothorax
    (b) Pericardial tamponade
    (c) Myocarditis
    (d) Acute pulmonary edema

14. Most pulmonary emboli originate from venous thrombi in the _____.

    (a) Calf
    (b) Upper extremities
    (c) Lower extremities and pelvis
    (d) Heart

15. All of the following statements regarding the use of aortography in the evaluation of acute aortic dissections are true except:

    (a) It can miss dissection if the false lumen is thrombosed.
    (b) It has been the traditional diagnostic gold standard.
    (c) It is 100% accurate.
    (d) Unlike rapid-sequence CT scanning with contrast, aortography also assesses the aortic valves and branches.

16. All of the following statements regarding Debakey Type III aortic dissections are accurate except:

    (a) Initial management of these dissections is medical.
    (b) They are equivalent to Stanford Type B dissections.
    (c) They are the most common type of dissection.
    (d) Long-term management of these dissections is usually medical.

17. Medical therapy for aortic dissections is aimed at controlling the forces that propagate the dissection. The first-line agent (or combination of agents) used to accomplish this goal is/are:

    (a) Beta blockers and Nitroprusside
    (b) Beta blockers and Nitroglycerin
    (c) Nitroprusside alone
    (d) Trimethaphan

18. A 30-year-old female presents with palpitations of sudden onset and a feeling of nervousness. The patient denies drug use of any type and has had no other episodes of palpitations or anxiety. The nurse hands you a rhythm strip demonstrating an irregular wide-complex tachycardia (QRS=0.13 secs.) at 250 beats/minute. There is no evidence of torsades. The likely etiology of this rhythm is:

    (a) Wolff-Parkinson-White syndrome
    (b) Mitral valve prolapse
    (c) Cocaine use (despite the history)
    (d) Anxiety

19. Atypical chest pain associated with mitral valve prolapse is treated with:
    (a) Nitroglycerin
    (b) Beta blockers
    (c) Morphine
    (d) Oxygen

20. The treatment of choice for hypertension associated with eclampsia is:
    (a) Magnesium sulfate and hydralazine
    (b) Diuretics
    (c) Nitroprusside
    (d) Labetalol

21. The primary difference between hypertensive urgencies and hypertensive emergencies is that, in hypertensive emergencies:
    (a) The patient's diastolic BP is ≥ 130mmHg.
    (b) The patient has no history of hypertension.
    (c) The patient is usually treated with oral medications.
    (d) The patient has evidence of end-organ dysfunction or damage.

22. Which of the following statements is incorrect?
    (a) A capillary refill > 2 secs. occurs with a volume deficit that is ≥ 15%.
    (b) The estimated blood volume of an adult is 70mL/kg.
    (c) A CVP monitor accurately measures the fluid volume status in patients with right ventricular failure.
    (d) The presence of tachycardia > 120 in an adult is associated with a volume deficit of 30 - 40%.

23. The ideal location of the catheter tip for temporary transvenous pacing is in the _____.
    (a) Right atrium
    (b) Superior vena cava
    (c) Apex of the right ventricle
    (d) None of the above

24. Successful placement of a temporary transvenous pacemaker under ECG guidance is indicated by the observation of _____ on the cardiac monitor.
    (a) ST depression
    (b) ST elevation
    (c) Small positive P waves and near-normal QRS complexes
    (d) Prominent inverted P waves and smaller negative QRS complexes

25. Placement of a pacemaker magnet over most permanent pacemakers results in _____.
    (a) Conversion from a demand to a fixed-rate mode
    (b) Conversion from a fixed-rate to a demand mode
    (c) Permanent disabling of the pacemaker
    (d) Temporary disabling of the pacemaker

26. All of the following statements regarding the coding system used for permanent pacemakers are accurate except:
    (a) It consists of a series of 3 to 5 letters.
    (b) The first letter represents the chamber paced.
    (c) The second letter represents the chamber sensed.
    (d) The third letter represents the shock/antitachydysrhythmia pacing functions.

27. A 31-year-old male is brought in by ambulance for evaluation of a syncopal episode that occurred while he was playing basketball with some very competitive friends. Exam reveals a rapid biphasic carotid pulse and a prominent systolic ejection murmur along the left sternal border and at the apex. You suspect the diagnosis of hypertrophic cardiomyopathy and ask the patient to perform the Valsalva maneuver while you auscultate his heart. Assuming your diagnosis is correct, you would expect the intensity of the murmur to _____ with this maneuver.
    (a) Increase
    (b) Decrease
    (c) Remain unchanged
    (d) Disappear

28. All of the following statements regarding hypertrophic cardiomyopathy are accurate except:
    (a) This disorder is inherited in > 50% of patients.
    (b) It is characterized by left ventricular hypertrophy (often asymmetrical) without associated ventricular dilatation.
    (c) Digitalis and vasodilators are typically the most useful agents in the management of this disorder.
    (d) Amiodarone is the treatment of choice for the ventricular dysrhythmias that occur in patients with this disorder.

29. Which of the following CXR findings best fits the description of an uncommon finding, but one that is very suggestive of pulmonary embolism?
    (a) Elevated hemidiaphragm
    (b) Atelectasis
    (c) Pleural effusion
    (d) Hampton's hump

30. The most common symptoms in patients presenting with pulmonary embolism are dyspnea and:

    (a) Pleuritic chest pain
    (b) Hemoptysis
    (c) Apprehension
    (d) Syncope

31. Which of the following findings can, by itself, reliably rule out the presence of a pulmonary embolus?

    (a) A normal PO_2
    (b) A normal CXR
    (c) A normal A-a gradient
    (d) None of the above

32. Antibiotic prophylaxis for bacterial endocarditis is warranted in high-risk patients when all of the following procedures are performed except:

    (a) I and D of an abscess
    (b) Suturing of a laceration
    (c) Placement of nasal packing
    (d) Dental procedures associated with gingival bleeding

33. Antibiotic prophylaxis for endocarditis is indicated in patients with all of the following conditions except:

    (a) History of bacterial endocarditis
    (b) Mitral valve prolapse without murmur (regurgitation) or thickened valve leaflets
    (c) Rheumatic heart disease
    (d) Prosthetic heart valves

34. All of the following statements regarding prosthetic heart valves are accurate except:

    (a) Mechanical valves require life-long systemic anticoagulation.
    (b) Patients with valve dysfunction secondary to thrombus formation usually present with acute onset of CHF, hypotension and muting (or loss) of the prosthetic valve sound.
    (c) Endocarditis should be suspected in any patient with a prosthetic valve who presents with fever, especially if a new regurgitation heart murmur is heard.
    (d) Tissue valves cause greater hemolysis and are more thrombogenic than mechanical valves.

35. In patients with automatic implantable cardioverter-defibrillators (AICDs) in place who require CPR:

    (a) CPR is performed in the usual manner.
    (b) The provider may perceive an AICD shock if the device has not been deactivated.
    (c) Perception of an AICD shock by a provider is neither dangerous nor uncomfortable.
    (d) All of the above are correct.

36. Janeway lesions are most accurately described as:

    (a) Retinal hemorrhages with central clearing
    (b) Nontender, erythematous macular lesions on the fingers, palms, soles
    (c) Tender, erythematous nodules on the volar aspect of the fingertips
    (d) Nontender erythematous nodules on the dorsal aspect of the fingertips

37. The most productive test for making the diagnosis of endocarditis is:

    (a) Blood culture
    (b) ESR
    (c) ECG
    (d) CBC

38. The organism responsible for most cases of right-sided endocarditis is:

    (a) *Staph. epi*
    (b) *Staph. aureus*
    (c) *Strep. viridans*
    (d) *Enterococci*

39. Which of the following statements regarding mitral stenosis is the least accurate?

    (a) Most cases are the result of rheumatic heart disease.
    (b) Common presenting symptoms include dyspnea on exertion and hemoptysis.
    (c) Common ECG findings are left atrial enlargement and atrial fibrillation.
    (d) The most common complication is infective endocarditis.

40. The type of congestive heart failure that occurs in association with beriberi is most accurately characterized as:

    (a) Low-output left ventricular failure
    (b) High-output left ventricular failure
    (c) Low-output right ventricular failure
    (d) High-output right ventricular failure

41. When compared with the ST elevation that occurs in association with acute MI, the ST elevation that occurs in association with acute pericarditis is:

    (a) More diffuse
    (b) Nonanatomic in distribution
    (c) Concave upward in configuration
    (d) All of the above

Answers: 1. a, 2. a, 3. d, 4. c, 5. b, 6. c, 7. d, 8. a, 9. b, 10. a, 11. c, 12. d, 13. c, 14. c, 15. c, 16. c, 17. a, 18. a, 19. b, 20. a, 21. d, 22. c, 23. c, 24. b, 25. a, 26. d, 27. a, 28. c, 29. d, 30. a, 31. d, 32. b, 33. b, 34. d., 35. d, 36. b, 37. a, 38. b, 39. d, 40. b, 41. d

Use the pre-chapter multiple choice question worksheet (p. xxv) to record and determine the percentage of correct answers for this section.

DYSRHYTHMIAS

I. Basic Principles of Cardiac Conduction Disturbances

A. Standard ECG and Rhythm Strips

1. Recordings are obtained at a paper speed of 25mm/sec.
2. The vertical axis measures distance; the smallest divisions are 1mm long and 1mm high.
3. The horizontal axis measures time; each small division is .04 sec./mm.

B. Normal Morphology

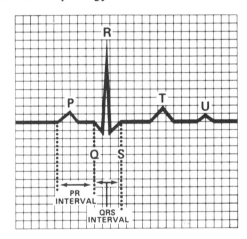

Reproduced with permission. <u>Textbook of Advanced Cardiac Life Support</u>, *1987,1990. Copyright American Heart Association.*

1. P wave = atrial depolarization
   a. Upright in Leads I, II, AVF, V_4-V_6; inverted in Lead AVR
   b. Measures < .10 secs. wide and < 3mm high
   c. PR interval is .12-.20 secs.

2. QRS complex = ventricular depolarization
   a. Measures .06 - .10 secs. wide
   b. Q wave is < .04 sec. wide and < 3mm deep; the Q wave is abnormal if it is > 3mm deep or > 1/3 of the QRS complex.
   c. R wave is ≤ (equal to or less than) 7.5mm high

3. QT interval varies with rate and sex but is usually .33 - .42 secs.; at normal heart rates, it is normally < 1/2 the preceding R-R interval.

4. T wave = ventricular repolarization
   a. Upright in Leads I, II, V_3-V_6; inverted in AVR
   b. Slightly rounded and asymmetric in configuration
   c. Measures ≤ 5mm high in limb leads and ≤ 10mm high in the V leads

5. U wave = a ventricular afterpotential
   a. Any deflection after the T wave (usually low voltage)
   b. Same polarity as the T wave
   c. Most easily detected in lead V_3
   d. Can be a normal component of the ECG
   e. Prominent U waves may indicate one of the following:
      (1) Hypokalemia (< 3mEq/L)
      (2) Hypercalcemia
      (3) Therapy with digitalis, phenothiazines, quinidine, epinephrine, inotropic agents or amiodarone
      (4) Thyrotoxicosis
   f. Inverted (negative) U waves may indicate one of the following:
      (1) Acute coronary ischemia
      (2) Ventricular strain / dilation / overload
      (3) Hypertension
      (4) Intracranial or subarachnoid hemorrhage

C. *Causes of Abnormal Morphologies*

1. Hypothermia: core temperature < 35°C (95°F)
   a. ECG findings
      (1) "J wave" (also referred to as an "Osborn wave"): a broad upright deflection at the end of an upright QRS complex.

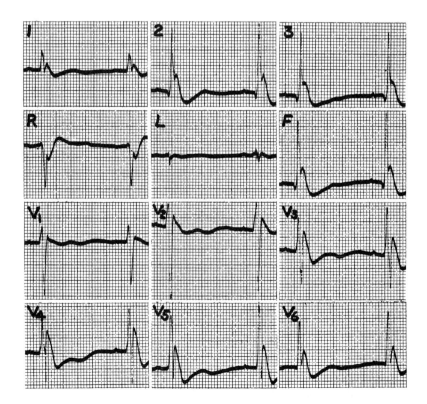

Marriott: Practical Electrocardiography, ed. 8, Williams & Wilkins, 1988.

(2) Conduction delays: PR, QRS and QT intervals are all prolonged.

(3) Dysrhythmias: sinus bradycardia and atrial fibrillation with a slow ventricular response are the most commonly encountered in this setting; the risk for developing dysrhythmias increases as the core temperature falls below 30°C (86°F); at core temperatures below 25°C (77°F), spontaneous ventricular fibrillation and asystole may occur. (Gentle handling of these patients is a must since dysrhythmias are easily introduced).

b. Treatment of dysrhythmias

(1) "Most rhythm disturbances [in hypothermia]. . . require no therapy and revert spontaneously with rewarming." [Tintinalli's Text, 6th ed., p. 1181].

(2) Rewarming — the modalities used to correct hypothermia are determined by the degree of hypothermia, the patient's cardiovascular status, the skills of the physician and the resources at one's disposal. The three modalities available are: passive external rewarming (PER), active external rewarming (AER) and active core rewarming (ACR).

(a) If a pulse is present, and the patient is mildly hypothermic (34 - 36°C), PER (dry clothes, blankets) is usually adequate but can be supplemented with AER (hot water bottles, radiant heat) and noninvasive ACR (warmed humidified O_2 and heated IV fluids).

(b) If a pulse is present and the patient is moderately hypothermic (30 - 34°C), a combination of PER, AER and noninvasive ACR should be used. In these patients, however, AER measures should be applied only to the trunk.

(c) If a pulse is present and the patient is severely hypothermic (< 30°C), rewarming should be accomplished with PER and ACR. In these patients, noninvasive ACR measures should be supplemented with invasive ACR measures (peritoneal lavage, extracorporeal rewarming).

(d) If cardiac arrest is present, invasive ACR measures (in addition to PER and noninvasive ACR) should be initiated; extracorporeal rewarming by cardiac bypass is the rewarming method of choice.

(3) Cardiac arrest

(a) CPR is indicated in all monitored patients with ventricular fibrillation or asystole.

(b) In unmonitored patients who appear to be profoundly hypothermic and in cardiac arrest, rescuers should take 30 - 45 secs. to confirm the absence of respirations and a pulse before commencing CPR.

(4) Ventricular fibrillation
  (a) V-Fib is often refractory to therapy until the patient is re-warmed.
  (b) Defibrillation should be attempted up to three shocks but, if unsuccessful, CPR and rapid rewarming measures should be instituted. Further attempts at defibrillation should be withheld until the patient's temperature rises above 30°C (86°F).
  (c) As the myocardium rewarms, V-Fib may convert spontaneously or in response to defibrillation.
  (d) Magnesium sulfate has been shown to be effective in producing spontaneous defibrillation in these patients.
(5) If narcotic abuse is suspected, naloxone should be considered because it may act on central opiate receptors to decrease the severity of hypothermia seen in overdoses.
(6) In general, a patient is not considered "dead" until "warm and dead," warm being ≥ 35°C (95°F).

2. Hypokalemia

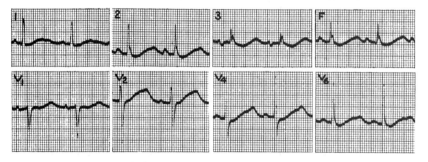

Marriott: Practical Electrocardiography, ed. 8, Williams & Wilkins, 1988.

a. Progressively more prominent U wave (best seen in V_3)

b. Flattening of T wave (earlier) followed by inversion (later)

c. Depression of ST segment

d. Prominent P wave

e. Prolongation of the PR and QT (U) interval

f. V-Tach / Torsades

Note: In the presence of hypokalemia, susceptibility to digitalis toxicity and its associated dysrhythmias is increased.

3. Hyperkalemia
   $[K^+ = 6.1mEq]$

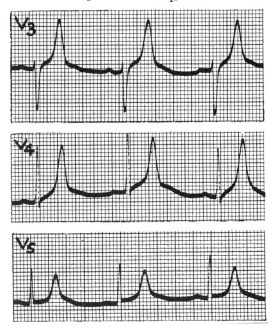

Marriott: Practical Electrocardiography, ed. 8, Williams & Wilkins, 1988.

$[K^+ = 8.1mEq]$

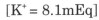
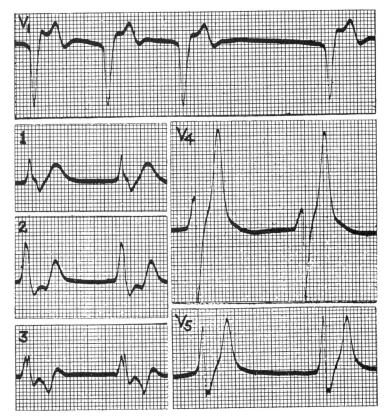

Marriott: Practical Electrocardiography, ed. 8, Williams & Wilkins, 1988.

a. Tall hyperacute T wave (earliest ECG finding)
b. Prolonged PR interval
c. Flattened or absent P wave
d. Wide QRS complex that eventually blends with the T wave to assume a "sine wave" appearance.
e. Heart blocks
f. QT interval normal or shortened

Hyperkalemia Level	ECG Changes
5.5 - 6.5	Large amplitude T waves, peaked, tented, symmetric
6.5 - 8.0	PR interval prolongation P wave flattening/disappearance QRS widening Conduction block with escape beats
> 8.0	Sine wave appearance Ventricular fibrillation Asystole

4. Hypocalcemia

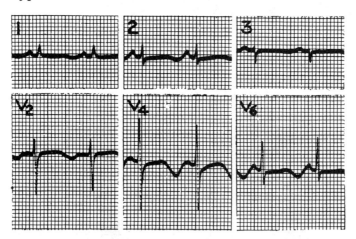

Marriott: Practical Electrocardiography, ed. 8, Williams & Wilkins, 1988.

a. Prolonged QT interval
b. Terminal T wave inversion (less consistent finding)
c. Ventricular dysrhythmias (including Torsades de Pointes)

5. Hypercalcemia

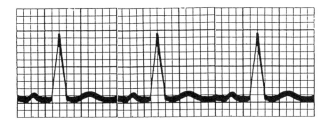

Reproduced with permission. Dubin, Rapid Interpretation of EKGs, ed. 4, 1989.
COVER Publishing Co., P.O. Box 1092, Tampa FL 33601.

"The most reliable ECG change of hypercalcemia is shortening of the QT interval, which is nearly always seen when the calcium concentration exceeds 13mg/100mL." [Rosen's Text, 3rd ed., p. 2157]

"Characteristic ECG changes include shortening of the QT interval and, to a lesser degree, prolongation of the PR interval and QRS widening." [Rosen's Text, 4th ed., p.2443 and 5th edition, p.1735].

6. Hypomagnesemia
   a. Prolonged PR and QT intervals
   b. Widened QRS complex
   c. ST segment abnormalities
   d. Flattened or inverted T waves (especially in the precordial leads)
   e. Ventricular dysrhythmias (PVCs, V-Tach, torsades de pointes, V-Fib)
   Note: (1) Hypomagnesemia usually occurs in association with other electrolyte abnormalities (particularly hypokalemia), and many of the ECG findings are similar to those seen with hypokalemia and hypocalcemia as pictured above. (2) In the presence of hypomagnesemia, susceptibility to digitalis toxicity and its associated dysrhythmias is increased.

7. Digitalis effects

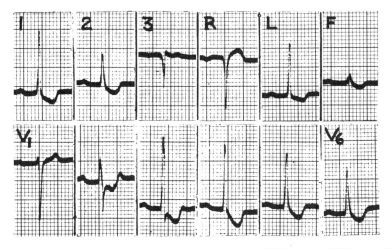

Marriott: Practical Electrocardiography, ed. 8, Williams & Wilkins, 1988.

a. Sagging ST segment with its concavity directed upward — resembles a hockey stick.
b. Short QT interval
c. Flattened or inverted T wave
d. Modestly prolonged PR interval

[Note: These effects are especially prominent in the lateral leads and occur in most patients who are adequately digitalized; they are not an indication of digitalis toxicity.]

8. Digitalis toxicity
   a. Pathophysiology — digitalis produces toxicity by:
      (1) Poisoning the Na^+-K^+-ATPase pump → increased intracellular entry of Na^+ and Ca^{++} and egress of K^+ → increased excitability → ectopy and tachydysrhythmias.
      (2) Increasing vagal tone and automaticity → decreased conduction in the AV node → bradydysrhythmias and AV blocks.
   b. Factors that increase sensitivity to digitalis and predispose to toxicity include:
      (1) Electrolyte abnormalities (hypokalemia, hypomagnesemia, hypercalcemia and hyperkalemia)
      (2) Hypoxia
      (3) Metabolic alkalosis
      (4) Increasing age
      (5) Presence of underlying cardiac disease (ischemia, CHF, congenital heart disease)
      (6) Presence of chronic underlying systemic illness (COPD, renal failure, hypothyroidism)
      (7) Drug interactions (quinidine, calcium-channel blockers, erythromycin, amiodarone, captopril and ibuprofen)
   c. ECG findings
      (1) PVCs (often bigeminal and multiform) — the most common Dig-induced rhythm disturbance
      (2) Paroxysmal atrial tachycardia with AV block is pathognomonic for Dig toxicity — see sample tracing in Tintinalli's Text, 5th ed., p.175, Fig. 24-11 (not in the 6th edition) or ECG in Emergency Medicine and Acute Care 2005: (Chan, et. al., p. 258, Figure 50-4).
      (3) Atrial fibrillation with a slow ventricular response
      (4) Sinus arrest
      (5) Junctional tachycardia (common)
      (6) V-Tach
      (7) Bidirectional V-Tach (highly suggestive of Dig toxicity, but rare)
      (8) V-Fib
      (9) Sinus bradycardia
      (10) SA and AV nodal blocks

d. Clinical symptoms
   (1) Flu-like syndrome with profound malaise, anorexia, nausea, vomiting and diarrhea
   (2) Visual disturbances (blurred vision, halos around objects and yellow or green color aberrations)
   (3) Mental status changes including confusion, drowsiness and psychosis

[Note: Acute digitalis toxicity is usually seen in young and otherwise healthy patients as a result of either accidental or intentional overdose; it is commonly associated with hyperkalemia, high digoxin levels and bradydysrhythmias as well as AV blocks. Toxicity in these patients is most closely correlated with the degree of hyperkalemia (not the serum digoxin level). Chronic digitalis toxicity generally occurs in the elderly cardiac patient with reduced renal function who is taking diuretics. These patients are usually normo- or hypokalemic, have digoxin levels that are minimally elevated or normal and most commonly have a ventricular dysrhythmia.]

e. **Clinical Pictures**
   (1) Acute intoxication — a 3-year-old is brought in by his parents for evaluation following accidental ingestion of grandpa's "heart pills." Based on information obtained from the parents, he has ingested 10.7mg of digoxin sometime within the past two hours and has vomited twice. The cardiac monitor shows a junctional rhythm with sinus block and Type I Second-Degree AV block; lab evaluation reveals a potassium of 6.2 along with a markedly elevated digoxin level (61). The child is on no medications and is otherwise healthy.
   (2) Chronic intoxication — A-65-year old woman with a PMH of CAD, CHF and renal insufficiency is brought in by ambulance for evaluation. Her medications include furosemide, digitalis, sublingual nitroglycerin and baby ASA. According to family members, she has become progressively more confused and weak over the past few days and has not been eating well. The ECG shows a regular wide complex tachycardia with alternating QRS polarity (bidirectional ventricular tachycardia) and lab evaluation reveals a digoxin level of 3.5 and a potassium of 3.0.

f. Treatment
   (1) IV, O_2, pulse oximeter and cardiac monitor.
   (2) If digitalis toxicity is acute, i.e. due to a massive ingestion within the past hour, consider gut decontamination via gastric lavage (controversial because of the vagal stimulation associated with this procedure → profound bradycardia or asystole).
   (3) Administer multiple doses of activated charcoal to all patients with potentially toxic ingestions; activated charcoal prevents systemic absorption and, when multiple doses are given, enhances elimination by interrupting digitalis' prominent enterohepatic circulation.

(4) Seek and treat factors which may contribute to digitalis toxicity:
    (a) Hypokalemia (correct cautiously in the presence of AV blocks; correction can actually exacerbate AV conduction defects).
    (b) Hyperkalemia — is best treated with Fab fragments (do <u>not</u> administer calcium; it can potentiate cardiotoxicity).
    (c) Hypomagnesemia
    (d) Hypoxia
    (e) Dehydration

(5) Control tachydysrhythmias
    (a) Phenytoin or lidocaine — are the drugs of choice.
    (b) Magnesium sulfate — may also be useful in suppressing ventricular irritability.
    (c) Avoid cardioversion (digoxin decreases the fibrillatory threshold); restrict its use to situations of last resort and use the <u>lowest</u> possible energy level.
    (d) Avoid use of bretylium, Class IA antidysrhythmics (procainamide, isoproterenol) and propranolol; these agents can exacerbate dysrhythmias and AV conduction disturbances.

(6) Manage symptomatic bradycardia or AV block with atropine. If atropine is unsuccessful, cardiac pacing (external or transvenous) may be used while waiting for Fab fragments to take effect. External pacing is preferred because transvenous pacemaker insertion can induce tachydysrhythmias in these patients.

(7) Fab fragments (digoxin-specific antibody fragments)
    (a) Should be administered to patients with:
        <u>1</u> Ventricular dysrhythmias (V-Fib, V-Tach)
        <u>2</u> Symptomatic bradycardias unresponsive to atropine
        <u>3</u> Hyperkalemia ($K^+ > 5.0$ mEq/L) secondary to digitalis intoxication
        <u>4</u> Coingestions of cardiotoxic drugs (beta-blockers, cyclic antidepressants)
        <u>5</u> Large, potentially lethal digitalis intoxications
        <u>6</u> Ingestions of plants known to contain cardiac glycosides (Oleander, Lilly of the Valley) with severe dysrhythmias
    (b) Fab fragments bind free digoxin in the vascular and interstitial spaces and form an inert compound that is eliminated by the kidneys. Treatment rapidly corrects conduction defects, ventricular dysrhythmias and hyperkalemia.
    (c) Dosage
        <u>1</u> If the serum digoxin level or the total amount of digoxin ingested are known, use the formulas found in the package insert to calculate the # of vials of Fab fragments to be administered.
        <u>2</u> If the amount of digoxin ingested is unknown, the initial dose of Fab fragments should be 5 - 10 vials (titrated incrementally).

(d) Following the administration of Fab fragments, conventional assays for determining digoxin levels (which measure both bound and unbound digoxin) are unreliable for at least a week.

	ST	PR	QRS	QT	P wave	T wave	Special Features
Hypothermia		Long	Wide	Long			"J" wave, Osborne
Hypokalemia	Down	Long		Long	Peaked	Flat	Progressively more prominent "U" wave
Hyperkalemia		Long	Wide	Short	Flat	Peaked	May be associated with Dig toxicity
Hypocalcemia				Long		Inverted	
Hypercalcemia				Short			
Hypomagnesemia	Abnormal	Long	Wide	Long		Flat	↑ Susceptibility to Dig toxicity
Digoxin Effects	Scooped			Short		Flat	
Digoxin Toxicity							PVCs = most common

II. Specific Rhythm Assessments

A. Sinus Rhythm

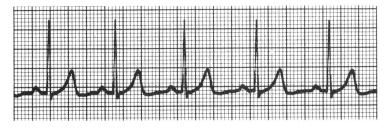

Reproduced with permission. Textbook of Advanced Cardiac Life Support, 1987,1990. Copyright American Heart Association.

1. Sinus rhythm is 60 - 100.
2. The rhythm is regular with 1:1 relationship of the P to QRS; the PR interval is .12 - .20 secs; QRS complex is .06 - .10 secs.
3. P waves are upright in Leads I, II and AVF. (Lead II is a favorite lead for a rhythm strip.)
4. There are no extra beats.

B. *Premature Atrial Contractions (PACs)* — are extra beats that originate outside the sinus node from ectopic atrial pacemakers. They appear interspersed throughout an underlying rhythm (usually sinus).

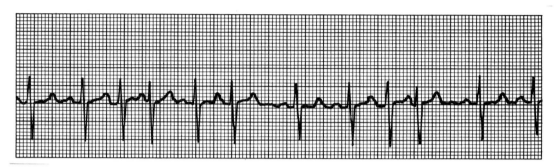

Reproduced with permission. Textbook of Advanced Cardiac Life Support, 1987, 1990. Copyright American Heart Association.

1. These ectopic P waves are upright in Lead II and appear earlier than the next expected sinus beat; they are different in configuration from normal P waves and may or may not be conducted through the AV node.
2. The QRS complex is usually normal but may be widened due to aberrant conduction.
3. They are generally followed by a <u>noncompensatory</u> pause; the SA node is reset and the returning sinus beat occurs ahead of schedule.

C. *Sinus Tachycardia* — is exactly like a sinus rhythm except that the rate is > 100 (and usually < 160).

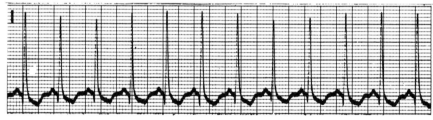

Marriott: Practical Electrocardiography, ed. 8, Williams & Wilkins, 1988.

D. *Sinus Bradycardia* — is exactly like a sinus rhythm except that the rate is < 60 (and usually > 45).

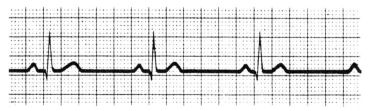

Reproduced with permission. Textbook of Advanced Cardiac Life Support, 1987, 1990. Copyright American Heart Association.

E. Paroxysmal Supraventricular Tachycardia (PSVT)

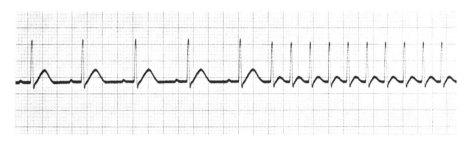

Reproduced with permission. Dubin, Rapid Interpretation of EKGs, ed. 4, 1989.
COVER Publishing Co., P.O. Box 1092, Tampa FL 33601.

1. P waves are abnormal and may not be visible (often hidden in the preceding T wave); atrial rate is 120 - 200.
2. Rhythm is regular.
3. QRS complexes are usually narrow but may be wide due to aberrant conduction through a bypass tract or pre-existing BBB; ventricular rate is 120 - 200 (usually around 150).
4. If P waves are visible, there is a 1:1 relationship of P to QRS.
5. There are no extra beats.

F. Atrial Fibrillation — is an irregularly irregular rhythm due to uncoordinated atrial activation and random occurrence of ventricular depolarization. The atria are not pumping but they do discharge electrical impulses to the ventricles; however, no single impulse depolarizes the atria completely, so only an occasional impulse gets through to the AV node. It is the most common sustained dysrhythmia in clinical practice; it occurs in 2% of the general population and in 5% of people > 60 years old.

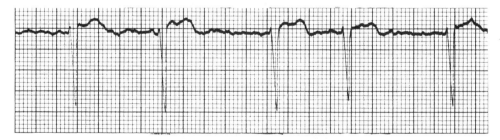

Reproduced with permission. Dubin, Rapid Interpretation of EKGs, ed. 4, 1989.
COVER Publishing Co., P.O. Box 1092, Tampa FL 33601.

1. P waves are absent but small irregular deflections in the baseline ("f waves") may be seen. They are most easily detected in the inferior leads (II, III and AVF) and in V_1 - V_3. The atrial rate is 400 - 700.
2. Since P waves are not visible, there is no PR interval.
3. QRS complexes are normal in configuration, unless there is aberrant conduction.
4. The rhythm is irregularly irregular.

5. Ventricular response rate is variable but is generally 160 - 180 in the undigitalized patient; a rate > 200 with a wide QRS complex suggests WPW syndrome with antegrade conduction through the accessory pathway; a <u>regular</u>, slow ventricular rate may be Dig toxicity.

6. There are no extra beats.

G. Atrial Flutter — is a very rapid atrial rhythm but, because of nodal delay, ventricular responses are slower. Therefore, atrial flutter always occurs with some sort of AV block (not all impulses are conducted); the resulting block is often variable (2:1, 3:1, 4:1, etc.).

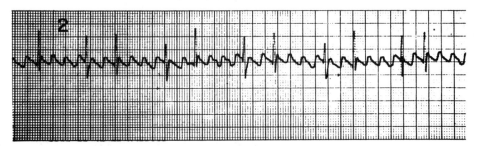

Reproduced with permission. Tintinalli, <u>Emergency Medicine: A Comprehensive Study Guide</u>, 1988. McGraw-Hill, Inc.

1. P waves have a characteristic sawtooth pattern and are called "F" or flutter waves; they are usually best seen in the inferior leads and Leads V_1 - V_2; atrial rate is 250 - 350.

2. The PR interval (when it is present) is always normal, but not every P wave is followed by a QRS complex.

3. QRS complexes are normal in configuration.

4. The ventricular rate is often 100 - 150, but depends on the degree of block present, and may be variable. Suspect atrial flutter with a 2:1 block in patients who present with a regular ventricular rate of 150.[*]

H. Multifocal Atrial Tachycardia (MAT) — is an irregular rhythm that is sometimes mistaken for atrial fibrillation. It originates from many different atrial sites and is characterized by P waves of varying shape.

[*]Easy to confuse with PSVT

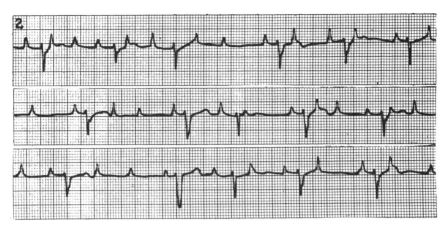

Marriott: Practical Electrocardiography, ed. 8, Williams & Wilkins, 1988.

1. There are at least three different types of P waves in one lead; atrial rate is 100 - 180.

2. The rhythm is irregularly irregular.

3. The PP, PR and RR intervals vary.

4. QRS complexes are normal in configuration.

5. Nonconducted (blocked) P waves are frequently present, particularly when the atrial rate is rapid.

I. ***Junctional Premature Contractions (JPCs)*** — are impulses that originate from an ectopic focus within the AV node or the bundle of His above the bifurcation. They may be isolated, multiple or multifocal.

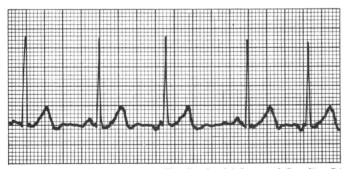

Reproduced with permission. Textbook of Advanced Cardiac Life Support, 1987, 1990. Copyright American Heart Association.

1. The ectopic P wave has a different shape and deflection (usually inverted in Leads II, III and AVF) and it may occur before, during or after the QRS complex.
2. When the P wave precedes the QRS, the PR interval is shorter than normal (often < .12 sec).
3. The ectopic QRS complex is premature, but has a normal shape unless there has been aberrant conduction.
4. They are generally followed by a <u>compensatory</u> pause; the SA node is <u>not</u> reset and the next P wave occurs at its usual time.

J. *Premature Ventricular Contractions (PVCs)* — appear as abnormal QRS complexes and T waves that occur in another underlying rhythm.

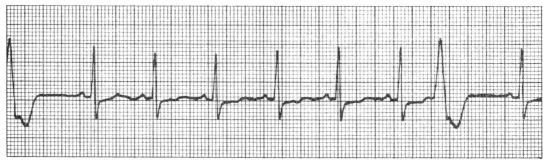

Reproduced with permission. Textbook of Advanced Cardiac Life Support, 1987, 1990. Copyright American Heart Association.

PVCs have six characteristics:
1. They occur earlier than the next expected normal QRS.
2. They are wider than a normal QRS (usually ≥ .12 sec.)
3. The QRS morphology is generally bizarre.
4. A preceding P wave is absent; however, retrograde conduction of a PVC can occasionally result in an inverted P wave following the QRS complex.
5. The deflection of the ST segment and T wave is opposite that of the QRS.
6. They are generally followed by a compensatory pause; the SA node is not reset and the next P wave occurs at its usual time.

K. *Ventricular Tachycardia* — is present when there are three or more consecutive PVCs occurring at a rate > 100.

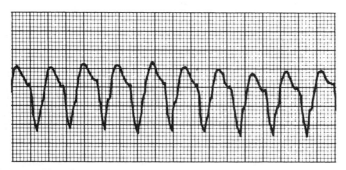

Reproduced with permission. Textbook of Advanced Cardiac Life Support, 1987, 1990. Copyright American Heart Association.

1. P waves are usually absent; when present, they are either retrogradely conducted or have no relationship to the QRS (atrioventricular — AV — dissociation).

2. QRS complexes are wide (≥ .12 sec.) and may be bizarre.

3. Fusion beats may be present; these are intermediate in appearance between a bizarre QRS complex and a normal QRS. When present, the diagnosis of V-Tach is certain.

4. Capture beats may also be seen; they are rare but, when present, confirm the diagnosis of ventricular tachycardia. Capture beats are the result of an atrial impulse penetrating the AV node from above to stimulate ("capture") the ventricles. Since ventricular conduction occurs over the normal pathways, the resulting QRS of the captured beat looks normal (narrow) in appearance.

5. Deflection of the ST segment and T wave is generally opposite that of the QRS complex.

6. Rate is > 100 (usually 150 - 200).

7. Rhythm is generally regular, although beat-to-beat variation may occur.

8. QRS axis is generally constant.

9. V-Tach is classified as "monomorphic" (QRS complexes look the same) or "polymorphic" (QRS complexes have varying morphology). Current therapeutic modalities are based on this classification; they are discussed in section III, Etiologies and Treatment of Dysrhythmias.

10. Differentiation of SVT with aberrancy from V-Tach:
    a. P waves preceding QRS complexes favor aberrancy.
    b. A fully compensatory pause is more likely to occur with V-Tach.
    c. Response to vagal maneuvers (Valsalva maneuver, carotid sinus massage*) may occur with aberrant SVT, whereas V-Tach is unaffected.
    d. Marked left axis deviation (> 30 degrees) suggests V-Tach; any QRS axis deviation > 40° in either direction (or an upright QRS in aVR) favors V-Tach.
    e. QRS duration > 0.14 sec. favors V-Tach.
    f. QRS concordance (all the QRS complexes from V_1 to V_6 are either positive or negative) strongly favors V-Tach.
    g. QRS morphology in Lead V_1: an RS, R or qR with left "rabbit ear" taller than the right suggests V-Tach, whereas an rsR′ pattern is more likely SVT with aberrancy; negative QRS morphology in this lead with a wide R wave (> 0.03 sec.), RS interval > 0.07 sec. and a slurred or notched S wave favors V-Tach.
    h. QRS morphology in Lead V_6: R/S ratio < 1, a qS or QR favors V-Tach
    i. Fusion and capture beats indicate AV dissociation and are practically diagnostic of V-Tach.

*Carotid sinus massage is contraindicated in elderly patients with a history of carotid disease/CVA or the presence of a carotid bruit.

    j. A bundle branch pattern that varies suggests SVT with aberrancy.

    k. A history of prior heart disease (MI, CHF, CABG) strongly favors V-Tach (likelihood ≥ 85%), as does a prior history of V-Tach.

    l. Age ≥ 50 years favors V-Tach, whereas age ≤ 35 years favors an aberrant SVT.

11. <u>Torsades de pointes</u> ("twisting of the pointes") is an atypical ventricular tachycardia in which the QRS axis swings from a positive to a negative direction in a single lead creating a "sine-wave" appearance. It originates from a <u>single</u> focus and is usually precipitated by drugs which prolong the QT interval such as Class IA antidysrhythmics (procainamide, quinidine), Class IC (propafenone, flecainide), cyclic antidepressants, droperidol and the phenothiazines. The combined use of certain drugs such as terfenadine plus ketoconazole or erythromycin also prolong the QT interval and may, therefore, precipitate torsades. Other causes include hypomagnesemia and hypokalemia. The rate is typically 200 - 240. [See <u>Tintinalli's Text</u>, 6th ed., p. 203, Table 29-1 if you need to review the "classes" of antidysrhythmic agents.]

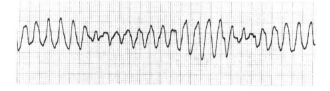

Reproduced with permission. Dubin, Rapid Interpretation of EKGs, ed. 4, 1989. COVER Publishing Co., P.O. Box 1092, Tampa FL 33601.

L. Ventricular Fibrillation

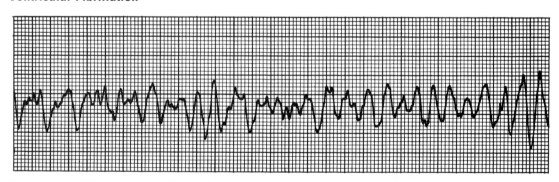

Reproduced with permission. <u>Textbook of Advanced Cardiac Life Support</u>, 1987, 1990. Copyright American Heart Association.

1. Most commonly recognized as a fine or coarse zigzag pattern without discernible P waves, QRS complexes or T waves.

2. Sometimes the rhythm may look like V-Tach. The point is moot if the patient has no pulse and is unresponsive since the treatment is the same.

M. *Pulseless Electrical Activity (PEA)* — is a term that refers to a heterogeneous group of rhythms characterized by the presence of some type of electrical activity other than V-Tach or V-Fib in the absence of a perceptible pulse. PEA includes electromechanical dissociation (EMD), pseudo-EMD, idio-ventricular rhythms, ventricular escape rhythms, bradyasystolic rhythms and postdefibrillation idioventricular rhythms. These dysrhythmias often occur in association with specific clinical conditions (hypovolemia, hypoxia, tension pneumothorax, cardiac tamponade, massive drug overdose, etc.) that can be reversed if promptly identified and appropriately treated.

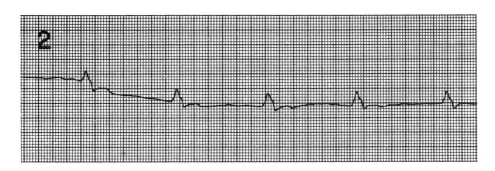

Reproduced with permission. Tintinalli, Emergency Medicine: A Comprehensive Study Guide, 1988. McGraw-Hill, Inc.

N. *Bundle Branch Blocks* — are abnormal conduction abnormalities (not rhythm disturbances) in which the ventricles depolarize in sequence (rather than simultaneously), thus producing a <u>wide</u> QRS complex (0.09-0.11 → incomplete BBB; ≥ 0.12 sec. → complete BBB) and an ST segment with a slope opposite that of the terminal half of the QRS complex.

   1. **RBBB** is a unifascicular block in which ventricular activation is by way of the <u>left</u> bundle branch; the impulse travels down the left bundle, thus activating the septum from the left side (as it normally does in the absence of RBBB). This is followed by activation of the free wall of the left ventricle (LV) and, finally, the free wall of the right ventricle (RV). Because of the two changes in direction, there is a tendency toward <u>triphasic</u> complexes in RBBB.

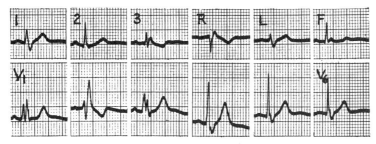

Marriott: Practical Electrocardiography, ed. 8, Williams & Wilkins, 1988.

     a. Wide QRS complex (≥ 0.12 sec.)
     b. Triphasic QRS complex (RSR′ variant) in Lead V_1
     c. Wide S waves in Leads I, V_5 and V_6

    d. Normal septal Q waves in Leads I and V_6 (because the initial activation of the ventricle occurs in the normal manner)

    e. T wave has a deflection opposite that of the terminal half of the QRS complex

    f. Associated axis is variable; a normal axis, left axis deviation (LAD) or even right deviation (RAD) may be present.

2. **LBBB** is a bifascicular block in which ventricular activation is by way of the <u>right</u> bundle branch; the impulse travels down the right bundle, activating the septum and the free wall of the RV, and then continues on in the same direction to activate the free wall of the LV. Because the dominant forces are traveling in the same direction, there is a tendency toward monophasic QRS complexes.

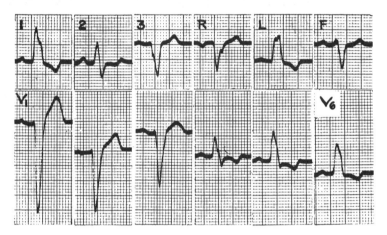

Marriott: <u>Practical Electrocardiography</u>, ed. 8, Williams & Wilkins, 1988.

    a. Wide QRS complex (≥ 0.12 sec)

    b. Negative wave (QS or rS) in Lead V_1

    c. Large wide R waves in Leads I, aVL, V_5 and V_6

    d. Absence of normal septal Q waves in Leads I and V_6

    e. T wave has a deflection opposite that of the terminal half of the QRS complex.

    f. Associated LAD is most common and implies the presence of additional myocardial disease.

O. ***Sinoatrial (SA) Block*** — occurs when there is abnormal conduction between the sinus node and atrial muscle; it is recognized by the <u>unexpected absence</u> of a P wave and its associated QRS complex. Like AV block, SA block is also divided into first, second and third degree varieties.

1. **First-degree SA block**
    a. The impulse is <u>delayed</u> in its conduction from the SA node to the atria.
    b. It cannot be diagnosed from a surface ECG.

2. **Second-degree SA block**
   a. <u>Some</u> of the sinus node discharges are blocked.
   b. It is recognized on ECG as the absence of an expected P wave and its associated QRS complex (see <u>Tintinalli's Text</u>, 6th ed., p.192, Figs. 28-21 and 28-22).

3. **Third-degree SA block (sinus arrest)**
   a. <u>All</u> of the sinus node discharges are blocked.
   b. On ECG, it may appear as a long sinus pause/arrest or junctional escape rhythm.

P. ***Sick Sinus Syndrome (SSS)*** — is an abnormality of cardiac impulse formation as well as intra-atrial and AV nodal conduction. It manifests as a wide variety of (or combinations of) bradyarrhythmias and tachyarrhythmias, and is most commonly seen in the elderly. Presenting symptoms may include dizziness, palpitations, dyspnea, fatigue, lethargy or syncope. Documentation of a bradyarrhythmia or tachyarrhythmia in association with these symptoms is the cornerstone of diagnosis.

Q. ***Atrioventricular (AV) Blocks*** — occur when the conduction between the atria and ventricles is abnormal. The conduction delay can occur in the atria, the AV node or the proximal His-Purkinje system.

1. **First-Degree AV Block**: normal AV conduction is slightly prolonged.

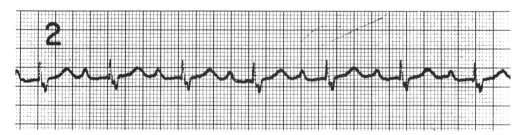

Reproduced with permission. Tintinalli, <u>Emergency Medicine: A Comprehensive Study Guide</u>, 1988. McGraw-Hill, Inc.

   a. P waves and QRS complexes are normal.
   b. There is a 1:1 relationship between the P and QRS.
   c. PR interval is prolonged (> 0.20 sec.)
   d. The block is most often at the level of the AV node.

2. **Second-Degree AV Block**: some atrial impulses are not conducted.
   a. Mobitz I (Wenckebach)

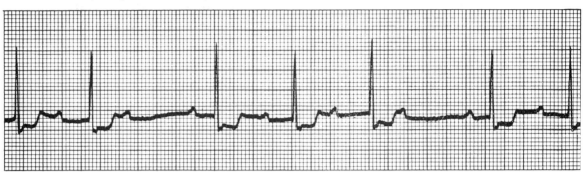

Reproduced with permission. Textbook of Advanced Cardiac Life Support, 1987, 1990. Copyright American Heart Association.

(1) P waves and QRS complexes are normal but there are <u>dropped</u> beats (P waves without QRS complexes).
(2) PR interval <u>progressively lengthens</u> and the R-R interval <u>progressively shortens</u> until a beat is dropped. This cycle repeats itself, producing a pattern referred to as "group beating."
(3) The longest cycles (those of the dropped beats) are less than twice the length of the shortest cycles (those of the impulses following the dropped beats).
(4) The block is almost always within the AV node.

   b. Mobitz II

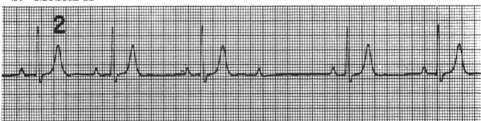

Reproduced with permission. Tintinalli, Emergency Medicine: A Comprehensive Study Guide, 1988. McGraw-Hill, Inc.

(1) P waves are normal.
(2) QRS complexes are usually (but not always) wide due to the common occurrence of a coexisting bundle branch block.
(3) PR intervals (when they occur) are always the <u>same duration</u>.
(4) There are dropped beats.
(5) The block is <u>below</u> the level of the AV node, generally in the His-Purkinje system.

3. **Third-Degree AV Block**: <u>no atrial impulses are conducted</u>; the atria and ventricles beat independently of one another.

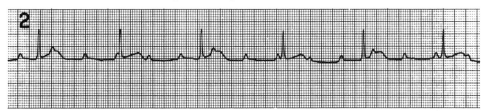

Reproduced with permission. Tintinalli, <u>Emergency Medicine: A Comprehensive Study Guide</u> 1988. McGraw-Hill, Inc.

   a. P waves appear normal.
   b. The block can occur at the level of the AV node, the bundle of His or the bundle branches.
   c. QRS complexes may be narrow or wide depending on the location of the block; if it is located above the His bundle, the QRS complexes will be narrow whereas, if it is located at or below the bundle of His, the QRS complexes will be wide.
   d. There is <u>no</u> relationship between P waves and QRS complexes.
      (1) There is an independent and regular atrial rate (constant PP interval) and a slower independent and constant ventricular rate (constant RR interval).
      (2) The P waves are <u>not</u> related (not conducted) to the QRS complexes but, rather, march through them as if they were not there.
      (3) The PR interval is <u>variable</u>.

R. *Pre-excitation Syndromes* — result from abnormal connections (<u>accessory pathways</u>) between the atria and ventricles. Impulses traveling down these pathways bypass all or part of the normal conduction system. This results in the ventricles being activated by atrial impulses sooner than would normally be anticipated (pre-excitation) and is reflected by changes in the surface ECG. The ECG changes seen are determined by the exact pathway the impulse travels. WPW (Wolff-Parkinson-White) syndrome and LGL (Lown-Ganong-Levine) syndrome are the two major variants of pre-excitation. Their characteristic ECG findings are listed below. Patients with pre-excitation syndromes are prone to tachydysrhythmias (especially PSVT and atrial fibrillation) with <u>very rapid</u> ventricular rates (up to 300).

1. WPW: the accessory pathway (Kent bundle) connects the atria directly to the <u>ventricles</u>, completely bypassing the AV node and the infranodal conduction system.

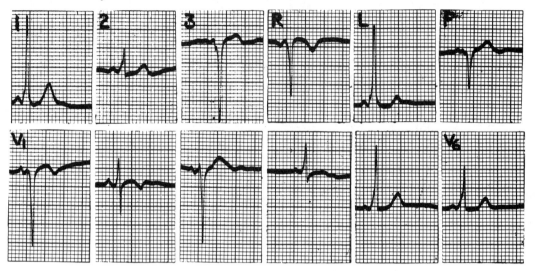

Marriott: <u>Practical Electrocardiography</u>, ed. 8, Williams & Wilkins, 1988.

   a.   Short PR interval (< .12 sec.)
   b.   Delta wave (a slurred upstroke to the QRS)
   c.   Wide QRS
   d.   Secondary ST-T wave changes; deflection of the T wave may be opposite that of the QRS vector if the classic triad is present. (Otherwise, the QRS -T may appear normal.)

2. LGL: the accessory pathway (James fibers) connects the atria directly to the <u>proximal His bundle</u>, completely bypassing the AV node.

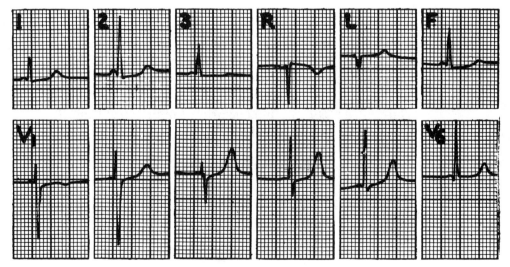

Marriott: <u>Practical Electrocardiography</u>, ed. 8, Williams & Wilkins, 1988.

   a.   Short PR interval (< .12 sec.)
   b.   No delta wave
   c.   Normal QRS

III. Etiologies and Treatment of Dysrhythmias

A. *PACs*

1. There are multiple causes (drugs or underlying disease) but they may also occur as a normal variant.

2. Clinical Significance
   a. PACs can precipitate SVT, A-Fib and A-Flutter.
   b. They are the most frequent cause of a pause on the ECG.

3. In general, no treatment is indicated. If, however, the PACs are frequent or symptomatic, treatment should be directed toward correcting the underlying cause.

B. *Sinus Tachycardia*

1. There are multiple causes; common ones include:
   a. Anxiety (diagnosis of exclusion)
   b. Drugs (e.g. cocaine)
   c. Fever
   d. Hypovolemia
   e. Hyperthyroidism
   f. Pulmonary embolism
   g. Anemia
   h. Hypoxia
   i. Pain

2. Treatment (in most instances) should be directed at finding and correcting the underlying cause. However, in the presence of an AMI, patients with "inappropriate" tachycardia may benefit from the administration of beta blockers to slow the heart rate and, in the setting of cocaine toxicity, administration of a benzodiazepine may be helpful.

C. *Sinus Bradycardia*

1. Common causes
   a. Acute inferior wall MI
   b. Vasovagal events (e.g. vomiting)
   c. Drug effect (e.g. beta-blockers, calcium-channel blockers)
   d. Sick sinus syndrome
   e. A normal variant (especially in those individuals who exercise aerobically on a regular basis)
   f. Hypothermia
   g. Hypothyroidism

2. Treatment
    a. Is indicated for those patients who are symptomatic: those with shock, hypotension, shortness of breath, chest pain, decreased mentation, CHF or PVCs in the setting of an acute MI.
    b. Intervention sequence
        (1) Atropine 0.5 - 1mg Q 5 mins. prn until a response is noted or a total of 0.03 - 0.04mg/kg has been administered.
            (a) Should be used cautiously in patients with an Acute MI as it may worsen ischemia or precipitate V-Tach or V-Fib.
            (b) Should also be used with caution in patients with Mobitz II Second-Degree AV Block and new Third-Degree AV Block with <u>wide</u> complexes → ↑the atrial rate → ↑AV Block → ↓ventricular rate and ↓BP)
            (c) Is ineffective in patients with heart transplants; go directly to transcutaneous pacing and/or catecholamine infusion.
            (d) Can be parasympathomimetic in doses < 0.5mg producing a further decrease in heart rate.
        (2) Transcutaneous pacing (TCP)
            (a) Is the treatment of choice for patients who are unresponsive to atropine and for those with severe symptoms.
            (b) Analgesics or sedatives may be required by some patients in order to be able to tolerate the pacing stimulus.
        (3) Dopamine 5 - 20mcg/kg/min.
            (a) Should be used when bradycardia is unresponsive to atropine and a transcutaneous pacer is not readily available.
            (b) It is also useful when associated hypotension is present.
        (4) Epinephrine 2 - 10mcg/min. — is the next agent of choice and is particularly useful in the presence of significant hypotension.
        (5) Isoproterenol 2 - 10mcg/min.
            (a) Can produce significant negative effects (increased myocardial oxygen consumption, peripheral vasodilatation, serious dysrhythmias).
            (b) It should only be used in low doses and as a <u>LAST RESORT</u>.
        (6) Transvenous pacing — may be required if symptomatic bradycardia persists.

D. SVT — is a generic term that refers to all dysrhythmias arising above the bifurcation of the bundle of His including sinus tachycardia, atrial fibrillation, atrial flutter, multifocal atrial tachycardia, paroxysmal supraventricular tachycardia (PSVT) and nonparoxysmal junctional tachycardia. It arises from re-entry or an ectopic pacemaker in the atria. Most physicians, however, use the term SVT to refer to AV nodal re-entry tachycardia and other undetermined supraventricular rhythms. In the discussion that follows, we are using the term SVT in this sense of the word. Treatment of other specific forms of SVT such as atrial fibrillation will be discussed separately.

1. Causes include:
   a. Pre-excitation syndromes (WPW and LGL)
   b. Mitral disease (prolapse, stenosis)
   c. Digitalis toxicity
   d. Drugs (alcohol, tobacco, caffeine)
   e. Acute MI and pericarditis
   f. Hyperthyroidism
   g. Rheumatic heart disease

2. Treatment is determined primarily by the patient's hemodynamic stability and secondarily by the width of the QRS complex.

   a. Hemodynamically <u>compromised</u> patients (those with hypotension, chest pain, a change in mental status or pulmonary edema) with a narrow complex SVT should be sedated (if possible) and treated with synchronized cardioversion. Start with 50 joules. [<u>Note</u>: In the digitalis toxic patient, cardioversion is potentially hazardous and should be avoided if at all possible. Use it only in situations of last resort and start with the lowest possible energy level (10 joules).]

   b. Vagal maneuvers and pharmacologic therapy may be used in the hemodynamically <u>stable</u> patient with <u>narrow</u> complex SVT.
      (1) Vagal maneuvers (such as carotid sinus massage* or Valsalva maneuver) increase vagal tone and may be effective in either terminating the dysrhythmia or slowing the ventricular rate enough to uncover the actual underlying rhythm. These maneuvers should be attempted prior to initiating pharmacologic therapy and may also be used to supplement it. The vagal maneuver of choice, i.e. the most effective, is the Valsalva maneuver.
      (2) Adenosine, because of its safety profile, is the drug of choice for the hemodynamically stable patient with narrow complex SVT. It is an ultra-short-acting AV nodal blocker that is very effective in converting SVT. Its major advantages over verapamil are its short half-life (< 10 secs.) and its lack of hypotensive and myocardial depressant effects. Although it does produce side effects (flushing, dyspnea, chest pain) they are transient. Recurrence of SVT, however, is common (occurs in up to 50 - 60% of patients). [<u>Note</u>: Adenosine does have several significant drug interactions. Its effects are antagonized by the methylxanthines (theophylline, caffeine) and potentiated by dipyridamole and carbamazepine. Therefore, large doses of adenosine may be required in the presence of methylxanthines, whereas smaller doses (or an alternative agent) should be used in the presence of dipyridamole and carbamazepine.]

---

*Should not be done if Dig toxicity is not ruled out.

(3) Calcium-channel blockers (such as diltiazem and verapamil) are as effective as adenosine, but slower in onset and produce more significant side effects (decreased myocardial contractility and peripheral vasodilation.) Calcium-channel blockers should <u>not</u> be used concomitantly with IV beta-blockers and should be <u>avoided</u> in patients with wide-complex tachycardias, A-Fib with WPW, Sick Sinus syndrome and advanced AV block.

    (a) Pretreatment with a fluid bolus and calcium chloride (0.5 - 1gm IV over several minutes) are useful in preventing the hypotension induced by verapamil's vasodilatory effects.

    (b) Diltiazem seems to be as effective as verapamil in the treatment of narrow-complex SVT and has the advantage of producing less myocardial depression.

(4) Beta blockers such as esmolol and propranolol are also effective in the treatment of narrow complex SVT. Esmolol has the advantage of being cardioselective as well as having a very short half-life. Propranolol is the drug of choice for SVT secondary to thyrotoxicosis because it partially blocks the conversion of T_4 and T_3. Avoid these drugs in patients with COPD, asthma or CHF as well as those who have received IV calcium-channel blockers.

(5) Digoxin is vagotonic. Compared with the other agents listed above, its effects are mild and have a much slower onset (may take several hours or more to work). Digoxin should be avoided if cardioversion is being considered.

(6) Magnesium sulfate, phenytoin and lidocaine are the drugs of choice for ectopic SVT due to digitalis toxicity. Treatment should also include correction of hypokalemia (if present) and discontinuation of digitalis. In the presence of hemodynamic instability (or potentially lethal digitalis intoxication), administration of digoxin-specific antibody fragments should be considered.

(7) Other antidysrhythmic agents, (e.g. procainamide, amiodarone,* sotalol) may also be effective.

(8) Vasopressors (norepinephrine, methoxamine, phenylephrine) and cholinergic drugs (edrophonium) are no longer recommended. Compared with agents such as calcium-channel blockers, adenosine and beta blockers, these drugs are effective but are associated with significant side effects/risks.

[<u>Note</u>: Patients who fail to respond to drug therapy may be treated with synchronized cardioversion (as described above) or overdrive cardiac pacing].

c. Drug dosages and administration:

    (1) <u>Adenosine</u> 6mg rapid IVP in a proximal vein followed by a 20mL bolus of normal saline. If there is no response after 1 - 2 mins., double the dose to 12mg.

    (2) <u>Verapamil</u> 2.5 - 5mg IV over 2 - 3 mins. A second dose of 5 - 10mg may be given in 15 - 30 mins. if necessary.

---

*Amiodarone is a good choice if the ejection fraction is < 40% or the patient is in CHF.

(3) Esmolol 300 - 500mcg/kg bolus over 1 min. followed by an infusion of 50mcg/kg/min. The loading dose may need to be repeated and the infusion rate increased by 50mcg/kg/min Q 5 mins. prn to a maximum of 200mcg/kg/min.

(4) Propranolol 1mg IV over 1 min. This dose may be repeated Q 5 mins. up to a total dose of 0.1 - 0.5mg/kg.

(5) Digoxin 0.5mg IVP initially, with repeated doses of 0.25mg Q 30 - 60 mins. prn. Total dose should not exceed 0.02mg/kg.

(6) Diltiazem 0.25mg/kg IV over 2 mins. followed in 15 mins. by a second bolus of 0.35mg/kg if the first bolus was tolerated, but ineffective.

(7) Magnesium sulfate 1 - 2gm slow IVP over 1 - 2 mins. followed by an infusion of 1 - 2gm/hr.

(8) Phenytoin 18mg/kg IVPB. Dissolve dose in normal saline and administer at a rate of 50mg/min or less.

d. Patients with wide complex tachycardia should be presumed to have ventricular tachycardia.

(1) If they are unstable → synchronized cardioversion.

(2) If they are stable → procainamide or amiodarone*

(a) Both convert SVT or V-Tach.

(b) Procainamide is contraindicated in patients with cyclic anti-depressant overdose.

(c) Adenosine may initially slow either rhythm, but it may recur (short therapeutic effect of the drug).

(d) If drug therapy fails → synchronized cardioversion

E. Atrial Fibrillation (most common supraventricular dysrhythmia)

1. Identify the type of A-Fib the patient has by determining the probable duration of the dysrhythmia:

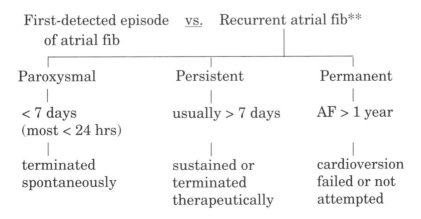

First-detected episode vs. Recurrent atrial fib**
of atrial fib

Paroxysmal	Persistent	Permanent
< 7 days (most < 24 hrs)	usually > 7 days	AF > 1 year
terminated spontaneously	sustained or terminated therapeutically	cardioversion failed or not attempted

*Amiodarone is a good choice if the ejection fraction is < 40% or the patient is in CHF.

**Ischemic stroke risk for recurrent AF is 5%/yr. or 2-7 times the risk for patients without AF.

2. Search for reversible <u>causes</u> and treat any <u>underlying medical condition;</u> then determine the <u>risk</u> for subsequent <u>stroke</u>.
   a. High risk for cardiogenic thromboembolism
      (1) Cardiac surgery
      (2) AMI
      (3) Hyperthyroidism
      (4) Myocarditis
      (5) Acute pulmonary disease
   b. Other risks of having a stroke

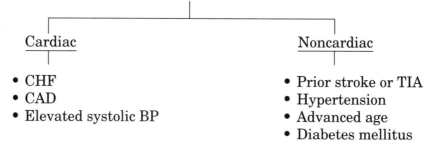

Cardiac	Noncardiac
• CHF	• Prior stroke or TIA
• CAD	• Hypertension
• Elevated systolic BP	• Advanced age
	• Diabetes mellitus

3. Plan the treatment using the following criteria:
   a. Cardiovascular stability
   b. Duration of the dysrhythmia
   c. Underlying cause/condition
   d. Presence/absence of an accessory pathway

4. There are fundamentally two ways to manage AF: restore and maintain sinus rhythm <u>or</u> allow AF to continue and ensure that the ventricular rate is controlled.
   a. Unstable patients → immediate electrical cardioversion
   b. Stable patients with significant symptoms → pharmacologic therapy
      (1) <u>Control the ventricular rate first</u>
         (a) Normal cardiac function (choose <u>one</u>)
            <u>1</u> Calcium-channel blocker (verapamil, diltiazem)
            <u>2</u> Beta-blocker (esmolol, atenolol, metoprolol)
            *Avoid these blockers in patients with WPW syndrome. Use one of the following instead:
            • Amiodarone or lidocaine*
            • Flecainide
            • Procainamide
            • Propafenone
         (b) Compromised cardiac function: EF < 40% (choose <u>one</u>)
            <u>1</u> Digoxin ⎤
            <u>2</u> Diltiazem ⎬ These agents will not promote further depression of cardiac function.
            <u>3</u> Amiodarone ⎦

         [<u>Note</u>: For patients treated with Dig, addition of MgSO$_4$ (2.5gm IV × 20 mins., then 2.5gm infused over 2 hrs.) may slow the heart rate even more and/or convert AF to sinus rhythm;** for WPW, use only amiodarone.]

*ACLS first-line recommended agents
**Consult with a cardiologist prior to administration.

(2) <u>Cardiovert the dysrhythmia</u> based on the <u>duration</u> of AF
   (a) < 48 hrs. duration
      <u>1</u> Normal cardiac function: perform DC cardioversion or use one of the following agents:
         <u>a</u> Amiodarone
         <u>b</u> Ibutilide
         <u>c</u> Flecainide
         <u>d</u> Propafenone
         <u>e</u> Procainamide
      <u>2</u> Compromised cardiac function: perform DC cardioversion or use amiodarone
   (b) > 48 hrs. duration (higher risk of systemic embolization)
      <u>1</u> Avoid <u>immediate</u> cardioversion if possible.
      <u>2</u> If <u>early</u> cardioversion (within 24 hrs.) is anticipated, consider starting heparin and consulting cardiology for TEE to exclude an atrial clot.
      <u>3</u> If <u>delayed</u> cardioversion is the best option, anticoagulation for 3 wks. is indicated prior to cardioversion.

5. Discussion of selected treatment options
   a. Hemodynamically <u>compromised</u> patients should be sedated (if possible) and treated with synchronized cardioversion. Start with 100 joules. (<u>Note</u>: In patients who are dig. toxic or hypokalemic, cardioversion is potentially hazardous; use only as a last resort and start with 10 joules.) If the patient has hypertrophic cardiomyopathy (or has been in A-Fib > 48 hours) immediate systemic heparinization is also indicated.
   b. Hemodynamically <u>stable</u> patients with A-Fib of <u>acute</u> (< 48 hours) onset (paroxysmal or persistent atrial fib.) should be managed with pharmacologic therapy, the primary goal of which is to slow the ventricular response rate to 100 beats/min. or less.
      (1) First-line agents include calcium-channel blockers (diltiazem, verapamil) and beta blockers (esmolol, metoprolol). Of these agents, diltiazem is the agent of first choice; it is rapid in onset and has fewer negative inotropic effects than either verapamil or the beta-blocking agents.[*]
      (2) Digoxin may also be used, but it is much slower in onset and is not likely to be effective if the sympathetic tone is high; it should, therefore, be considered a second-line agent.
      (3) Magnesium is also effective in slowing the ventricular rate and may be used in combination with one of the above agents as adjunctive therapy.
      (4) Once the ventricular rate is controlled, a pharmacologic agent can be given to chemically convert the patient to sinus rhythm. Ibutilide is effective, but is associated with a significant risk of inducing torsades de pointes.

---

[*]A special circumstance is the hemodynamically stable patient with atrial fib-or-flutter of acute onset and known ejection fraction < 40% or CHF. These patients should be treated with amiodarone and then cardioverted.

c. In patients with pre-excitation syndromes, synchronized cardioversion is often required, and is considered by some authors to be the preferred treatment modality regardless of the presence or absence of hemodynamic stability. Procainamide prolongs the refractory period of the accessory pathway and is the alternative therapy of choice in patients who are hemodynamically stable. Calcium channel and beta-blockers, digoxin and adenosine are <u>contraindicated</u> in these patients; by blocking AV nodal conduction, these agents can increase conduction down the accessory pathway, producing an increase in the ventricular response and, occasionally, V-Fib.

[<u>Note</u>: Presence of an accessory pathway should be suspected in any patient who presents with a ventricular rate > 200/min. because the normal AV node does not conduct impulses at a rate > 150 - 180/min.]

d. Patients with atrial fibrillation longer than 2 days duration should, when stable, receive anticoagulation before pharmacologic or electric cardioversion is attempted in order to decrease the risk of arterial embolization of an intra-atrial thrombus.

F. Atrial Flutter

1. Causes are essentially the same as for atrial fibrillation, but it is most often associated with post-cardiac surgery and peri-infarction periods.

2. Atrial flutter is usually a transitional rhythm between sinus rhythm and atrial fibrillation.

3. Treatment — is determined by the patient's cardiovascular stability, duration of the dysrhythmia and whether or not the patient has an accessory pathway.
   a. Hemodynamically <u>unstable</u> patients should be sedated (if time permits) and treated with synchronized cardioversion. Start with 50 joules.
   b. Vagal maneuvers and pharmacologic therapy should be used in the hemodynamically <u>stable</u> patient. [*See "footnote" on previous page.]
      (1) Vagal maneuvers or adenosine may be of diagnostic value; by inducing a transient AV nodal blockade, they may reveal the characteristic flutter waves of this rhythm and confirm the Dx.
      (2) Once the diagnosis is confirmed, rate control should be accomplished with a calcium-channel blocker (diltiazem, verapamil) or a beta blocker (esmolol, metoprolol). Of these drugs, diltiazem is the preferred agent. Digoxin may also be used, but is considered a second-line drug. Magnesium may be used in combination with one of the above agents as adjunctive therapy.
      (3) Once the ventricular response rate is controlled, chemical conversion to sinus rhythm can be achieved with procainamide or quinidine.

c. Patients with pre-excitation syndromes and <u>acute</u> onset should be treated with synchronized cardioversion or, if hemodynamically stable, with procainamide; if the duration of the dysrhythmia is unknown or > 48 hours, anticoagulation is recommended prior to cardioversion. As discussed above, calcium-channel blockers, digoxin, adenosine and beta blockers should be avoided in these patients.

G. Multifocal Atrial Tachycardia (MAT)

1. Causes include:
    a. Decompensated COPD (most common cause)
    b. CHF
    c. Sepsis
    d. Theophylline toxicity

2. Treatment
    a. Is primarily aimed at correcting the underlying disease process.
        (1) Hypoxia should be corrected with supplemental oxygen (and bronchodilator therapy) in a patient with COPD <u>and</u>
        (2) Evaluation for theophylline toxicity should be performed.
    b. If the above measures are unsuccessful and the patient is symptomatic, other modalities that may be used include:
        (1) Calcium-channel blockers (diltiazem, verapamil) — are usually effective in slowing the ventricular rate, decreasing atrial ectopy, and may produce conversion to a sinus rhythm in some patients.
        (2) Magnesium sulfate — decreases atrial ectopy.
        (3) Metoprolol — is effective in slowing the ventricular rate and produces conversion to a sinus rhythm in most patients. However, like all beta-blockers, this agent must be used cautiously in the presence of bronchospastic disease and CHF.
        <u>Note</u>: Digoxin and cardioversion are usually <u>ineffective</u> in the treatment of MAT.

H. JPCs (junctional premature contractions)

1. Primary causes are:
    a. Digitalis toxicity
    b. Coronary artery disease
    c. CHF
    d. Acute MIs (especially inferior wall MIs)

2. Treat the underlying cause; if JPCs precipitate more lethal dysrhythmias, consider using IV procainamide.

I. **PVCs** (premature ventricular contractions)

1. Causes include the following:
    a. Hypokalemia
    b. Hypomagnesemia
    c. Hypoxia
    d. Myocardial infarction
    e. Drugs
        (1) Alcohol-tobacco-caffeine
        (2) Cocaine
        (3) Digitalis or quinidine toxicity (PVCs are the most common dysrhythmia seen with Dig toxicity)
        (4) Methylxanthines (commonly used by patients with asthma or COPD)
    f. Hyperthyroidism
    g. CHF
    h. Cardiomyopathy
    i. Mechanical — PVCs are not uncommon when a catheter is placed in the right ventricle.
    j. Myocardial contusion

2. Treatment — is dictated by the underlying cause and is not indicated in all cases.
    a. Patients who are asymptomatic and have PVCs of unknown cause should <u>not</u> be treated (particularly when the PVCs are found as an incidental finding); PVCs in this setting may represent a normal variant; isolated PVCs occur in as many as 50% of young healthy subjects and increase in frequency with age.
    b. When an underlying cause is identified (hypokalemia, hypomagnesemia, hypoxia, etc.) therapy should be directed toward correcting the underlying problem (rather than suppressing PVCs). This is usually sufficient.
    c. Mechanical causes, if present, should also be corrected:
        (1) A central line catheter that is located in the right ventricle may induce PVCs; withdraw the catheter or advance it out of the ventricle.
        (2) To reduce the likelihood of inducing PVCs during Swan-Ganz placement, inflate the balloon to cover the catheter tip while advancing into the right ventricle; then deflate the balloon to avoid floating into the ventricular outflow tract.
        (3) If these measures fail to ameliorate the PVCs, use lidocaine.
    d. "Escape PVCs" (those associated with bradycardia) should be treated with atropine (<u>not</u> lidocaine), since administration of lidocaine under these circumstances may suppress the existing functioning rhythm.
    e. Treatment of PVCs occurring in association with an Acute MI or ischemia is more controversial. Optimal treatment of the underlying ischemia/infarction with oxygen, nitroglycerine, morphine, ASA and fibrinolytic therapy is clearly the first priority. If these measures fail, most authors currently recommend a conservative course of watchful waiting, while a few advocate treatment if the PVCs:

(1) Are frequent (> 30/hr.), multiform (multifocal) or associated with short runs of V-Tach

(2) Occur in couplets or display the R-on-T phenomenon (which occurs during ventricular depolarization)

[Note: The use of lidocaine as prophylaxis against the development of PVCs in these patients is <u>not</u> recommended.]

f. Pharmacologic agents

(1) Lidocaine — is the drug of first choice. Administer a 1 - 1.5mg/kg bolus followed by a 2 - 4mg/min. drip. Repeat boluses of 0.5 - .75 mg/kg may be given Q 5 - 10 mins. prn to a maximum total dose of 3mg/kg.

(2) Procainamide — may be tried if lidocaine is ineffective or is contraindicated. It is administered at an infusion rate of 20 - 30mg per min. until a favorable response is noted, the QRS widens by 50% of its original width, hypotension develops or a total dose of 17mg/kg has been administered. This should be followed by a maintenance drip of 1 - 4mg/min.

(3) Magnesium sulfate — is also effective in decreasing the frequency of PVCs. The dose is 1 - 2gms slow IVP over 1 - 2 mins. followed by an infusion of 1 - 2gms/hr.

J. *Ventricular Tachycardia*

1. The causes are basically the same as those for PVCs. The most common causes are ischemic heart disease and acute myocardial infarction.

2. Treatment depends on the status of the patient and QRS morphology.

a. If the patient is clinically <u>stable</u> (awake, pain-free and has a good blood pressure) pharmacologic therapy is appropriate. Patients who fail to convert with these agents should be cardioverted; start with 100 joules.

(1) Monomorphic V-Tach: amiodarone, lidocaine, procainamide or sotalol.

(2) Polymorphic V-Tach

(a) If the baseline QT interval is normal, all of the above agents are considered first-line.

(b) If the QT interval is prolonged,* it should be assumed that the dysrhythmia is torsades de pointes (atypical V-Tach):

<u>1</u> The therapy of choice is magnesium sulfate 1 - 2gms IV over 1 - 2 mins. followed by an infusion of 1 - 2gms/hour; it is nondysrhythmogenic and rapidly effective.

---

*Class IA and IC antidysrhythmic agents are <u>contraindicated</u>; they prolong ventricular repolarization which can worsen torsades.

        <u>2</u>   Overdrive electrical pacing (transcutaneous or transvenous) and isoproterenol are also effective; they work by increasing the heart rate, thereby shortening ventricular repolarization.

        <u>3</u>   Sustained torsades should be treated with cardioversion; start with 200 joules.

    (3) Mono-or-polymorphic V-Tach with impaired cardiac function (EF < 40% or CHF): amiodarone or lidocaine may be used.

  b. If the patient is compromised (but has a pulse) cardioversion is indicated. Synchronized cardioversion should be attempted initially. Start with 100 joules and pretreat with a sedating agent such as Versed or Fentanyl. If delays in synchronization occur, switch to unsynchronized shocks using equivalent energy. Once cardioversion is achieved, antidysrhythmic therapy with lidocaine should be given.

  c. If there is <u>no</u> pulse, treat like ventricular fibrillation and defibrillate immediately; start with 200 joules.

3. It is a common misconception that all patients with ventricular tachycardia will appear to be clinically unstable. Stable patients with a wide complex tachycardia are frequently assumed to have SVT with aberrancy rather than V-Tach. This is an <u>inaccurate</u> assumption.

  a. V-Tach can<u>not</u> be differentiated from SVT with aberrancy on the basis of clinical symptoms and vital signs.

  b. <u>Unstable patients with either rhythm should be cardioverted</u>; it is effective in both cases.

  c. An ECG should be obtained in all stable patients.

    (1) Examine for evidence that favors one dysrhythmia over the other and treat accordingly.

    (2) If unable to decide, assume it is V-Tach and treat as above based on QRS morphology and cardiac function.

  d. Verapamil is <u>harmful</u> in most patients with V-Tach because it accelerates the heart rate, drops the blood pressure and does not convert the rhythm.

  e. Adenosine will not convert V-Tach to a sinus rhythm unless it is a catecholamine-induced dysrhythmia (which is rare); therefore, use of this drug as a diagnostic/therapeutic measure to distinguish V-Tach from SVT with aberrancy is not valid.

K. *Ventricular Fibrillation* (and pulseless ventricular tachycardia)

1. Causes — Easy to remember if organized by letter:

—— The Five "H*s*" —— and —— The Five "T*s*" ——

• Hypovolemia (most common)	• Tablets (drug OD)
• Hypoxemia	• Tamponade (cardiac)
• Hydrogen ion (acidosis)	• Tension pneumothorax
• Hyper/Hypokalemia	• Thrombosis, coronary (ACS)
• Hypothermia	• Thrombosis, pulmonary (embolism)

2. Treatment
    a. <u>Initial</u> therapy is <u>IMMEDIATE DEFIBRILLATION</u>. Time is of the essence. Deliver 3 successive shocks in a "stacked" fashion, checking only the monitor between shocks (do not pause for pulse checks). Start with 200 joules. If the <u>monitor</u> continues to display persistent V-Fib/V-Tach, immediately defibrillate again with 200 - 300 joules and, then, 360 joules.
    b. If defibrillation is unsuccessful, follow the "ABCs" as summarized in the ACLS 2000 Guidelines.
        (1) Airway → intubate
        (2) Breathing → confirm ET tube placement, secure the tube and confirm oxygenation and ventilation
        (3) Circulation → establish IV, put on monitor/identify rhythm and administer epinephrine or vasopressin:
            ▲ Epi is still the drug of choice for cardiac arrest: 1mg IVP
            ▲ Vasopressin can be used instead of Epi as a one-time-single-dose of 40 units IV; however, because of the large dose and long half-life (10-20 mins.), it can cause dose-related adverse effects (if given too soon) or reduce the chance of a positive outcome (if given too late). Therefore, the ACLS 2000 Guidelines (check website www.emeeinc.com for after printing updates) do not confirm an <u>active</u> recommendation for its use.
    c. 30 to 60 secs. following the dose of epinephrine, the patient's rhythm should be reassessed; if V-Fib/pulseless V-Tach persists, defibrillate with 360 joules. (Multiple sequential shocks may be used here and with subsequent defibrillations.)
    d. Epinephrine should be repeated every 3 - 5 mins. as needed in 1mg doses. At this point, an <u>active</u> search for one of the reversible causes listed above should be sought and, if found, treated.
    e. If V-Fib/pulseless V-Tach persist despite defibrillation treatment of a reversible cause and one or more doses of epinephrine, an <u>anti-fibrillatory</u> agent should be administered. Lidocaine is no longer considered the agent of first choice in the arrest situation according to the ACLS 2000 Guidelines. Amiodarone is a better choice unless the patient has an atypical V-Tach (torsades-de-pointes) or hypomagnesemia, in which case, magnesium sulfate is the drug of choice. Procainamide is also preferred over lidocaine especially in the presence of recurrent V-Fib. If all else fails, then lidocaine may be given.
    f. Whatever agent is selected, continue shocking every 30 - 60 secs. while the med is being drawn up. For any med used, defibrillate with 360 joules after each dose; the pattern should be drug-shock, drug-shock.
    g. Doses of these agents are as follows:
        (1) Amiodarone 300 mg IVP; may repeat at 150mg IVP followed by a 1mg/min. infusion for 6 hrs., then 0.5mg/min. for 18 hrs. prn.
        (2) Magnesium sulfate 1 - 2 gms IVP for torsades de pointes, known or suspected hypomagnesemia or severe refractory V-Fib.
        (3) Procainamide 30mg/min. to a max. total dose of 17mg/kg.
        (4) Lidocaine 1 - 1.5mg/kg/IVP; may repeat at 1.5mg/kg up to a total of 3mg/kg. Follow with an infusion (1 - 4mg/min.)

L. *Pulseless Electrical Activity (PEA)* — refers to a heterogeneous group of rhythms characterized by the presence of some sort of electrical activity (other than V-Tach or V-Fib) in the absence of a detectable pulse.

1. Causes... are the same as those for V-Fib/pulseless V-Tach.

2. Treatment
    a. Initiate resuscitation — perform CPR, intubate, start an IV.
    b. <u>Search for and treat the underlying cause</u> when possible. Your approach will be guided by your clinical findings, the medical history and the circumstances that preceded the development of the rhythm. Appropriate measures include:
        (1) Ventilating the patient with 100% O_2 (to treat hypoxia)
        (2) Listening for breath sounds in both lung fields and assessing the ease of manual ventilation (to R/O tension pneumothorax)
        (3) Administering a fluid bolus (to correct hypovolemia)
        (4) Assessing the patient's ECG for evidence of an Acute MI and hyperkalemia
        (5) Checking a core body temperature (to R/O hypothermia)
        (6) Looking for distended neck veins (R/O tension pneumothorax and cardiac tamponade)
        (7) Obtaining a brief history from the patient's family/friends regarding the possibility of drug overdose
    c. Administer epinephrine (see previous page for dosing); atropine 1mg IVP (for bradycardia) may be repeated Q 3 - 5 mins. up to a total dose of 0.04mg/kg.

M. *Sinoatrial (SA) Block*

1. Causes
    a. Ischemia
    b. Hyperkalemia
    c. Drugs (e.g. digitalis, beta-blockers, calcium channel blockers)
    d. Vagal stimulation

2. Treatment — is determined by the patient's cardiovascular stability. Patients with symptoms of hypoperfusion should be treated with atropine, isoproterenol or cardiac pacing. In the absence of these symptoms, observation alone is adequate.

N. *Sick Sinus Syndrome (SSS)*

1. Causes
    a. Ischemia
    b. Cardiomyopathies
    c. Myocarditis
    d. Trauma
    e. Atherosclerosis
    f. Aging

2. Treatment — depends on the hemodynamic stability of the patient. If symptoms of hypoperfusion are present, rate <u>stimulation</u> with atropine, isoproterenol or pacemaker (for bradydysrhythmias) or rate <u>control</u> with a calcium channel blocker, beta-blocker or digoxin (for tachydysrhythmias) can be <u>cautiously</u> attempted (excessive tachycardia or bradycardia may result). Hemodynamically stable patients should be referred to a cardiologist for demand pacemaker insertion and antidysrhythmic therapy.

O. Atrioventricular (AV) Blocks

1. Causes of impaired conduction:
   a. Acute MI (inferior wall or anterior wall)
   b. Drugs: digitalis, lidocaine, phenytoin, procainamide, quinidine, beta-blockers and calcium-channel blockers (including $MgSO_4$)
   c. Inflammation: myocarditis, endocarditis
   d. Hyperkalemia > 7mEq/L
   e. Hypermagnesemia > 5mEq/L
   f. Hypothermia < 30°C (86°F)
   g. Congenital conduction defects

2. Treatment:
   a. First-Degree AV Block — is often a normal variant. Other causes include increased vagal tone, digitalis toxicity and myocarditis. It does not require specific therapy.
   b. Second-Degree AV Block
      (1) Mobitz I (Wenckebach)
         (a) Is usually <u>transient</u>.
         (b) Is often seen in the setting of an acute inferior wall MI but can also be caused by digitalis toxicity, increased vagal tone and myocarditis.
         (c) Unless the patient is symptomatic, this rhythm does not generally require specific therapy.
         (d) Symptomatic patients should be treated with atropine; if this fails, transcutaneous pacing is indicated.
      (2) Mobitz II
         (a) Is a more severe form of block; it implies an organic lesion in the infranodal conduction system and is often <u>permanent</u>.
         (b) It usually occurs in association with an acute anteroseptal MI and can abruptly progress to complete block.
         (c) These patients require pacing. Transcutaneous pacing may be used as a bridging device while preparations are made for insertion of a transvenous pacemaker. Atropine should be avoided (it can accelerate the atrial rate and produce an increased AV block → ↓ventricular response rate and ↓BP).
   c. Third-Degree (complete) AV Block
      (1) Nodal (<u>narrow complex</u>) third-degree AV block — occurs in association with an acute <u>inferior</u> wall MI or drug toxicity and is usually transient. It should be treated like Second-Degree Mobitz I AV Block with atropine or transcutaneous pacing.

(2) Infranodal (<u>wide complex</u>) Third-Degree AV Block — often occurs in association with an acute <u>anterior</u> wall MI and implies significant structural damage to the infranodal conduction system. It almost always requires the insertion of a transvenous pacemaker. Transcutaneous pacing or catecholamines may be used as a bridging device while awaiting pacemaker insertion. Atropine should be used cautiously (if at all) in this setting and is probably best avoided (see discussion above under 2. b. (2) (c)).

P. *Wolff-Parkinson-White Syndrome (WPW)*

1. Recognition:
   a. PR interval < .12 secs.
   b. Delta wave — a slurred initial upstroke of the QRS complex
   c. Wide and/or bizarre QRS complex (≥ .10 secs.)
   d. An episodic tachycardia > 200 in an adult — is very suspicious of an accessory pathway syndrome.
   <u>Note</u>: Patients with WPW frequently do <u>not</u> have all of the classic features described above on their surface ECG, particularly if they are in sinus rhythm at the time of evaluation and conduction is occurring through the AV node in the normal fashion (concealed tract).

2. Importance — The primary significance of WPW syndrome is that it predisposes patients to the development of tachydysrhythmias (particularly atrial fibrillation).
   a. Patients with WPW have two parallel conducting pathways with different refractory periods (the AV node and an accessory pathway called the Kent Bundle). This predisposes them to the development of circus-movement tachycardias where an impulse is conducted anterograde to the ventricles by one pathway and retrograde back up to the atria by the other.
   b. When conduction is occurring anterograde down the AV node and retrograde back up the accessory pathway (<u>orthodromic</u> tachycardia), the ECG will appear normal. However, when the impulse is being conducted anterograde through the accessory pathway and retrograde through the AV node (<u>antidromic</u> tachycardia), the QRS complex will be wide.
   c. In the presence of antidromic conduction, the normal restraining effect of the AV node on conduction is lost and rapid ventricular response rates (>200/min.) can occur. This is particularly dangerous in atrial fibrillation, where ventricular response rates can exceed 300 per minute and degeneration to V-Fib can occur.

3. Treatment of supraventricular tachydysrhythmias in patients with WPW is determined by the patient's cardiovascular stability, specific presenting dysrhythmia, the width of the QRS complex and (with A-fib) how long they have been in it.

a. WPW with a narrow complex SVT* (orthodromic tachycardia) is treated in the same manner as other re-entrant SVT.
  (1) If the patient is hemodynamically compromised, treat with synchronized cardioversion. Start with 50 joules and pretreat with a sedating agent.
  (2) In the hemodynamically stable patient, vagal maneuvers and drugs which slow conduction through the AV node (adenosine, calcium channel or beta blockers, procainamide or amiodarone) should be used. Adenosine and verapamil are the most effective agents given their rapid onset and strong AV nodal blocking effects. IV procainamide is also effective, but is slower in onset. Amiodarone is the preferred agent if the ejection fraction is < 40% or the patient is in CHF.
b. WPW with a wide complex SVT (antidromic tachycardia)
  (1) If the patient is hemodynamically compromised, treat with cardioversion.
  (2) In stable patients, IV procainamide or amiodarone is the drug of choice depending on whether or not the heart is impaired. [Note: All AV nodal blocking agents (especially the calcium channel and beta blockers, but also digitalis and adenosine) are CONTRAINDICATED and should be avoided.]
c. WPW with atrial fibrillation or flutter (regardless of QRS duration)
  (1) In hemodynamically compromised patients and those with a fast** ventricular response rate, cardioversion is the treatment of choice. Start with 100 joules for A-Fib and 50 joules for atrial flutter.
  (2) In the hemodynamically stable patient, IV procainamide (or amiodarone) is the drug of choice; cardioversion is also acceptable if < 48 hrs. duration.
  (3) As discussed above, calcium-channel blockers, digitalis, adenosine and beta blockers should not be used in these patients.
d. In summary, drugs of choice in WPW-associated tachydysrhythmias are procainamide (normal pump function) or amiodarone (impaired pump function). Avoid AV nodal blocking agents in the presence of a wide or bizarre-looking QRS complex or A-Fib/flutter.

Specific abnormalities on ECG may differ in appearance from one tracing to the next. The sample tracings in this section may not look like the ones you will see in practice or on the exam. Therefore, it is important that you review other tracings. ECG abnormalities that you must be able to recognize include the following:
- U Waves
- Junctional escape rhythm and JPCs
- Atrial tachydysrhythmias (Sinus Tach, MAT, A-Fib/flutter, SVT with and without aberrancy)
- AV Blocks (Mobitz I / II, complete)
- Ventricular dysrhythmias (V-Tach/V-Fib and torsades)
- WPW syndrome

*Most common presentation of WPW
**Over 200 BPM

- MIs (anterior/inferior)
- ECG abnormalities secondary to hypo/hyperkalemia, bretylium and digitalis
- Epicardial injury current produced by pericardiocentesis
- Brugada Syndrome — RBBB with coved or saddle-back shaped ST segments in the anteroseptal leads (V_1 + V_2).

More examples of these rhythms can be found in <u>Rosen's Text,</u> <u>Tintinalli's Text</u> or <u>ECG in Emergency Medicine and Acute Care 2005</u> (Chan, et.al.).

If you have trouble with dysrhythmias, review the ACLS manual. Better yet, take an ACLS course. If you need more exposure to specific ECG abnormalities, do the following:

(1) Gain access to an ECG teaching file. All hospitals with residency programs in Emergency Medicine or Internal Medicine have them. Coronary Care Units frequently have them too. Ask to borrow or copy those tracings that demonstrate abnormalities you need to review. If you have trouble recognizing any of them, find an emergency physician, internist or cardiologist who can help you.

(2) On a 3"x 5" card list those tracings you want to see and put a number after each one to designate how many you think you need to see to feel comfortable. You may need to see only one tracing of A-Fib with a slow ventricular rate. On the other hand, you may want to see ten tracings of SVT with aberrancy that look like V-Tach. Put a check mark down every time you see a specific tracing.

(3) Don't worry about doing this "all at once." It's not necessary. Just get started by finding a teaching file and letting other physicians know what you need to see. You will learn best by reviewing the tracings in piecemeal fashion (just a few a week) and this can be done easily during those "odd moments" in the Emergency Department.

Most Written Board Courses and residency programs provide dozens of ECG samples. A discussion of Written Board Courses is included in this text under the section entitled, "Additional Tips for Good Performance."

IV. Pacemakers — When to pace and problems with pacers

A. *Emergency Pacing Techniques* — emergency cardiac pacing can be accomplished via transcutaneous, transesophageal or transvenous electrodes. Transcutaneous pacing (TCP) is the technique of choice in the emergency care setting, particularly in the presence of an Acute MI in patients who have received (or may receive) thrombolytic therapy. It is the most easily and rapidly applied technique as well as the least invasive.

B. Indications for Temporary Cardiac Pacing

1. Emergent
   a. Hemodynamically unstable bradycardias
   b. Bradycardias associated with malignant escape rhythms that fail to respond to pharmacologic therapy
   c. Overdrive of refractory tachydysrhythmias
   d. <u>Early</u> bradyasystolic arrest (within 10 - 20 mins. of arrest)

2. Prophylactic (standby kit at bedside)
   a. Stable bradycardias (asymptomatic or those that responded to initial drug therapy)
   b. The presence of one of the following in the setting of an acute MI:
      (1) Symptomatic sinus node dysfunction
      (2) Mobitz II Second-Degree AV Block
      (3) Complete heart block
      (4) Newly acquired or age-indeterminate LBBB, RBBB, alternating BBB or bifascicular block.

C. Tips for Temporary Transvenous Pacemaker Placement

1. The ideal location of the catheter tip is lodged in the trabeculae of the apex of the <u>right ventricle</u>.

2. The <u>right internal jugular</u> is the preferred access site because it provides the most direct route to the right ventricle.

3. Although more time consuming and not always possible, insertion using fluoroscopic or ECG guidance is preferred to blind placement (which is less reliable in achieving proper catheter positioning).

4. When ECG guidance is used, the V lead is connected to the distal lead of the pacing catheter with a standard connector or alligator clip. Then, while monitoring the V lead, the pacing catheter is advanced and the size of the P wave and QRS complex is observed to determine location of the catheter tip; the size of these wave forms will increase when the corresponding heart chambers are entered. The development of ST elevation ("current of injury") signals successful placement of the catheter tip.

5. Pacing results in an abnormal QRS morphology. When the catheter tip is properly placed in the right ventricle, this ventricle is stimulated first, while stimulation of the left ventricle is delayed. This produces a <u>left bundle branch block</u> pattern on the surface ECG.

6. Following pacemaker placement, a CXR (AP and lateral) should be obtained to confirm appropriate placement and r/o a procedural pneumothorax.

D. Coding System for Permanent Pacemakers

1. A series of 3 - 5 letters, designating the specific capabilities of each pacemaker, is used to describe the many types of permanent pacemakers currently available today:

- **First letter (VADO) = chamber <u>paced</u>**
  V - ventricle
  A - atrium
  D - dual (V + A)
  O - none

- **Second letter (VADO) = chamber <u>sensed</u>**
  V - ventricle
  A - atrium
  D - dual (V + A)
  O - none

- **Third letter (TIDO) = response to sensing of electrical activity**
  T - triggers
  I - inhibits
  D - dual (T + I)
  O - none

- **Fourth letter (PMCRO) = program functions**
  P - programmable rate, output or both
  M - multiprogrammability of rate, output, sensitivity, etc.
  C - communication function (telemetry)
  R - rate modulation
  O - none

- **Fifth letter (PSDO) = antitachydysrhythmia function**
  P - antitachydysrhythmia pacing
  S - shock
  D - dual (P + S)
  O - none

2. Referring to the above table, a pacemaker coded with the series of VVIR both paces and senses the ventricle (V V), responds to spontaneous electrical activity sensed (in the ventricle) by inhibiting pacing (I), and has biosensors that allow for an increase in the pacing rate to match the patient's level of physical activity (R).

E. Pacemaker Failure

1. Tools for evaluating pacemaker malfunction:
   a. ECG — to confirm that appropriate sensing and capture are occurring and to indirectly assess the position of the pacing catheter by evaluating QRS morphology.

    b. CXR (PA and lateral) — to evaluate lead position, R/O cardiac perforation and look for lead fracture (not always visible).

    c. Pacemaker magnet — application of the magnet over the pacemaker turns off the sensing function (via the Reed switch) and thereby temporarily converts the pacemaker from the demand (synchronous) mode to the fixed-rate (asynchronous) mode → continuous asynchronous pacing at a specified rate (the magnet rate) which is usually around 70. This allows assessment of whether the pacing function is intact and whether the pacing stimulus can capture the myocardium. This maneuver is especially helpful in cases in which the baseline ECG does not reveal any pacemaker spikes. Moreover, it also allows assessment of the battery status; a decrease in the magnet rate suggests battery depletion.

2. Signs of pacemaker failure:

    a. Slowing of the pacing rate — is due to battery depletion. Replacement is urgent if the rate is 10% below the setpoint.

    b. A rapidly paced rhythm resembling V-Tach ("runaway pacemaker") — is usually due to battery depletion or circuitry malfunction.

3. Specific problems:

    a. Failure to pace — is detected clinically by the absence of pacemaker spikes in a patient whose intrinsic cardiac rhythm is slower than the programmed pacemaker rate. Causes include:

        (1) Wire fracture — is accompanied by acute onset of symptoms that may be sustained or intermittent. It usually occurs at one of 3 sites: (1) close to the pulse generator; (2) where the lead enters the vein; or (3) within the heart where the lead makes a sharp bend. Check the CXR; it will demonstrate lead placement and may also reveal wire fracture.

        (2) Battery depletion — is rare with the lithium batteries used today if the patient is being monitored often enough.

        (3) Oversensing (sensing electrical events not associated with atrial or ventricular depolarizations) — suppresses impulse generation in pacemakers in the <u>inhibit</u> mode. It is more common in patients with unipolar leads and the most common cause of failure to pace.

    b. Failure to sense or capture — is detected clinically by the presence of pacemaker spikes occurring at the wrong time (failure to sense) or the presence of pacemaker spikes without associated QRS complexes (failure to capture). [Be able to recognize on monitor strip] Causes include:

        (1) Lead malposition

            (a) Lead displacement — usually occurs in the first month post-implantation.

            (b) Cardiac perforation — usually occurs within 4 days of insertion.

        (2) Wire or insulation fracture

        (3) Battery depletion

   (4) Elevated myocardial threshold — due to:
    (a) Fibrosis or inflammation at the electrode tip
    (b) Lead displacement
    (c) Metabolic and physiologic causes
     <u>1</u> Metabolic acidosis
     <u>2</u> Hypoxia
     <u>3</u> Hyperkalemia
     <u>4</u> Antidysrhythmic drugs (particularly ones which prolong the QRS)
     <u>5</u> Ischemia
     <u>6</u> MI
   (5) Undersensing (which means voltage of the patient's own intrinsic QRS complex is too low for the pacemaker to sense) — is more common with bipolar pacemakers. Sensitivity may be increased by converting to a unipolar pacemaker.
   (6) Oversensing (in pacemakers in the <u>triggered</u> mode) — pacemaker spikes appear when none are expected because the pacemaker senses and reacts to events other than true cardiac events.
  c. Pacemaker-mediated tachycardia (PMT)
   (1) Only occurs in patients with <u>dual-chamber</u> pacemakers that are programmed for synchronous atrioventricular pacing.
   (2) Requires the presence of ventriculoatrial conduction; is a form of re-entrant tachycardia.
   (3) Can be precipitated by a PAC or PVC.
   (4) Treatment
    (a) May be terminated by using a pacemaker magnet to briefly turn off the sensing function.
    (b) Definitive therapy requires reprogramming of the atrial refractory period by a pacemaker specialist.
  d. Runaway pacemaker
   (1) May be triggered by battery depletion.
   (2) Rarely occurs today because most newer pacemakers have built-in safety circuits.
   (3) Heart rate is frequently > 200 beats/min.
   (4) Treatment
    (a) Placement of a pacemaker magnet over the pacemaker may convert the pacemaker to the magnet rate and break the tachycardia.
    (b) If this is unsuccessful, and the patient is hemodynamically unstable, the pacemaker must be disconnected. To do this, exteriorize the pacer and cut the electrode wires. These wires may be reconnected to a temporary pacer if the patient's underlying rhythm is unstable.

V. Automatic Implantable Cardioverter - Defibrillators (AICDs)

A. *Indications* — AICDs are placed in patients who are at high risk for fatal dys-rhythmias (V-Tach, V-Fib) and sudden cardiac death (SCD). Included in this high-risk group are patients who survived an episode of SCD and those with a prior MI or Brugada Syndrome. In these patients, AICDs decrease the risk of SCD remarkably from 30 - 45% per year to < 2% per year.

B. *Biomechanics*

    1. AICD components include:
       a. A lead system with both sensing and shocking electrodes
       b. Logic circuitry — to analyze the signal sensed
       c. A pulse generator — generate high voltage (shock)
       d. A capacitor — to deliver the shock

    2. Longevity of AICDs — varies with the generation of the AICD and the frequency of its use; the newer, third-generation devices can deliver approximately 300 shocks and have a projected life-span of 7 - 8 years.

C. *AICD Issues in the Emergency Department*

    1. Device ineffectiveness — may result from lead fracture (is sometimes detectable on x-ray) or failure of one of the other components of the device (e.g. battery depletion); malfunctions have also been reported from strong electromagnetic fields and interference from appliances and security/anti-theft devices.

    2. Frequent and recurrent AICD discharge
       a. May be reported or result from:
          (1) More frequent episodes of V-Fib/V-Tach
          (2) Sensing malfunction/false sensing (e.g. sensing and shocking of SVT or muscular contractions)
          (3) "Ghost shocks" (patient reports shocks when none have occurred)
       b. Evaluation of these patients should include:
          (1) Continuous cardiac monitoring
          (2) ECG and CXR
          (3) Cardiac markers and drug levels
          (4) Potassium, magnesium* and calcium levels
          (5) Telemetry interrogation of the AICD
          (6) Consultation with the patient's cardiologist
       c. Inactivation — placement of a magnet over the AICD generator will inactivate it and thereby prevent further shocks (see next page)

---

*Hypomagnesemia is a common cause of dysrhythmias in AICD patients

3. Performance of CPR and defibrillation with an AICD in place
   a. CPR — is performed in the usual manner; while the provider may perceive an AICD shock, it is neither uncomfortable nor dangerous.
   b. External transthoracic defibrillation — may also be performed in the standard manner. The paddles should <u>not</u> be placed close to the AICD generator; paddle placement is otherwise unchanged. Following successful external cardioversion/defibrillation, the AICD should be tested to confirm that sensing and therapy parameters have not been altered.

4. AICD inactivation — AICDs are generally inactivated by the presence of a magnet; however, some device-to-device variability exists:
   a. With second-generation AICDs, the placement of a donut-shaped magnet over the upper right quadrant of the pulse generator for 30 seconds will inactivate the antitachycardic pacing and shock therapy components of the AICD. Reapplication of the magnet for thirty seconds reactivates it.
   b. With the newer third-generation AICDs, placement of the magnet over the pulse generator inactivates antitachycardic pacing therapy and shocks for as long as the magnet remains in place over the AICD. Removal of the magnet reactivates the device.

5. Infection — Patients who present with erythema, induration or drainage at the generator site require hospitalization for IV antibiotics. Early infections are usually caused by Staph species.

ACUTE CORONARY SYNDROMES

I. **Definition** — Acute coronary syndromes are defined as a continuum or pro-gression of coronary artery disease from myocardial ischemia to necrosis: stable angina → unstable angina → acute myocardial infarction.

II. **Clinical Presentations, Risk Factors and Predictive Factors**

A. *Classic Presentations* of an acute coronary syndrome (ACS):

1. Stable angina: transient, episodic chest discomfort that is predictable and reproducible, i.e. familiar symptoms occur from a characteristic stimulus that improve with rest or sublingual nitroglycerin within a few minutes. [These patients are usually sent home or observed briefly in the ED.]

2. Unstable angina: angina that is new in onset, occurs at rest or is simi-lar but somewhat "different" than previous episodes, and is severely limiting or lasts longer than a few minutes. Other signs are an increased frequency of attacks or resistance to prescribed meds that previously relieved the symptoms (e.g. NTG, the "blockers"). [These patients are admitted for observation or coronary care.]

3. Acute myocardial infarction: substernal chest discomfort > 15 minutes duration associated with dyspnea, diaphoresis, light-headedness, palpi-tations, nausea and/or vomiting; pain radiation to the inner aspect of one or both arms, shoulders, neck or jaw is not uncommon and increases the probability the pain/pressure is ischemic in origin; most patients experience these signs and symptoms in the morning within a few hours of awakening. An AMI is classified as a non-ST-segment elevation MI (NSTEMI) or an ST-segment elevation MI (STEMI). [These patients are admitted to CCU after appropriate treatment.]

B. *Atypical Presentations* (more common in the elderly)

1. Chest pain or discomfort (not substernal chest pain/pressure) with or without any of the classic associated symptoms; a history of angina is often absent.

2. Epigastric discomfort/indigestion or nausea and vomiting (which may be the only complaint in female patients or those with an inferior wall MI)

3. Shortness of breath (which may progress to pulmonary edema)

4. Syncope or confusion

5. Fatigue, dizziness or generalized weakness

6. Women with prodromal symptoms (unusual fatigue, sleep disturbances, shortness of breath) for a month or more *

7. No chest or abdominal pain or discomfort; associated symptoms may or may not be present; patient frequently has vague complaints — "Silent MI".
   a. Approximately 12.5% of all MIs
   b. The following patients should be suspect:
      (1) The elderly
      (2) Diabetics
      (3) Those with spinal cord injuries or disease
      (4) Alcoholics
      (5) Hypertensive patients or those with hypotensive insults
      (6) Post-op patients receiving analgesics and post-coronary artery bypass graft patients

   Note: These patients generally have a worse prognosis than those with a classic presentation.

C. Risk Factors

1. Major
   - Cigarette smoking
   - Hypertension
   - Diabetes Mellitus
   - Hypercholesterolemia
   - Family history of coronary artery disease prior to age 55 in a first-degree relative
   - Previous history of coronary artery disease, peripheral vascular disease, hypercoagulability or carotid arteriosclerosis

2. Other
   - Male sex
   - Advanced age
   - Methamphetamine use
   - Cocaine use (especially within an hour of presentation or when combined with ingestion of ETOH → cocaethylene; a longer-acting and more toxic by-product)
   - Obesity
   - Inactive lifestyle
   - Postmenopausal state

D. Predictive Factors of an Evolving AMI**

1. Prior history of ischemic heart disease

2. Chest pain/discomfort that is worse than usual angina

3. Pain that is similar to a prior AMI, lasting longer than an hour or radiates to the left shoulder/arm

---

*LLSA 2006 reading list: "Women's Early Warning Symptoms of Acute Myocardial Infarction."
**Are of greater clinical significance than risk factors

III. Diagnosis (<u>Note</u>: A patient without chest pain whose initial ECG and cardiac enzymes are normal may still have an MI)

A. *History:* A thorough history is the most important tool for identifying patients with cardiac ischemia and is adequate by itself to initiate hospital admission. Patients with a suspicious history, normal initial ECG and cardiac enzymes should be admitted to the hospital or chest pain evaluation/observation unit with a diagnosis of "Rule out MI"; typically, only 25% or fewer of these patients will have a diagnosis of "Acute MI" on discharge.

B. *Response To Medication:* Clinical improvement after administration of nitroglycerin or an antacid does not rule out an acute MI.

C. *ECG* *

1. Single most important adjunctive diagnostic test for assessing patients suspected of having acute myocardial ischemia. The <u>initial</u> ECG is diagnostic, however, in only 25 - 50% of patients presenting with an AMI. Therefore, the finding of a normal or nondiagnostic ECG in a patient with chest pain does <u>not</u> R/O the presence of an ACS.
    a. ECG findings suggestive of the presence of an acute <u>STEMI</u> include the presence of ST segment elevation, Q waves and inverted T waves. Increased amplitude of the R and T waves ("giant" R waves and "hyperacute" T waves) is actually the first change to occur in an evolving MI, but this finding is transient and has usually resolved by the time the patient arrives in the ED. ST segment elevation (representing the current of injury) is usually the earliest sign to be <u>recorded</u> and may be accompanied by associated reciprocal changes. The initial upsloping portion of the ST segment is <u>usually</u> convex or flat (horizontally or obliquely) in STEMI; exceptions, however, do occur. This is followed over the next few hours by the development of Q waves (representing myocardial necrosis but not the severity of the infarct) and, finally, T wave inversion.
        (1) Isolated ST segment elevation (no Q waves or T wave changes) may occur in the absence of an ACS (especially if it does not occur in characteristic leads); this is seen most often with ECG evidence of left ventricular hypertrophy (most common) and LBBB; however, a <u>new</u> LBBB in this setting may indicate an ACS. [Note: an isolated ST segment elevation may also occur with a ventricular aneurysm.]
        (2) Q waves without associated ST and T wave changes may be due to an old (not new) MI in the presence of LBBB; however, Q waves in Leads I, AVL, V_5 and V_6 suggest AMI.
        (3) Isolated T wave inversion (no Q waves or ST changes) indicates ischemia (not acute infarction).

*Should be obtained and reviewed within 10 minutes of patient's arrival in ED.

    b. Reciprocal changes: ST segment depression (horizontal or down-sloping) that occurs in leads opposite to those with ST segment elevation. The presence of these changes increases the positive predictive value for the ECG diagnosis of STEMI to > 90% and denotes a patient at higher risk for later complications.

    c. ECG localization of the site of infarction

       (1) ST segment elevation in Leads I, aVL and V_1 - V_4 (with ST segment depression in Leads II, III and aVF) represents an <u>acute anterior wall MI (LAD)</u> → greater risk for development of conduction abnormalities (AV, bundle branch, fascicular and infranodal blocks) and LV dysfunction (CHF).

       (2) ST segment elevation in Leads I, aVL and V_5 - V_6 (with ST segment depression in Leads V_1, V_{3R} and V_{4R}) represents an <u>acute lateral wall MI(LAD)</u> → risk for development of LV dysfunction.

       (3) ST segment elevation in Leads II, III and aVF (with ST depression in I, aVL and V_1 - V_4) represents <u>an acute inferior wall MI</u> (right CA) → greater incidence of increased vagal tone-mediated dysrhythmias such as sinus bradycardia and varying degrees of AV block.

       (4) ST segment elevation in Leads V_{3R} and V_{4R} represents an <u>acute right ventricular wall MI (right CA)</u> → greater risk for developing hypotension and cardiogenic shock. Most right ventricular wall MIs occur in association with an inferior wall MI; ST elevation will be mild.

       (5) Because none of the "routine" ECG leads face the posterior surface of the heart, the presence of an <u>acute posterior wall MI (circumflex art. off right CA)</u> is usually inferred from the finding of reciprocal changes in the anterior leads, particularly V_1 and V_2; ST segment <u>depression</u> in association with abnormally tall R waves in these leads is the main ECG feature of this diagnosis. When a posterior wall MI is suspected, obtain "additional" posterior leads (V_8 and V_9); the presence of ST segment elevation in these leads confirms the diagnosis.[*]

    d. Additional-lead (15-lead) ECGs

       (1) Allow more accurate characterization of acute inferior wall MIs by improving identification of associated right ventricular (RV) and posterior wall involvement.

       (2) They incorporate three additional leads to better visualize the right ventricle (V_{4R}) and posterior wall of the left ventricle (V_8 and V_9), areas that are poorly defined on standard 12-lead ECGs.

       (3) These ECGs should be obtained in patients being admitted for suspected acute ischemia who have:
- ST segment <u>depression</u> or suspicious isoelectric ST segments in leads V_1 - V_3 (posterior infarct)
- ST segment elevation in leads II, III, and aVF (inferior wall infarct) → screen for right ventricular infarction as well (V_{4R}).

---

[*]ACEP Clinical Policy for "The initial approach to patients with suspected acute myocardial infarction or unstable angina"

- Isolated ST segment elevation in V_1 or ST segment elevation in leads V_1 and V_2 (right ventricular infarct)
- Borderline ST segment elevation in leads II, III and aVF or in leads V_5 and V_6 (inferior wall infarct)
- Symptoms consistent with RV ischemia (e.g. epigastric pain, significant hypotension following administration of NTG.)

(4) Clinical Significance

    (a) Patients with an acute posteroinferior wall MI or right ventricular infarction usually have larger-sized MIs, lower ejection fractions and higher morbidity/mortality rates.

    (b) Associated hypotension in patients with right ventricular infarction will likely respond to IV fluids; morphine, nitrates and diuretics may further compound the situation.

Note: Use of 15-lead ECGs should be restricted to the patient population described above; obtaining additional-lead ECGs in all ED patients with chest pain does not appear to have therapeutic or diagnostic benefits, and results in an unacceptable increase in false-positive diagnosis.

2. The initial ECG* is also useful in the following situations:
   a. Screening for nonischemic (but potentially serious) causes of chest pain such as pericarditis and pulmonary embolism.
   b. Stratifying the risk of an adverse outcome in association with in-hospital disposition:

      (1) Patients at high risk for complications and death should be admitted to a CCU or ICU bed. Included in this group are patients with any of the following ECG findings:
      - Ischemic ST or T wave changes (in characteristic leads)
      - Pathologic Q waves (are > .04 sec. long or ≥ 25% of R wave height)
      - Left ventricular hypertrophy
      - LBBB (new or age uncertain)
      - RBBB and ST changes (R/O Brugada Syndrome)
      - Paced rhythm

      (2) Patients at low risk for complications can safely be admitted to a step-down unit. Included in this group are patients whose initial ECG is either normal or has nonspecific ST - T wave changes.
   c. Establishing the criteria that determine which therapeutic interventions will be employed (beta blockers, thrombolytic therapy, etc.)

3. Serial ECGs
   a. Are indicated in patients with nondiagnostic ECGs in whom there is concern for possible ongoing ischemia.
   b. Capture ischemic ECG changes, demonstrate ECG stability and detect silent ischemia; ST segment trend-monitoring may improve detection.

   [Note: Patients demonstrating normal or nonspecific initial ECGs with subsequent confirmed AMIs within 72 hrs. still have a high rate of mortality and life-threatening complications.]

*2006 LLSA Reading List   "Prognostic Value of a Normal of Nonspecific Initial Electrocardiogram in Acute Myocardial Infarctions."

A visual glossary entitled "Radiographic Diagnosis of Acute Coronary Syndromes" (which appeared in *Emergency Medicine Reports*, April 23, 2001) contains ECG tracings that depict the characteristic findings of each coronary syndrome. This glossary may be viewed or downloaded from the homepage of our website (emeeinc.com). For enhanced clarity in viewing some ECGs, be sure to enlarge the view of the document to correctly interpret its recording. It is an excellent addendum to this section of the cardiovascular chapter.

D. Serum Markers of Acute MI

1. Myoglobin — rises within 2 - 3 hours of symptom onset and peaks within 4 - 24 hours. It is more sensitive than the total CK and CK-MB but is <u>not</u> specific for cardiac muscle and, therefore, has a high false-positive rate. Therefore, it cannot reliably identify or exclude an MI at any time junction; it is best used in conjunction with other markers.

2. CK — rises within 4 - 8 hours of an infarction and peaks within 12 - 24 hours. However, it is <u>not</u> specific for an Acute MI; in addition to heart muscle, it is also found in skeletal muscle and brain tissue, so elevations can be due to disorders of any of these organ systems.

3. CK-MB — rises within 4 - 10 hours of an infarction, peaks within 20 hours and is fairly specific. The newer monoclonal assays which directly measure CK-MB mass (and subforms) are more sensitive and more rapidly performed than the old electrophoretic assays and have essentially replaced them.

4. Troponin T and I — appear in the serum within 6 hours of symptom onset and remain elevated for 1 - 2 weeks. Troponin I is the most specific cardiac marker available (almost 100%). Troponin T is not as specific as Troponin I (but far more than CK-MB) and is valuable in predicting cardiovascular complications in unstable angina and AMI.

5. Appropriate use of serum markers
   a. The decision to admit or discharge a patient should be based <u>primarily</u> on the patient's history and clinical presentation, not on the presence or absence of elevated cardiac enzymes.
      (1) Detection of these markers requires that sufficient myocardial cell damage has occurred and that enough time has passed for these markers to be released into the serum.
      (2) Initial determination of these markers has a low sensitivity for detecting ischemia and <u>cannot</u> be used to reliably diagnose or exclude the presence of an acute coronary syndrome.
      (3) No <u>single</u> determination of <u>one</u> serum biomarker of myoneurosis reliably identifies or excludes AMI in < 6 hours of symptom onset.

b. As you can see from the summary table below, the lab result reported for each serum marker is not as valuable as the <u>pattern</u> of the results as well as an accurate history of the onset of signs and symptoms in a patient with a nondiagnostic ECG.
   (1) When did the signs/symptoms begin (today and before today)?
   (2) What's been going on in the past two weeks that was new or different (changes in meds, doses, habits, activities, other illnesses or complaints)?
   (3) Pinpointing the <u>time</u> when things changed and signs/symptoms appeared allows you to plot the timing of enzyme activity and interpret the results more accurately.

Summary table of cardiac serum markers

Serum marker	Rises	Peaks	Remains elevated
Myoglobin	2 - 3 hrs.	4 - 24 hrs.	< 1 day
CK	4 - 8 hrs.	12 - 24 hrs.	< 3 - 4 days
CK-MB*	4 - 10 hrs.	20 hrs.*	< 2 days
Troponins** (T + I)	6 hrs.	12 - 18 hrs.	TnI = 7 - 10 days TnT = 10 - 14 days

*A CKMB2:CKMB1 ratio > 1.5 at this time is diagnostic of AMI.

**The markers of choice, especially if there is a delayed presentation; their presence is positive proof a problem exists.

E. **Two-dimensional Echocardiography**: Is effective in detecting the regional wall abnormalities that occur in association with an acute MI but is unable to distinguish between ischemia, acute infarction and old infarction. Moreover, it is operator-dependent and not readily available. However, it has been used recently with stress testing ("Stress Echo") in selected patients.

F. **Radionuclide Scanning**

1. Technetium 99m sestamibi imaging
   a. Technetium 99 is a myocardial perfusion tracer that is taken up by the myocardium in proportion to blood flow; sestamibi is a small protein that is labeled with radio-pharmaceutical technetium 99.
   b. It can detect perfusion defects and segmental wall abnormalities such as hypokinesia.
   c. In patients with <u>active</u> chest pain and a nondiagnostic ECG, it has 100% sensitivity and 83 - 92% specificity; in painfree patients, however, its sensitivity is only 65%.

2. Thallium 201 scintigraphy
   a. Thallium 201 is reversibly taken up by normally perfused cells, thus areas of decreased uptake indicate regions of severe ischemia or infarction.

    b. In patients presenting <u>within 6 hours</u> of infarction, it identifies AMI with a sensitivity of 100% but has specificity of only 80%.

    c. Unfortunately, it ca<u>nnot</u> distinguish new from old infarct; its accuracy decreases over time and its sensitivity is decreased in patients with small infarcts, non-Q-wave infarcts and unstable angina.

Although these studies can be helpful in evaluating patients who have chest pain suggestive of myocardial ischemia and a nondiagnostic ECG, they are expensive, have limited availability and poor specificity; therefore, they have a limited role in the ED setting.

G. Chest Pain Evaluation Unit

1. A safe, effective alternative to routine admission of low-intermediate risk patients with chest pain.
2. Protocols vary but usually involve serial studies (ECGs, markers) and selective stress testing for evaluation of risk stratification.

IV. Treatment

A. IV (NS) — O₂ (2 - 4L/min) — Cardiac Monitor — Pulse Oximeter

B. Antiplatelet Agents

1. Aspirin (ASA)
   a. ASA, through its antiplatelet activity, is beneficial in the treatment of angina (reduces the <u>risk</u> of AMI) and infarction itself. It decreases mortality, infarct size and rate of reinfarction associated with unstable angina (UA) and AMI whether or not thrombolytic therapy is given. Maximum benefit occurs if given in the first 4 hours of chest pain onset.
   b. ASA <u>irreversibly</u> acetylates platelet cyclo-oxygenase and has a <u>rapid</u> onset of action (within 60 minutes).
   c. Unless contraindications exist, administer 160 - 325mg on arrival in the ED and continue indefinitely. It should be chewed so as to maximize bioavailability. If vomiting is present, it may be given as a rectal suppository.

2. Platelet Receptor Inhibitors
   a. Available agents: ticlopidine (Ticlid®) and clopidogrel (Plavix®).
   b. Mechanism of action: affect platelet activity (including aggregation) through inhibition of ADP platelet activation.
   c. Indication: "second-line" antiplatelet therapy for patients who can not take ASA (poor tolerance, allergy) or who have failures on ASA therapy; they are less effective than ASA; due to their <u>delayed</u> onset of action, they are not ideal agents for the initial management of UA/AMI.

d. Clopidogrel is the agent of choice because its onset of action is 2 - 3 hours versus 3 - 5 days for ticlopidine. In addition, ticlopidine has significant toxic (even potentially life-threatening) side effects (e.g. agranulocytosis, thrombocytopenia); clopidogrel, however, has relatively few side effects and is similar to ASA in its safety profile. [Note: There is an increased morbidity/mortality rate when clopidogrel is used in patients undergoing coronary bypass surgery after admission.]

e. Current status: patients with unstable angina or NSTEMI (in whom an early noninvasive approach is planned) clopidogrel should be given soon after ASA administration; this combination has been associated with a reduced risk of cardiovascular events in these patients; however, there is also a higher risk of major bleeding.

3. Glycoprotein (GP) IIb/IIIa Receptor Antagonists
   a. Available agents include: abciximab (ReoPro®), eptifibatide (Integrilin®) and tirofiban (Aggrastat®)
   b. These agents represent the latest generation of powerful platelet inhibitors; there are multiple trials investigating the adjunctive role of these agents in combination with fibrinolytic therapies (incl. TPA).
   c. Mechanism of action: in the presence of platelet activation, the GP IIb/IIIa receptor inhibitors block the final common pathway for platelet aggregation.
   d. Current indications:
      (1) Patients in whom catheterization and a procedural coronary intervention is planned, but they are not recommended after PCI due to an increased rate of thrombotic complications.
      (2) Patients with ACS and refractory symptoms, a confirmed NSTEMI or an elevated troponin level.

C. Anticoagulant (anti-thrombotic) Therapy

1. Heparin
   a. Is indicated for all patients presenting with an ACS (AMI, UA) except those with a low-risk presentation.
   b. Acts as an indirect thrombin inhibitor by accelerating the action of antithrombin III (a thrombin inhibitor) and activated factors IX, X + XI. Its antithrombotic activity complements the antiplatelet activity of ASA to prevent progression of ischemia to AMI; when used together, heparin + ASA are more effective than when either one is used alone.
   c. Has the following beneficial effects:
      (1) In the Acute MI setting, it decreases the incidence of DVT, reinfarction, nonhemorrhagic CVA and the formation (as well as embolization) of left ventricular thrombus.
      (2) When administered to patients receiving thrombolytic agents, it prevents/decreases the incidence of reocclusion. (Note: It should not be administered after APSAC because it significantly increases bleeding complications when used in combination with this agent; it should also be avoided in patients who received streptokinase since it may increase the risk of bleeding complications.)

    (3) In patients with unstable angina, it may be useful in decreasing the rate of subsequent transmural infarction.

    (4) It may be preferred by cardiologists who are taking patients to the cath lab because you can turn it off.

  d. Low molecular weight heparins may be considered acceptable in patients < 75 yrs. old without significant renal dysfunction; in addition, enoxaparin (Lovenox) is preferred to unfractionated heparin in patients with UA/NSTEMI in the absence of renal failure or planned CABG within 24 hours.

    (1) Produce less bleeding than unfractionated heparin with equivalent or better antithrombotic effects.

    (2) Are also the agents of choice when unfractionated heparin is contraindicated due to non-availability of an aPTT (or PTT) measurement.

    (3) Provide simple administration and dosing, limited blood monitoring, better bioavailability and a more predictable anticoagulation effect.

    (4) Reduce the incidence of recurrent angina and AMI, the need for urgent revascularization and the mortality rate.

    (5) Are more expensive than standard heparin.

  e. Dosage: bolus of 60U/kg (maximum 4000U) followed by an initial infusion of 12U/kg/hr. (maximum 1000U/hr.) adjusted to maintain a PTT 1.5 - 2.0 times control (~50 - 70 seconds).

2. <u>Direct</u> thrombin inhibitors (Hirudin, Hirulog, Argatroban): can inactivate thrombin already bound to fibrin (clot-bound thrombin) which unfractionated heparin cannot do as effectively.

D. Nitroglycerin (NTG)

1. Limits infarct size, preserves ventricular function, prevents aneurysm formation, reduces pain (and consequently catecholamine release) -- all of which subsequently reduces mortality in patients with acute infarction.

2. Pathophysiology

  a. Dilates collateral coronary vessels and increases collateral blood flow to ischemic myocardium.

  b. Has antiplatelet effects and reduces infarct size and mortality.

  c. Decreases myocardial oxygen demand by decreasing preload, left ventricular end-diastolic volume and afterload (which makes it the drug of choice when there is coexisting left ventricular failure).

  d. May also reduce myocardial susceptibility to ventricular dysrhythmias during ischemia and reperfusion.

3. Should be administered to patients with ischemic chest pain whose BP is > 90mmHg. Start with sublingual nitroglycerin 0.4mg Q 3 - 5 mins. prn pain. Follow with an infusion of 10 - 20mcg/min. and increase it by 5 - 10mcg/min. Q 5 - 10 mins. until pain is controlled or the systolic BP is decreased by 10%.

4. Adverse reactions
   a. Hypotension — usually responds to a fluid bolus and leg elevation; it is particularly common when NTG is given to patients with inferior wall MIs with associated RV infarction as well as to those with hypovolemia or bradycardia; caution should be exercised when administering NTG to these patients.
   b. Reflex tachycardia — may be moderated by the concomitant use of beta blockers.

Note: Administration of NTG to patients taking sildenafil citrate (Viagra®) is CONTRAINDICATED. In these patients, NTG can precipitate a sudden and profound decrease in BP → decreased coronary perfusion and conversion of myocardial ischemia to myocardial infarction with all of its potential consequences; it should be avoided for 12 - 24 hours after using this agent. Morphine can be used instead, followed by a trip to the Cath Lab or administration of thrombolytics.

E. Beta Blockers

1. Early intravenous administration of beta-blocking agents (metoprolol, atenolol or esmolol) dramatically decreases the mortality rate associated with acute infarction; these agents decrease infarct size, reduce the incidence of reinfarction, recurrent ischemia and fatal dysrhythmias and are associated with less intracranial bleeding. Most authors recommend their use as early as possible (within two hours of presentation) in all patients with AMI (without contraindications) whether or not they receive reperfusion therapy; those with the largest infarctions benefit most from beta blockers.

2. Pathophysiology
   a. Decrease myocardial oxygen demand by reducing the heart rate and myocardial contractility.
   b. Increase coronary blood flow by prolonging the time of diastole and reducing myocardial wall tension.
   c. Markedly decrease the rate of myocardial rupture (particularly in the elderly).
   d. Decrease the incidence of V-Fib and cardiac rupture.
   e. Reduce platelet aggregation.

3. Most useful in patients with tachycardia, hypertension or those with recurrent/unrelenting chest pain, with the greatest benefit in patients > 65 yrs. old; they should be given early in the clinical management of AMI to achieve maximum results.

4. Contraindications include:
   a. Bradycardia (HR < 60/min.)
   b. Hypotension (systolic BP < 100mmHg)
   c. Moderate to severe left ventricular dysfunction (CHF, pulmonary edema)
   d. Signs of hypoperfusion

        e. Infarction precipitated by cocaine use

        f. PR interval > 0.24 secs.

        g. Second-or-third degree AV block

        h. Active bronochospasm

5. Precautions

    a. Avoid in patients with cocaine-induced chest pain (↑HTN)

    b. Use cautiously in patients with bronchospastic lung disease (COPD or asthma) or moderate LV dysfunction.

    c. 2nd and 3rd Degree AV block (inferior and right ventricular wall AMIs are where these occur most often)

6. Unless contraindications exist, administer the following:

    a. Metoprolol 5mg IV Q 5 mins. to a total dose of 15mg followed 15 minutes later by 100mg PO as tolerated or

    b. Atenolol 5mg IV Q 10 mins. to a total dose of 15mg, followed 15 minutes later by 50mg PO as tolerated.

    c. Esmolol 500mcg/kg IV (over a minute) followed by a 50mcg/kg/min. infusion titrated to a maximum dose of 200mcg/kg/min.

        (1) Can be given to patients with <u>mild</u> CHF or COPD since it is an ultrashort-acting beta blocker, i.e.; there is less beta-adrenergic antagonism than with the other agents.

        (2) May be considered in patients with left ventricular failure (when this is a concern) since its effects can be terminated rapidly.

F. Morphine

1. Should be administered if chest pain persists despite adequate treatment with antiplatelet, anticoagulant and anti-ischemic agents.

2. Pathophysiology

    a. Decreases pain and anxiety → reduction in circulating catecholamines → decreases tendency toward dysrhythmias.

    b. Reduces both preload and afterload → decreases myocardial oxygen demand.

3. Administer 2 - 5mg Q 5 - 10 mins. prn pain.

4. Adverse effects

    a. Hypotension and bradycardia — respond to fluid bolus and atropine (<u>Note</u>: Do <u>not</u> administer morphine to patients with a HR < 50/min. or those with symptomatic hypotension).

    b. Respiratory depression — responds to naloxone.

G. Reperfusion Therapy

1. Thrombolytic (fibrinolytic) therapy
   a. Available agents include:
      (1) Streptokinase (SK)
      (2) Anisoylated Plasminogen Streptokinase Activator Complex (APSAC, Eminase, Anistreplase)
      (3) Tissue Plasminogen Activator (TPA, Activase, Alteplase)
      (4) Reteplase (RPA, Reptilase, Retavase)
      (5) Tenecteplase (TNK)
   b. These agents convert plasminogen to plasmin (its active form) which, in turn, lyses the fibrin content of acute intracoronary thromboses → reperfusion of coronary arteries → reduced infarction size, improved residual left ventricular function and increased survival. The fibrin specificity of these agents varies.
   c. Thrombolytic therapy should be initiated as quickly as possible (preferably within 30 minutes of arrival in the ED) in patients who meet selection criteria (~33% of patients with Acute MI) and have no absolute contraindications; the shorter the time period between symptom onset and initiation of thrombolytic therapy, the greater the reduction in mortality.
   d. Agent availability and administration protocols vary from hospital to hospital. Familiarize yourself with the agent(s) and protocol(s) used at your institution.
   e. AHA/ACC criteria for thrombolysis
      (1) *Class I* (treatment benefit has been established)
         • ST elevation > 0.1mV in two or more contiguous leads
            Time to therapy ≤ 12 hours
            Age < 75 years
         • Bundle branch block (old) obscuring ST segment analysis
            History suggesting AMI
      (2) *Class IIa* (likely benefit)   *Class IIb* (may be beneficial)
         • ST elevation   • ST elevation
            Age > 75 years   Time to therapy > 12 - 24 hours
                                           • BP > 180 systolic or > 110 diastolic
                                              associated with high-risk of MI
      (3) *Class III* (not indicated, may be harmful)
         • ST elevation
            Time to therapy > 24 hours
            Ischemic pain resolved
         • ST depression only
         • No ST elevation
         • A true posterior MI
         • A presumed <u>new</u> bundle branch block
   f. Absolute contraindications:
      (1) Any prior cerebral hemorrhage
      (2) Known structural CNS lesion (AV malformation, tumor, etc.)
      (3) Ischemic stroke within 3 months (unless TIA < 3 hrs. onset)
      (4) Significant closed head/facial injury within 3 months
      (5) Suspicion of aortic dissection
      (6) Active bleeding (excluding menses) or bleeding disorders

    g. Relative contraindications
        (1) History of chronic, severe, poorly controlled hypertension or severe hypertension on admission (systolic BP > 180 mmHg or diastolic BP > 119mmHg)
        (2) Traumatic/prolonged (> 10 mins.) CPR or noncompressible vascular punctures
        (3) Major surgery or internal bleeding within 3-4 weeks
        (4) Any other CNS disease (structural or functional, e.g. dementia) not noted above
        (5) Pregnancy
        (6) Active peptic ulcer
        (7) Current use of anticoagulants (the higher the INR, the greater the risk of bleeding)
        (8) Prior exposure/allergic reaction to SK or anistreplase (if using these agents)

    h. Complications
        (1) Systemic bleeding — incidence 2 - 10%; usually occurs in the setting of invasive procedures.
        (2) Cerebral hemorrhage — incidence < 1% (greater with TPA); associated with high mortality rate (48%).
        (3) Hypotension — incidence 3 - 10%; more common with streptokinase and APSAC than TPA; usually responds to a fluid bolus and a temporary reduction of the infusion rate.
        (4) Allergic phenomena — incidence 1.5 - 20%; usually minor (anaphylaxis is rare); most commonly occur with streptokinase and APSAC.
        (5) Reperfusion dysrhythmias (PVCs, accelerated idioventricular rhythm, V-Tach, V-Fib) — incidence is > 50%; other than V-Fib, most do not require treatment.
        (6) Failure to open occluded coronary arteries (incidence ~ 20%)

2. Percutaneous coronary intervention (PCI) — When the needed facilities and personnel are available (within 60 - 90 minutes per guidelines). PCI is an attractive alternative to thrombolytic therapy in all patients. According to the 2000 AHA guidelines, angioplasty or stent placement is a Class I recommendation for patients < 75 with ACS and signs of cardiogenic shock and Class IIa for patients > 75. When compared to thrombolysis, immediate angioplasty is the primary treatment modality for these patients because it: (1) appears to be more effective than thrombolysis in opening occluded arteries because it can treat the underlying fixed obstructed coronary artery lesion as well as relieve the acute thrombosis; (2) is associated with a lower incidence of recurrent ischemia, reinfarction, intracranial hemorrhage and death and (3) results in similar left ventricular function. It also has the advantage of allowing the operator to determine the site and extent of coronary artery stenosis. In many institutions today, however, PCI is not available on a 24-hour basis and, when it is, performance varies based on the center's volume and operator's experience; facilities with established protocols and experienced interventionalists (but without cardiac surgery capability) appear to offer safe and effective management for AMI patients.

H. Intravenous Magnesium

On the basis of existing evidence, current recommendations are that magnesium not be given routinely to patients who undergo reperfusion therapy. While it is possible that magnesium is of benefit (particularly in patients <u>not</u> receiving perfusion therapy) further studies are required to evaluate its use in the UA/AMI setting.

I. Angiotensin Converting Enzyme (ACE) Inhibitors

1. When administered within the first 24 hours, these agents decrease the incidence of severe ventricular dysfunction and death. Unless specific contraindications exist, all patients with an AMI should receive an ACE inhibitor, but <u>not</u> until 6 hours after initial therapy has been started in the ED and the patient is stable. If given too early, ACE-inhibitors can potentiate hypotension.

2. One of the following agents should be administered in the first 24 hours post-infarction:
   a. Captopril 12.5mg PO bid (a test dose of 6.25mg may be given)
   b. Lisinopril 5mg PO QD (if systolic BP is < 120, use 2mg PO QD.)

3. Contraindications include:
   a. ACE-inhibitor allergy
   b. Killip Class III or IV heart failure
   c. Hypotension (systolic BP < 100)
   d. Creatinine > 2.5mg/dL
   e. Renal artery stenosis

J. Glucose-Insulin-Potassium (GIK) Therapy

1. May reduce mortality during an AMI because of its anti-free-fatty acid (FFA) activity. (FFAs are toxic to the ischemic myocardium.)

2. The results of a large, controlled, multinational study (published in 2005) refuted earlier studies claiming a reduced mortality rate with GIK therapy. Its use in this setting is not recommended at this time.

V. Complications — Myocardial ischemia produces altered electrical depolarization and contractility (which are the major complications of an acute MI, i.e. dysrhythmias and left ventricular failure).

A. Dysrhythmias

1. The prehospital phase is the period associated with the highest incidence of lethal dysrhythmias; the occurrence of primary V-Fib (no evidence of CHF or hypotension) is greatest in the first hour of infarction.

---

2. Treatment is indicated if the dysrhythmia:
   a. Exacerbates myocardial ischemia <u>or</u>
   b. Could potentially deteriorate into cardiac arrest

3. Specific treatment guidelines have already been discussed. Review the ACLS protocols if you need an algorithmic approach to clinical therapy.

4. Lidocaine is <u>no longer recommended</u> as a prophylactic antidysrhythmic for uncomplicated Acute MI or ischemia; its use in this setting has been associated with an increased mortality rate.

5. PVCs occurring in association with an Acute MI should be treated only if they are frequent (> 30/hr.), multifocal, associated with short runs of V-Tach, occur in couplets or display R-on-T phenomenon. However, even in these instances, treatment of PVCs with lidocaine (the drug of first choice) is controversial. The initial treatment priority should be to optimally manage the underlying ischemia/infarction with oxygen, ASA, NTG, morphine, beta-blockers or thrombolytic therapy. If these measures fail, administration of lidocaine may be considered; procainamide and amiodarone* are alternative first-line agents.

6. Endotracheal administration of medications:
   a. Certain medications (Remember the acronym "**LEAN**") may safely be administered through the endotracheal tube in the event that an IV line has not yet been established:
      (1) **L**idocaine
      (2) **E**pinephrine
      (3) **A**tropine
      (4) **N**alaxone
      <u>Note</u>: Do NOT give sodium bicarb or calcium chloride by this route.
   b. When the endotracheal route is used, administer 2 - 2.5 times the recommended IV dose and dilute it in 10mL of normal saline.

B. Left Ventricular Failure (CHF, pulmonary edema, cardiogenic shock)

1. Acute MI → impaired contractility of the left ventricle (LV)
   a. Impairment ≥ 25% of the LV → CHF/pulmonary edema
   b. Impairment ≥ 40% of the LV → cardiogenic shock

2. Pathogenesis: pump failure = CHF; over time, this leads to increased pulmonary vascular congestion → pulmonary edema. Cardiogenic shock can occur with either acute, severe pump failure or acute, severe pulmonary edema (each of which further impairs left ventricular function).

3. Treatment - (see section on CHF/Pulmonary Edema, pp. 81 - 84)

*A good choice if patient in cardiogenic shock.

C. Conduction Disturbances

1. AV Blocks
   a. First-Degree AV Block and Mobitz I Second-Degree AV block
      (1) Generally due to increased vagal tone
      (2) Rarely progress to complete AV block
      (3) Usually associated with an inferior MI
      (4) Generally respond to drug therapy (atropine)
   b. Mobitz II Second-Degree AV Block
      (1) Generally due to destruction of infranodal conduction tissue
      (2) Sudden progression to complete AV Block may occur
      (3) Usually associated with an anterior MI
      (4) Prophylactic pacemaker therapy is indicated

2. Bundle Branch Blocks (BBBs)
   a. In general, BBBs (old or new) associated with an AMI identify patients who are more likely to develop CHF, AV block and V-Fib.
   b. In patients with an acute anterior wall MI and a new RBBB, there is a high risk of developing complete AV Block and/or cardiogenic shock.

D. Other less common complications of Acute MI include cardiac rupture, ventricular septal rupture, papillary muscle dysfunction/rupture, mitral regurgitation, left ventricular aneurysm, thromboembolism and pericarditis. Most of these complications are delayed in onset, occurring one or more days post-infarction.

CONGESTIVE HEART FAILURE (CHF)

ACUTE CARDIOGENIC PULMONARY EDEMA (ACPE)

I. Causes

A. Causes of _Left_ Ventricular Failure (LVF)

1. Ischemic heart disease (most common cause)
2. Idiopathic dilated cardiomyopathy
3. Hypertension (HTN)
4. Valvular disease (aortic or mitral)
5. High-output states (anemia, thyrotoxicosis, A-V fistula, beriberi, Paget's disease)
6. Congenital heart disease
7. Coarctation of the aorta

B. Causes of _Right_ Ventricular Failure (RVF)

1. Left ventricular failure (most common cause)
2. Pulmonary arterial HTN (+ RVF = cor pulmonale)
3. Valvular disease (tricuspid or pulmonic)
4. Restrictive or infiltrative cardiomyopathies
5. Myocarditis and some forms of congenital heart disease
6. Right ventricular infarction
7. Pulmonary embolism
8. Chronic pulmonary disease

II. Precipitating Factors

1. Myocardial ischemia or infarction

2. Noncompliance with medications

3. Tachydysrhythmias (e.g. atrial fibrillation) and severe bradydysrhythmias

4. Dietary indiscretion (sodium overload)

5. Administration of drugs which impair cardiac function (beta blockers or Ca^{++} channel blockers) or result in sodium retention (glucocorticoids, NSAIDs, nasal decongestants, vasodilators)

6. Increased hemodynamic demand due to infection, trauma, physical overexertion, environmental stress or pregnancy

7. Hypoxia (due to pulmonary embolism or pneumonia)

8. Cardiac disease progression (coronary insufficiency and CHF are the most common precipitating causes of ACPE)

9. Severe hypertension

10. COPD (the leading cause of chronic cor pulmonale)

11. Acute myocarditis or endocarditis

12. Acute valvular dysfunction

III. Signs and Symptoms

- Shortness of breath (most common symptom)
- Paroxysmal nocturnal dyspnea (PND)/orthopnea
- Nocturnal angina
- Moist rales and/or wheezing ("cardiac asthma")
- Cough
- Fatigue and/or weakness
- Pleural effusion (usually right-sided)
- Tachypnea and tachycardia
- S_3 gallop (due to reduced left ventricular compliance)
- S_4 gallop (not heard in patients with atrial fibrillation)
- Hepatojugular reflux → JVD (RVF)
- Pulsus alternans
- Ascites (RVF)
- Hepatic enlargement/tenderness (RVF)
- Pale, clammy skin or diaphoresis
- Neck vein distention (RVF)
- Anxiety
- Nocturia
- Dependent edema (RVF)

IV. Radiologic and Respiratory Progression

A. Stage I: pulmonary vascular redistribution to upper lung fields ("cephalization")

1. CXR → fullness or prominence of the pulmonary vessels in the apices.

2. Predominate symptom (if any are present) is dyspnea.

3. PAWP = 12 - 18mmHg

B. Stage II: interstitial edema

1. On CXR the pulmonary vessels are enlarged and their shadows are blurred; Kerley B lines (1cm horizontal markings at the periphery of lung fields) are also present.

2. Predominate symptom is dry cough.

3. PAWP = 18 - 25mmHg

C. Stage III: alveolar edema (frank pulmonary edema)

1. On CXR, there are bilateral confluent perihilar infiltrates creating a "butterfly" pattern.

2. Predominate symptom is a wet cough with production of a frothy, pink sputum.

3. PAWP > 25mmHg

<u>Note</u>: (1) The cardiac silhouette is generally enlarged (although it may be normal size) in all 3 stages; (2) associated pleural effusions (usually right-sided) are common; and (3) CXR findings may be delayed up to 12 hours relative to symptom onset.

V. Brain-type natriuretic peptide (BNP)

• Is gaining use as a serum marker for acute CHF.

• Pathogenesis: cardiac hypertrophy/wall stress and volume overload → release of endogenous BNP by atrial + ventricular myocytes → smooth muscle relaxation and vasodilation, diuresis and natriuresis.

• Acute CHF can lead to <u>high</u> serum levels which are especially significant in the absence of pulmonary disease and advancing age (where moderate elevations can occur).

• Recent studies suggest that a serum BNP level < 100 pg/ml reliably excludes the diagnosis of acute CHF (sensitivity 90%, specificity 76%).

VI. Treatment of Acute Cardiogenic Pulmonary Edema

A. *First-line Therapy* (for all patients who are not hypotensive)

1. Place the patient in the <u>sitting</u> position with the legs dependent, attach a cardiac monitor and pulse oximeter, start an IV, check the vital signs and review a monitor strip.

2. Oxygen
   a. All of these patients are hypoxemic and should immediately be given supplemental oxygen; it is the most important agent in the treatment of pulmonary edema.
   b. Administer high-flow via a nonrebreather mask at 10 - 15 L/min. to deliver 100% O_2; maintain adequate arterial saturation.
   c. Early application of noninvasive positive pressure ventilation (NPPV) improves oxygenation and dyspnea and also reduces the likelihood of intubation in hypercapneic patients. It can be applied with a tight-fitting facial mask — a method called continuous positive airway pressure (CPAP) or with a nasal mask — a method known as bi-level PAP (BiPAP). BiPAP has the advantage of being able to separately regulate inspiratory (IPAP) and expiratory (EPAP) pressures and is better tolerated than CPAP.
   d. If the patient is (or becomes) obtunded, cannot maintain a PaO_2 above 60mmHg despite receiving 100% O_2, displays a progressive increase in pCO_2 or demonstrates increasing acidosis, he should be intubated.[*] Positive-pressure ventilation can then be applied via the endotracheal tube — a method called positive end-expiratory pressure (PEEP).
   <u>Note</u>: Since positive-pressure ventilation decreases preload, it can produce a decrease in cardiac output and BP. So start with 5 - 10cm water and monitor the BP carefully.

3. Initial medications
   a. Nitroglycerin (NTG)
      (1) At low doses, nitroglycerin is primarily a venodilator and rapidly acts to decrease <u>preload</u>. Its effects on arterial dilation are less profound and are usually associated with higher doses. NTG also acts to <u>increase coronary blood flow</u> by promoting dilation of large epicardial vessels and is, therefore, the vasodilator of choice in the presence of ischemia or an Acute MI.
      (2) Give the patient sublingual nitroglycerin 0.8-1.2mg Q 5-10 mins. (use higher dose if BP is moderately - severely elevated).
   b. Furosemide
      (1) Induces diuresis and has a direct venodilatory effect (to ↓ preload) but it has been associated with initial adverse hemodynamic effects; prior administration of nitroglycerin (↓ preload) and an ACE-inhibitor such as captopril (↓ afterload) may blunt these effects.
      (2) Dose: 0.5 - 1mg/kg IV push over 1 - 2 mins. (use lower dose if the patient is not taking furosemide; use higher dose if he is).

---

[*]Do not wait for ABGs if patient's clinical condition is deteriorating.

c. Morphine sulfate (MS)

(1) Is a potent sedative and analgesic agent that acts to calm the patient down, relieve ischemic chest pain and reduce circulating catecholamine levels (thereby reducing myocardial oxygen consumption and diminishing the tendency toward fatal dysrhythmias). Its effects on preload and afterload are mild when compared with those of nitroglycerin and other vasodilators and it has undesirable side-effects (e.g. vomiting) that can exacerbate afterload; low-dose benzodiazepines are preferred by some authors if anxiety reduction is desired.

(2) Dose: 2 - 5mg IV Q 5 mins. prn unless it induces hypotension or further depresses respiration.

B. *Second-line Therapy* — is based on the patients systolic blood pressure and the presence or absence of clinical shock.

1. Systolic BP > 100 (no signs/symptoms of shock)

a. Nitroglycerin IV at 10 - 20mcg/minute; titrate the drip upward in 5 - 10mcg/min. increments Q 5 mins. until the desired effect is attained or the BP decreases to < 100 mmHg. (A reduction in preload is usually achieved at 50 - 80mcg/min.)

b. Nitroprusside

(1) Is a mixed venous and arteriolar dilator; it reduces both preload and afterload, thereby decreasing pulmonary congestion and reducing cardiac output.

(2) It is usually reserved for patients with a systolic BP > 100mmHg who fail to respond to adequate doses of the standard preload reducers (nitroglycerin, furosemide, morphine) or for those with low output who require controlled afterload reduction.

(3) Dose: 0.1 - 5mcg/kg/min. IV; hemodynamic monitoring is advisable.

2. Systolic BP 70-100

a. No signs/symptoms of shock → dobutamine

(1) Is a direct-acting inotropic agent that is effective in increasing the cardiac output and decreasing the PCWP.

(2) Dose: 2 - 20mcg/kg/min. IV*

(3) Hemodynamic monitoring is advisable.

(4) If there is severe pulmonary congestion, dobutamine should be used in combination with a vasodilator (nitroglycerin or nitroprusside).

(5) <u>Pretreatment</u> with diltiazem (0.25mg/kg, followed by a second dose of 0.35mg/kg IV) is recommended for patients in A-Fib without signs/symptoms of shock; dobutamine facilitates AV conduction and may increase the ventricular response rate.

b. Signs/symptoms of shock are present → dopamine

(1) Provides indirect inotropic support as an effective pressor agent. It is the preferred agent when persistent oliguria or shock is present (systolic BP < 100mmHg) and should be administered <u>prior to</u> venodilating agents and diuretics when hypotension is present on arrival. Dose: 5 - 15mcg/kg/minute IV.*

*Patients on beta-blockers may need the higher dose.

(2) Hemodynamic monitoring is advisable.

(3) Combination therapy with a vasodilating agent (nitroglycerin or nitroprusside) is strongly recommended for patients with severe pulmonary congestion; the vasodilating agent decreases preload and improves cardiac output by countering the dopamine-induced increase in vascular resistance. The hemodynamic effects of dopamine + nitroprusside approximate those of dobutamine.

(4) Dopamine may also be used in combination with dobutamine; dopamine maintains the BP while dobutamine prevents further increase in pulmonary congestion.

3. Systolic BP < 70 with obvious signs/symptoms of shock → norepinephrine
   a. Is a potent vasoconstrictor and inotropic agent.
   b. Dose: 0.1 - 0.5mcg/kg/min.
   c. Hemodynamic monitoring is advisable.

C. Third-line Therapy: — is reserved for patients who are resistant to first- and second-line agents and for those who develop specific complications.

1. Amrinone
   a. Is a phosphodiesterase inhibitor with hemodynamic properties similar to those of dobutamine; it improves myocardial contractility via its positive inotropic action and reduces preload and afterload by its direct vasodilatory effect on vascular smooth muscle.
   b. It is indicated for the treatment of severe pulmonary edema unresponsive to diuretics, vasodilators and conventional inotropic agents.
   c. Dose: 0.75mg/kg IV × 2 - 3 mins. followed by an infusion (5 - 10mcg/kg/min.)
   d. Requires hemodynamic monitoring to titrate the dose properly since hemodynamic improvement is not necessarily associated with either changes in heart rate or BP.
   e. Prior treatment with diltiazem is recommended for stable patients with atrial fibrillation, as amrinone enhances AV conduction and may increase the ventricular response rate; unstable patients with A-Fib should be cardioverted.
   f. When used in combination with dobutamine, the positive inotropic effects are additive; "concomitant use of both drugs appears to be better tolerated than aggressive dosing with dobutamine alone." [Rosen's Text, 5th ed., p. 1125]
   g. May be cardiotoxic.

2. Nesiritide
   a. This drug has multiple physiologic effects:
      (1) Hemodynamic (vasodilation, reduction in preload and afterload)
      (2) Diuretic (promotes free water and sodium loss)
      (3) Neurohormonal (vasodilation, reduced aldosterone levels, inhibition of the renin-angiotensin system)
   b. Clinical trials do not clearly demonstrate efficacy of this drug as a third-line agent. In addition, recent studies have demonstrated an increased mortality rate + impaired renal function after a single infusion of this drug; therefore, its use is not recommended at this time.

3. Thrombolytic therapy
   a. Is indicated for patients with an acute MI diagnosed within twelve hours of symptom onset who meet the inclusion criteria and have no known contraindications.
   b. Agents: Streptokinase, TPA, APSAC and Reteplase.
   Note: Angioplasty is the preferred modality for patients with an acute MI in cardiogenic shock.

4. Intra-aortic balloon counter pulsation
   a. Is indicated for cardiogenic shock refractory to inotropes.
   b. It works by "unloading" the heart during systole as well as increasing coronary and cerebral blood flow during diastole.
   c. Can be a life-saving intervention for patient stabilization prior to thrombolytic therapy or angioplasty.

5. Norepinephrine
   a. Is the pressor agent of choice for those in profound cardiogenic shock unresponsive to inotropic therapy. If not administered prior to this time (i.e. as second-line therapy) for hypotension, consider it now.
   b. Its use should be viewed as a necessary temporizing measure to maintain coronary perfusion while other rescue strategies (angioplasty, balloon pumping, surgery) are being arranged.
   c. Concomittant use of additional agents should be considered:
      (1) Dopamine → in lower doses, may blunt renal vasoconstriction → ↑ renal perfusion → ↑ urine output
      (2) Dobutamine → once BP is restored, may ↑ cardiac output
   d. Dose: start at 1 - 4mcg/min. IV and titrate upward as needed.

VII. Treatment of Heart Failure Without Pulmonary Congestion

A. Patients present with hypotension, JVD and clear lung fields.

B. This presentation is common in patients with inferior wall MIs associated with right ventricular infarction (which is present in one-third of inferior wall MIs)

C. Hypotension in these patients is due to a decrease in left ventricular preload and should be treated with small boluses (250mL) of an isotonic crystalloid solution (up to 2 liters). Multiple fluid boluses as well as inotropic support may be needed to provide sufficient preload and correct the blood pressure.

D. Nitrates and diuretics can produce a significant and rapid decline in BP and should be used with caution (if at all) in these patients.

CARDIOMYOPATHIES AND SPECIFIC HEART MUSCLE DISEASES

I. **Cardiomyopathies** — are diseases of the heart muscle of <u>unknown</u> etiology that produce both structural and functional damage to the myocardium. They are classified as dilated (most common), restrictive or hypertrophic on the basis of differences in their pathophysiology and clinical presentation. However, there is some overlap.

A. *Idiopathic Dilated (congestive) Cardiomyopathy [IDC]*

   1. Is characterized by <u>dilatation</u> of all four chambers (ventricles > atria), increased myocardial mass (hypertrophy) and <u>systolic</u> pump failure. [Note: There is a high association of IDC with viral myocarditis; unexplained heart failure is commonly the only manifestation.]

   2. Clinical profile
      a. Patients usually present with:
         (1) Signs and symptoms of left-and-right-ventricular CHF (dyspnea on exertion and fatigue [the two most common complaints], PND, orthopnea, palpitations, dependent edema, ascites) <u>and/or</u>
         (2) Manifestations of systemic or peripheral embolization (acute neurologic deficit, flank pain and hematuria, pulseless cyanotic extremity)
      b. Physical findings
         (1) Bibasilar rales
         (2) Peripheral edema, JVD and hepatomegaly [-- when associated with a pulsatile liver, tricuspid regurgitation is also present]
         (3) Abnormal heart sounds
            (a) S_3 and S_4 gallop (most common auscultatory findings)
            (b) High-pitched systolic ejection murmur of mitral regurgitation (best heard at the apex)
            (c) Holosystolic ejection murmur of tricuspid regurgitation (best heard at the lower left sternal border)
            (d) Tachycardia (often with a narrow pulse pressure) when CHF is present

   3. Diagnostic studies
      a. ECG
         (1) Left ventricular or biventricular hypertrophy
         (2) Left atrial or biatrial enlargement
         (3) Poor R wave progression
         (4) A new BBB (may occur prior to any signs of chamber dilation or pump dysfunction)
         (5) AV block (usually First or Second-Degree)
         (6) Atrial fibrillation (most common dysrhythmia)

    b. CXR
      (1) Cardiomegaly with enlargement of all four chambers
      (2) Pulmonary venous congestion
    c. Echocardiography
      (1) Enlargement of ventricles and atria
      (2) Increased systolic and diastolic volumes
      (3) Decreased ejection fraction (< 45%)
      (4) Abnormal ventricular contractility (the *sine qua non* of IDC)
      (5) Mitral and tricuspid valve regurgitation
      (6) Mural thrombi

4. Treatment
    a. Is aimed at alleviating symptoms and generally includes a regimen of diuretics, digitalis and vasodilators (nitroprusside, nitrates, prazocin, hydralazine, angiotensin-converting enzyme inhibitors).
    b. Anticoagulants should be administered to patients with:
      (1) Intracardiac thrombi
      (2) Evidence of pulmonary or systemic thromboembolism
      (3) Chronic atrial fibrillation

B. Restrictive Cardiomyopathy (RC)

1. Is characterized by <u>diastolic restriction</u> of ventricular filling; the end-diastolic ventricular volume is low, the end-diastolic ventricular pressure is high and cardiac output is decreased...a hemodynamic picture that mimics constrictive pericarditis (CP).

2. Clinical profile
    a. Is similar to patients with dilated cardiomyopathy. Patients with restrictive disease also present with signs and symptoms of systemic and pulmonary venous congestion; however, evidence of right-sided CHF often predominates. Exercise intolerance is a common complaint.
    b. Physical exam (is similar to IDC)
      (1) Bibasilar rales
      (2) Peripheral edema, JVD, hepatomegaly
      (3) Abnormal heart sounds
        (a) S_3 and S_4 gallop (common)
        (b) Systolic ejection murmur of mitral or tricuspid regurgitation
        (c) Tachycardia
      (4) The apex impulse is usually easily palpable and mitral regurgitation is more common (in contrast to constrictive pericarditis). Other signs that are not present in constrictive pericarditis are a gallop rhythm and a positive Kussmaul's sign (JVD on inspiration).

3. Diagnostic studies (biopsy is the gold standard to R/O CP if all else fails)
    a. ECG
      (1) Chamber enlargement (atria > ventricles)
      (2) Nonspecific ST-T-wave changes
      (3) Low-voltage
      (4) Dysrhythmias (especially A-Fib) are common

b. CXR
   (1) May be normal initially (a small heart suggests CP)
   (2) Cardiomegaly with pulmonary venous congestion is seen with disease progression.
c. Echocardiography
   (1) Thickened walls
   (2) Normal or slightly enlarged ventricular cavity and moderate to markedly dilated atria
   (3) Normal or slightly decreased systolic function
   (4) Mitral and tricuspid regurgitation

   [Note: If differentiation from constrictive pericarditis is still uncertain after this study, then CT, MRI or combined Doppler and 2D-echo may be required to make the diagnosis → thickened pericardium in constrictive pericarditis.]

4. Treatment — is aimed at alleviating symptoms and usually includes a regimen of diuretics and digitalis. However, in the absence of left ventricular enlargement, administration of digitalis may be without beneficial effect. Vasodilators reduce afterload but produce hypotension and have not been found to be beneficial.

C. Hypertrophic Cardiomyopathy (HCM)

1. Is characterized by <u>left</u> ventricular hypertrophy without associated ventricular dilatation. The hypertrophy is generally asymmetric, involving the septum to a greater extent than the free wall; on histologic exam, the myocardial fibers have a marked and extensive disorganized whorled pattern (particularly in the septum). Other common features include: ventricular cavities that are reduced in size, atrial dilatation, mitral valve thickening, impaired diastolic relaxation and restricted LV filling.

2. In more than 50% of cases, this disorder is inherited via an autosomal dominant transmission pattern with variable penetration. The remaining cases appear to be sporadic.

3. Clinical Profile
   a. Symptoms
      (1) Dyspnea on exertion (most common <u>initial</u> complaint)
      (2) Ischemic chest pain (poor response to NTG is common)
         [Chest pain that is relieved by assuming the recumbent position is pathognomonic of HCM ... but rarely encountered]
      (3) Palpitations
         (a) Ventricular and atrial dysrhythmias are common.
         (b) Tachydysrhythmias (particularly atrial fibrillation) are poorly tolerated and may require emergent intervention (see "Therapeutic guidelines" on p. 89).
      (4) Syncope and pre-syncope (dizziness)
         (a) Usually exertion-related
         (b) Due to dysrhythmias or a sudden decrease in cardiac output
      (5) Sudden death (is usually due to dysrhythmias that occur with exercise, especially V-Tach)

<u>Note</u>: Symptom severity correlates with the degree of hypertrophy which, in turn, correlates with the patient's age; thus, the older the patient, the more severe the symptoms.

    b. Physical exam

        (1) A prominent "a wave" may be noted on inspection of the neck veins, i.e. a pulse wave that reflects the powerful systolic pressure of the hypertrophied left ventricle; this should not be confused with JVD, since jugular venous pressure is not usually elevated.

        (2) Rapid biphasic carotid pulse (pulsus biferiens)

        (3) Abnormal heart sounds

            (a) S_4 gallop

            (b) Prominent systolic ejection murmur along the lower left sternal border and at the apex with radiation to the axilla. This murmur is the result of LV outflow obstruction and mitral regurgitation; it is <u>increased</u> with maneuvers that <u>decrease</u> left ventricular end-diastolic volume: the Valsalva maneuver, sudden standing, exercise, amyl nitrate inhalation and administration of isoproterenol. (<u>Note</u>: Remember to perform one of these maneuvers when evaluating young patients presenting with exertional syncope or chest pain.)

    4. Diagnostic studies

        a. ECG... is almost always abnormal

            (1) Left ventricular hypertrophy and left atrial enlargement

            (2) Changes in the anterior, lateral or inferior leads:

                (a) "Septal Q waves" > 0.3mV (represent septal depolarization) [Note: The diagnosis of hypertrophic myocardiopathy should be considered in any young patient whose ECG suggests myocardial infarction but who does not have a history of infarction.]

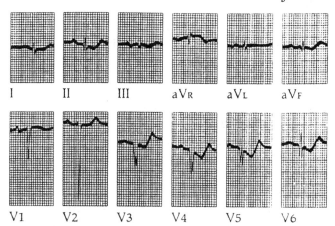

Abnormal Q waves suggestive of an old anterior myocardial infarct are observed in leads V3 through V6 in an ECG recorded in a 45-year-old woman with obstructive hypertrophic cardiomyopathy.

Abnormal Q Waves, from Dec GW, DeSanctis RW: Cardiomyopathies, in Wilmore DW, Cheung LY, Harken A, et al (eds) Scientific American Surgery. New York, Scientific American Inc., 2000, vol 1, sec I, chap 14.

      (b) Upright T waves in leads with QR or QS complexes (represent mid-ventricular obstruction)

      (c) Giant negative T waves (represent obstruction that is primarily localized in the ventricular apex)

    (3) Paroxysmal or sustained atrial fibrillation and PVCs are the most common dysrhythmias.

  b. CXR: usually normal

  c. Echocardiography

    (1) Left ventricular hypertrophy with disproportionate septal hypertrophy

    (2) Small left ventricular cavity

    (3) Systolic anterior motion (SAM) of the mitral valve (a highly specific finding ... but not very sensitive)

5. Therapeutic guidelines

  a. Patients with HCM who present with unstable atrial fibrillation (severe CHF, cardiogenic shock) require immediate cardioversion and heparinization (preferably with a LMWH such as enoxaparin 1mg/kg SQ). Risk of sudden death is high, not only from hemodynamic compromise, but from thromboembolism as well. Rate control and anticoagulation are of paramount importance in this situation. The reason that A-Fib can cause such dramatic hemodynamic compromise is because HCM patients have restricted left ventricular filling and, therefore, depend on atrial contraction to maintain efficient flow; when A-Fib occurs, there is a sudden drop in cardiac output.

  b. Beta-blockers (propranolol 160 - 320mg/day)

    (1) Improve most symptoms of this disease (dyspnea, chest pain, dizziness and syncope) and are, therefore, the mainstay of therapy.

    (2) They work by decreasing myocardial oxygen consumption by reducing exertion-related outflow obstruction.

  c. Calcium-channel blockers (verapamil, nifedipine)

    (1) May be useful in select patients who fail to respond to beta blockers.

    (2) These agents reduce outflow obstruction, increase exercise capacity and decrease myocardial oxygen consumption as well as the incidence of angina.

    (3) They should be avoided in patients with conduction blocks and in those with elevated pulmonary venous pressures (CHF).

  d. Amiodarone

    (1) Is the treatment of choice for ventricular dysrhythmias and is also indicated for patients who fail to respond to beta blockers and calcium-channel blockers.

    (2) It controls most atrial and ventricular dysrhythmias and it appears to prevent sudden cardiac death (the most common cause of death in these patients).

e. Diuretics — are useful in the setting of pulmonary and venous congestion but must be used with caution to avoid hypotension.

f. Agents which either increase myocardial contractility (digitalis, beta-adrenergic agents) and/or reduce ventricular volume (nitrates, other vasodilators) should be avoided as they can increase outflow obstruction.

g. Surgical management (most common procedure is septal myomectomy)
   (1) Is reserved for very symptomatic patients with large systolic gradients (> 50mmHg) who do not respond to drug therapy.
   (2) It effectively relieves LV outflow obstruction in 95% of patients but has a mortality rate of 3-8%.

h. Antibiotic prophylaxis is indicated for dental and potentially unsterile surgical procedures to reduce risk of bacterial endocarditis.

i. Anticoagulation is indicated for stable patients in atrial fibrillation (sustained or intermittent) and for those who have had a prior embolic event; systemic embolization is a common complication of atrial fibrillation in this disease; it can even occur from bacterial endocarditis (which most commonly affects the mitral valve).

j. Avoidance of competitive athletics is advised as sudden death can follow vigorous exertion.

II. **Specific Heart Muscle Diseases** — disorders of the heart muscle associated with a single known cause or systemic disease. These diseases were previously referred to as secondary cardiomyopathies, but this terminology is no longer used. They can be divided into several categories and include:

A. *Toxins*

- Ethanol
- Cobalt, cocaine
- Lithium
- Doxorubicin (Adriamycin)
- Daunorubicin
- Emetine
- Heavy Metals
- Amphetamines

most commonly associated with dilated cardiomyopathy

B. *Nutritional Deficiencies*

- Thiamine deficiency (beriberi)
- Vitamin C deficiency (scurvy)
- Vitamin B_6 deficiency (pellagra)
- Selenium deficiency (Keshan's disease)
- Kwashiorkor

C. Metabolic

- Hemochromatosis ⎫ most commonly associated with
- Glycogen storage disease Type II ⎭ <u>restrictive</u> cardiomyopathy
- Hypothyroidism (myxedema)
- Hyperthyroidism (thyrotoxicosis)
- Uremia
- Pheochromocytoma
- Hypophosphatemia

D. Infiltrative (most commonly associated with <u>restrictive</u> cardiomyopathy)

- Amyloidosis (most common cause in the Western Hemisphere)
- Sarcoidosis
- Endomyocardial fibrosis (most common cause worldwide)

E. Collagen Vascular Diseases

F. Neuromuscular

- Muscular dystrophies
- Friedreich's ataxia
- Myasthenia gravis

G. Myocarditis

- Viral
- Bacterial
- Parasitic (Chagas' disease due to *Trypanosoma cruzi*)
- HIV-associated

H. Peripartum (associated with <u>dilated</u> cardiomyopathy)

I. Ischemia

J. Radiation

DEEP VENOUS THROMBOSIS (DVT)

I. **Pathogenesis** — DVTs have their origin in Virchow's triad of:

- Venostasis
- Hypercoagulability
- Vessel wall injury/abnormality

II. **Clinical Presentation**

A. *Acute Deep Vein Thrombosis*

1. The physical manifestations of DVT are determined by the degree of thrombosis present (partial vs totally occluding), its location and the extent of collaterals at the level of the occlusion; physical findings may be minimal or absent and, therefore, may <u>not</u> be relied upon by themselves to make or exclude the diagnosis.

2. Common signs and symptoms include unilateral pain, swelling, edema (most reliable sign) and tenderness. Other findings may include the presence of a palpable cord (most often detected in the popliteal fossa), superficial venous dilatation, discoloration and Homans' sign (the least reliable finding).

3. Unilateral swelling is the most specific physical finding (especially if the measured difference is > 3cm).

4. Tenderness, erythema or induration in the groin and popliteal fossa (where the femoral and popliteal veins are quite superficially located) are also highly suggestive of acute thrombosis of the underlying vessel.

B. *Massive Deep Vein Thrombosis*

1. Phlegmasia cerulea dolens (painful blue inflammation)
    a. Occurs in < 1% of patients with symptomatic venous thrombosis.
    b. Is an <u>ischemic</u> form of venous occlusion due to massive iliofemoral thrombosis that also involves most of the venous collateral system.
    c. The leg is tensely swollen, painful and cyanotic; petechiae and skin bullae may also be present.
    d. Occasionally results in venous gangrene (irreversible ischemia).

2. Phlegmasia alba dolens (milk leg)
   a. Is due to massive iliofemoral thrombosis associated with arterial spasm.
   b. The entire leg is swollen (but not tense) and the pulse may be diminished.
   c. The skin is doughy and white; petechiae are often present.
   d. This is a temporary condition; as the arterial spasm resolves, the leg takes on the cyanotic appearance of phlegmasia cerulea dolens.

III. Risk Factors

- Prior DVT (highest <u>risk</u>)*

- Carcinoma

- Age > 40

- MI/CHF/CVA

- Obesity

- Estrogen therapy

- Polycythemia vera

- Thrombocytosis

- Pregnancy or postpartum state

- Immobility or prolonged bedrest

- Recent trauma (including burns) or surgery*

- Inherited abnormalities of coagulation (deficiency of antithrombin III, protein C or protein S) or fibrinolysis

- Catheter placement (central venous, Swan-Ganz) + IV drug abuse

  - Immune (e.g. AIDS) and autoimmune (e.g. SLE) deficiencies

The prevalence of DVT is directly correlated with the number of risk factors present; the greater the number of risk factors, the greater the risk for DVT. Thus, patients can be stratified into high- and low-risk groups based on the <u>number</u> of risk factors they possess; this, in turn, can facilitate the decision-making process. Low-risk patients are those with one or no risk factors plus equivocal findings on physical exam; high-risk patients are those with multiple risk factors and highly suggestive exam findings.

*The highest <u>incidence</u> of DVT is in patients undergoing surgical repair of a fractured hip.

IV. Predicting Pretest Probability for DVT: The Well's Clinical Criteria

A. Clinical features and scoring

- Active cancer (palliative, within 6 mos. or ongoing Tx)   1
- Paralysis, paresis or recent immobilization   1
- Recently bedridden (> 3 days) or major surgery   1
  (within 4 weeks)
- Localized tenderness along deep venous system   1
- Entire leg swollen   1
- Calf swelling > 3cm when compared with opposite leg   1
  (10cm below tibial tuberosity)
- Pitting edema (greater in suspected leg)   1
- Collateral superficial veins (nonvaricose)   1
- Alternative diagnosis as likely as (or greater than) DVT   -2

B. Total score interpretation

- ≥ 12 hours 3 = high pretest probability (> 65% risk)
- 1 - 2 = moderate pretest probability
- ≤ 0 = low pretest probability (< 10% risk)

V. Diagnosis

A. A DVT should be suspected from the patient's signs, symptoms and history of risk factors. However, a clinical diagnosis of DVT is insensitive and inaccurate; therefore, the diagnosis must be confirmed (with one of the diagnostic tests described on the next page) prior to treatment.

B. The trend today is to use a noninvasive test (duplex ultrasonography or impedance plethysmography) as the initial modality of choice for evaluating these patients.

C. If duplex Doppler or impedance plethysmography (IPG) results are clearly positive for proximal DVT, the patient should be anticoagulated. If IPG was done initially and a false-positive result is suspected, the diagnosis should be confirmed with either duplex ultrasonography or venography.

D. If the results of duplex ultrasonography are clearly <u>negative</u>, the patient may be discharged with close follow-up, as it is unlikely that he has a significant proximal venous thrombosis (a thrombosis involving the popliteal vein or more proximal vessels). Arrangements should be made for the patient to undergo repeat ultrasound testing on days 3, 5 and 7 to look for proximal extension of the thrombus. If the repeat duplex scan studies are negative, the diagnosis is excluded. If one is positive, the patient should be anti-coagulated.

*An exception is the patient who has a <u>high clinical probability</u> of thrombosis and a negative ultrasound; in this case, <u>immediate</u> venography is strongly recommended (unless there is a contraindication to do so) because duplex scanning only detects about 80% of distal thrombi.

E. If duplex Doppler or IPG are unavailable, or the results of these studies are nondiagnostic or equivocal, venography should be performed.

<u>NOTE</u>: The treatment of isolated calf deep vein thromboses remains controversial even though these thrombi <u>do</u> propagate and subsequently embolize. If an isolated calf deep vein thrombosis is detected, the patient should be anti-coagulated and, if the tibial veins are involved, treated as a proximal deep vein thrombosis.

VI. Ancillary Testing Modalities for DVT

A. *Duplex Ultrasonography (B-mode, i.e. two-dimensional)*

1. Is the <u>initial</u> diagnostic test of choice in most institutions where it is available; it is also the ideal study for evaluating pregnant patients in their first trimester as well as those with renal insufficiency, diabetes, CHF or an allergy to contrast dye.

2. It combines real-time ultrasonographic two-dimensional imaging with simultaneous Doppler flow evaluation with color-flow mapping...a process called, "duplex scanning" (which is the best method of differentiating cellulitis from DVT).

3. It is noninvasive and inexpensive, has a sensitivity of 93% and a specificity of 98% for detecting proximal DVTs and can also identify other causes of calf pain and swelling (Baker's cyst, abscess or hematoma).

4. Disadvantages — it is less sensitive than venography in detecting isolated deep calf vein thrombosis and thrombosis above the groin i.e. pelvic or inferior vena caval thrombosis. [<u>Note</u>: It is also less accurate in the second and third trimesters of pregnancy.]

5. Reliability — In patients with a low pretest probability, a single, negative, lower extremity venous ultrasound scan is sufficient to R/O "clinically significant" proximal DVT; patients with a moderate/high pretest probability require serial ultrasound scans if the initial one is negative.

B. Contrast Venography

1. Is the accepted <u>standard</u> against which all other diagnostic tests are measured, but has largely been replaced by duplex ultrasonography. In fact, venography is now used primarily in patients with uncertain ultrasound results.

2. It has a sensitivity and specificity of nearly 100% and outlines the entire venous system.

3. Disadvantages — it is invasive, painful, expensive, limited in availability and associated with the risk of contrast-related allergic reactions and post-venography phlebitis/DVT. Moreover, up to one-quarter of patients with suspected DVT have contraindications to venography (renal failure, dye allergy, pregnancy) or nondiagnostic studies.

C. Impedance Plethysmography (IPG)

1. Measures blood volume changes in the leg in response to temporary venous occlusion with a pneumatic cuff.

2. It is a noninvasive study and has a sensitivity of approximately 65 - 85% for proximal DVTs (the major source of pulmonary emboli).

3. Disadvantages — it is insensitive to isolated calf vein thrombosis and nonoccluding proximal deep vein thrombosis; it does not distinguish a thrombotic occlusion from extravascular compression. Furthermore, a <u>false-positive</u> result may be obtained in the presence of conditions that interfere with peripheral blood flow (hypotension, increased central venous pressure, severe peripheral vascular disease).

4. It may be the most useful in patients with a history of <u>recurrent</u> DVT in whom the affected veins often remain "incompressible" (which renders real-time B-mode ultrasonography less reliable since it measures compressibility of a vein, i.e. it can't differentiate between an old DVT and an acute DVT.

D. Hand-held Doppler Ultrasonography

1. Evaluates changes in venous blood flow with respiration and distal compression.

2. It is noninvasive, inexpensive, portable, readily available in the ED and can provide immediate information to the examiner regarding the presence of a DVT.

3. Disadvantages — it is subjective, requires significant skill and expertise on the part of the examiner and has a lower accuracy rate than IPG, duplex ultrasonography or venography.

4. It should <u>not</u> be used by itself to diagnose deep vein thrombosis.

E. Magnetic Resonance Imaging (MRI)

1. Detects calf, thigh, pelvic, renal and pulmonary thrombi; it can also diagnose other anatomic causes of leg pain and swelling.

2. It is noninvasive, 97% sensitive and 95% specific for DVT.

3. Disadvantages — it is expensive, not readily available and requires significant patient cooperation, so it should not replace ultrasound as the primary screening tool.

4. It is most useful during the second and third trimesters of pregnancy when ultrasound is less accurate.

F. D-dimer Assay

1. D-dimer is a fibrin degradation product which is elevated in patients with DVT and PE. Unfortunately, it is also elevated in many other conditions (poor specificity) such as AMI, CVA, trauma and pregnancy.

2. There are a number of rapid D-dimer assays including <u>qualitative</u> whole blood agglutination tests (SimpliRED) and <u>quantitative</u> turbidimetric or ELISA tests where levels > 500mg/L are abnormal.

3. Like duplex ultrasonography and IPG, it is more sensitive for proximal clots (93%) than distal ones (70%).

4. Interpretation of D-dimer assay results
   a. In low pretest probability patients, a negative test result can R/O proximal or distal DVT using quantitative ELISA or turbidimetric assay alone <u>or</u> the qualitative whole blood assay when used in conjunction with the Wells Criteria.*
   b. In moderate/high pretest probability patients, a positive D-dimer does <u>not</u> diagnose DVT; further testing is required.

*ACEP clinical policy: Critical issues in the evaluation and management of adult patients presenting with suspected lower-extremity DVT.

VII. Pharmacologic Therapy — is aimed at preventing pulmonary embolism, reducing the morbidity associated with the acute event and preventing (or minimizing) the post-phlebitic syndrome.

A. Anticoagulation

1. IV heparin (unfractionated) is no longer the treatment of choice. Low-molecular-weight heparin (LMWH) is at least as effective as IV unfractionated heparin in the treatment of DVT and has several advantages: it requires little or no laboratory monitoring, can be given subcutaneously once or twice daily, has better bioavailability and is associated with fewer bleeding complications than unfractionated heparin. However, LMWH and unfractionated heparin are contraindicated in patients with a history of heparin-induced thrombocytopenia; these patients should receive alternative agents (danaparoid, lepirudin or argatroban). There are four LMWHs approved for therapy:
    a. Enoxaparin
        (1) 1mg/kg SQ Q12 hours (inpatient or outpatient)
        (2) 1.5mg/kg SQ QD (inpatient only) <u>or</u>
    b. Tinzaparin 175 units/kg SQ QD <u>or</u>
    c. Dalteparin
        (1) 100 units/kg SQ Q12 hours (inpatient or outpatient)
        (2) 200 units/kg SQ QD (inpatient only) <u>or</u>
    d. Nadroparin
        (1) 86 units/kg SQ Q12 hours (inpatient or outpatient)
        (2) 171 units/kg SQ QD (inpatient only)

    • Fondaparinux (not yet approved by the FDA at this printing)
        (1) An antithrombotic agent that is a specific inhibitor of Factor X
        (2) Has been found to be as effective as enoxaparin in the treatment of DVT
            (a) Advantage is once a day dose (enoxaparin is twice a day)
            (b) Disadvantage is that fondaparinux does not have a specific antidote for bleeding complications (although it is considered as safe as enoxaparin)
        (3) Dose is 7.5 - 10mg SQ daily

2. Patients with antithrombin III deficiency require pretreatment with antithrombin III concentrate or FFP to replenish this factor prior to heparinization.

3. Warfarin 5mg QD should generally be initiated on the first day of treatment; anticoagulation parameters should be checked on day 3.

4. Outpatient treatment may be considered for carefully selected patients:
    a. Those without serious concomitant disease requiring hospitalization
    b. Those with whom communication and transportation is adequate
    c. Those who will have their INR blood level checked in 2 - 3 days

B. Thrombolytic Therapy

1. Compared with heparin therapy, lytic therapy produces a more rapid resolution of symptoms, preserves valve integrity and may decrease the incidence of post-phlebitic syndrome. However, indications for thrombolytics in patients with DVT are unclear.

2. It is usually reserved for patients < 60 yrs. old with massive or limb-threatening iliofemoral thrombosis (such as those with phlegmasia cerulea dolens) and for those with upper extremity DVT* who have had symptoms < 1 wk. and who have a low risk of bleeding.**

3. Before thrombolytic therapy is administered, the diagnosis must be confirmed with an objective diagnostic study and contraindications must be ruled out (see discussion of reperfusion therapy in section on Myocardial Infarction pp. 73 - 74).

4. It is administered in conjunction with heparin therapy.

5. It is associated with an increased risk of bleeding (about three times greater than heparin -- which is greater than the risk of bleeding associated with the use of lytic agents for the treatment of AMI).

6. Approved agents include streptokinase, urokinase and TPA.

C. Inferior Vena Caval Interruption with a Greenfield Filter

1. Primary indication → proximal DVT (above the level of the knee) in a patient with a contraindication to anticoagulation or thrombolytic therapy, those who require urgent surgery that precludes anticoagulation or those in whom treatment has failed.**

2. Other indications include:
   a. Recurrent DVT despite adequate anticoagulation
   b. Presence of a large free-floating caval thrombus
   c. Chronic recurring embolization in a patient with pulmonary hypertension

3. Patients with malignancies seem to benefit most from this procedure.

VIII. Indications for Admission

- Extensive ileofemoral deep-vein thrombosis with circulatory compromise
- Increased risk of bleeding requiring close monitoring of therapy
- Limited cardiorespiratory reserve
- Risk of poor compliance with home therapy or inadequate assistive support
- Contraindications to LMWH heparin necessitating IV heparin therapy

*ACEP clinical policy: Critical issues in the evaluation and management of adult patients presenting with suspected lower-extremity DVT.
**LLSA 2006 reading list: "Treatment of deep-vein thrombosis."

PULMONARY EMBOLISM (PE)

I. **Definition** — Pulmonary embolism is primarily a complication of deep venous thrombosis in which a thrombus from one of the deep veins migrates through the right heart and subsequently lodges in and occludes vessels of the pulmonary arterial circulation.

A. The majority of pulmonary emboli originate from venous thrombi in the lower extremities and pelvis; except for major trauma and postsurgery (Gyn) patients, lower extremity venous thrombi almost <u>always</u> start in the calf veins.

B. Other less common sources include: hepatic, renal and ovarian veins, right side of the heart, paradoxical left-to-right cardiac shunts, vena cava and neck veins (especially central venous catheter sites).

C. < 10% of pulmonary emboli cause pulmonary infarction and most of them occur in patients with left ventricular failure (LVF) and underlying pulmonary disease (in combination). Since therapy is the same for both entities, clinical distinction is unimportant.

II. Clinical Importance

A. PE is the third most common cause of death in the U.S. and progressive right ventricular failure is the most common cause of death in these patients (usually secondary to massive embolization).

B. The diagnosis is missed antemortem in up to 70% of cases (> 400,000/year); one-third of these patients die, while the other two-thirds are at risk for recurrent PE and the development of pulmonary HTN.

C. A significant percentage of patients with DVT will develop (or already have) PE and many of these cases will go unrecognized because clinicians see it more often than they think. The so-called "clinically silent" calf vein thrombus can be deadly. In fact, clinically significant embolization from calf vein DVT is not uncommon.

III. Risk Factors

A. All known risk factors for PE (and DVT) have their basis in Virchow's triad of venostasis, hypercoagulability and vessel wall injury or abnormality; they include:
- Current DVT* (high risk for occult cancer)
- Prior DVT or PE*
- Carcinoma* or chemotherapy
- MI/CHF/COPD/CVA
- Obesity*
- Estrogen therapy
- Hypercoagulable settings (use of oral contraceptives, pregnancy, post-partum period)
- Immobility (including travel) or prolonged bedrest*
- Recent trauma (including burns) or surgery (especially orthopedic)*
- Inherited abnormalities of coagulation or fibrinolysis
- Indwelling central venous catheter
- Autoimmune (e.g. SLE) and immune (e.g. AIDS) disorders
- Intravenous drug abuse
- Polycythemia vera

B. Most patients (≥ 90%) with thromboembolic disease possess at least one of these risk factors although some (those with cancer, inherited abnormalities of coagulation) may not be apparent at the time of presentation. Furthermore, the risk represented by these factors is additive: the greater the number of risk factors present, the greater the risk for PE. Thus, knowledge of whether or not a patient has risk factors for PE can be used to increase or decrease one's clinical suspicion for the diagnosis. For example: A patient with at least one common risk factor or two or more other risk factors should be considered to have a moderate-to-high risk of having a PE.

IV. Signs and Symptoms

A. Presenting signs and symptoms of acute PE are determined by the extent of pulmonary vascular occlusion (massive vs. submassive) and the patient's baseline cardiopulmonary status.

B. Symptoms (in decreasing order of frequency)

- Dyspnea (by far, the most common symptom)

- Pleuritic chest pain

- Apprehension

*These are the most common risk factors in patients with proven PE.

- Cough

- Hemoptysis

- Sweating

- Nonpleuritic chest pain

- Syncope (more common with massive than submassive emboli)

C. Signs (in decreasing order of frequency)

- Tachypnea (RR > 16/min) — most common sign

- Rales

- Accentuated S_2

- Tachycardia (HR > 100 beats/min)

- Elevated temp (> 37.8° C)

- Diaphoresis

- S_3 or S_4 gallop

- Clinically evident thrombophlebitis

- Decreased breath sounds

- Lower extremity edema

- Cardiac murmur

- Cyanosis

- Hypotension (more common with massive emboli)

D. Dyspnea, pleuritic chest pain or tachypnea are present in 95% of patients; if all three of these findings are absent, PE is unlikely (especially if there are no risk factors). The "classic triad" of dyspnea, pleuritic chest pain and hemoptysis is uncommon (present in < 25 % of patients).

E. Predicting Pretest probability for PE: The Well's Clinical Criteria

1. Clinical features and scoring

• Suspected DVT	3.0
• Alternative diagnosis is less likely than PE	3.0
• Pulse > 100/min.	1.5
• Immobilization (or surgery) within 4 weeks	1.5
• Hx of previous DVT/PE	1.5
• Hx of hemoptysis	1.0
• Hx of malignancy (Tx within 6 mos. or palliative)	1.0

2. Total score interpretation

    - > 6 = high pretest probability (66.7% risk)

    - $2 - 6$ = moderate pretest probability (20.5% risk)

    - < 2 = low pretest probability (3.6% risk)

3. "The clinical gestalt of experienced clinicians and the clinical prediction rules used by physicians of varying experience have shown similar accuracy in discriminiating among patients who have a low, moderate and high pretest probability of PE." [JAMA 2003, 290 (21): 2849]

V. Routine Screening Tests — are most useful in excluding other disease processes (MI, pneumothorax, pneumonia, acute pulmonary edema). These tests can also function as data that increase or decrease one's suspicion of PE but, of themselves, do not rule in or rule out the diagnosis.

A. *Arterial Blood Gas (ABG)*

1. Usually reveals hypoxemia; a $PO_2 < 80mmHg$ is present in 80% of these patients and is often associated with a mild respiratory alkalosis ($\downarrow PCO_2$ + $\uparrow$ pH) due to hyperventilation / tachypnea .

2. The finding of hypoxemia increases the likelihood that a PE is present, but a normal PO_2 does <u>not</u> exclude the diagnosis.

3. The alveolar-arterial (A-a) gradient — is a more sensitive indicator of systemic hypoxemia than the PO_2 alone.
    a. The formula for calculating the A-a gradient at sea level is:

$$A\text{-a gradient} = 150 - (PO_2 + \frac{PCO_2}{0.8})$$

    b. The normal A-a gradient for a patient is age-dependent (increases with age) and can be calculated with the following formula:

$$normal\ A\text{-a gradient} = \frac{Age}{4} + 4$$

    c. The A-a gradient is abnormally <u>elevated</u> in 95% of patients with PE.
    d. The finding of an increased A-a gradient increases the probability a PE is present, but a normal gradient does <u>not</u> exclude the diagnosis; therefore, it should not be used as a "screening" test for PE.

B. Chest x-ray (CXR)

1. The CXR is useful in ruling out other disease processes and is also needed to interpret the ventilation/perfusion scan.

2. It is <u>abnormal</u> in > 80% of patients with PE, but the findings are neither sensitive nor specific. They may include:

   - Atelectasis or pulmonary parenchymal abnormalities (consolidation or patchy infiltrates)

   - Elevated hemidiaphragm

   - Pleural effusion

   - Hampton's hump — a triangular pleural-based density with a rounded apex that points toward the hilum.

   - Westermark's sign — dilatation of pulmonary vessels proximal to the embolus in association with regional oligemia distally.

   a. The most common radiographic abnormalities are atelectasis, pulmonary parenchymal abnormalities, an elevated hemidiaphragm and small unexplained pleural effusions.
   b. Hampton's hump and Westermark's sign are rare but, when present, are very suggestive of PE.

3. The presence of a normal CXR (present in < 20% of patients) does <u>not</u> rule out the diagnosis. In fact, in the setting of dyspnea and hypoxia, a normal CXR is very suggestive of PE.

C. Electrocardiogram (ECG)

1. A normal ECG is seen in 9 - 26% of patients; abnormalities are nonspecific and may include:
   a. Transient nonspecific ST-T wave changes (most common finding)
   b. Sinus tachycardia
   c. Evidence of right heart strain (high correlation in the presence of PE):

   - P pulmonale (peaked P wave in Lead II)

   - Left or right axis deviation

   - Atrial fibrillation

   - RBBB ⎤
   - $S_1 Q_3 T_3$ ⎦ classic but uncommon findings

   - Shift in transition zone to V_5 (R and S waves are equivalent)

2. These findings (if new onset) are suggestive of PE.

3. A normal ECG is found in up to 15% of patients and does <u>not</u> rule out the diagnosis.

D. Alveolar Dead Space Determination

1. May become an important diagnostic test since studies suggest that it compares favorably to V/Q scanning as a screening tool; it can also determine the size of the PE and it is inexpensive.

2. Measurement of expired CO_2 provides an indirect assessment of alveolar dead space; if there is diminished/absent perfusion in an area of lung, there will be a low CO_2 or none at all.

E. D-Dimer

1. Should only be used as a screening tool in <u>low</u> pretest probability patients; it cannot be used to make the diagnosis of PE.

2. Value of a negative D-dimer
   a. Can exclude PE in patients with low pretest probability using turbidimetric or ELISA quantitative D-dimer < 500 alone <u>or</u>
   b. Cannot exclude PE in patients with moderate or high pretest probability without further study, e.g. V/Q scan*

VI. Specific Diagnostic Tests

A. Ventilation - Perfusion (V/Q) Scan

1. Is essentially a screening test; it is occasionally diagnostic of PE (or excludes the diagnosis with near certainty) but is most often non-diagnostic.

2. Is usually the preferred initial diagnostic test of choice for evaluating patients with suspected PE, but this is changing; at least 70% of V/Q scans will not provide the <u>quality</u> of info needed to make appropriate clinical decisions.

3. A PE typically produces an area that is ventilated (V) but <u>not</u> perfused (Q), referred to as a V/Q mismatch; the larger the V/Q mismatch, the greater the likelihood that a PE is present. Therefore, V/Q scans are classified as normal, or near-normal, indeterminate (most common reading) low, intermediate or high probability for PE based on the number and size of V/Q mismatches present.

4. The V/Q scan result should be interpreted in the context of the physician's clinical suspicion for PE because it increases the predictive value of this test (especially if there is a commitment to a <u>level</u> of clinical suspicion for PE <u>prior to</u> obtaining the V/Q scan results).

*ACEP Clinical Policy: Critical issues in the evaluation and management of adult patients presenting with suspected pulmonary embolism.

5. In patients with low-moderate pretest probability, a normal perfusion scan excludes clinically significant PE 98% of the time. A normal perfusion scan also decreases the probability that an angiographically provable PE is present, at least to the point where further workup is indicated only in the presence of high clinical suspicion

6. An indeterminate or nondiagnostic (low or intermediate probability) scan neither confirms nor eliminates the diagnosis of PE and should not be taken as a diagnostic end point.

7. A high probability scan in a patient with high pretest clinical probability for PE is considered confirmatory and should result in treatment; no further workup is required.

8. Advantages — V/Q scanning is relatively noninvasive, can be performed in critically ill patients and is safe during pregnancy (where, following duplex Doppler, it is considered the diagnostic test of choice — it is less invasive and has less fetal exposure than angiography).

9. Disadvantages — V/Q scanning is nondiagnostic most of the time, less useful in patients with lung disease (or abnormal chest x-ray); it also takes time to perform and requires isotope injection.

B. Spiral CT Angiography (sCTA)

1. Has emerged as the most extensively studied new confirmatory test with a good overall test performance that is equal to or slightly better than that of the V/Q scan. However, an sCT scan read as negative for PE is not as sensitive as a V/Q scan read as normal; therefore, a negative sCTA in a patient with high probability for PE requires pulmonary angiography.

2. In settings where a V/Q scan reading is "indeterminate" (or likely to be so in patients with pulmonary pathology, e.g. COPD, pneumonia, etc.), an sCTA with contrast is the procedure of choice.

3. An intraluminal-filling defect or vascular occlusion characterizes a positive result; the sensitivity and specifity of the sCTA are higher for PE in the central vessels than in peripheral vessels (95% sensitivity for segmental or large PE, 75% sensitivity for subsegmental PE).*

4. Advantages over V/Q scanning — can be performed within minutes, has a marked reduction of indeterminate readings and is useful for its ability to identify a convincing diagnostic alternative to PE.

5. Disadvantages — cost, need for patient transport, use of iodinated contrast material, radiation exposure and availability of radiologists with special expertise in performing and interpreting the test are serious drawbacks for its routine use as a screening test for PE.

*Newer generation sCTA (thin collimation-spiral CT) may increase diagnostic accuracy.

C. Pulmonary Angiography

1. Is the gold standard for diagnosing PE. Although false-positive and false-negative results do occur occasionally, angiography offers the best available combination of sensitivity and specificity for diagnosing thromboembolic disease.

    a. Current techniques are unable to detect obstruction in small, subsegmental arterial branches, so many small peripheral emboli may be missed.

    b. Augmentation techniques (subselective injections, magnification, radiography, balloon occlusion angiography) are able to visualize emboli as small as 1mm in diameter.

    c. Standard angiography (without augmentation techniques) may completely miss emboli as large as 2.5mm in diameter.

2. A positive study demonstrates an embolus obstructing a vessel (a dye "cut-off" sign) or an intraluminal filling defect (in more than one projection).

3. Advantages — pulmonary angiography is currently the most reliable test available for diagnosing PE.

4. Disadvantages — it is invasive, not universally available, has a mortality rate of 0.1 - 0.5%, a morbidity rate of 1 - 5% and is relatively contraindicated in patients with pulmonary HTN.

5. Complications are more common in elderly patients with underlying cardiopulmonary disease. They include anaphylactoid reactions, dysrhythmias, cardiac arrest, endocardial injury and perforation.

D. Color-Flow Duplex Ultrasonography

1. In patients with nondiagnostic V/Q scans, this is the next study of choice in ruling out PE since a lower extremity DVT confirmed by duplex US is considered defacto evidence that PE also exists.

2. Demonstration of a DVT in the setting of suspected PE is an indication for initiating appropriate therapy.

3. Negative lower extremity vascular studies cannot eliminate the possibility of PE and, therefore, do not change the clinical management. A single negative lower extremity US duplex study should not be used to exclude PE in patients with moderate-high pretest probability and a nondiagnostic V/Q scan. (ACEP clinical policy).

Note: In pregnant patients, duplex Doppler is the initial diagnostic study of choice for the evaluation of PE because it is the least invasive. In these patients, duplex Doppler is performed first and, if it's positive, treatment is initiated. If it's negative, then a V/Q scan is performed.

E. **Other Diagnostic Modalities** — that are currently under investigation include fiberoptic angioscopy, ECG-gated spinecho MRI, monoclonal antibodies, computer-assisted V/Q scan interpretation and dielectric imaging. Although most of these tests show promise, they are not widely available and their role in the evaluation of thromboembolic disease has not as yet been clearly defined.

F. **Echocardiography**

1. Should be considered for the patient with shock of uncertain etiology in whom the diagnosis of PE is suspected but who is not stable enough for other diagnostic tests.

2. The finding of right ventricular dysfunction in the absence of an AMI, pericardial tamponade or aortic dissection supports the diagnosis of right ventricular failure (RVF) secondary to PE.

3. Bedside techniques
   a. Transthoracic echocardiography (TTE) — rarely provides image resolution adequate enough to visualize the inferior vena cava or cardiac chambers, but it can detect RV strain.
   b. Transesophageal echocardiography (TEE) — has more consistent cardiac imaging, but it is invasive and requires specialty consultation and equipment.

VII. Diagnostic Approach

A. The diagnosis of PE begins with a clinical suspicion drawn from the patient's clinical presentation, history, risk factors and physical exam findings.

B. The workup then proceeds to include an ECG, ABG and CXR. These tests may uncover another diagnosis and, thus, eliminate the need for further workup or, they may provide additional evidence to support the suspicion for PE.

C. If these tests do not reveal another diagnosis (pneumothorax, MI) that explains the patient's signs and symptoms, then the patient's pretest probability for PE should be determined and a screening test should be performed.

D. Further management decisions must incorporate both the physician's assessment of the patient's pretest probability of having a PE and the test results (screening and diagnostic).

E. If pulmonary angiography reveals PE, the patient should be treated.

F. If pulmonary angiography is negative and the study was technically adequate, another diagnosis should be considered.

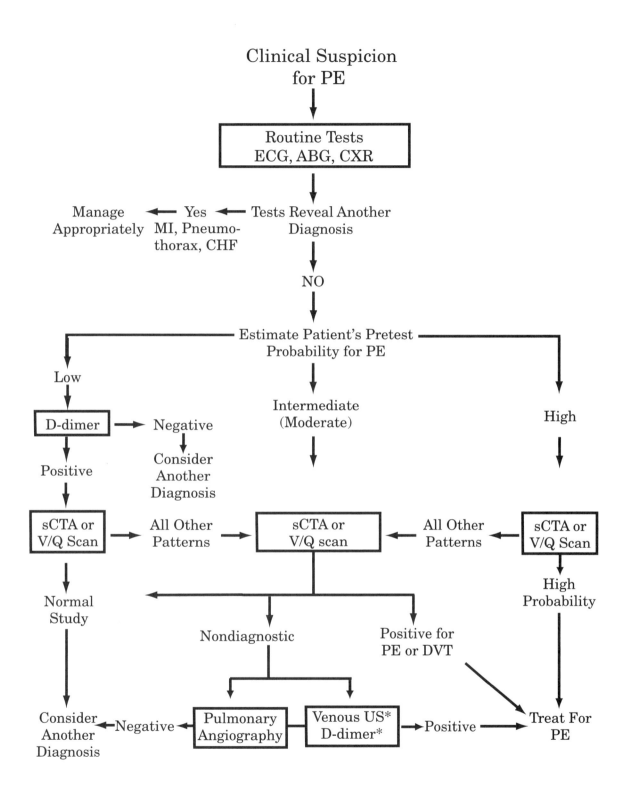

Algorithm For Evaluating Patients With Suspected PE

*Low-moderate pretest probability patients only

VIII. Treatment

A. *Objectives*

1. Short term — prevent thromboembolic propagation, additional embolic events and eliminate thromboemboli from the pulmonary vasculature.

2. Long term — prevent or minimize recurrence of PE, chronic venous insufficiency and the development of chronic pulmonary hypertension.

B. *Basic Supportive Measures*

1. Assess and stabilize the ABCs — establish an IV of NS or LR, provide supplemental O_2, place the patient on a cardiac monitor and check a rhythm strip.

2. Manage shock with fluid resuscitation and the administration of a cardiotropic agent (one that improves "pump function"). Isoproterenol, a pure beta agonist is preferred over dopamine because it is a more effective dilator of pulmonary arterioles; it decreases right ventricular outflow resistance while improving right ventricular contractility. However, if the cardiac output does not rise enough to compensate for the reduced peripheral vascular resistance, hypotension may actually worsen. In these patients, norepinephrine may be required. Volume loading can worsen right ventricular function and, therefore is not usually helpful.

C. *Anticoagulation with IV Unfractionated Heparin or SQ LMWH*

1. The cornerstone of therapy for PE, heparinization should be started as soon as the diagnosis is strongly suspected (unless contraindications exist); do not wait for confirmatory test results.

2. The decision to use UF heparin or a LMWH is an arbitrary one since both appear to be equally effective and safe for the initial treatment of submassive PE. The choice is often made by the admitting/consulting cardiologist based on his/her personal preference.
   a. Since PE is not (yet) treated on an outpatient basis, some cardiologists still prefer IV UF heparin because they can monitor the anticoagulation effect more accurately and the cost is less than an LMWH.
   b. Others prefer using a SQ LMWH until the patient can become therapeutic on coumadin. Again, better bio-availability, less lab draws + no need for a continuous infusion pump are reasons for this choice.

3. Heparin prevents propagation of the clot and decreases the risk of further embolic events, but does not dissolve clots that are already present. It works by binding to (and enhancing) the activity of <u>antithrombin III</u>, a naturally occurring substance which prevents thrombosis by inhibiting <u>activated</u> coagulation factors of the intrinsic and common pathways, particularly thrombin and Factor Xa.

4. If UF heparin is the agent selected, administer a bolus of 100 units/kg IV (7,000 units/70kg patient) followed by a continuous infusion of 18 units/kg/hr. Draw an aPTT in six hrs. and adjust the infusion rate as needed to maintain the aPTT at 1.5 - 2.5 times the control value. This weight-adjusted heparin regimen minimizes the time needed to achieve a therapeutic PTT without increasing the likelihood of bleeding complications.

5. Enoxaparin is the LMWH of choice and is rapidly becoming the therapeutic modality preferred by many clinicians; the dose is 1mg/kg SQ Q 12 hours or 1.5mg/kg SQ daily.*

6. Both UF Heparin and LMWHs are safe to use in pregnancy as neither crosses the placenta.

7. Complications
   a. Hemorrhage — which can be reversed by turning off the infusion and administering protamine sulfate (1 mg neutralizes 100 units of heparin but not enoxaparn or other LMWHs).
   b. Thrombocytopenia — which requires discontinuation of all forms of heparin. It is immune-mediated and generally develops 7 - 10 days following the initiation of therapy.

8. Low-molecular-weight heparins have a number of advantages over unfractionated heparin; when these agents become more widely used for treatment of PE and DVT, they are likely to replace current anticoagulant therapy with unfractionated heparin.

D. *Thrombolytic (Fibrinolytic) Therapy*

1. Current indications**
   a. Hemodynamic instability in patients with confirmed PE
   b. Hemodynamic instability in patients with a high clinical index of suspicion (especially with RV dysfunction on bedside echo)
   c. RV dysfunction on echo in hemodynamically stable patients with confirmed PE

2. Lytic agents work by directly lysing clot.

3. Before administering these agents, the diagnosis of PE should ideally be established with a high degree of certainty. If, however, there is a high suspicion for PE in a patient who is hemodynamically compromised, thrombolytic therapy may be administered prior to diagnostic testing.

4. Administration of these agents should be followed immediately by full-dose heparin anticoagulation (There is no increase in bleeding complications when heparin is administered concurrently with TPA).

*Tinzaparin, dalteparin and nadroparin are acceptable alternatives.
**ACEP clinical policy: Critical issues in the evaluation and management of adult patients presenting with suspected pulmonary embolism.

5. Advantages — in contrast to heparin, thrombolytic therapy has been shown to prevent the postphlebitic syndrome, reduce the risk of recurrent PE/DVT, restore normal myocardial and valvular function, normalize pulmonary vascular resistance and pulmonary arterial pressure, improve long-term exercise capacity, and normalize pulmonary capillary volume and pulmonary gas diffusion. There is also some evidence that it does decrease mortality but, as yet this has not been clearly demonstrated; this will require multicenter trials.

6. Contraindications — are identical to those for acute MI (see discussion of reperfusion therapy in section on Myocardial Infarction pp. 73-74).

7. Complications
   a. Lytic therapy and anticoagulant therapy produce a similar incidence of systemic bleeding complications. However, the risk of hemorrhage increases directly with the duration of infusion of the lytic agent: urokinase and streptokinase are usually infused over a 12 - 24 hour period, whereas the usual TPA protocol is a 2-hour infusion.
   b. If serious bleeding complications occur, the lytic infusion should be discontinued and aminocaproic acid (Amicar) should be administered along with transfusions of fresh frozen plasma and cryoprecipitate.

8. Lytic agents approved for treatment of PE include streptokinase and TPA; TPA is preferred because it produces significant improvement of hemodynamic parameters in < 2 hrs. (hemodynamic effects are more delayed with streptokinase) and, as indicated above, is associated with a lower risk of hemorrhage. The dose of TPA is 100mg over 2 hrs.

E. Surgery

1. Pulmonary embolectomy
   a. Is rarely performed today (except on NBC's "ER"); it has, for the most part, been supplanted by lytic therapy.
   b. It is currently reserved for patients in whom thrombolytic therapy is contraindicated or unsuccessful.
   c. The operative mortality is 25%.

2. Vena caval filter placement to prevent recurrent PE — is indicated in patients with:
   a. Contraindications to anticoagulation (or major bleeding while receiving anticoagulant therapy)
   b. Recurrence despite adequate anticoagulation
   c. Septic emboli arising from the pelvis
   d. Right heart failure in those who are not candidates for thrombolysis

PERICARDIAL DISORDERS

I. Pericarditis

A. Causes

1. Idiopathic
2. Infectious agents — most common causes
   a. Viral
   - Coxsackie viruses A and B
   - Echovirus
   - Adenovirus
   - HIV
   - Epstein-Barr virus
   - Influenza
   - Hepatitis B
   b. Bacterial — uncommon cause
   - Staphylococcus
   - Pneumococcus
   - Streptococcus
   - Meningococcus
   - Mycobacterium sp.
   - Rickettsia sp.
   - Borrelia burgdorferi
   - Mycoplasma
   c. Fungal
   - Histoplasmosis
   - Blastomycosis
   - Coccidiomycosis

3. Malignancies
   a. Metastatic
   - Breast
   - Lung
   - Melanoma
   - Leukemia
   - Lymphoma
   b. Primary pericardial tumors (mesotheliomas) - rare cause

4. Systemic illnesses
   a. Systemic lupus erythematosus (SLE)
   b. Acute rheumatic fever
   c. Rheumatoid arthritis (RA)
   d. Scleroderma

   e. Polyarteritis nodosa
   f. Sarcoidosis
   g. Myxedema
   h. Amyloidosis

5. Medications
   a. Anticoagulants
   b. Procainamide
   c. Hydralazine
   d. Isoniazid

6. Radiation

7. Cardiac injury
   a. Acute MI
   b. Dressler's syndrome (late post-MI pericarditis)
   c. Posttraumatic (including postsurgical) → <u>constrictive</u> pericarditis

B. Diagnosis

1. History
   a. Sharp precordial or retrosternal chest pain exacerbated by inspiration, swallowing or movement of the upper torso (pain is increased in the supine position but relieved by sitting up and leaning forward). Radiation to the trapezius muscle ridge (especially the left) is common and is a distinctive characteristic.
   b. Dyspnea
   c. Low-grade, intermittent fever

2. Physical exam: a pericardial friction rub is pathognomonic
   a. May be positional and intermittent.
   b. Is best appreciated when the patient is sitting and leaning forward or is in the hands-and-knees position.
   c. Is scratchy in character; best heard with the <u>diaphragm</u> of the stethoscope positioned along the lower left sternal border or cardiac apex.
   d. Is classically triphasic (with presystolic, systolic and diastolic components) but may be biphasic or monophasic.

3. ECG
   a. Normal sinus rhythm or sinus tachycardia; dysrhythmias are <u>un</u>common.
   b. Diffuse, <u>non</u>anatomic ST segment elevation with <u>upward concavity</u> is seen acutely in all leads except aVR and V_1. [<u>Note</u>: ST segment elevation due to AMI is, by comparison, obliquely flat or <u>convex</u> in configuration and has a <u>non</u>diffuse, anatomic distribution (e.g. inferior or anterior wall pattern)].
   c. Reciprocal ST segment depression in leads aVR and V_1.
   d. PR segment depression (very specific for pericarditis); most prominent in lead II; often the earliest ECG manifestation.
   e. Diffuse T wave inversion (occurs after ST elevation has resolved) — a late sign.

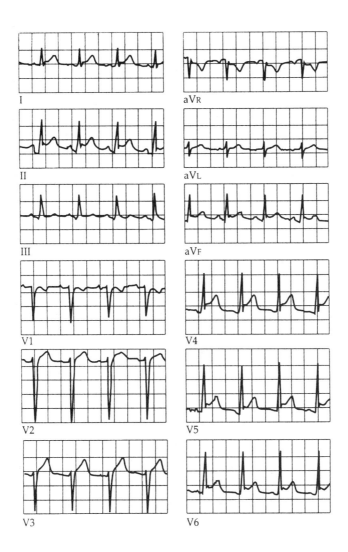

4. CXR — usually normal, but in the presence of a large pericardial effusion (> 200mL) it may reveal an enlarged cardiac silhouette.

5. Echocardiography — is the most sensitive and most specific procedure for detecting the presence and size of an associated pericardial effusion; it is considered to be the diagnostic modality of choice. Two dimensional

(2D) echocardiography can detect as little as 15mL of fluid and has the advantage of being able to provide information about cardiac function. Transesophageal echocardiography (TEE) and chest CT are superior to transthoracic echocardiography (TTE) for the demonstration of pericardial thickening (seen in constrictive pericarditis).

6. CT scan
   a. Can define the presence and extent of pericardial effusion but, unlike echocardiography, it cannot assess cardiac function and may miss hemopericardium due to similar densities of blood and myocardium.
   b. It is usually reserved for those times when echocardiography is unavailable or yields equivocal results.

7. Lab studies
   a. CBC — an elevated WBC count with a left shift is common.
   b. ESR — is usually elevated.
   c. BUN/creatinine — are useful in ruling out uremia.
   d. Cardiac enzymes — are often minimally elevated.
   e. Other specific tests (blood cultures, viral titers, TFTs, etc.) — should be obtained as appropriate, depending on the suspected underlying etiology.

C. Treatment

1. Patients with viral or idiopathic pericarditis may be treated as outpatients if reliable follow-up can be assured as they tend to follow a benign, self-limited course. All others, particularly those with severe intractable pain or an underlying precipitant which requires specific treatment (MI, uremia, bacterial infection, etc.) should be hospitalized.

2. Pain relief
   a. Anti-inflammatory agents — generally provide symptomatic relief within 24 hours of initiation. Use one of the following:
      (1) Aspirin (650mg PO Q6 hrs.)
      (2) Ibuprofen (600 - 800mg PO Q6 - 8hrs.)
      (3) Indomethacin (25 - 75mg PO Q6 - 8hrs.)
      (4) Prednisone (60mg PO QD) — should be reserved for patients who fail to respond to the above agents (since 25% of patients will experience relapsing pericarditis when it is discontinued) and should not be used until the presence of bacterial or mycobacterial infection has been excluded.
   b. Narcotic agents (morphine, meperidine) — may be used when immediate pain relief is needed.

3. Treat the underlying disorder:
   a. Antimicrobial agents for patients with underlying infections
   b. Dialysis for uremic patients
   c. Cessation of the causative agent for medication-induced pericarditis

4. Pericardiocentesis for tamponade

II. Pericardial Tamponade

A. Classic Clinical Findings

1. Beck's triad:
   - Hypotension
   - Jugular venous distention
   - Distant heart tones (quiet heart)

   are late findings occurring just prior to cardiac arrest

2. Narrow pulse pressure

3. Dyspnea

4. Tachycardia (earliest sign)

5. Pulsus paradoxus > 10mmHg

6. ECG findings:
   a. Low QRS voltage — a nonspecific finding of pericardial effusion
   b. Total electrical alternans (a beat-to-beat alternating pattern primarily affecting the QRS complex that occurs from shifting pericardial fluid and heart position — is pathognomonic for cardiac tamponade but not always present.) [See Rosen, 5th. ed., page 399, Fig. 38-11]

7. Kussmaul's sign — a rise in central venous pressure (by observation of jugular venous pulsation) with spontaneous inspiration.

8. CXR — in patients with chronic effusions, the CXR may reveal an enlarged "water bottle" shaped cardiac silhouette without associated pulmonary redistribution. This is not true in acute traumatic tamponade where the cardiac silhouette is typically normal.

9. Echocardiography
   a. Is the gold standard for diagnosing pericardial effusion; it can quickly and accurately confirm the presence of tamponade.
   b. If it is rapidly available and if the patient's condition allows, it should be performed whenever this diagnosis is suspected.
   c. Findings consistent with tamponade include:
      (1) A large pericardial effusion (visualized as an echo-free space behind the left ventricle and in front of the right ventricle)
      (2) Diastolic collapse of the right ventricle and the right atrium
      (3) Swinging motion of the heart in the effusion (producing electrical alternans)

B. Differential Diagnosis (in patients with neck vein distention and hypotension)

1. Tension pneumothorax

2. Massive pulmonary embolism

3. Acute pulmonary edema

C. Clinical Picture of a Patient Who Needs Immediate Pericardiocentesis

1. Air-hunger + drowsiness or confusion

2. Thready pulse + pulsus paradoxus that is > 50% of the pulse pressure

3. ↑ JVD + ↓ systolic BP

4. ECG finding of total electrical alternans in a symptomatic patient

D. Treatment of Pericardial Tamponade

1. Stabilizing/temporizing measures — these steps should be performed while arrangements for pericardiocentesis are being set-up.
   a. Establish two large-bore IVs, provide supplemental oxygen (5 - 10 Liters/min.) and attach patient to cardiac monitor.
   b. Provide aggressive volume resuscitation with crystalloid solution or blood.
   c. Administer dobutamine or dopamine as needed for inotropic support.
   d. Obtain immediate cardiothoracic surgery consult regarding pericardiotomy and thoracotomy.

2. Definitive therapy → pericardiocentesis. Although this procedure can be performed blindly or by using ECG guidance, 2D echocardiographic guidance is safer and is the technique of choice if it can be performed in a timely manner.

MYOCARDITIS

I. **Definition:** Myocarditis is an inflammation of the heart muscle. It often presents in association with acute pericarditis.

II. **Diagnosis**

A. *Clinical Presentation* — is determined by the degree of cardiac involvement and ranges from nonspecific symptoms of fatigue and dyspnea to florid CHF, significant dysrhythmias and sudden death. History of a preceding or concurrent viral illness is common. Signs and symptoms may include:

1. Fever and retrosternal or precordial chest pain (frequent complaints)

2. Fatigue, palpitations, dizziness and/or syncope

3. Signs and symptoms of CHF (dyspnea, rales, peripheral edema, JVD)

4. Sinus tachycardia disproportionate to the degree of fever (>101°F) present and probably secondary to associated heart failure

5. Cardiac dysrhythmias or conduction disturbances

6. Abnormal heart sounds:
    a. Pericardial friction rub (when associated pericarditis is present)
    b. Soft S_1
    c. S_3 or S_4 gallop
    d. Murmurs of mitral or tricuspid regurgitation

B. *Lab Studies*

1. ECG
    a. Nonspecific ST-T wave changes (may be localized or diffuse)
    b. Dysrhythmias ranging from sinus tachycardia (most common) to atrial or ventricular dysrhythmias
    c. Conduction disturbances (AV Block, BBB)
    d. Low QRS voltage
    e. Pseudoinfarction patterns, nonspecific ST/T wave changes

2. CXR — Although it is generally normal, cardiomegaly, pulmonary venous HTN and/or pulmonary edema may be present.

3. Echocardiography — demonstrates dilated chambers with either diffuse hypokinesis or focal wall motion abnormalities.

4. CBC — reveals mild to moderate leukocytosis.

5. ESR — is elevated.

6. Cardiac enzymes
   a. Characteristically rise and fall slowly over a period of days (unlike the rapid rise seen in AMI).
   b. Troponin I levels are more sensitive and specific than CK-MB levels.

7. Gallium 67 imaging and indium-III antimyosin antibodies — may demonstrate areas of myocardial inflammation or necrosis but they are nonspecific.

8. Endomyocardial biopsy — can provide definitive diagnosis but suffers from problems of sampling error and interobserver variability.

III. Causes

A. Viruses — most common cause of myocarditis

1. Coxsackie A and B

2. Echovirus

3. Poliovirus

4. HIV

5. Cytomegalovirus

6. Influenza

7. Epstein-Barr

8. Hepatitis B

9. Adenovirus

B. Bacteria

1. *Beta-hemolytic strep.* (rheumatic fever)

2. *Corynebacterium diphtheriae*

3. *Neisseria meningitidis*

4. *Borrelia burgdorferi*

5. *Mycoplasma pneumoniae*

C. *Parasites*

1. Chagas' disease

2. Toxoplasmosis

3. Trichinosis

D. *Systemic Diseases*

1. Kawasaki syndrome

2. Systemic lupus erythematosus (SLE)

3. Sarcoidosis

4. Inflammatory disorders

E. *Drug Hypersensitivity*

1. Sulfonamides

2. Penicillins

3. Methyldopa

F. *Toxins*

1. Cocaine

2. Inhalants (e.g. toluene)

IV. Treatment — is primarily supportive

A. Admit to ICU setting.

B. Bed rest (strenuous activity should be avoided).

C. Administer antibiotics if an underlying bacterial cause is present.

D. Immunosuppressive agents (steroids, cyclosporin) and NSAIDs are contraindicated in early myocarditis.

E. High-dose IV gamma-globulin (IVIG) has been shown to be beneficial in preliminary studies of the pediatric population (especially kids with Kawasaki's syndrome).

F. Antiviral agents (e.g. interferon) are currently under investigation and may also prove to be effective.

G. CHF should be managed with the usual drug protocols; however, it should be noted that:

1. Digoxin should be used with caution because the inflamed myocardium is very sensitive to it.

2. ACE inhibitors (e.g. captopril) have been shown to be particularly beneficial in that they decrease cellular necrosis and inflammation.

H. Dysrhythmias should be managed with the usual antidysrhythmic agents.

ENDOCARDITIS

I. **Definition:** Endocarditis is a localized infection of the endocardium, the hall-mark of which is vegetation. It can involve the valve leaflets, the walls of the heart cavities or the tissue surrounding prosthetic heart valves.

II. Pathophysiology

A. Injury to the endothelium results in formation of a platelet-fibrin complex which is subsequently colonized by micro-organisms during periods of transient bacteremia.

B. Although endocarditis does occur in patients with normal valves, patients with congenital/acquired valvular disease and prosthetic valves are most commonly affected.

C. Risk Factors Include:

- Prosthetic valve(s)

- Congenital valvular heart disease (e.g. mitral valve prolapse)

- Acquired valvular heart disease (e.g. rheumatic heart disease)

- Intravenous drug abuse (IVDA)

- Calcific valve degeneration

- Indwelling venous catheters, vascular shunts

- Hemodialysis

- Peritoneal dialysis

- Cardiac surgery

- HIV infection

- History of endocarditis

- Extensive burn injury

D. **Causative Organisms:** Although endocarditis is most commonly caused by bacteria, it may also be caused by fungi, rickettsiae and viruses. The causative organism varies with the <u>type</u> of valve involved (native versus prosthetic) and in the presence of IVDA/immunocompromise. Common bacterial pathogens include the following:

1. Native valves
   a. *Non-viridans streptococci* (most common)
   b. *Staph. aureus*
   c. *Strep. viridans*
   d. *Enterococci*

2. Prosthetic valves
   a. *Coagulase-neg. Staph.* (early - - < 60 days post-op)
   b. *Staph. aureus* / epidermidis (late - - > 60 days post-op)
   c. *Strep. viridans*
   d. *Enterococci*

3. IV drug abusers/immunocompromised
   a. Staph. aureus
   b. Strep. species
   c. Gram-negative bacilli

E. **Left - versus Right-sided Disease**

1. Left-sided endocarditis → <u>systemic</u> vascular involvement
   a. Most commonly occurs in patients with acquired valvular disease and congenital heart disease (and is more common than right-sided disease).
   b. Depending on the virulence of the infecting organism, it can present as an acute or subacute illness.
   c. The mitral valve is most commonly affected.
   d. *Strep. viridans* and *Staph. aureus* are the most frequent pathogens.

2. Right-sided endocarditis → <u>pulmonary</u> vascular involvement
   a. Is primarily a disease of intravenous drug abusers.
   b. Usually has an acute presentation.
   c. Most commonly involves the tricuspid valve.
   d. Is caused by *Staph. aureus* in approximately 75% of cases.

III. Clinical Presentation

A. *Symptoms* — are protean and nonspecific and may include intermittent fever, chills, sweats, malaise, fatigue, weight loss, chest pain, cough and neurologic complaints/focal deficits; the most common presentation in kids is malaise and weight loss.

B. *Physical Findings* — may include:

1. Fever (most common finding)

2. Heart murmur

3. Signs of CHF

4. Signs of metastatic infection (e.g. meningitis, pneumonia)

5. Opthalmologic signs
   a. Conjunctival hemorrhages
   b. Roth spots (retinal hemorrhages with central clearing)

6. Cutaneous signs
   a. Splinter hemorrhages
   b. Osler's nodes — tender erythematous nodules found on the volar surface of the fingertip
   c. Janeway lesions — nontender erythematous macular lesions appearing on the fingers, palms and soles
   d. Petechiae

7. Neurologic findings
   a. Focal motor deficits
   b. Altered level of consciousness

IV. Lab Studies

A. *CBC* — reveals leukocytosis with a left shift and a mild normocytic anemia.

B. *ESR/C-reactive protein and serum rheumatoid factor* — are elevated.

C. *U/A* — reveals microscopic hematuria in > 50% of patients.

D. *CXR* — is often unremarkable, but may reveal septic emboli in patients with right-sided endocarditis.

E. ECG — is usually normal, but may demonstrate conductive deficits in the presence of extensive myocardial damage.

F. Blood Cultures

1. Are the <u>most useful</u> test for making the diagnosis; they are positive in > 90% of patients with bacterial endocarditis.

2. Three blood cultures from 3 different sites should be obtained and each should be evaluated for aerobic, anaerobic and fungal pathogens.

G. Echocardiography

1. Is useful if positive for vegetations, but a negative exam does <u>not</u> rule out the diagnosis.

2. Transesophageal echo (TEE) is more sensitive in revealing vegetations than transthoracic echo (TTE), especially in the patients with prosthetic valves.
    a. TTE is recommended as the initial study for low-risk patients.
    b. TEE is recommended as the initial study for high-risk patients and as the follow-up study for the low-risk patients with a negative or technically inadequate TTE.

V. Diagnosis

A. A presumptive diagnosis of endocarditis should be made in the patient presenting with risk factors and clinical findings (e.g. a patient with a prosthetic valve or a recent history of IV drug use and fever).

B. Positive blood cultures and evidence of valvular injury/vegetations usually confirm the diagnosis; if there is any doubt, a tissue biopsy is still considered the gold standard (best diagnostic modality).

VI. Treatment

A. Antibiotic Therapy

1. Ideally, empiric antibiotic therapy should be initiated <u>after</u> appropriate blood cultures have been obtained. In hemodynamically unstable patients, however, antibiotic therapy should not be delayed to obtain cultures but, rather, should be started immediately.

2. The initial antibiotic regimen selected should reflect the susceptibilities of the suspected organism, the acuteness of the presentation and local resistance patterns.

3. Acceptable empiric antibiotic regimens are as follows:
    a. In patients with <u>native</u> valves and a subacute presentation:
        (1) PCN G (or ampicillin) IV plus nafcillin (or oxacillin) IV plus gentamicin IM or IV <u>or</u>
        (2) Vancomycin IV plus gentamicin IM or IV in PCN allergic patients
    b. In patients with a <u>prosthetic</u> valve:* vancomycin IV plus gentamicin IV plus rifampin PO.

    [Note: Vancomycin-resistant enterococcal infections are occurring, especially in IV drug abusers, patients with prosthetic valves and those recently hospitalized or taking antimicrobial agents. Current suggested therapy for these patients: quinupristin/dalfopristin combination plus doxycyline and rifampin.]

B. Although ambulatory treatment is possible in certain select cardiovascularly stable patients, patients with endocarditis should generally be admitted to the hospital for treatment, particularly those with prosthetic valves and a history of IVDA.

VII. Conditions Requiring Prophylaxis for Endocarditis:

- Prosthetic heart valves
- History of bacterial endocarditis
- Complex cyanotic congenital heart lesions
- Surgically constructed systemic pulmonary shunts or conduits
- Mitral valve prolapse with regurgitation or thickened leaflets
- Acquired valvular disease (e.g. rheumatic heart disease)
- Hypertrophic cardiomyopathy
- Most other congenital cardiac malformations

The oral cavity and the genitourinary tract are the most frequent sites of entry for bacteria causing endocarditis, thus antibiotic prophylaxis is especially important for procedures involving manipulation of these areas.

---

*Early consultation with a cardiothoracic surgeon should be obtained in all patients with a prosthetic valve.

THORACIC AORTIC DISSECTIONS AND ABDOMINAL AORTIC ANEURYSMS

I. **Thoracic Aortic Dissections (most common lethal disease of the aorta)**

A. Epidemiology

1. TADs are 2 - 3 times more common than abdominal aortic aneurysm (AAA) ruptures.

2. Males are affected more commonly than females (ratio 3:1)

3. Most patients are 50 - 70 years of age.

4. Risk factors (more than one increases the overall risk):
   a. A history of systemic <u>hypertension</u> — this is the <u>most common predisposing factor</u>; it is present in 70 - 90% of patients.
   b. Connective tissue disorders
      (1) Ehlers-Danlos syndrome
      (2) Marfan's syndrome ⎤
      (3) Lupus Erythematosus ⎬ Patients may present
      (4) Giant cell arteritis ⎦ younger than 50 yrs.
      (5) Cystic medial necrosis
   c. Pregnancy (3rd trimester)
   d. Congenital heart disease
      (1) Bicuspid aortic valve
      (2) Coarctation of the aorta
   e. Turner's syndrome
   f. Trauma
   g. Cocaine and methamphetamine use (cause hypertension)
   h. Epstein's anomaly
   i. Aortic valve stenosis
   j. Infectious disease (syphilis, endocarditis)
   k. Tobacco use

B. Pathophysiology

1. Starts with an intimal tear that allows blood to leak into the media and cleave it longitudinally from the adventitia.*

2. Once the dissection begins, its propagation is dependent upon the BP and the steepness of the pulse wave (dP/dT)**; high blood pressure and rapid ventricular contractions enhance migration of the dissection.

*An important variant of aortic dissection is an intimal tear that arises without classic dissection into the media and produces only a localized bulge in the aortic wall. It is just as deadly as classic dissection and, unfortunately, is not typically seen with the usual tests used to diagnose TAD.
**Rate of change in pressure/time

C. *Natural History* — untreated, the mortality rate is:

- ~33% within 24 hours
- 50% within 48 hours
- >75% within 2 weeks
- 90% within 1 - 3 months

D. *Classification System* — aortic dissections are classified according to the location of the dissecting process. There are two major classification systems: Debakey and Stanford. The complications, prognosis and treatment protocols vary with the location of the dissection. Dissections involving the proximal aorta are more common and more lethal than those confined to the distal aorta.

1. Debakey Classification
   a. Type I: ascending aorta and part of distal aorta (most common type)
   b. Type II: ascending aorta only
   c. Type III: descending aorta only
      (1) Subtype IIIA (extension limited to the diaphragm)
      (2) Subtype IIIB (continuation beyond the diaphragm)

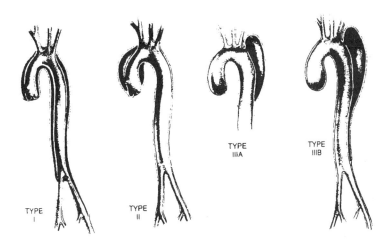

Reproduced with permission from: Galloway AC, Miller JS, Spencer FC, et al. Thoracic aneurysms and aortic dissection. In: Schwartz GR, et al, eds. Principles and Practice of Emergency Medicine. Philadelphia: Lea & Febiger; 1992:924

2. Stanford Classification
   a. Type A: ascending aorta (= Debakey Type I and Type II)
   b. Type B: descending aorta (= Debakey Type III)

E. Presentation

1. <u>Pain</u> — is the <u>most common</u> presenting symptom.
    a. The pain is excruciating, <u>starts abruptly</u>, is <u>maximal from its onset</u> and <u>migrates</u> as the dissection propagates. It generally (but not always) has a tearing or ripping quality and is most commonly located in the chest, upper back or abdomen.
    b. The location of pain provides a clue to the location of the dissection; anterior chest pain (± radiation into the neck, jaw or arms) is typical of ascending (proximal) dissections; arch dissections cause pain in the neck and jaw; and interscapular back pain (± radiation into the abdomen or lumbar area) is typical of descending (distal) dissections.

2. Based on the location of the dissection, patients may also present with:
    a. Acute CVA, visual changes
    b. Acute paraplegia, spinal cord deficits
    c. A cold <u>pulseless</u> extremity
    d. CHF and pulmonary edema
    e. Abdominal pain (mesenteric ischemia), nausea/vomiting
    f. Flank pain, hematuria or oliguria (impaired renal blood flow)
    g. Syncope
    h. Acute MI (if dissection involves a coronary artery or ostia)
    i. Aortic regurgitation

3. A significant number of patients present <u>only</u> with ischemic or neurologic complications of a "silent" (painless) aortic dissection.* This is an important point since inadvertent administration of a thrombolytic agent to a patient who seems to be having a "stroke" or an "MI" would be disastrous.

F. Clinical Findings

1. Blood Pressure Findings
    a. Ⓝ or ↓ → ascending aorta
    b. ↑BP → descending aorta
    c. A 20mmHg extremity blood pressure difference

2. Shock-like appearance (cool, clammy skin) despite elevated BP

3. Focal neurologic deficits

4. Unequal or absent pulses (hallmark of aortic dissection) between extremities

5. Diastolic murmur of aortic insufficiency (with Types I, II and A)

6. Signs of cardiac tamponade (with Types I, II and A)

---

*Most frequently encountered in Type A dissection that has extended to involve the descending aorta (similar to a Debakey Type I dissection)

G. Diagnostic Studies

1. Initial studies
    a. Chest x-ray
        (1) Should be taken immediately.
        (2) The patient should be in the <u>upright position</u>.
        (3) It is <u>usually abnormal</u> <u>but</u> the findings are <u>nonspecific</u>; a normal chest x-ray does <u>not</u> rule out the diagnosis.
        (4) Suggestive findings:
            (a) Mediastinal widening > 8cm (most common finding)
            (b) A change in the configuration or size of the thoracic aorta when compared with older films; loss of space between the aorta and pulmonary artery.
            (c) "Eggshell" or "calcium" sign → extension of the aortic shadow by more than 5mm beyond its calcified aortic wall (most specific sign; when present, is pathognomonic for dissection.)
            (d) A blurred aortic knob or one with a localized hump
            (e) A "double density" appearance of the aorta which suggests the presence of true and false channels; the false lumen is less radiopaque than the true lumen.
            (f) On the <u>right side</u> of the film:
                • Deviation of the trachea/NG tube
                • Shift and elevation of the right mainstem bronchus
                • Deviation of the right paraspinous line
            (g) On the <u>left side</u> of the film:
                • A pleurapical cap
                • Depressed left mainstem bronchus
                • Pleural effusion
    b. ECG...is abnormal in most patients with aortic dissection.
        (1) Changes consistent with AMI/ischemia have been reported in up to 40% of cases (the most common misdiagnosis in these patients).* A dissection-induced MI should be ruled out (with a TEE or CT) in patients who are candidates for thrombolytic therapy and have clinical findings that suggest the possibility of TAD.
        (2) Varying degrees of AV Block can be produced by propagation of the dissection into the ventricular septum.
        (3) Left ventricular hypertrophy (due to long-standing hypertension) is a frequent finding.

2. Definitive studies — One (or more) of the following tests may be used to confirm the diagnosis. Each has certain advantages and disadvantages (and their 24-hour availability is variable). The diagnostic approach chosen will vary from institution to institution and patient to patient depending on the technology available, the speed of obtaining each diagnostic test, the experience of the radiologist in interpreting each test, the preference of the surgeon, the probability of the diagnosis and comorbid disease of the specific patient. When the probability of dissection is high, the most readily available study should be the initial study of choice.

---

*Inferior wall MI patterns are most common since they involve the <u>right</u> coronary artery.

a. Transesophageal echocardiography (with color-coded Doppler imaging)
   (1) Is the most expedient technique for confirming the diagnosis of aortic dissection and has become the diagnostic study of choice in many hospitals.
   (2) It has a sensitivity and specificity of nearly 100%.
   (3) All the information required for decision-making regarding emergency surgical intervention can be obtained with this study; in addition to identifying the dissection, it detects the intimal tear site, flow in the proximal coronary arteries, aortic regurgitation and pericardial effusion; it also differentiates true from false lumens.
   (4) Advantages — it is only minimally invasive, requires only 10 - 15 minutes to complete, does <u>not</u> necessitate exposure to IV contrast and can be performed at the bedside in the ED while the patient is being treated and appropriately monitored.
   (5) Disadvantages — it is contraindicated in patients with esophageal disease (e.g. strictures, varices) and the necessary equipment/expertise are not readily available in all hospitals.
b. Aortography
   (1) Has been the traditional diagnostic gold standard.
   (2) It has a sensitivity and specificity of about 90%.
   (3) In addition to confirming the diagnosis, it defines the intimal tear site, the extent of the dissection and also assesses the aortic valves and branches.
   (4) Disadvantages — it is invasive, time-consuming, requires special personnel, can<u>not</u> be performed in the ED, necessitates exposure to IV contrast and is <u>not</u> 100% accurate (can miss dissection if the false lumen is thrombosed).
   (5) It is best reserved for situations in which TEE is not available or is nondiagnostic.
c. Magnetic Resonance Imaging (MRI)
   (1) It has a sensitivity and specificity of 100%.
   (2) It delineates the desired anatomy: type and extent of dissection, site of the intimal tear, presence of aortic insufficiency and differential flow velocities in the true and false channels and in aortic branch vessels.
   (3) Advantages — it is noninvasive and does <u>not</u> require IV contrast material or ionizing radiation.
   (4) Disadvantages — it is time-consuming (requires more than 60 minutes to perform), cannot be performed in the ED or on patients with metallic implants, allows only limited access to the patient during the exam, some patients cannot tolerate the scanner and most units cannot accommodate monitoring or advanced life support equipment.

    d. Rapid-sequence (Dynamic) CT Scanning with contrast
       (1) The newer helical CT scans have almost 100% specificity and sensitivity; they are becoming the preferred diagnostic technique.
       (2) It can confirm the diagnosis, define the extent of the dissection and distinguish between Type A and Type B dissections, but cannot identify aortic insufficiency or extension to the aortic branches.
       (3) Advantages — it is less invasive and provides greater contrast resolution than aortography and may reveal other abnormalities in cases where dissection is ruled out.
       (4) Disadvantages — it is time-consuming, cannot be performed in the ED, exposes the patient to IV contrast and may miss a dissection flap (if it is moving rapidly).
       (5) It is a good choice for EDs without access to TEE because of its high sensitivity.

H. Treatment

1. All patients require 10 - 15 units of blood on stand-by and immediate consultation with a thoracic surgeon.

2. Initial management for all types of dissections is medical and involves controlling the forces that propagate the dissection: pulse rate, systolic BP and rate of elevation of the aortic pulse pressure (dP/dT). If your suspicion for dissection is high, begin treatment immediately; it should not be delayed to await confirmatory study results.
    a. Intravenous beta-blockers (propranolol, metoprolol, atenolol or esmolol) are administered first and titrated to a HR of 60 - 80.
    b. Nitroprusside is then initiated and titrated to a systolic BP of 100 - 120mmHg.
    c. Another alternative to the beta-blocker and nitroprusside combination is single-agent therapy with IV labetalol.

3. Hypotensive patients should be managed with small boluses of a crystalloid solution or blood.

4. Pain should be treated with IV narcotics.

5. Long-term management
    a. Dissections involving the ascending aorta (Types A, I and II) — are treated surgically.
    b. Dissections involving only the descending aorta (Types B and III) — are treated medically unless complications are present.

II. Expanding and Ruptured Abdominal Aortic Aneurysms (AAA)

A. ***Definition and Anatomic Location*** — Aortic aneurysms are <u>true</u> aneurysms (they involve all three layers of the arterial wall) and the vast majority (97%) are <u>infra</u>renal in location.

B. ***Pathogenesis***

1. Although AAAs often occur in patients with atherosclerotic disease, athero-sclerosis is no longer believed to be the primary etiologic factor in the development of these aneurysms.

2. They are currently theorized to be due to a combination of genetic, structural and metabolic factors including:
   a. Genetic predisposition
   b. Increased levels of elastase and collagenase
   c. Failure or loss of blood vessel elastin
   d. Copper deficiency
   e. Infection (mycotic aneurysms)
   f. Inflammatory disorders
   g. Local mechanical forces

C. ***Risk Factors for the Development of an AAA***

1. Advanced age (75% of AAAs occur in patients > 60 yrs. old)

2. Male sex (particularly Caucasian males)

3. Family history of an AAA in a first-degree (blood) relative

4. Smoking history

5. Hypertensive history

6. History of coronary artery disease or peripheral vascular disease

7. Elevated serum cholesterol levels

D. ***Clinical Presentation***

1. The patient is frequently a middle-aged or elderly male (and a heavy smoker) who had a syncopal episode at home with transient improvement.

2. Sudden onset of severe abdominal, back or flank pain with or without an associated syncopal episode (due to sudden hemorrhage) is the classic presentation in the Emergency Department: retroperitoneal bleeding with hematoma formation occurs in the majority of patients (usually on the left) and accounts for the variety of clinical presentations that are possible...and confusing.
   a. Flank pain (usually on the left side) may radiate to the groin and be accompanied by hematuria, thus simulating a kidney stone (the most common misdiagnosis).

b. Low back pain may be dull and radiate into the legs, thus mimicking musculoskeletal back pain.

c. Abdominal pain that is localized to the LLQ and accompanied by guaiac-positive stools is common in patients with diverticulitis, but it's also seen in a ruptured AAA (and may be associated with a non-pulsatile mass).

d. A scrotal hematoma can be interpreted as a "mass" in the scrotum and thus simulate an incarcerated hernia.

e. Ecchymoses can result from significant bleeding and may be seen on the abdominal wall, flank, scrotum, penis, inguinal region, perineum or perianal area.

f. Femoral neuropathy (pain in the hip and thigh, quadricep muscle weakness, diminished sensation over the antero-medial thigh and a weakened patellar reflex) may be from femoral nerve compression due to a hematoma.

3. Physical exam findings are variable.

a. A pulsatile (and occasionally tender) mass is palpable in the epigastric area in 77% of patients with a ruptured AAA; unruptured aneurysms are smaller in size and less frequently detected; in the presence of obesity or abdominal distention, a pulsatile mass may not be felt.

b. A tender (pulsatile) mass is highly suggestive of a rapidly expanding or recently ruptured AAA; most intact aneurysms are not tender.

c. Bruits may be heard over the abdominal aorta or femoral arteries.

d. Signs of distal extremity ischemia (not always present): unequal or unsynchronized distal pulses and cool, pale skin.

E. Diagnosis and Management

1. Presence of a symptomatic AAA is usually suggested by the patient's clinical presentation and physical exam. This information alone is sufficient evidence in many patients to take them immediately to the OR (particularly the hemodynamically unstable ones).

2. Once this diagnosis is suspected, the following measures should be undertaken immediately:

a. Establish 2 large bore IVs (NS or LR), place the patient on a cardiac monitor and pulse oximeter, and administer supplemental O_2.

b. Draw blood for preoperative lab evaluation and type and cross for at least 10 units of blood.

c. Order an ECG.

d. Obtain immediate surgical consultation (preferably with a vascular surgeon).

3. Further evaluation is determined by the hemodynamic stability of the patient.

a. Hemodynamically unstable patients with a suspected AAA require prompt surgical repair. Fluid and blood resuscitation should be initiated in the ED and the patient should be transferred to the OR for definitive treatment as soon as the surgeon is available. Any delay for further diagnostic testing increases the risk of death from exsanguination.

b. Hemodynamically <u>stable patients</u> in whom this diagnosis is suspected may undergo further diagnostic testing (<u>under close medical supervision</u>) prior to surgical intervention. The various imaging modalities available are described below. Of these, ultrasonography or CT are the most appropriate studies in this setting.

(1) Plain abdominal x-rays (AP and lateral films) — Although most patients with an AAA (75%) have suspicious findings on plain film evaluation (aneurysmal calcification, soft-tissue mass, loss of renal shadow, renal displacement and/or change in the posterior peritoneal flank stripe) with the exception of aneurysmal calcification, none of these findings are specific for AAA and their absence does not reliably exclude the presence of an AAA. Furthermore, plain films are not very accurate in determining the extent of the aneurysm, rupture or associated vascular pathology.

(2) Ultrasonography — has a sensitivity of nearly 100% in detecting an AAA and has the advantage of being quick, readily available, noninvasive and portable. It cannot, however, accurately detect aneurysmal leaking and complications such as visceral or renal artery involvement. Moreover, the study may be limited in the presence of obesity or intestinal gas. Thus, US is most useful in determining whether or not an aneurysm is <u>present</u>, which may be more than enough information in the appropriate setting.

(3) CT with contrast — also has a sensitivity of ~ 100% in detecting an AAA but is more accurate than US in detecting aneurysmal rupture and visceral artery involvement; also, it is not limited by obesity or intestinal gas. Visualization of the retroperitoneal structures and diagnosis of other pathology are also superior with this modality. Disadvantages include exposure to IV contrast material and longer study time.

(4) MRI — is excellent at imaging the aorta and is superior to CT in assessing branch vessel involvement. However, it is of limited use in this setting because it is time-consuming, has limited availability, cannot be performed in the ED or in the patient with metallic implants and allows only limited access to the patient during the study. This modality is usually reserved for evaluation of <u>asymptomatic</u> patients.

(5) Angiography — Although useful in determining the anatomy of the aorta and demonstrating occlusive lesions, angiography is not entirely reliable in detecting the presence (has a high false-negative rate) or diameter of an AAA. Furthermore, this study is time-consuming, invasive, requires specialized personnel and necessitates exposure to IV contrast. For these reasons, angiography is the least desirable study for emergent diagnostic evaluation of these patients.

HYPERTENSIVE EMERGENCIES AND URGENCIES

I. Hypertensive Emergencies

A. *Definition* — Patients with severely elevated diastolic BP (> 140mmHg) and evidence of acute end-organ dysfunction or damage. It is the presence of end-organ damage (<u>not</u> the absolute blood pressure) that determines a patient with a hypertensive emergency. The heart, brain and kidneys are the organs most often affected.

B. *Clinical Presentations*

1. Malignant HTN

2. Hypertensive encephalopathy

3. HTN with acute intracranial events (hemorrhagic CVA, thrombotic CVA, SAH)

4. Aortic dissection

5. Acute pulmonary edema

6. Acute myocardial ischemia or injury

7. Eclampsia

8. Acute hypertensive renal insufficiency

9. Catecholamine-induced hypertensive crisis — an acute elevation of circulating catecholamines that produces an elevated BP with headache, palpitations, sweating and tachycardia. Causes include:
   a. Pheochromocytoma (adrenal tumor)
   b. Concomitant use of monoamine oxidase inhibitors (MAOIs) and sympathomimetic agents. Commonly implicated sympathomimetics include:
      (1) Tyramine (Chianti wine, aged cheese, beer, pickled herring, chicken liver)
      (2) Ephedrine and phenylpropanolamine (found in OTC cold and cough preparations)
      (3) Diet pills
   c. Acute cocaine intoxication
   d. Acute clonidine withdrawal (particularly when withdrawn simultaneously with a beta-blocking agent)

C. Treatment

1. The goal of therapy is to arrest and reverse the progression of end-organ dysfunction while maintaining organ perfusion and avoiding complications. To do this, the BP must be lowered rapidly and in a controlled manner. The exact extent of BP reduction is determined by the clinical situation; however, a reasonable target is to reduce the BP by 30% of pretreatment levels over the first hour of therapy.

2. Medications are usually given by the <u>intravenous</u> route which provides a faster onset of action and is more easily titrated.

3. The antihypertensive agent of choice varies with the specific hypertensive emergency as follows:
   a. <u>Malignant HTN and hypertensive encephalopathy</u> → nitroprusside is the drug of choice. IV labetalol is a good alternative, particularly when intra-arterial pressure monitoring is not available. IV Nicardipine is also effective.
   b. <u>HTN with an ischemic CVA</u> → treatment of HTN in the immediate poststroke period can be detrimental in these patients and should <u>not</u> be initiated in most instances; acute reduction in BP can reduce perfusion to the surrounding watershed areas and may thereby extend the infarction. Therefore, BP reduction should <u>only</u> be considered in patients with extremely high blood pressures (> 220/120). Short-acting agents with few CNS effects (such as IV nitroprusside or IV labetalol) are the drugs of choice.
   c. <u>HTN with hemorrhagic CVA</u> → Although somewhat more controversial, most authors agree that mild to moderate HTN is generally well-tolerated in these patients, but that severe HTN (BP > 220/120) may promote further hemorrhage and should be judiciously controlled with a titratable agent such as IV labetalol.*
   d. <u>HTN with subarachnoid hemorrhage</u> → nimodipine or nicardipine (calcium channel-blockers) is the initial therapeutic agent of choice. In addition to its antihypertensive effect, it also decreases the cerebral vasospasm that occurs following SAH. The goal of treatment is to reduce the MAP to prehemorrhagic levels. BP reduction is associated with a decrease in the risk of rebleeding in these patients.
   e. <u>Aortic dissection</u> → nitroprusside in combination with an intravenous beta-blocker (propranolol or esmolol) is the therapy of choice; the beta-blocking agent should be administered first to prevent the reflex tachycardia that can occur in association with nitroprusside. IV labetalol is the alternative agent of choice.
   f. <u>Acute myocardial ischemia or injury</u> → IV nitroglycerine is the primary agent of choice because of its beneficial effects on coronary perfusion. However, an intravenous beta blocker should also be given to reduce myocardial oxygen demand. If the BP remains elevated, nitroprusside is the alternative of choice; however, it can increase myocardial ischemia via the coronary steal syndrome.

*Other acceptable agents: esmolol, enalapril, nicardipine.

g. <u>Acute pulmonary edema</u> → if standard treatment measures for pulmonary edema (e.g., IV furosemide, IV morphine, CPAP) fail to adequately reduce the BP, specific antihypertensive therapy should be initiated. IV nitroglycerine is the drug of choice. If the BP remains elevated, nitroprusside is the alternative agent.

h. <u>Eclampsia</u> → IV or IM magnesium sulfate in combination with IV or IM hydralazine (available as a generic) are the first-line agents. IV labetalol is also safe and effective. Nitroprusside may be used in postpartum eclampsia but, due to the risk for fetal cyanide poisoning, is relatively contraindicated antepartum; it should be reserved for those patients who fail to respond to the above-mentioned treatment regimens.

i. <u>Acute hypertensive renal insufficiency</u> → nitroprusside is the drug of choice, but patients must be carefully monitored for thiocyanate toxicity (which is more common in this setting). Nifedipine or labetalol are good alternatives.

j. <u>Catecholamine-induced hypertensive crisis</u> due to:
   (1) Pheochromocytoma or MAOI interaction → IV labetalol as a single agent or phentolamine <u>followed by</u> an IV beta-blocker are first-line agents. Nitroprusside <u>followed by</u> an IV beta-blocker is also effective.
   (2) Acute clonidine withdrawal → restart clonidine. IV labetalol or phentolamine <u>followed by</u> an IV beta-blocker are also effective.
   (3) Acute cocaine intoxication → sedation with a benzodiazepine such as diazepam is usually very effective. If HTN persists despite adequate sedation, administer IV labetalol or phentolamine (<u>followed by</u> an IV beta-blocker if severe tachycardia is present).

4. Medications to <u>AVOID</u> in hypertensive emergencies:
   a. Malignant HTN/Hypertensive encephalopathy
      • ACE inhibitors
      • Clonidine
      • Pure beta-blockers
   b. Acute myocardial ischemia or injury/aortic dissection
      • Diazoxide
      • Hydralazine
      • Minoxidil
   c. Acute pulmonary edema
      • Diazoxide
      • Hydralazine
      • Minoxidil
   d. Eclampsia
      • Diuretics (furosemide, bumetanide, hydrochlorothiazide)
      • ACE inhibitors
      • Nitroprusside — relatively contraindicated antepartum
   e. Acute hypertensive renal insufficiency
      • Diazoxide
      • Pure beta-blockers as single agents

      f. Catecholamine-induced hypertensive crisis
- Minoxidil
- Pure beta-blockers as single agents

II. Hypertensive Urgencies

A. Definition — patients with a diastolic BP ≥ 115mmHg <u>without</u> evidence of end-organ dysfunction or damage. These patients are asymptomatic and usually come to our attention when they present to the ED for an unrelated problem.

B. Cause — This condition most commonly occurs in patients with chronic hypertension who are noncompliant with their medications.

C. Treatment

1. Goal of therapy is to lower the BP <u>gradually</u> over a period of 24 - 48 hrs. with oral medications. Catastrophic consequences may occur with IV administration; this practice should be condemned.

2. Commonly used agents include:
   a. Nifedipine
   b. Labetalol
   c. Clonidine
   d. ACE inhibitors
   e. Minoxidil (can be used if other meds fail)

VALVULAR HEART DISEASE

I. Prosthetic Valves

A. *Types and Characteristics* — There are two types of prosthetic valves (mechanical and bioprosthetic) each with its own particular characteristics.

1. Mechanical (nontissue) valves
    a. Are constructed from man-made materials.
    b. Have a life span > 20 years.
    c. Typically make a loud metallic closure sound and softer opening click and, when located in the aortic position, an associated <u>systolic</u> ejection murmur is normally present.
    d. Require life-long systemic anticoagulation.
    e. Cause greater hemolysis and are more thrombogenic than tissue prostheses.
    f. Common designs include the tilting disc variety, e.g. Björk-Shiley, Medtronic-Hall, the caged ball variety (e.g. Starr-Edwards) and the bileaflet variety (e.g. St. Jude).

2. Bioprosthetic (tissue) valves
    a. Are made with human, porcine or bovine tissue cups.
    b. Have a life span of only 8 - 10 years.
    c. Make opening and closing sounds that are similar to (but louder than) those of native valves.
    d. With the exception of the initial post-operative period and patients in atrial fibrillation, anticoagulation is optional; aspirin is sufficient in most patients.
    e. Cause less hemolysis and are less thrombogenic than mechanical valves.

B. *Complications and their Clinical Presentations*

1. Thromboembolic events
    a. Are the most serious complication of prosthetic valves.
    b. Occur more frequently with mechanical valves than with bioprosthetic ones.
    c. Patients with <u>valve dysfunction</u> secondary to thrombus formation typically present with acute onset of CHF, hypotension and muting or loss of the prosthetic valve sounds. The signs and symptoms of patients with embolic events will depend on the location of the emboli and may include paralysis, aphasia, abdominal pain, chest pain or a cold extremity.

2. Primary valve failure
   a. Is a significant cause of morbidity and mortality.
   b. Can result in regurgitant blood flow, acute valvular occlusion, embolization of a prosthetic fragment or severe hemolysis.
   c. The Björk-Shiley 60° and 70° convexoconcave valves were taken off the market because they were associated with a high incidence of strut fracture with resultant embolization of the disc. Patients with this complication present with sudden onset of CHF, hypotension, <u>loss</u> of the metallic valve sound and a new <u>regurgitant</u> murmur. Although these valves are no longer manufactured, many patients still have them.

3. Paravalvular leak
   a. Occurs when a portion of the prosthetic valve becomes unseated from the valve annulus.
   b. When it occurs immediately after surgery, it is usually due to suture disruption, whereas delayed leaks are generally due to endocarditis.
   c. Is more common with mechanical valves.
   d. Patients typically present with sudden onset of pulmonary edema or severe hemolytic anemia. Physical exam reveals a <u>regurgitant</u> murmur.

4. Endocarditis
   a. The causative organism varies with the length of time the valve has been present. During the first two months following surgery, Staph. aureus and Staph. epidermidis are the most common organisms. After this time period, non-viridans streptococcus is the most frequent organism.
   b. The diagnosis should be suspected in any patient with a prosthetic valve who presents with fever, particularly if a new regurgitant murmur is present. Lab evaluation typically reveals a leukocytosis with a left shift, anemia (hematocrit < 34%) and an elevated Sed rate.

5. Hemolysis
   a. Is a common problem with mechanical valves but rarely occurs with tissue valves.
   b. Is usually low-grade in nature and easily treated with iron and folate supplementation.
   c. The presence of severe hemolysis suggests the possibility of a paravalvular leak. These patients typically complain of fatigue, demonstrate orthostatic changes and/or they are jaundiced on exam.

6. Degeneration
   a. Results in the valve becoming incompetent.
   b. Presenting symptoms are those of ongoing or accelerating CHF.

C. Evaluation and Treatment of Complications

1. Assess and stabilize the ABCs — establish an IV (NS or LR), provide supplemental O_2, place the patient on a cardiac monitor and check a rhythm strip.

2. Determine the type, location and age of the prosthetic valve (most patients carry a card containing this information).

3. Order appropriate lab studies:
   - CBC — to detect hemolysis
   - LDH — to assess the severity of hemolysis; the degree of LDH elevation correlates closely with the degree of hemolysis.
   - PT (INR)/PTT — to assess adequacy of anticoagulation, especially in patients presenting with thromboembolic events.
   - CXR — to assess valve position and look for evidence of vascular congestion
   - Sed rate + C-reactive protein ─┐ if a fever is present, to
   - Blood cultures ────────────┴─ evaluate for endocarditis
   - Emergency echocardiography or cinefluoroscopy — if there is any question of valvular dysfunction

4. Obtain immediate cardiothoracic surgery consultation for patients presenting with prosthetic valve dysfunction secondary to thrombus, primary valve failure, paravalvular leak, endocarditis, abscess (perivalvular, intracardiac) or a vegetation that is fungal or large in size.

5. Provide specific therapy for the particular presentation:
   - Endocarditis → IV antibiotics
   - Severe anemia → blood transfusion
   - Thromboembolic event → anticoagulation/thrombolytic therapy
   - CHF → diuretics

II. Mitral Valve Prolapse ("Click Murmur Syndrome")

A. Epidemiology and Etiology

1. Mitral valve prolapse (MVP) is the most common valvular heart disease. It is present in 5 - 10% of the population; young women are the most frequently affected (female-to-male ratio of 2:1).

2. MVP can occur as an autosomal dominant congenital disorder, as part of a connective tissue disorder (Ehlers-Danlos syndrome, Marfan's syndrome) in association with skeletal abnormalities (such as severe scoliosis, "straight" back, pectus excavatum) or it may occur sporadically in otherwise normal people.

B. Common Clinical Presentations

1. Young woman with palpitations

2. Young athlete passed out during a training or practice session. She is anxious and complains of chest pain and palpitations. On physical exam, you find a tachydysrhythmia and orthostatic hypotension.

3. Elderly male with a syncopal episode at home

C. Clinical Diagnosis

1. Physical exam findings
   a. The murmur of MVP is a high-pitched, late <u>systolic</u> regurgitant murmur heard best at the apex using the diaphragm of the stethoscope. One or more mid - or late-systolic clicks may also be heard.
   b. Maneuvers that <u>decrease</u> left ventricular volume (Valsalva maneuver, sudden standing, inhalation of amyl nitrate, isoproterenol infusion) → earlier and greater prolapse → movement of the click <u>closer</u> to S_1 and an <u>increase</u> in the <u>duration</u> of the murmur.
   c. Maneuvers that <u>increase</u> left ventricular volume (passive leg raising, maximal isometric handgrip, squatting, phenylephrine infusion) → delay of prolapse until late in systole → movement of the click and murmur away from S_1 and a <u>decrease</u> in the duration of the murmur.

2. ECG — Although most often normal, findings may include flattened or inverted T waves in the inferior leads (II, III and AVF) and prolongation of the QT interval.

3. CXR — unless significant mitral regurgitation is present, the lungs and cardiac silhouette are usually normal.

4. Echocardiography — confirms the diagnosis; 2-D echo is more sensitive than M-mode.

D. Complications — Although most patients are asymptomatic and without complications, patients may present with any of the following:

1. Atypical (nonexertional, sharp) chest pain — thought to be due to localized ischemia from tension on the papillary muscles or to coronary artery spasm.

2. Palpitations, light-headedness or syncope — due to dysrhythmias (PACs, PVCs, PSVT, V-Tach)

3. Sudden death (rare) — due to V-Tach or V-Fib

4. TIAs or CVAs — believed to result from embolization of leaflet thrombi

5. CHF — due to severe mitral valve regurgitation associated with MVP

6. Infective endocarditis — occurs in patients who have mitral valve <u>regurgitation</u> (murmur) and/or thickened valve leaflets in association with MVP.

E. *Treatment* — is reserved for <u>symptomatic</u> patients.

1. Beta blockers — for patients with chest pain and dysrhythmias

2. Antibiotic prophylaxis (during dental and other procedures) — for patients with mitral valve <u>regurgitation</u> and/or thickened valve leaflets in association with MVP.

3. Antiplatelet (aspirin) or anticoagulant therapy — for patients with a history of systemic embolization (TIA or CVA)

III. Mitral Stenosis

A. *Etiology*

1. Rheumatic heart disease — is responsible for ≥ 90% of cases of isolated mitral stenosis.

2. Congenital malformations

3. Calcification of the mitral annulus and leaflets

4. Left atrial myxoma

B. *Diagnosis*

1. Symptoms
    a. Exertional dyspnea (most common symptom)
    b. Hemoptysis (second most common symptom)
    c. Orthopnea and paroxysmal nocturnal dyspnea
    d. Palpitations (PACs, paroxysmal atrial fibrillation)
    e. Fatigue
    f. Systemic emboli

2. Physical exam findings
    a. Mitral facies (malar rash)
    b. Palpable diastolic thrill at the apex
    c. Loud S_1
    d. Early diastolic opening snap followed by a low-pitched, rumbling diastolic murmur heard best at the apex

3. ECG
    a. Left atrial enlargement (P mitrale)
    b. Atrial fibrillation
    c. Right ventricular hypertrophy (if marked pulmonary HTN is present)

    4. CXR
- a. Straightening of the left heart border due to left atrial enlargement
- b. Calcification of the mitral annulus and leaflets
- c. Findings of pulmonary congestion
- d. Right ventricular lift (or hypertrophy) if pulmonary HTN is present

C. *Complications*

1. Atrial fibrillation (most common complication)

2. Embolic events, especially with atrial fibrillation

3. Frequent respiratory infections

4. Infective endocarditis (rare)

5. Massive pulmonary hemorrhage from rupture of pulmonary bronchial venous connections

D. *Management*

1. Antibiotic prophylaxis against endocarditis for procedures prone to bacteremia

2. Rate control with IV diltiazem or digoxin for atrial fibrillation with rapid ventricular response

3. Blood transfusion and, possibly, surgery for massive hemoptysis

4. Diuretics for pulmonary congestion

5. Anticoagulation for patients with systemic embolization and atrial fibrillation

---

IV. Mitral Regurgitation — can be acute or chronic; these two disease entities differ significantly in terms of their causation, disease course, presentation and management.

A. *Acute Mitral Regurgitation* — is the result of chordae tendineae, papillary muscle or valve leaflet rupture and is <u>abrupt</u> in onset.

1. Etiology
- a. Acute myocardial infarction (AMI)
- b. Infectious endocarditis
- c. Trauma

---

2. Diagnosis
   a. Symptoms — are those of fulminant CHF/pulmonary edema (e.g. dyspnea) and those of the disease process that precipitated the event (e.g. chest pain in the AMI patient)
   b. Physical exam findings
      (1) Tachycardia, tachypnea and rales
      (2) Hypotension
      (3) JVD with a prominent *a wave*
      (4) Palpable thrill at apex
      (5) Soft S_1
      (6) Loud apical systolic murmur (radiating to the axilla) that can be holosystolic, late systolic or crescendo-decrescendo.
      (7) S_3 and S_4 (a common finding)
   c. ECG
      (1) <u>Absence</u> of left atrial enlargement and left ventricular hypertrophy
      (2) Sinus tachycardia
   d. CXR — normal cardiac silhouette and severe pulmonary edema

3. Management
   a. Airway and hemodynamic support (may include intraaortic balloon pump to augment cardiac output)
   b. Supplemental O_2
   c. Afterload reduction
   d. Emergent consultation with a cardiothoracic surgeon
   e. Treatment of underlying cause (e.g. antibiotics for infectious endocarditis)

B. *Chronic Mitral Regurgitation* — evolves slowly and frequently coexists with mitral stenosis.

   1. Etiology
      a. Rheumatic heart disease — most common cause
      b. Mitral valve prolapse (MVP)
      c. Connective tissue disorders (e.g. Marfan's syndrome)

   2. Diagnosis
      a. Symptoms
         (1) Exertional fatigue or dyspnea
         (2) Orthopnea and paroxysmal nocturnal dyspnea (PND)
         (3) Systemic emboli
      b. Physical exam findings
         (1) Left parasternal heave and thrill
         (2) High-pitched holosystolic murmur that radiates to the axilla
         (3) Soft S_1 that is often obscured by the murmur
         (4) Wide-split S_2
         (5) S_3 and S_4 — common with severe regurgitation
      c. ECG
         (1) Left atrial enlargement
         (2) Left ventricular hypertrophy with strain
         (3) Atrial fibrillation (75% of patients)

       d. CXR
          (1) Left atrial enlargement
          (2) Left ventricular enlargement
          (3) Pulmonary congestion

   3. Management
       a. Antibiotic prophylaxis against endocarditis for procedures (dental, renal) prone to bacteremia.
       b. Rate control of atrial fibrillation with diltiazem or digoxin
       c. Diuretics for symptoms of pulmonary congestion
       d. Anticoagulation if atrial fibrillation is present

V. Aortic Stenosis

A. Etiology

1. Congenital bicuspid valve (most common cause in patients < 65 yrs. old)

2. Rheumatic heart disease (associated mitral valve disease is common in these patients)

3. Calcific aortic stenosis (most common cause in patients > 65 yrs. of age)

B. Diagnosis

1. Symptoms — appear late in the disease process; patients remain relatively asymptomatic until the valve opening decreases to < 1 cm.
       a. Dyspnea on exertion
       b. Angina
       c. Exertional syncope
       d. Symptoms of heart failure
       e. Sudden death

2. Physical exam findings
       a. Carotid pulse is <u>diminished</u> and delayed (pulsus parvus and tardus)
       b. Pulse pressure may be narrowed (< 30mm Hg)
       c. Palpable left chest heave
       d. Harsh systolic crescendo-decrescendo murmur heard best at base with radiation into the carotids; also heard on auscultation:
          (1) Absent S_2 component
          (2) Ejection click
          (3) S_4 gallop

3. ECG
       a. Left ventricular hypertrophy
       b. Left or right bundle branch block

4. CXR
   a. Left ventricular enlargement
   b. Poststenotic dilatation of the ascending aorta (is a characteristic finding)
   c. Pulmonary vascular congestion (if heart failure is present)
   d. Aortic valve calcification

C. Management

1. Antibiotic prophylaxis against endocarditis is indicated for bacteremia-prone procedures (especially dental and renal).

2. Patients with mild symptoms should be advised to avoid strenuous activities.

3. Patients with CHF require hospital admission; administration of medications which decrease preload or afterload in these patients can produce sudden decompensation and should be administered with caution.

4. Symptomatic patients are at high risk for sudden death. They should be referred for valve replacement (definitive therapy) or valvuloplasty (temporizing measure).

VI. Aortic Regurgitation — can be acute and fulminant or chronic and slowly progressive.

A. Acute Aortic Regurgitation

1. Etiology — most common causes are:
   a. Infective endocarditis
   b. Aortic dissection
   c. Trauma

2. Diagnosis
   a. Symptoms
      (1) Severe dyspnea (most common symptom)
      (2) Apprehension
      (3) Other signs of heart failure (e.g. paroxysmal nocturnal dyspnea, orthopnea)
      (4) Chest pain
   b. Physical exam findings
      (1) Tachypnea, tachycardia and inspiratory rales
      (2) Normal or low systolic and diastolic pressures

        (3) <u>Normal</u> pulse pressure*

        (4) Signs of decreased cardiac output (cool, pale extremities, peripheral cyanosis, hypotension, diaphoresis, confusion)

        (5) Diminished or absent S_1

        (6) Loud S_3

        (7) Short <u>diastolic</u> murmur of aortic regurgitation best heard at the left sternal border with the diaphragm of the stethescope.

        (8) Midsystolic flow murmur

  c. ECG

        (1) Sinus tachycardia

        (2) Nonspecific ST-T wave changes

        (3) LV strain

  d. CXR

        (1) Normal cardiac silhouette

        (2) Signs of increased pulmonary venous pressure and pulmonary edema.

3. Management

  a. Determine and treat the underlying cause (e.g. administer IV antibiotics to patients with bacterial endocarditis).

  b. Treat CHF with supplemental O_2, diuretics, digitalis and vasodilators (nitroglycerine, nitroprusside).

  c. Obtain immediate cardiothoracic surgery consult for emergent valve replacement.

B. Chronic Aortic Regurgitation

1. Etiology

  a. Rheumatic heart disease

  b. Congenital (bicuspid) valve

  c. Prior infective endocarditis

  d. Diseases that dilate the aortic wall (e.g. Marfan's syndrome, ankylosing spondylitis)

2. Diagnosis

  a. Symptoms

        (1) Exertional fatigue and dyspnea

        (2) Orthopnea, paroxysmal nocturnal dyspnea (PND)

        (3) Palpitations

        (4) Angina

        (5) Pulmonary edema

  b. Physical exam findings

        (1) <u>Wide</u> pulse pressure

        (2) Displaced, hyperdynamic PMI

        (3) Soft S_1

        (4) High-pitched, decrescendo <u>diastolic</u> blowing murmur best heard along the left sternal border (sine qua non of aortic regurgitation)

*30 - 40 mmHg difference between systolic & diastolic BP

(5) Rapid and forceful carotid upstroke with dramatic collapse (Corrigan's or water-hammer pulse)

(6) Head bobbing with each heartbeat (deMusset's sign)

(7) Prominent nail pulsations (Quincke's pulse)

(8) Singsong murmur over the femoral artery (Duroziez's murmur)

(9) A presystolic or mid-diastolic murmur (Austin-Flint murmur) — may be present with severe aortic regurgitation.

   c. ECG

     (1) LVH

     (2) Conduction abnormalities such as LBBB

   d. CXR

     (1) Cardiomegaly

     (2) Aortic root dilatation

     (3) Pulmonary vascular congestion

3. Management

   a. Administer antibiotic prophylaxis against endocarditis for procedures prone to bacteremia.

   b. Treat CHF with supplemental oxygen, diuretics, vasodilators and digitalis.

VII. Tricuspid Stenosis

A. Etiology

1. Rheumatic heart disease

2. Endocarditis secondary to intravenous drug abuse (IVDA)

B. Diagnosis

1. Symptoms — patients complain of fatigue and symptoms due to increased systemic venous pressure (e.g. edema).

2. Physical exam findings

   a. <u>Diastolic</u> murmur best heard along the left sternal border and accentuated with inspiration

   b. Peripheral edema

   c. Hepatosplenomegaly

   d. Ascites

   e. JVD and giant jugular *a waves*

3. ECG

   a. Tall, pointed P waves if sinus rhythm is present

   b. Atrial fibrillation

4. CXR — enlarged right atrium

C. Management

1. Rate control with IV diltiazem for atrial fibrillation with rapid ventricular response

2. Anticoagulation for chronic atrial fibrillation

3. Treatment of underlying cause (e.g. IV antibiotics for infectious endocarditis)

<u>Note</u>: Tricuspid stenosis rarely exists in isolation. Coexisting mitral and aortic valve disease are common and, when present, they typically dominate and determine the clinical course.

VIII. Tricuspid Regurgitation

A. Etiology

1. Right ventricular dilatation secondary to pulmonary HTN

2. Rheumatic heart disease

3. Infective endocarditis

4. Trauma

B. Diagnosis

1. Symptoms
   a. Fatigue and dyspnea on exertion
   b. Peripheral edema
   c. Throbbing in the neck and abdomen
   d. Anorexia

2. Physical exam findings
   a. Palpable left ventricular heave
   b. Prominent c-v wave in the jugular veins
   c. Holosystolic murmur best heard at the xiphoid area adjacent to the left sternal border

3. ECG
   a. Right atrial enlargement
   b. Right ventricular enlargement
   c. Atrial fibrillation (80% of patients)

4. CXR
   a. Right atrial enlargement
   b. Right ventricular enlargement
   c. Normal pulmonary vasculature

C. Management — patients in atrial fibrillation require rate control with IV diltiazem and long-term anticoagulation.

IX. Conditions Necessitating Antibiotic Prophylaxis for Infective Endocarditis

- Prosthetic heart valves ─────────┐
- History of bacterial endocarditis ────────┤ high risk of infection
- Complex cyanotic congenital heart lesions ───┤
- Surgically constructed systemic pulmonary───┘ shunts or conduits
- Mitral valve prolapse with regurgitation or thickened leaflets
- Hypertrophic cardiomyopathy
- Most other congenital cardiac malformations

Emergency department procedures that merit prophylaxis include incision and drainage of abscesses, nasal packing and dental procedures associated with gingival bleeding. Clean procedures (e.g. suturing of lacerations, placement of central lines under sterile conditions) do not warrant prophylaxis.

ADULT FLUID VOLUMES

I. Normal Values

A. Extracellular Fluid = 200mL/kg

B. Estimated Blood Volume = 70mL/kg

C. Plasma Volume = 35.5mL/kg*

II. Patient Assessment

A. Normal capillary refill (of nailbeds) ≤ 2 seconds. If it is delayed more than 2 seconds, a volume deficit ≥ 15% is present.

B. Acute onset tachycardia
  1. > 100 = 15 - 30% vol. deficit
  2. > 120 = 30 - 40% vol. deficit
  3. > 140 = > 40% vol. deficit

C. Orthostatic pulse and BP changes = at least a 20% volume deficit.

D. Hypotension = at least a 30% volume deficit

E. PAWP monitoring is the most accurate method of determining fluid volume status, especially in patients with pulmonary disease, right ventricular failure and cardiac tamponade. CVP monitoring is an acceptable alternative in patients without these disorders. The use of CVP in shock states continues to be a controversial issue.

*Is approximately half of the blood volume.

Journal References

ACCID EMERG MED, Richell-Herren, K. J., January 2000, "Immediate Anticoagulant Management of Unstable Angina." (at http://ccme.org)

AJR, Blachere, H., Latrabe, V., Montaudon, M., et. al., 2000, Vol. 174, (1041-1047), "Pulmonary Embolism Revealed on Helical CT Angiography: Comparison with Ventilation — Perfusion Radionuclide Lung Scanning."

AM COLL CARD / AM HEART ASSOC, Ryan, T. J., Antman, E. M., Brooks, N. H., Califf, R. M., Hillis, L. D., Hiratzka, L. F., Rapaport, E., Riefel, B., Russell, R. O., Smith, E. E. III, Weaver, W. D., "ACC/AHA Guidelines for the Management of Patients with Acute Myocardial Infarction", 1999 update: a report of the ACC/AHA Task Force on Practice Guidelines.

AM J CARDIOL, Antman, E. M., February 15, 1995, "Randomized Trials of Magnesium in Acute Myocardial Infarction: Big Numbers Do Not Tell the Whole Story." (in Emer. Med. Abstracts, 1995)

AM J CARDIOL, Barron, H. V., February 2000, "Intracranial Hemorrhage Rates and Effect of Immediate Beta-Blocker Use in Patients with Acute Myocardial Infarction Treated with Tissue Plasminogen Activator." (at http://ccme.org)

AM J CARDIOL, Brodsky, M. A., et. al., June 15, 1994, "Magnesium Therapy in New-Onset Atrial Fibrillation." (in Emer. Med. Abstracts, 1994)

AM J CARDIOL, Chandra-Strobos, N., 2001, "Magnesium Use in the Treatment of Acute Myocardial Infarction in the United States (Observation From the Second National Registry of Myocardial Infarction.)"

AM J CARDIOL, Freimark, D., et. al., February 15, 2002, "Timing of Aspirin Administration as a Determinant of Survival of Patients with Acute Myocardial Infarction Treated with Thrombolysis."

AM J CARDIOL, Morrow, D.A., et.al., September 15, 2004, 94:774, "Usefulness of Tirofiban Among Patients Treated Without Percutaneous Coronary Intervention (TIMI High Risk Patients in Prism-Plus)."

AM J CARDIOL, Schecter, M. et. al., February 15, 1995, "Magnesium Therapy in Acute Myocardial Infarction When Patients are not Candidates for Thrombolytic Therapy." (in Emer. Med. Abstracts, 1995)

AM J CARDIOL, Vakili, B.A., et.al, April 15, 2003, 91:946, "Inhibitor Therapy on In-Hospital Outcomes After Percutaneous Coronary Intervention."

AM J EMERG MED, Khan, I. A., Tun, A., Wattanasauwan, N., et. al., 1999, "Elevation of Serum Cardiac Troponin I in Noncardiac and Cardiac Diseases Other Than Acute Coronary Syndromes."

AM J GASTROENT, Akhtar, A. J., et. al., June 2000, "Safety and Efficacy of Digital Retal Examination in Patients with Acute Myocardial Infarction." (at http://www.ccme.org).

AM J RESP CRIT CARE MED, Nava, S., et.al., 2003, 168:1432, "Noninvasive Ventilation in Cardiogenic Pulmonary Edema."

ANN EMER MED, Davey, M.J., et. al., April 2005, 45(4):347, "A Randomized Controlled Trial of Magnesium Sulfate in Addition to Usual Care, for Rate Control in Atrial Fibrillation."

ANN EMER MED, Farrell, S., Hayes, T., Shaw, M., February 2000, "A Negative SimpliRED D-Dimer Assay Result Does Not Exclude the Diagnosis of Deep Vein Thrombosis or Pulmonary Embolus in Emergency Department Patients."

ANN EMER MED, Gallagher, E. J., February 2000, "Clots in the Lung."

ANN EMER MED, Gallagher, E. J., April 2000, 41(4):530, "Hypertensive Urgencies: Treating the Mercury?"

ANN EMER MED, Gupta, M., Tabas, J. A., Kohn, M. A., August 2000, "Presenting Complaint Among Patients with Myocardial Infarction who Present to an Urban, Public Hospital Emergency Department."

ANN EMER MED, Hotchkiss, J. R., and Marini, J. J., October 1998, "Noninvasive Ventilation: An Emerging Supportive Technique for the Emergency Department."

ANN EMER MED, Ioannidis, J. P. A., et. al., May 2001, "Accuracy of Imaging Technologies in the Diagnosis of Acute Cardiac Ischemia in the Emergency Department: A Meta-Analysis."

ANN EMER MED, Kline, J., Johns, K. L., Colucciello, S. A., Israel, E. G., February 2000, "New Diagnostic Tests for Pulmonary Embolism."

ANN EMER MED, Rathbun, S. W., Raskob, G. E., Whitsett, T. L., 2000, "Sensitivity and Specificity of Helical Computed Tomography in the Diagnosis of Pulmonary Embolism: A Systematic Review."

ANN EMER MED, Sarasin, F. P., et. al., September 1996, "Detecting Acute Thoracic Aortic Dissection in the Emergency Department: Time Constraints and Choice of the Optimal Diagnostic Test."

ANN EMER MED, Schriger, D. L., et. al., September 2001, "Medically Managed Acute Coronary Syndrome: Does the Enthusiasm Exceed the Science?"

ANN EMER MED, Vinson, D. R., Berman, D. A., March 2001, "Outpatient Treatment of Deep Venous Thrombosis: A Clinical Care Pathway Managed by the Emergency Department."

ANN INTERNAL MED, Krumholz, H. M., et. al., 1999, "Early Beta-Blocker Therapy for Acute Myocardial Infarction in Elderly Patients." (at http://www.ccme.org).

ANN INTERNAL MED, Buller, H.R., et. al., July, 2004, "Fondaparinux or Enoxapsarin for Initial Treatment of Symptomatic Deep Venous Thrombosis."

ANN INTERNAL MED, Turkstra, F., et. al., May 1997, "Diagnostic Utility of Ultrasonography of Leg Veins in Patients Suspected of Having Pulmonary Embolism."

ANN INTERNAL MED, Wells, P. S., et. al., December 1998, "Use of a Clinical Model for Safe Management of Patients with Suspected Pulmonary Embolism."

ANN THORAC SURG, Ascione, R., et. al., April 2005, 79(4):1210, "In-Hospital Patients Exposed to Clopidogrel Before Coronary Artery Bypass Graft Surgery: A Word of Caution."

ARCHIVES OF INTERNAL MEDICINE, Dolovich, L. R., et. al., January 2000, "A Meta-Analysis Comparing Low-Molecular-Weight Heparins with Unfarctionated Heparin in the Treatment of Venous Thromboembolism: Examining Some Unanswered Questions Regarding Location of Treatment, Product Type and Dosing Frequency."

ARCHIVES OF INTERNAL MEDICINE, Hull, R. D., et. al., January 2000, "Low-Molecular-Weight Heparin vs. Heparin in the Treatment of Patients with Pulmonary Embolism."

ARCHIVES OF INTERNAL MEDICINE, Lensing, A. W. A., et. al., March 27, 1995, "Treatment of Deep Venous Thrombosis with Low-Molecular-Weight Heparins: A Meta-Analysis." (in Emer. Med. Abstracts, 1995)

ARCHIVES OF INTERNAL MEDICINE, Meignan, M., et. al., January 2000, "Systematic Lung Scans Reveal a High Frequency of Silent Pulmonary Embolism in Patients with Proximal Deep Venous Thrombosis."

AUDIO-DIGEST: EMER MED, Birnbaumer, D., June 1996, "Abdominal Aortic Aneurysm."

AUDIO-DIGEST: EMER MED, Galli, R., September 1999, "Cocaine Intoxication."

AUDIO-DIGEST: EMER MED, Levine, Robert L., December 18, 1995, "Respiratory Disorders; EM Board Review: Pulmonary Infections." (CME activity)

AUDIO-DIGEST: EMER MED, Lex, Jr., Joseph R., October 21, 2002, "New Drugs and Devices." (CME activity)

AUDIO-DIGEST: EMER MED, Panacek, Edward, October 15, 1998, "Update of the Diagnosis and Treatment of Pulmonary Embolism." (CME activity)

AUDIO-DIGEST: EMER MED, Ryan, C., April 1997, "Individualized Treatment of Hypertension." (CME activity)

AUDIO-DIGEST: EMER MED, Tabas, J. A., October 7, 2001, "Acute Coronary Insufficiency." (CME Activity)

AUDIO-DIGEST: EMER MED., Tabas, J. A., August 21, 2002, "Pulmonary Embolism." (CME Activity)

CAN J CARD, Novak, P. G., et. al., September 1999, "Survey of British Columbia Cardiologists' and Emergency Physicians' Practice of Using Non-Standard ECG Leads (V4R to V6R and V7 to V9) in the Diagnosis and Treatment of Acute Myocardial Infarction."

CARDIOL CLIN, Wijffels, M.C., Crijns H.J., February 2004, 22 (1): 63-9, "Rate Versus Rhythm Control in Atrial Fibrillation".

CARDIOVASC DRUG THER, Jonassen, A. K., et. al., December 2000, "Glucose-Insulin-Potassium Reduces Infarct Size when Administered During Reperfusion."

CHEST, Agnelli, G., January 1995, "Anticoagulation in the Prevention and Treatment of Pulmonary Embolism."

CHEST, Goldhaber, S. Z., April 1991, "Recent Advances in the Diagnosis and Lytic Therapy of Pulmonary Embolism."

CHEST, Henry, J. W., et. al., May 1995, "Continuing Risk of Thromboemboli Among Patients with Normal Pulmonary Angiograms."

CHEST, Morpurgo, M. and C. Schmid, January 1995, "The Spectrum of Pulmonary Embolism: Clinicopathologic Correlations."

CIRCULATION, 2000, Vol. 102 (suppl I), (I-112-I-128), "Part 6: Advanced Cardiovascular Life Support: Section 5: Pharmacology I: Agents for Arrhythmias."

CIRCULATION, Antman, E. M., et. al., October 1999, (1593), "Enoxaparin Prevents Death and Cardiac Ischemic Events in Unstable Angina/Non-Q-Wave Myocardial Infarction: Results of the Thrombolysis in Myocardial Infarction." (at http://www.ccme.org)

CIRCULATION, Hirsch, J., October 1992, "Oral Anticoagulant for Standardization." (in Emer. Med. Abstracts, 1993)

CIRCULATION, Kontos, M. C., et. al., April 2000, (2003), "Comparison of Myocardial Perfusion Imaging and Cardiac Troponin I in Patients Admitted to the Emergency Department with Chest Pain." (at http://www.ccme.org)

CIRCULATION, Mehta, S. R., et. al., August 2000, "Risk of Intracranial Hemorrhage with Bolus Versus Infusion Thrombolytic Therapy: A Meta-Analysis." (at http://www.ccme.org)

CIRCULATION, Mittal, S., et. al., March 21, 2000, Vol. 101, (1282-1287), "Transthoracic Cardio-version of Atrial Fibrillation: Comparison of Rectilinear Biphasic Versus Damped Sine Wave Monophasic Shocks."

CIRCULATION, Mittleman, M. A., Mintzer, D., Maclure, M., et. al., 1999, "Triggering of Myocardial Infarction by Cocaine."

CIRCULATION, Sackner-Bernstein, J.D., et.al., March 29, 2005, 111:1487, "Risk of Worsening Renal Function with Nesiritide in Patients with Acutely Decompensated Heart Failure."

CIRCULATION, Thiemann, D. R., et, al., May 2000, (2239), "Lack of Benefit for Intravenous Thrombolysis in Patients with Myocardial Infarction who are Older Than 75 Years." (at http://www.ccme.org)

CIRCULATION, ACC/AHA/NASPE Committee to Update the 1998 Pacemaker Guidelines, 2002, 106: 2145 "ACC/AHA/NASPE 2002 Guideline Update for Implantation of Cardiac Pacemakers and Antiarrhythmia Devices: Summary Article".

CLINICAL CARDIOLOGY, Vaitku, Paul, January 1995, "Percutaneous Transluminal Coronary Angioplasty versus Thrombolysis in Acute Myocardial Infarction: A Meta-Analysis."

CLINICS IN FAMILY PRACTICE, Rodgers, P. E., Green, L. A., December 2001, Vol. 3, No. 4, "Management of Acute Coronary Syndromes."

CONCISE REVIEW FOR CLINICIANS, Rabatin, J. T., and Gay, P. C., August 1999, "Noninvasive Ventilation."

CRITICAL PATHWAYS IN EMERGENCY MEDICINE, Huott, M., February 1999, "Treatment of Deep Venous Thrombosis for the Emergency Department Physician."

CRITICAL PATHWAYS IN EMERGENCY MEDICINE, Manthey, D., Hemphill, R., September 1997, "Aspirin Therapy in Unstable Angina: Alone or with Heparin?"

CUSTOMER ADVOCACY OF PFIZER, INC., Siegal, R. L., March 1998, "Important Prescribing Information - Viagra."

DICP, THE ANNALS OF PHARMACOTHERAPY, Allen, Nancy M. and Gary D. Dunham, October 1990, "Treatment of Digitalis Intoxication with Emphasis on the Clinical Use of Digoxin Immune Fab."

EMERGENCY DEPARTMENT: RAPID IDENTIFICATION AND TREATMENT OF PATIENTS WITH ACUTE MYOCARDIAL INFARCTION, U. S. Department of Health and Human Services, NIH Publication, no. 93-3278 (September 1993)

EMERGENCY MANAGEMENT OF ACUTE CORONARY SYNDROMES, The Department of Emergency Medicine and The Office of Continuing Education, University of Massachusetts Medical School, Eighteenth Annual Series: Series 12, "Emergency Medicine and Acute Care."

EMERGENCY MEDICAL ABSTRACTS, Brewer, D., January 1999, "Should Low-Molecular-Weight Heparins Replace Unfractionated Heparin as the Agent of Choice for Adults with Deep Venous Thrombosis?"

EMERGENCY MEDICAL ABSTRACTS, Bukata, R., August, 2004, "Pulmonary Embolism, BTS Guidelines, Part 1"

EMERGENCY MEDICAL ABSTRACTS, Harrison, L., et. al., October 1998, "Assessment of Outpatient Treatment of Deep-Vein-Thrombosis with Low-Molecular-Weight-Heparin."

EMERGENCY MEDICAL ABSTRACTS, June 1999, "Effects of Recombinant Hirudin (Lepirudin) Compared with Heparin on Death, Myocardial Infarction, Refractory Angina and Revascularisation Procedures in Patients with Acute Myocardial Ischaemia Without ST Elevation: A Randomized Trial Oasis-2." (Investigators Lancet 353:429, February 1999)

EMERGENCY MEDICAL ABSTRACTS, O'Shaughnessy, D. F., et al, September 1998, "Outpatient Management of Deep Vein Thrombosis."

EMERGENCY MEDICAL ABSTRACTS, Shlipak, M. G., et. al., June 1999, "Should the Electrocardiogram be Used to Guide Therapy for Patients with Left Bundle Branch Block and Suspected Myocardial Infarction?"

EMERGENCY MEDICAL ABSTRACTS, Wells, P. S., et. al., September 1998, "Expanding Eligibility for Outpatient Treatment of Deep Venous Thrombosis and Pulmonary Embolism with Low-Molecular-Weight Heparin: A Comparison of Patient Self-injection with Homecare Injection."

EMERGENCY MEDICINE, (no author listed), September 1995, "An Alternative to Angiography in Suspected Aortic Rupture."

EMERGENCY MEDICINE, Idell, S., February 2001, "Recognition and Treatment of Recurrent Venous Thromboembolism."

EMERGENCY MEDICINE ALERT, Ufberg, J. W., February 2001, "Does Emergency Department Trauma Care Affect Evaluation of Chest Pain Patients?"

EMERGENCY MEDICINE AND ACUTE CARE ESSAYS, Bukata, W. R., May 2000, "Unstable Angina Pectoris."

EMERGENCY MEDICINE AND ACUTE CARE ESSAYS, Herbert, M., November 1999, Vol. 23, No. 11, "Glycoprotein IIb/IIIa Receptor Antagonists for Coronary Syndromes."

EMERGENCY MEDICINE AND ACUTE CARE ESSAYS, Herbert, Mel E., February 2000, Vol. 24, No. 2, "Atrial Fibrillation, Part I."

EMERGENCY MEDICINE AND ACUTE CARE ESSAYS, Herbert, Mel E., March 2000, Vol. 24, No. 3, "Atrial Fibrillation, Part II."

EMERGENCY MEDICINE CLINICS OF NORTH AMERICA, Mattu, A., et. al., November 2005, "Modern Management of Cardiogenic Pulmonary Edema."

EMERGENCY MEDICINE CLINICS OF NORTH AMERICA, Stack, L. B., et. al., November 1995, "Advances in the Use of Ancillary Diagnostic Testing in the Emergency Department Evaluation of Chest Pain."

EMERGENCY MEDICINE CLINICS OF NORTH AMERICA, Thakur, R. K., Reisdorff, E. J., August 1998, "Selected Topics in Emergency Cardiac Care."

EMERGENCY MEDICINE CLINICS OF NORTH AMERICA, Wellford, L. A., Young, G. P., November 1995, "Advances and Updates in Cardiovascular Emergencies."

EMERGENCY MEDICINE CONSENSUS REPORTS, Peacock, W. F., Freda, B. J., May 1, 2002, "The Clinical Challenge of Heart Failure: Comprehensive, Evidence-Based Management of the Hospitalized Patient with Acute Myocardial Decompensation — Diagnosis, Risk Stratification and Outcome-Effective Treatment - Part I: Presentation, Differential Diagnosis, Laboratory Examination and Prophylaxis Against Venous Thromboembolic Disease (VTED)."

EMERGENCY MEDICINE CONSENSUS REPORTS, Peacock, W. F., Freda, B. J., May 15, 2002, "The Clinical Challenge of Heart Failure: Comprehensive, Evidence-Based Management of the Hospitalized Patient with Acute Myocardial Decompensation - Part II: Outcome-Effective Treatment and Prophylaxis Against Venous Thromboembolic Disease (VTED)."

EMERGENCY MEDICINE CONSENSUS REPORTS, Poponick, J., Bosker, G., July 1, 2002, "The Current Challenge of Venous Thromboembolism (VTE) in the Hospitalized Patient: Optimizing Recognition, Evaluation, and Prophylaxis of Deep Venous Thrombosis (DVT) and Pulmonary Embolism (PE) - Part 1: Patient Identification, Risk Factor Assessment, and Diagnostic Strategies."

EMERGENCY MEDICINE NEWS, Brady, W., Chan, T., Harrigan, R., March 2001, "Left Bundle Branch Block and the Electrocardiographic Diagnosis of AMI."

EMERGENCY MEDICINE NEWS, Gillard, J. M., March 2001, "Bedside Cardiac Markers Identify Patients at High Risk for Mortality."

EMERGENCY MEDICINE PRACTICE, Kosowsky, J. M., Kobayashi, L., February 2002, Vol. 4, No. 2, "Acutely Decompensated Heart Failure: Diagnostic and Therapeutic Strategies for the New Millennium."

EMERGENCY MEDICINE REPORTS, Ahluwalia, M., Quest, T., February 2002, Vol. 23, No. 4, "Supraventricular Tachycardia (SVT): Strategies for Diagnosis, Risk Stratification, and Management in the Emergency Department Setting."

EMERGENCY MEDICINE REPORTS, Albrich, J. M., August 1997, "Congestive Heart Failure: A State-of-the-Art Review of Clinical Pitfalls, Evaluation Strategies, and Recent Advances in Drug Therapy (Part I)."

EMERGENCY MEDICINE REPORTS, Albrich, J. Michael, August 18, 1997, "Congestive Heart Failure: Critical Clinical Issues in Cardiogenic Shock, Hemodialysis, and Maintenance Drug Therapy (Part II)."

EMERGENCY MEDICINE REPORTS, Anderson E., Glauser J., 2003, 24, "Noncardiac Causes of Chest Pain in the ED. Parts I & II."

EMERGENCY MEDICINE REPORTS, Bosker, G., 1999, "Thrombolysis in Myocardial Infarction and Stroke: Patient Selection and Outcome-Effective Management."

EMERGENCY MEDICINE REPORTS, Bosker, Gideon, Robinson, David J., Jerrard, David A., Kuo, Dick C., July 5, 1999, "Acute Myocardial Infarction: Current Clinical Guidelines for Patients Evaluation, Thrombolysis, and Mortality Reduction (Part I)."

EMERGENCY MEDICINE REPORTS, Bosker, Gideon, Jerrard, David A., July 19, 1999, "Acute Myocardial Infarction: Current Clinical Guidelines for Patients Evaluation, Thrombolysis, and Mortality Reduction (Part II)."

EMERGENCY MEDICINE REPORTS, Bosker, G., Poponick, J., July 15, 2002, "Venous Thromboembolism (VTE) in the Hospitalized Patient: Treatment and Prevention of DVT and PE — Evolving Risk-Stratification and Prophylaxis Strategies for Emergency Medicine (Part II)."

EMERGENCY MEDICINE REPORTS, Brady, William J., May 12, 1997, "Missing the Diagnosis of Acute MI: Challenging Presentation, Electrocardiographic Pearls and Outcome-Effective Management Strategies."

EMERGENCY MEDICINE REPORTS, Brady, William J., April 13, 1998 "Mastering the Electrocardiogram: State-of-the-Art Techniques for Evaluating ST Segment Elevation in Acute Myocardial Infarction and Other Clinical Syndromes (Part I)."

EMERGENCY MEDICINE REPORTS, Brady, William J., April 27, 1998, "Mastering the Electrocardiogram: State-of-the-Art Techniques for Evaluating ST Segment Elevation in Acute Myocardial Infarction and Other Clinical Syndromes (Part II)."

EMERGENCY MEDICINE REPORTS, Brady, W. J., Bosker, G., Kleinschmidt, K., October 8, 2001, "Acute Myocardial Infarction and Coronary Syndromes: Optimizing Selection of Reperfusion and Revascularization Therapies in the ED. Part I: Fibrinolysis, Procedural Coronary Intervention (PCI), and the Central Role of the Low Molecular Weight Heparin, Enoxaparin, in Fibrinolysis-Mediated Myocardial Reperfusion."

EMERGENCY MEDICINE REPORTS, Brady, W. J., Bosker, G., Kleinschmidt, K., October 22, 2001, "Acute Myocardial Infarction and Coronary Syndromes: Optimizing Selection of Reperfusion and Revascularization Therapies in the ED. Part II: Procedural Coronary Intervention (PCI), GP IIb/IIIa Inhibitors, Combination Therapies, Fibrinolysis-Mediated Myocardial Reperfusion and the Paradigm Shift to Low Molecular Weight Heparin in Patients with Acute Coronary Syndrome."

EMERGENCY MEDICINE REPORTS, Brady, W. J., Perron, A. D., Ullman, E., April 23, 2001, "Electrocardiographic Diagnosis of Acute Coronary Syndromes (ACS): A Clinical Decision Support Tool for Optimizing Patient Management."

EMERGENCY MEDICINE REPORTS, Colucciello, S. A., June 10, 1996, "Pulmonary Embolism: A Rational Approach to the Patient with Suspected PE (Part I)."

EMERGENCY MEDICINE REPORTS, Colucciello, S. A., June 24, 1996, "Pulmonary Embolism: A Rational Approach to the Patient with Suspected PE (Part II)."

EMERGENCY MEDICINE REPORTS, Colucciello, S. A., January 1999, "Protocols for Deep Venous Thrombosis (DVT): A State-of-the-Art Review. Part I: Risk Factor Assessment, Physical Examination, and Current diagnostic Modalities."

EMERGENCY MEDICINE REPORTS, Colucciello, S. A., February 1999, "Protocols for Deep Venous Thrombosis (DVT): A State-of-the-Art Review Part II: Patient Management, Anticoagulation, and Special Considerations."

EMERGENCY MEDICINE REPORTS, Coyne, Michael A., November 2, 1992, "Avoiding Indecision and Hesitation in Hemophilia-Related Emergencies."

EMERGENCY MEDICINE REPORTS, Hagley, Michael T., January 25, 1993, "Emergency Intervention for Acute Myocardial Infarction: Thrombolytic Agents and Adjuvant Therapy."

EMERGENCY MEDICINE REPORTS, Hals, G. D., Carleton, S. C., August 1996, "Pericardial Disease and Tamponade."

EMERGENCY MEDICINE REPORTS, Hals, G., January 2000, "Acute Thoracic Aortic Dissection: Current Evaluation and Management - Part I: Pathophysiology, Risk Factors and Clinical Presentation."

EMERGENCY MEDICINE REPORTS, Hals, G., January 2000, "The Clinical Challenges of Acute Thoracic Aortic Dissection - Part II: Definitive Diagnosis, Patient Evaluation and Outcome Optimizing Management in Emergency Department."

EMERGENCY MEDICINE REPORTS, Hals, G., Pallaci, M., May 2000, "The Clinical Challenges of Abdominal Aortic Aneurysm: Rapid, Systematic Detection and Outcome-Effective Management Part I: Clinical Pathophysiology, Patient Presentation and Diagnostic Pitfalls."

EMERGENCY MEDICINE REPORTS, Hals, G., Pallaci, M., June 2000, "The Clinical Challenges of Abdominal Aortic Aneurysm: Rapid, Systematic Detection and Outcome-Effective Management Part II: Diagnosis, Management and Post-Operative Complications."

EMERGENCY MEDICINE REPORTS, Harrigan, R. A., Brady, W. J., September 11, 2000, Vol. 21, No. 19, "The Clinical Challenge of Bradycardia: Diagnosis, Evaluation, and Intervention in the Emergency Department."

EMERGENCY MEDICINE REPORTS, Johnson, David J., Rogers, B., June 7, 1999, "The Clinical Challenge of Congestive Heart Failure: Optimizing Outcomes in the Emergency Department and Outpatient Setting (Part I)."

EMERGENCY MEDICINE REPORTS, Jones, E. B., Robinson, D. J., May 8, 2000, "Unstable Angina: Year 2000 Update - Multi-Modal Strategies for Reducing Mortality, Urgent Revascularization, and Adverse Cardiovascular Events."

EMERGENCY MEDICINE REPORTS, Kleinschmidt, K., November 6, 2000, "Acute Coronary Syndromes (ACS): Pharmacotherapeutic Interventions — Treatment Guidelines for Patients With and Without Procedural Coronary Intervention (PCI) - Part I: Clinical Pathophysiology and Antiplatelet Agents."

EMERGENCY MEDICINE REPORTS, Kleinschmidt, K., November 20, 2000, "Acute Coronary Syndromes (ACS): Outcome-Optimizing Treatment Guidelines for Patients With and Without Procedural Coronary Intervention (PCI) - Part II: Evidence-Based Analysis of Antithrombin Therapy — Standard Heparin vs. Low Molecular Weight Heparins."

EMERGENCY MEDICINE REPORTS, Kleinschmidt, K., December 4, 2000, "Acute Coronary Syndromes: An Evidence-Based Review and Outcome-Optimizing Guidelines for Patients With and Without Procedural Coronary Intervention (PCI) - Part III: Fibrinolytic Therapy, Procedural Coronary Intervention, Multi-Modal Approaches, Low Molecular Weight Heparins, and Treatment Guidelines."

EMERGENCY MEDICINE REPORTS, Meyer, M.C., 2004, 25, "Reperfusion Strategies for ST Segment Elevation MI: An Overview of Current Therapeutic Options."

EMERGENCY MEDICINE REPORTS, Moffa, Jr., D. A., August 26, 2002, "Atrial Fibrillation Part I: Classification, Presentation and Diagnostic Evaluation."

EMERGENCY MEDICINE REPORTS, Moffa, Jr., D. A., September 9, 2002, "Atrial Fibrillation Part II: Management, Complications and Disposition."

EMERGENCY MEDICINE REPORTS, Peacock, W. F., Freda, B. J., March 25, 2002, "The Clinical Challenge of Heart Failure: Comprehensive, Evidence-Based Management of the Hospitalized Patient with Acute Myocardial Decompensation — Diagnosis, Risk Stratification and Outcome-Effective Treatment - Part I: Presentation, Differential Diagnosis, Laboratory Examination and Prophylaxis Against Venous Thromboembolic Disease (VTED)."

EMERGENCY MEDICINE REPORTS, Peacock, W. F., Freda, B. J., April 8, 2002, "The Clinical Challenge of Heart Failure: Comprehensive, Evidence-Based Management of the Hospitalized Patient with Acute Myocardial Decompensation - Part II: Outcome-Effective Treatment and Prophylaxis Against Venous Thromboembolic Disease (VTED)."

EMERGENCY MEDICINE CONSENSUS REPORTS, Peacock, W. F., Freda, B. J., May 1, 2002, "The Clinical Challenge of Heart Failure: Comprehensive, Evidence-Based Management of the Hospitalized Patient with Acute Myocardial Decompensation — Diagnosis, Risk Stratification and Outcome-Effective Treatment - Part I: Presentation, Differential Diagnosis, Laboratory Examination and Prophylaxis Against Venous Thromboembolic Disease (VTED)."

EMERGENCY MEDICINE REPORTS, Promes, S. B., Quest, T., Colucciello, S. A., Bosker, G., November 1998, "Anticoagulation and Antiplatelet Therapy in Emergency Medicine: An Evidence Based, State-of-the-Art Review. Part I: Aspirin, Glycoprotein IIb/IIIa Inhibitors, and ADP Platelet Receptor Antagonists."

EMERGENCY MEDICINE REPORTS, Promes, S. B., Quest, T., Bosker, G., December 7, 1998, "Anticoagulation and Antiplatelet Therapy in Emergency Medicine: An Evidence Based, State-of-the-Art Review (Part II)."

EMERGENCY MEDICINE REPORTS, Promes, S. B., Quest, T., Colucciello, S. A., Bosker, G., June 1999, "Low Molecular Weight Heparins (LMWHs) in Emergency Practice: Guidelines and Protocols for Thrombosis Management — Acute Ischemic Syndromes and Deep Venous Thrombosis."

EMERGENCY MEDICINE REPORTS, Robinson, D. J., Jerrard, D. A., Kuo, D. C., May 16, 1998, "Acute Myocardial Infarction: Clinical Guidelines for Patient Evaluation and Mortality Reduction."

EMERGENCY MEDICINE REPORTS, Robinson, D. J., Woolridge, D. P., December 1999, "Infectious Endocarditis: A Comprehensive Review for Emergency Physicians."

EMERGENCY MEDICINE REPORTS, Rogers, R., Robinson, D. J., June 1999, "The Clinical Challenge of Congestive Heart Failure: Optimizing Outcomes in the Emergency Department and Outpatient Setting Part II: Targeted Drug Therapy, Invasive Interventions, and Patient Disposition."

EMERGENCY MEDICINE REPORTS, Soria, David M. and Emerman, Charles L., March 18, 1996, "Chronic Obstructive Pulmonary Disease: Targeted Assessment Strategies and Emergency Management of Patients with Acute Exacerbations."

EMERGENCY PHYSICIANS' MONTHLY, Shapiro, N., June 1999, "Hypertensive Emergencies."

EUR. HEART J, Bonnefoy, E., et. al., May 2000, "Serum Cardiac Troponin I and ST-Segment Elevation in Patients with Acute Pericarditis." (at http://www.ccme.org)

EUR. HEART J, Cowie, M.R., Jourdain, P., Maisel, A., et.al., 2003, 24 (19): 1710-8, "Clinical Applications of B-Type Natriuretic Peptide (BNP) Testing."

EUR. HEART J, de Winter, R. J., Bholasingh, R., Nieuwenhuijs, A. B., et. al., 1999, "Ruling Out Acute Myocardial Infarction Early with two Serial Creatine Kinase-MB $_{mass}$ Determinations."

EUR. HEART J, Task Force on Aortic Dissection., September 2001, (18) 1642-81, "Diagnosis and Management of Aortic Dissection."

EUR. HEART J, Elizari, M. V., et. al., February 2000, Vol. 21, No. 3, (198), "Morbidity and Mortality Following Early Administration off Amiodarone in Acute Myocardial Infarction." (at http://www.ccme.org)

GERIATRIC EMERGENCY MEDICINE REPORTS, Glauser, J., February 2001, Vol. 2, No. 2, "Atrial Fibrillation Part I: Etiologies and Strategies for Ventricular Rate Control."

INTERNAT J CARDIO, Raghu, Co. et. al., December 1999, (209), "Protective Effect of Intravenous Magnesium in Acute Myocardial Infarction Following Thrombolytic Therapy." (at http://www.ccme.org).

INTERNAT J CARDIO, Thogersen, A. M., et. al., April 1995, "Effects of Intravenous Magnesium Sulfate in Suspected Acute Myocardial Infarction on Acute Arrhythmias and Long-term Outcome." (in Emer. Med. Abstracts, 1995)

JAMA, Dajani, Adnan S., et. al., June 1997, "Prevention of Bacterial Endocarditis."

JAMA, Hagan, P.G., et.al., 2000, 283:897-903, "The International Registry of Acute Aortic Dissection (IRAD). New Insights Into an Old Disease."

JAMA, Klompas, M., 2002, 287:2262-2272, "Does This Patient Have an Acute thoracic Aortic Dissection?"

JAMA, Mukherjee, D., et. al., August 2001, "Risk of Cardiovascular Events Associated with Selective Cox-2 Inhibitors."

JAMA, Randall, T., February 26, 1992, "Cocaine, Alcohol Mix in Body to Form Even Longer-Lasting, More Lethal Drug." (in Emer. Med. Abstracts, 1992)

JAMA, Sanjeev, D. C., et.al., 2003; 290(21): 2849-2858, "Does This Patient Have PE."

JAME, Trial Group Investigators, January 26, 2005, 293(4);437, "Effect of Glucose-Insulen-Potassium Infusion on Mortality in Patients with Acute ST-Segment Elevation Myocardial Infarction: the Create-ECLA Randomized Controlled Trial Create-ECLA."

JAMA, VMAC Investigators, 2002, 287:1531-40, "Intravenous Nesiritide vs Nitroglycerin for Treatment of Decompensated Congestive Heart Failure - a Randomized Trial."

J AM COLL CARDIOL, Fuster, V., et.al., 2001, 38: 2101-13, "ACC/AHA Guidelines for the Evaluation and Management of Chronic Heart Failure in the Adult: Executive Summary: A Report of the American College of Cardiology/American Heart Association Task Force on Practice Guidelines and the European Society of Cardiology Committee for Practice Guidelines and Policy Conferences (Committee to Revise the 1995 Guidelines for the Evaluation and Management of Heart Failure)."

J AM COLL CARDIOL, Hunt, S.A., et.al., 2001, 38: 1231-65, "ACC/AHA/ESC Guidelines for the Management of Patients with Atrial Fibrillation: Executive Summary: A Report of the American College of Cardiology/American Heart Association Task Force on Practice Guidelines and the European Society of Cardiology Committee for Practice Guidelines and Policy Conferences (Committee to Develop Guidelines for the Management of Patients with Atrial Fibrillation."

J AM COLL CARDIOL, Kontos, M. C., Anderson, F. P., Alimard, R., et. al., 2000, "Ability of Troponin I to Predict Cardiac Events in Patients Admitted from the Emergency Department."

J AM COLL CARDIOL, Ottesen, M. M., et. al., May 2001, "Consequences of Overutilization and Underutilization of Thrombolytic Therapy in Clinical Practice."

J AM COLL CARDIOL, Ravklide, J., et. al., March 1, 1995, "Independent Prognostic Value of Serum Creatine Kinase Isoenzyme MB Mass, Cardiac Tropinin T and Myosin Light Chain Levels in Suspected Acute Myocardial Infarction: Analysis of 28 Months of Follow-Up in 196 Patients." (in Emer. Med. Abstracts, 1995)

J AM COLL CARDIOL, Wharton, T.P., et.al., June 2, 2004, 43(11):1943, "Primary Angioplasty in Acute Myocardial Infarction at Hospitals with No Surgery On-Site (PAMI-NO SOS Study) Versus Transfer to Surgical Centers for Primary Angioplasty."

J EMERG MED, Carter, C. J., et. al., July-August 1999, "Rapid Fibrin D-Dimer Tests for Deep Venous Thrombosis: Factors Affecting Diagnostic Utility."

J EMERG MED, Chan, T.C., Brady, W.J., Pollack, M. L., 1999, 17(5):865-872, "Electrocardiographic Manifestations: Acute Myopericarditis."

J EMERG MED, Chan, T.C., Vilke, G.M., Pollack, M. L. Brady, W.J., 2001, 21(3): 263-270, "Electrocardiographic Manifestations: Pulmonary Embolism."

J EMERG MED, Harrigan, R.A. Pollack, W.J., Chan, T.C., 2003, 25(1): 67-77, "Electrocardiographic Manifestations: Bundle Branch Blocks and Fascicular Blocks."

J EMERG MED, Hudson, K.B., Brady, W.J., Chan, T.C., Pollack, M. L., Harrigan, R.A., 2003, 25(3): 303-314, "Electrocardiographic Manifestations: Ventricular Tachycardia."

J EMERG MED, Ma, G., Brady, W.J., Pollack, M., Chan, T.C., 2001, 20(2): 145-152 "Electrocardiographic Manifestations: Digitalis Toxicity."

J EMERG MED, Pollack, M. L. Brady, W.J., Chan, T.C., 2003, 24(1): 35-43, "Electrocardiographic Manifestations: Narrow QRS Complex Tachycardias."

J EMERG MED, Turnipseed S.D., 2003, 24(4): 369 "Frequency of Acute Coronary Syndrome in Patients Presenting to the Emergency Department with Chest Pain After Methamphetamine Use."

J. GEN INTERN MED, Lee, H. N., et. al., June 1995, "Inadequacy of Intravenous Heparin in the Initial Management of Venous Thromboembolism."

J TRAUMA, Dyer, D. S., et. al., April 2000, Volume 48, (673-83), "Thoracic Aortic Injury: How Predictive is Mechanism and is Chest Computed Tomography a Reliable Screening Tool? A Prospective Study of 1,561 Patients."

J VASC SURG, Aschwanden, M., et. al., 1999, "The Value of Rapid D-Dimer Testing Combined with Structured Clinical Evaluation for the Diagnosis of Deep vein Thrombosis."

J VASC SURG, Lennox, A. F., et. al., 1999, "Combination of a Clinical Risk Assessment Score and Rapid Whole Blood D-Dimer Testing in the Diagnosis of Deep Vein Thrombosis in Symptomatic Patients."

LANCET, Eikelboom, J. W., et. al., June 2000, "Unfractionated Heparin and Low-Molecular-Weight Heparin in Acute Coronary Syndrome without ST Elevation: A Meta-Analysis." (at http://www.ccme.org)

LANCET, Wells, P. S., et. al., May 27, 1995, "Accuracy of Clinical Assessment of Deep-Vein Thrombosis." (in Emer. Med. Abstracts, 1995)

LANCET, August 25, 2001, "Assessment of the Safety & Efficacy of a New Thrombolytic Regimen (ASSENT)-3 Investigators."

MASSACHUSETTS MEDICAL SOCIETY, Meaney, J. F. M., et. al., 1997, "Diagnosis of Pulmonary Embolism with Magnetic Resonance Angiography." (in The New England Journal of Medicine, May 1997)

MAYO CLIN PROCEEDINGS, Ryu, J. H., et. al., September 1998, "Clinical Recognition of Pulmonary Embolism: Problem of Unrecognized and Asymptomatic Cases."

MAYO CLIN PROCEEDINGS, Sohn, Dae-Won, et. al., October 1995, "Role of Transesophageal Echocardiography in Hemodynamically Unstable Patients."

NEUROL RES, Kraus, J.J., Metzler, M.D., Coplin, W.M., 2002, 24: S47-S57, "Critical Care Issues in Stroke and Subarachnoid Hemorrhage."

N ENGL J MED, Anderson, H.R., Nielsen, T.T., Rasmussen, K., 2003, 349(8): 733-42, "A Comparison of Coronary Angioplasty with Fibrinolytic Therapy in Acute Myocardial Infarction."

N ENGL J MED, Bates, S.M., Ginsberg, J.S., July 15, 2004, 351-3, "Treatment of Deep-Vein Thrombosis."

N ENGL J MED, DiMarco, J.P., 2003, 349: 1836-1847, "Implantable Cardioverter-Defibrillators.

N ENGL J MED, Dorian, P., Cass, D., et. al., March 21, 2002, Vol. 346, No. 12, "Amiodarone as Compared with Lidocaine for Shock-Resistant Ventricular Fibrillation."

N ENGL J MED, Montalescot, G., et. al., June 21, 2001, Vol. 344, "Platelet Glycoprotein IIb/IIIa Inhibition with Coronary Stenting for Acute Myocardial Infarction."

N ENGL J MED, Mylonakis, E., Calderwood, S.B., 2001, 345: 1318-30, "Infective Endocarditis in Adults."

N ENGL J MED, Topol, E. J., et. al., June 21, 2001, "Inhibitors Tirofiban and Abciximab, for the Prevention of Ischemic Events with Percutaneous Coronary Revascularization."

N ENGL J MED, Zimetbaum P.J., Josephson, M.E., March, 2003, 348(10): 933-40, "Use of the Electrocardiogram in Acute Myocardial Infarction."

N ENGL J MED, August 16, 2001, "Clopidogrel in Unstable Angina to Prevent Recurrent Events Trial Investigators."

PRIMARY CARE REPORTS, Donovan, P., January 23, 2000, Vol. 6, No. 2, "Atrial Fibrillation: Current Management."

PRIMARY CARE REPORTS, Pruitt, J. C., April 2000, "Practical Consideration for Vascular Screening."

QUICK CONSULTS IN EMERGENCY CARDIOLOGY, Crawford, M. H., December 2000, "Low Molecular Weight Heparin for Unstable Coronary Syndromes." (supplement to Emergency Medicine Reports, 2000)

RADIOLOGY, Mayo, J. R., et. al., November 1997, " Pulmonary Embolism: Prospective Comparison of Spiral CT with Ventilation-Perfusion Scintigraphy."

RESUSCITATION, Martens, P. R., 2001, Vol. 49, (233), "Optimal Response to Cardiac Arrest Study: Defibrillation Waveform Effects."

SCIENTIFIC AMERICAN, INC., Berger, P. B., April 1999, "Acute Myocardial Infarction."

SCIENTIFIC AMERICAN, INC., Dec, G. William., DeSanctis, Roman W., June 1998, "Cardiomyopathies."

SCIENTIFIC AMERICAN, INC., Dec, G. William., Hutter, Jr., Adolph M., May 1998, "Congestive Heart Failure."

SCIENTIFIC AMERICAN, INC., Dec, G. W., DeSanctis, R. W., September 2000, "Cardiomyopathies."

SCIENTIFIC AMERICAN, INC., Eagle, K. A., Armstrong, W. F., May 1999, "Diseases of the Aorta."

SCIENTIFIC AMERICAN, INC., Hancock, E. W., September 1999, "Diseases of the Pericardium, Cardiac Tumors, and Cardiac Trauma."

SCIENTIFIC AMERICAN, INC., Hirsh, J., April 1999, "Venous Thromboembolism."

SCIENTIFIC AMERICAN, INC., Langberg, J. J., DeLurgio, D. B., August 1999, "Ventricular Arrhythmias."

TOPICS IN HYPERTENSION, Phillips, R. A., Krakoff, L. R., 1997, "Hypertensive Emergencies - True and False."

THORACIC RADIOLOGY, Mayo, J. R., et. al., July 1997, "Pulmonary Embolism: Prospective Comparison of Spiral CT with Ventilation-Perfusion Scintigraphy."

Specific Text References

AHA 2000 Handbook of Emergency Cardiovascular Care for Healthcare Providers. Hazinski, M. F., Cummings, R. O., Field, J. M., (Dallas, TX, 2000).

Advanced Cardiac Life Support. American Heart Association (1997-1999).

ECG in Emergency Medicine and Acute Care. Chan, Brady, Harrigan, Ornato, Rosen, eds. (Mosby 2004).

ECG in Emergency Medicine and Acute Care. Chan, et.al., (Mosby 2005).

Emergency Cardiac Care. Gibler and Aufderheide (Mosby-Year Book Inc., St. Louis, 1994).

Emergency Medical Therapy. Mengert, Eisenberg, 4th ed., (W. B. Saunders, Philadelphia, 1996).

Emergency Medicine Clinics of North America: Emergency Department Diagnosis and Treatment of Acute Myocardial Infarction. Brady, Jr., W. J., Harrigan, R. A., (Saunders, Philadelphia, 2001).

Guidelines 2000 for Cardiopulmonary Resuscitation and Emergency Cardiovascular Care. International Consensus on Science / American Heart Association (Circulation 2000).

Practical Electrocardiography. Marriott (Williams & Wilkins, Baltimore, 1988).

Rapid Interpretation of EKGs. Dubin (Cover Publishing, Tampa, 1989).

Textbook of Advanced Cardiac Life Support. American Heart Association (1998).

Web and Other Sources

1997 SCIENTIFIC ASSEMBLY, Bessen, H. A., October 1997, "Aortic Disasters: Diagnosis Imaging Techniques and Management."

1997 SCIENTIFIC ASSEMBLY, Dunmire, S. M., October 1997, "Pulmonary Embolism: An Update in Diagnosis and Treatment."

1999 WRITTEN BOARD REVIEW COURSE PLUS, Gillespie, M., August 1999, "Cardiology, Pulmonary Edema/CHF/Syncope."

A CME WHITE PAPER, Topol, E. J., April 2000, "Finding the Optimal Fibrinolytic Agent."www.acc.org/, Antman, E.M., et. al., "ACC/AHA Guidelines for the Management of Patients with ST-elevation Myocardial Infarction; a Report of the ACC/AHA Task Force on Practice Guidelines 2004".

ACEP NEWS, Zoler, M.L. July 2005, Elsevier Global Medical News, "Expert Panel Calls for Limited Nesiritide Use."

www.eMedHome.com/, Jobe, K. A., University of Washington, "Implantable Cardioverter Defibrillators for the Emergency Physician."

www.eMedHome.com/, Mattu, A., University of Maryland School of Medicine, "Myths and Pitfalls in Advanced Cardiac Life Support."

ACLS QUICK REFERENCE CARD, American Heart Association, "Acute Coronary Syndromes and Stroke."

ADVANCES IN EMERGENCY CARDIAC AND NEUROVASCULAR CARE, May 2000, "Evolution of Treatment Options for Acute Coronary Syndromes and Neurovascular Disease." (monograph)

AMERICAN HEART ASSOCIATION, Broderick, J.P., Adams, H.P., Barsan, W., et.al. 1999, 30:905-15, "Guidelines for the Management of Spontaneous Intracerebral Hemorrhage: A Statement for Healthcare Professionals", from a special writing group of the Stroke Council.

CARDIOLOGY SCIENTIFIC UPDATE, August 2000, "National Investigators Collaborating on Enoxaparin (NICE-3)." (symposium)

EMER MED & ACUTE CARE ESSAYS, July 2003, Volume 27, No. 7, "ACC/AHA Guidelines: Unstable Angina/Non-ST Elevation MI."

FORESIGHT, Amer. Coll. of Emer. Physicians, Dunmire, Susan M., October 1995, "Thromboembolic Disease."

FORESIGHT, Joseph, A., June 2002, "Acute Coronary Syndromes."

FORESIGHT, Pennza, Paul T., January 1995, "Thrombolytic Therapy for Acute Myocardial Infarction."

MEDICAL EDUCATION RESOURCES, Van de Werf, F. J., December 2001, "GUSTO-V and ASSENT-3: What Lessons Can We Learn?"

MEDIVIEW EXPRESS REPORT, September 2001, "ASSENT 3: New Standard of Care in Acute Coronary Syndromes." (symposium)

General Text References, Acep Clinical Policies and LLSA Reading Lists *for all chapters located in the back of both volumes.*

NOTES

NOTES

NOTES

ENT, MAXILLOFACIAL AND DENTAL EMERGENCIES

1. All of the following are true of peripheral vertigo except:

   (a) Onset is gradual.
   (b) Nystagmus may be horizontal or horizontorotary in direction.
   (c) It may be associated with nausea, vomiting, hearing loss and tinnitus.
   (d) It is generally self-limited.

2. The most reliable sign of acute otitis media is:

   (a) A tympanic membrane that is erythematous
   (b) The presence of fever
   (c) Loss of mobility of the tympanic membrane on pneumatic otoscopy
   (d) The presence of a scarred and retracted tympanic membrane

3. Which of the following statements regarding malignant otitis externa is true?

   (a) It is a common complication of otitis externa that afflicts otherwise healthy patients.
   (b) It is treated on an outpatient basis with oral antibiotics.
   (c) It is caused by pseudomonas.
   (d) Patients with this disease process are generally afebrile and experience little pain.

4. Which of the following is least characteristic of croup?

   (a) Barking cough
   (b) High fever
   (c) Preceding URI
   (d) Insidious onset

5. All of the following are true of temporal arteritis except:

   (a) It is associated with a markedly elevated sedimentation rate.
   (b) It may present as sudden, painless, unilateral loss of vision.
   (c) It is treated with steroids.
   (d) It is a nonsegmental vasculitis.

6. Appropriate antibiotic therapy of GABH Strep pharyngitis can limit or prevent all of the following complications except:

   (a) Rheumatic fever
   (b) Glomerulonephritis
   (c) Pharyngeal space infections
   (d) Spread of the infection to others

7. _____ is/are the most common cause(s) of pharyngitis.
   (a) GABH Strep
   (b) Mycoplasma
   (c) Viruses
   (d) Gonorrhea

8. Which statement is most true regarding GABH Strep pharyngitis?
   (a) Accurate diagnosis can be made on the basis of clinical findings alone.
   (b) It commonly affects children less than 3 years of age.
   (c) Associated complaints of abdominal pain, vomiting and headache are common in children.
   (d) Patients classically have tender posterior cervical adenopathy, mild fever and exudative tonsillitis.

9. Which of the nerve blocks listed below is most appropriate when midfacial anesthesia is required?
   (a) Inferior alveolar nerve block
   (b) Infraorbital nerve block
   (c) Supraorbital nerve block
   (d) Posterior superior alveolar nerve block

10. All of the following statements regarding Ellis II fractures are true except:
    (a) They involve both the enamel and dentin.
    (b) They are associated with hot and cold sensitivity.
    (c) Bleeding from the tooth is characteristic.
    (d) Dental follow-up within 24 hours is recommended.

11. Which of the following descriptive statements is most consistent with alveolar osteitis?
    (a) It occurs within 24 hrs. of extraction and responds to oral analgesics.
    (b) It is seen several days post-extraction, after an initial pain-free time interval and is not relieved by oral analgesics.
    (c) It is associated with dental caries and treated by tooth extraction.
    (d) It is a periodontal lesion in which bacteria invade non-necrotic tissue.

12. Which is true regarding treatment of avulsed teeth:
    (a) The tooth should be wiped clean before replanting
    (b) Primary teeth should be replaced immediately
    (c) Handling the tooth by the root is preferred
    (d) Hanks solution + milk are better transport solutions than tap water

13. The most common arterial source of posterior epistaxis is:

   (a) Sphenopalatine artery
   (b) Anterior ethmoidal artery
   (c) Posterior ethmoidal artery
   (d) Kiesselbach's plexus

14. All the following statements regarding posterior epistaxis (including its treatment) are accurate except:

   (a) It is less common than anterior epistaxis.
   (b) Most commonly occurs in children and young adults.
   (c) Placement of a posterior pack can result in hypoxia and hypercarbia.
   (d) Patients treated with a posterior pack should be admitted.

15. The treatment of choice for simple Strep throat is:

   (a) Penicillin
   (b) Erythromycin
   (c) Cephalosporins
   (d) TMP/SMX

16. The following statements regarding glomerulonephritis are accurate except:

   (a) It is a suppurative complication of GABH Strep infection.
   (b) It can result from either pharyngeal or cutaneous infection with GABH Strep.
   (c) Patients usually present after a latent period of 1.5 - 3 weeks.
   (d) The most useful lab test for making the diagnosis is the U/A.

17. The following statements regarding rheumatic fever are accurate except:

   (a) The Jones Criteria (revised) are used to establish the diagnosis.
   (b) Evidence of a preceding GABH Strep infection plus the presence of one major and one minor criteria make the diagnosis highly probable.
   (c) Patients usually present with severe migratory joint pain.
   (d) Morbidity is most closely related to the development of carditis and valvular damage.

18. Bacterial tracheitis is most commonly caused by _____.

   (a) *H. influenza*
   (b) *Strep. pneumoniae*
   (c) *Staph. aureus*
   (d) GABH Strep

19. A mother brings in her 3-year-old child for evaluation. She states that he was playing on the floor while she was preparing dinner and he suddenly started coughing. As you evaluate the child, you note that he is playful, appropriate and in no acute distress. Which of the following statements is most accurate?

    (a) You should reassure the mother and send the child home; further work-up is unnecessary since foreign body (FB) aspiration is unlikely in this scenario.

    (b) You should obtain further history and perform PA and lateral CXRs; normal findings on these x-rays R/O the possibility of FB aspiration.

    (c) You should obtain further history and perform PA, lateral and (possibly) bilateral decubitus CXR films; if these films are negative (and your suspicion for FB aspiration remains high) bronchoscopy should be arranged.

    (d) You should immediately arrange for diagnostic bronchoscopy in every child with this presentation.

20. Which of the following is not true regarding peritonsillar abscesses?

    (a) Most commonly occurs subsequent to suppurative tonsillitis
    (b) Needle aspiration provides sufficient drainage for most abscesses
    (c) Is most common in young children
    (d) The causative organism(s) is/are polymicrobial

21. A patient presents with complaint of decreased hearing after being slapped on the ear by his brother. Exam reveals a small perforation of the tympanic membrane and a conductive hearing loss, but is otherwise entirely normal. The child is acting normally, appears to be comfortable and has normal vital signs. The most appropriate treatment for this patient is:

    (a) Emergent ENT referral for possible surgical repair.
    (b) A prescription for an oral antibiotic and referral for follow-up with ENT in 24 hrs.
    (c) A prescription for a topical antibiotic and referral for follow-up with ENT in one week.
    (d) Recommend the ear be kept dry and refer to ENT on a nonurgent basis.

22. Which of the following statements regarding the diagnosis of sinusitis is most accurate?

    (a) It requires diagnostic imaging in most instances.
    (b) Normal findings on plain x-rays (Waters, Caldwell, submental-vertex and lateral views) rule out the diagnosis.
    (c) Plain films are the most useful in diagnosing sphenoid and ethmoid sinusitis.
    (d) The "gold standard" for diagnosing sinus disease and its complications is CT of the sinuses.

23. Which of the following statements regarding hairy leukoplakia is false?
    (a) It is a white plaque-like lesion with hairy projections.
    (b) It is usually asymptomatic.
    (c) It is easily removed with a tongue blade.
    (d) 80% of patients presenting with this lesion go on to develop AIDS within the next three years.

24. The initial study of choice for confirming the presence of a retropharyngeal abscess is a soft-tissue lateral film of the neck. To avoid obtaining a false positive result, this film must be taken:
    (a) During expiration with the neck in slight extension
    (b) During expiration with the neck in slight flexion
    (c) During inspiration with the neck in slight extension
    (d) During inspiration with the neck in slight flexion

25. Croup (laryngotracheobronchitis) is most commonly caused by:
    (a) Respiratory syncytial virus (RSV)
    (b) Parainfluenza virus
    (c) Adenovirus
    (d) Influenza virus

26. A three-year-old is brought in for evaluation of sore throat, fever and refusal to eat. The child's voice is muffled. Exam reveals a unilateral bulging of the posterior pharyngeal wall, tender anterior cervical adenopathy and temperature of 102°F. The most likely diagnosis is:
    (a) Retropharyngeal abscess
    (b) Peritonsillar abscess
    (c) Ludwig's angina
    (d) Masticator space abscess

Answers: 1. a, 2. c, 3. c, 4. b, 5. d, 6. b, 7. c, 8. c, 9. b, 10. c, 11. b, 12. d, 13. a, 14. b, 15. a, 16. a, 17. b, 18. c, 19. c, 20. d, 21. d, 22. d, 23. c, 24. c, 25. b, 26. a

Use the pre-chapter multiple choice question worksheet (p. xxv) to record and determine the percentage of correct answers for this section.

OTOLOGIC EMERGENCIES

I. Anatomy

A. Sensory Supply to the Ear

1. Trigeminal nerve (third branch of the fifth cranial nerve) → anterior canal and auricle
2. Cranial VII → posterior canal
3. Cranial IX → lower canal
4. Cranial X → tympanic membrane
5. Cervical nerves 2 and 3 → posterior auricular region

B. Auditory Transmission

Sound waves enter ear canal → TM → ossicles → perilymph → endolymph → organ of Corti → spiral ganglion → cochlear nuclei → temporal lobes

II. Infections

A. Otitis Externa (Swimmer's Ear)

1. *Pseudomonas aeruginosa* and *Staphylococcus aureus* are responsible for most cases of otitis externa. Other pathogens include Proteus, Streptococcus and fungi (usually Aspergillus).

2. A major predisposing factor is exposure to a warm, moist environment so, most cases occur in the summer months and in patients exposed to tropical environments; foreign body trauma and water exposure are obvious risk factors.

3. Signs and symptoms
   - Itching (may be intense with severe fungal infections)
   - Pain (may be intense, constant and aggravated by motion of the jaw)
   - Sense of fullness in the ear
   - Redness/swelling of external ear and/or auditory canal
   - White, cheesy or watery green discharge
   - Pulling on the ear or pressing on the tragus causes pain
   - If the TM can be visualized, it is often red, thick and covered with flat vesicles or areas of desquamating epithelium.

4. Management
    a. Cleanse the ear canal of debris using suction, irrigation or gentle curettage; this is the most important part of therapy.
    b. Treat the infection with a topical agent as follows:
        (1) Mild nonpurulent infections → 2% acetic solution with hydrocortisone 1% (VoSol HC otic sol.)
        (2) When associated edema and discharge are present → a combination of polymyxin B and neomycin sulfate with hydrocortisone (Cortisporin otic suspension or solution); if TM perforation is present, use the suspension, as it is less toxic to structures of the middle ear.
        (3) If significant edema is present, a wick or ribbon gauze that is moistened with the desired medication, should be inserted in the external canal and left in place for 24 - 48 hours.
    c. Advise the patient to avoid getting water in his ear for 2 - 3 weeks.
    d. Cellulitis is often present in severe cases; a systemic antibiotic (i.e. dicloxacillin or amoxacillin/clavulanate) is required.

B. ***Malignant (necrotizing) Otitis Externa*** is a complication of otitis externa that is associated with a high mortality rate. It occurs primarily in adult diabetics, but is also seen in debilitated and immunocompromised patients. This is a Pseudomonas osteitis of the underlying bone of the external canal. Distinguishing features include: fever, excruciating pain, the presence of friable granulation tissue in the external auditory canal, edema/erythema of the pinna and periauricular tissues. Cranial nerve palsies and trismus may also be seen. These patients require immediate otolaryngology consultation and hospitalization for IV antibiotics (fluoroquinolones or antipseudomonal cephalosporins) and possible surgical debridement. CT and MRI are the most appropriate imaging studies to evaluate for osteomyelitis.

C. ***Post-Traumatic Perichondritis***

• Is an infection of the auricular cartilage.

• Clinical features: ear pain, swelling and fever are typical; exam reveals erythema and warmth/swelling of the pinna.

• Treatment consists of consultation with an otolaryngologist for surgical drainage and administration of parenteral antibiotics effective against Pseudomonas, Proteus and Staphylococcus.

D. ***Acute Otitis Media (AOM)***

1. Epidemiology, pathophysiology and microbiology
    a. Children 6 - 36 months of age are most often affected; peak incidence occurs at 6 - 13 months.
    b. It is more common in the winter and spring months and frequently occurs in association with a viral URI.

    c. Eustachian tube dysfunction plays a central role in the pathogenesis: eustachian tube dysfunction → retention of secretions → colonization (usually bacterial).

    d. The most common bacterial pathogens are:

       (1) *S. pneumoniae* — is the most common pathogen in all age groups; ampicillin-resistant strains have emerged and are becoming an increasing problem to treat.

       (2) *H. influenza* (predominantly nontypeable) — is the second most common pathogen; 30 - 40% of strains are ampicillin-resistant.

       (3) *Moraxella (Branhamella) catarrhalis* — is the third most common pathogen; most strains are resistant to ampicillin.

       (4) *Strep. pyogenes* — less common.

       (5) *Staph. aureus, Group B Strep* and gram-negative enteric bacilli may be seen as pathogens in the neonatal period.

2. The clinical entity known as "otitis media" represents a continuum of an illness that begins as an asymptomatic otitis media with effusion to acute otitis media with effusion plus signs and symptoms of an infection:

    a. Symptoms: vary from irritability, poor feeding and ear-pulling (infants), to otalgia and hearing loss (older child). Upper respiratory symptoms are often present as well.

    b. Signs: the tympanic membrane is usually red or opaque and may be full or bulging (bony landmarks are difficult to discern). Otorrhea may be present if spontaneous perforation has occurred. However, the <u>most reliable sign</u> of AOM is decreased mobility of the tympanic membrane on pneumatic otoscopy. Fever is present in only one-third of patients.

3. Treatment

    a. First-line antibiotics

       (1) Amoxicillin 80 - 90mg/kg/day — despite increasing resistance, is still considered to be the initial agent of choice by most authors.

       (2) Trimethoprim-sulfamethoxazole[*]

       (3) Erythromycin-sulfisoxazole[*]

    b. Second-line agents — are usually reserved for treatment failures. A broad-spectrum antibiotic that provides coverage of Beta-lactamase-producing species should be selected; choose one of the following:

       (1) Amoxicillin-clavulanate

       (2) Clindamycin

       (3) Cefuroxime axetil

       (4) Cefpodoxime proxetil

       (5) Cefprozil

       (6) Macrolides

    c. Patients should be advised to return in <u>48 - 72 hours</u> if signs and symptoms fail to improve and <u>immediately</u> if increasing temperature, lethargy or worsening irritability develop.

---

[*]Alternative agents for penicillin-allergic patients and for use in communities with a high rate of Beta-lactamase producing organisms.

d. The possibility of systemic infection should be considered in infants with acute otitis media (especially those less than 2 months old) who have a fever or appear toxic. These infants require a septic work-up and are often admitted for parenteral antibiotic therapy. In infants < 2 months old, broad spectrum coverage is recommended since there is a higher incidence of coliforms, *Group B Strep* and *S. aureus* encountered in this age group; use ampicillin <u>plus</u> gentamicin <u>or</u> ampicillin <u>plus</u> cefotaxime.

e. Antipyretics and analgesics such as acetaminophen or Pediaprofen should also be initiated.

<u>Note</u>: Further discussion of this topic can be found in the Pediatric chapter on pp. 661-663.

E. *Bullous Myringitis*

- Clinical characteristics: an acute otitis media with clear or hemorrhagic blisters within the layers of the tympanic membrane associated with ear pain and mild hearing loss.

- Etiology: viral or bacterial (same organisms that cause AOM): may also be caused by *Mycoplasma pneumoniae*.

- Treatment is with local heat applications, analgesics and antibiotics (same choices as for AOM).

III. Sudden Hearing Loss

A. *Pathophysiology* — Acute hearing loss may be associated with lesions of the external, middle or inner ear. Lesions of the external auditory canal, tympanic membrane (TM), middle ear and ossicles produce <u>conductive</u> hearing loss whereas lesions of the cochlea, the auditory nerve and brainstem auditory pathways produce <u>sensorineural</u> hearing loss.

B. *Causes of Sudden Hearing Loss*

1. Conductive loss
   a. Impacted cerumen or foreign body
   b. Otitis externa
   c. Middle ear effusion (otitis media, barotitis media)
   d. TM perforation
   e. Sclerosis of the TM or ossicles

2. Sensorineural loss
    a. Unilateral
        (1) Viral neuritis (of the cochlear branch of cranial nerve VIII)
        (2) Acoustic neuroma
        (3) Ménière's disease
        (4) Temporal bone fracture
    b. Bilateral
        (1) Ototoxic drug exposure
            • Antibiotics (aminoglycosides, erythromycin, vancomycin, antimalarials)
            • NSAIDs, ASA
            • Loop diuretics (furosemide, ethacrynic acid)
            • Antineoplastics (cisplatin, nitrogen mustard)
        (2) Exposure to loud noise

C. Clinical Evaluation

1. Otoscopic examination should distinguish the patients with conductive hearing loss (due to cerumen impaction, TM perforation or the presence of middle ear fluid) from those with sensorineural hearing loss.

2. The Rinne and Weber tests are also useful in distinguishing conductive from sensorineural hearing loss.
    a. Rinne test — compares air-vs-bone conduction and is performed by placing the base of a vibrating 512 Hz tuning fork against the mastoid process. Then, when the patient can no longer feel the vibration, the tuning fork tips are placed adjacent to the external auditory canal of the ear. In patients with normal hearing, the vibrations of the tuning fork will still be heard.
        (1) If there is unilateral <u>conductive</u> loss, vibrations will <u>not</u> be heard.
        (2) If there is a unilateral <u>sensorineural</u> loss, test will be normal.
    b. Weber test — is performed by placing the base of the vibrating tuning fork against the middle of the forehead and asking the patient in which ear the sound is loudest. Normally, it is equal in both ears.
        (1) If a unilateral <u>conductive</u> hearing loss is present, vibrations will be heard better in the ear with conductive loss.
        (2) If a unilateral <u>sensorineural</u> hearing loss is present, vibration will be heard better in the normal ear.
    <u>Note:</u> If bilateral sensorineural hearing loss is present, both of these tests will be normal despite a bilateral decrease in hearing acuity.

3. Physical exam should include a thorough HEENT exam including the cranial nerves; these patients frequently have associated deficits of adjacent cranial nerves, particularly V and VII (corneal reflex) as well as tinnitus, vertigo and disequilibrium.

4. CT of the brain (with and without contrast) should be considered if a tumor is suspected based on the history and exam.

D. Management — depends on the underlying disease process. Cerumen and foreign body impactions should be removed and infections (otitis media or externa) should be treated. Patients with tumors require admission and neurosurgical consultation. For other patients with sudden sensorineural hearing loss, referral to an otolaryngologist for follow-up (in 1 - 2 days) should be arranged. If an ototoxic drug is the presumed cause of hearing loss, it should be discontinued.

IV. Vertigo — A sensation of movement of oneself (subjective vertigo) or the environment (objective vertigo), most commonly described as a feeling of spinning. Vertigo may be either peripheral or central in origin. Peripheral vertigo accounts for 85 - 90% of cases and is considered less serious prognostically than central vertigo, which accounts for 10 - 15% of cases. Peripheral vertigo arises from diseases of the vestibular apparatus or Cranial Nerve VIII and is usually self-limited. Central vertigo originates from diseases of the CNS (brain stem or cerebellum). Distinguishing factors include onset, intensity, duration, the effect of position changes, associated symptoms and nystagmus.

A. Peripheral Vertigo is characterized by:

1. Abrupt onset

2. Severe intensity

3. Brief/intermittent duration

4. Worsening with change in position

5. Associated symptoms may include nausea/vomiting, diaphoresis, tinnitus and hearing loss.

6. Nystagmus that is:
   - Fatigable
   - Inhibited by visual fixation
   - Unidirectional; horizontal or horizontorotary (but <u>never</u> vertical)
   - <u>No</u> associated neurologic abnormalities

B. Central Vertigo is characterized by:

1. Insidious onset

2. Mild intensity

3. Prolonged/continuous duration

4. Little or no effect with change in position

5. Associated symptoms may include: headache, diplopia, dysarthria, dysphagia, ataxia, facial numbness and hemiparesis.

6. Nystagmus that is:
    *   Nonfatigable
    *   Not suppressed by visual fixation
    *   Multi-directional (changes direction with changes in position); horizontal, rotary or vertical

7. Not usually associated with hearing loss

V. Trauma

A. *Lacerations of the Auricle* must be carefully repaired to avoid cosmetic defects.

B. *Hematomas of the Auricle* should be drained and dressed with a compressive dressing which maintains normal ear contours; this will prevent formation of "cauliflower ear." Patients should be reassessed in 24 hours for reaccumulation of blood which, if present, will require repeat drainage and dressing replacement.

C. *Frostbite of the Auricle* should be treated by rapid rewarming using warm water irrigation (40 - 42°C).

D. *Foreign Body* located beyond the isthmus of the ear (the cartilaginous-bony junction) or in patients who are agitated and uncooperative may need to be removed by an ENT specialist under general anesthesia.

E. *Perforation of the TM* can result from a penetrating object, loud noise, infection, lightning strike or rapid changes in pressure, i.e. scuba diving accidents. Otoscopic exam usually reveals the tear and immobility of the TM on bulb insufflation confirms it. (Acute perforations → irregular borders with blood on the edges or in the canal; chronic perforations → smooth margins, no blood.) Patients with associated symptoms of complete hearing loss, nausea, vomiting, vertigo or facial palsy need immediate ENT referral. (These symptoms suggest the presence of concurrent injury to the ossicles, labyrinth or temporal bone.) Otherwise, most perforations generally heal spontaneously and follow-up with ENT can be on a less-urgent basis. In either case, the ear should be kept dry. If coexisting otitis externa is present, a topical antibiotic otic suspension should be prescribed.

F. *Severe Blunt Injury* to the ear may be associated with fracture of the temporal bone and hearing loss.

NASAL TRAUMA

In evaluating nasal trauma, it is important to elicit any history of previous nasal deformity or surgery.

I. Nasal Fractures

A. Diagnosis of an <u>uncomplicated</u> nasal fracture can be determined on clinical grounds alone. Suggestive findings include the presence of tenderness, swelling, ecchymosis, deformity or crepitance. X-rays add little or nothing to initial or subsequent management (other than cost) and need not be obtained in most cases.

  1. If swelling does not preclude an accurate assessment of nasal contour, early reduction is frequently possible.

  2. If swelling does not allow an accurate assessment, reduction is deferred until the swelling has subsided (usually 2 - 7 days).

  3. All patients with suspected or confirmed nasal fractures should be referred for re-evaluation once the edema has resolved.

B. Complex fractures (e.g. nasoethmoid fractures) and nasal fractures associated with other facial fractures (e.g. orbital floor fractures, tripod fractures of the zygomatic bone) may require CT scanning to assess the extent of injury present and establish a treatment plan. Nasoethmoid fractures are particularly complex and difficult injuries. These fractures are usually produced by a blow to the bridge of the nose and may require CT scanning, admission and neurosurgical consultation.

C. Prophylactic antibiotic therapy (anti-staphylococcal) is warranted in patients discharged with nasal packing and may be warranted for nasal fractures associated with a laceration of the nasal mucosa or skin (potential bacterial contamination). Nasal saline irrigation helps remove blood and cleanse the mucosa; cold compresses will help reduce swelling.

II. Major Complications of Nasal Trauma

A. *Septal Hematoma* – Patients with nasal trauma should always be carefully evaluated to rule out the presence of a septal hematoma (a bluish-purple, grapelike swelling of the nasal septum). These subperichondral hematomas should be vertically incised and drained. Following this, the anterior nasal cavity is packed to prevent blood from reaccumulating. The patient is then placed on an antistaphylococcal antibiotic and referred to ENT for followup in 24 - 48 hours. Failure to drain these hematomas can result in formation of a septal abscess or avascular necrosis of the nasal septum with subsequent development of a "saddle-nose" deformity.

B. CSF Rhinorrhea

1. Is due to fracture of the cribriform plate of the ethmoid bone.

2. It may not develop for days to weeks.

3. It should be suspected whenever a patient develops a clear nasal discharge following facial trauma and may be associated with hyposmia (or anosmia) and headache.

4. It is usually unilateral and may be increased by having the patient lean forward or by compression of the jugular vein.

5. If CSF rhinorrhea is suspected:
   a. Place the patient in the upright position.
   b. Obtain immediate neurosurgical consultation.
   c. Avoid nasal packing.
   d. Advise the patient to avoid coughing, sneezing and blowing the nose.

6. The diagnosis is most reliably confirmed by metrizamide CT cisternography. A positive dextrose test (in the absence of bleeding) is also suggestive; however, a negative result does not rule out the diagnosis.

7. The administration of prophylactic antibiotics (PCN, cephalosporins) remains controversial and should be determined by the neurosurgical consultant.

C. Hemorrhage

1. Bleeding may be profuse but is usually of short duration.

2. If bleeding does not subside spontaneously, and CSF rhinorrhea is not suspected, nasal packing may be required; if so, be sure to prescribe an antistaphylococcal antibody.

NASAL FOREIGN BODIES

I. Clinical Presentation
Nasal foreign bodies most commonly occur in children 2 - 3 years of age. Although the child sometimes presents with a nasal foreign body (FB), this history is frequently lacking. It is not uncommon for a child to be brought in for evaluation of a unilateral foul-smelling nasal discharge, persistent unilateral epistaxis or a foul body odor.

II. Diagnosis — is usually made by inspecting the nares with an otoscope or nasal speculum in combination with a head lamp. Application of a vasoconstrictor and topical anesthetic (1% phenylephrine and a small amount of 2 - 4% lidocaine) facilitates the exam (by providing patient comfort and improving the visual field) as well as subsequent treatment.

III. Treatment — Many nasal foreign bodies can be removed in the ED by using one of the techniques described below. The method selected will depend on the age and cooperativeness of the child as well as the characteristics of the foreign body. Patient restraint is frequently necessary. Options include:

- Positive pressure techniques — have the advantage of being simple, noninvasive and probably should be tried first.

  1. Have the child forcefully blow his nose while occluding the uninvolved nostril. This method works best in older, cooperative patients and may require several attempts.

  2. Have the parent blow a puff of air into the child's mouth using mouth-to-mouth technique while occluding the uninvolved nostril. If a parent is unwilling or unable to do this, the physician can blow into the child's mouth with an Ambu bag.

- A suction catheter with a phalange may also be used to remove the FB.

- Forceps (alligator, bayonet), right angle probes, wire loops or a small Fogarty catheter are acceptable alternatives but particular care must be exercised to avoid injuring the mucosa or pushing the object posteriorly with these instruments.

- Following removal, the nasal cavity should be inspected for the presence of additional foreign objects, infection and trauma.

- If the foreign body cannot be safely removed, the patient should be referred to an otolaryngologist. Follow-up on an outpatient basis in 24 hours is appropriate for most of these patients. However, immediate consultation (and possible admission) are required for patients with a lodged button battery, associated facial cellulitis or associated systemic symptoms.

EPISTAXIS

I. Vascular Supply to the Nose

A. **Upper Half of the Nose:** anterior and posterior ethmoidal arteries (internal carotid → ophthalmic artery → ethmoidal arteries).

B. **Lower Half of the Nose:** sphenopalatine and greater palatine arteries (both are distal branches of the external carotid).

C. **Anteroinferior Nasal Septum (Little's area):** KIESSELBACH'S PLEXUS → the most common source of anterior nosebleeds.

D. **PosteromedialTurbinate:** WOODRUFF'S PLEXUS → the most common venous source of posterior nosebleeds.

E. **Sphenopalatine Artery** → most common arterial source of posterior nosebleeds.

II. Etiologies of Epistaxis

A. **Anterior Bleeds (90% of all nosebleeds)** – more common in children[*] and young adults

  1. Trauma - look for septal hematoma

  2. Foreign body - especially children

  3. Nose picking - "epistaxis digitorum"

  4. "Winter syndrome" - dry air and URI

  5. Allergies

  6. Nasal irritants - cocaine, nasal sprays

  7. Pregnancy - epistaxis may be due to increased blood volume and venous engorgement

  8. Rapid changes in atmospheric pressure

  9. Infection - rhinitis, sinusitis

  10. Osler-Weber-Rendu syndrome (Hereditary hemorrhagic telengectasia)

[*]Have a high level of suspicion for blood dyscrasias (e.g. leukemia)

B. *Posterior Bleeds (10% of all nosebleeds)* – more common in the elderly

   1. Coagulopathy - either iatrogenic, blood dyscrasias or liver disease

   2. Atherosclerosis of nasal blood vessels

   3. Neoplasm

   4. Hypertension (debatable)

III. Evaluation of Epistaxis

A. *History*
   - Onset (spontaneous or precipitated), duration, severity
   - Isolated event or recurrent problem
   - Medications and illicit drug use
   - Underlying medical problems (e.g. clotting Factor abnormalities, thrombocytopenia, liver/renal failure)
   - Easy bruising and bleeding at other sites
   - Recent chemotherapy or prior history of neoplasm

B. *Physical*
   - Vital signs (note any orthostatic change)
   - Location of bleeding site
   - Signs of underlying bleeding disorder (ecchymoses, purpura, petechiae, spider angiomata)

IV. Management of Epistaxis
Assemble the necessary supplies and equipment at bedside; appropriately gown both the patient and yourself. Then, with the patient seated and his head in the sniffing position, evacuate accumulated blood and clots from the nose, apply a topical anesthetic and vasoconstrictor and ask him to pinch his nose firmly for ten minutes.

A. *Anterior Sites*

   1. Chemical cautery (silver nitrate sticks) — if the bleeding has stopped.

   2. A small piece of a hemostatic material (e.g. Surgicel, Gelfoam) on the bleeding site — if the bleeding is mild.

   3. Anterior nasal packing — if tamponade is needed to control the bleeding.

   4. Follow-up with ENT or PMD in 2 - 3 days.

B. Posterior Sites

1. Posterior packing is indicated; use a gauze pack, intranasal balloon device (Nasostat or Epistat) or a Foley catheter. The posterior gauze pack + Foley catheter are used in conjunction with a traditional anterior pack.

2. <u>Admit</u> posterior bleeds to an ENT specialist

3. Administer supplemental oxygen.

<u>Note</u>: Since packing impairs sinus drainage, <u>all patients who require anterior or posterior packing</u> should be started on an antibiotic (such as amoxicillin-clavulanate or a first-generation cephalosporin) as prophylaxis against sinusitis, otitis media and toxic shock syndrome. Analgesic agents and decongestants are also appropriate. ASA and NSAIDs should be avoided.

V. Complications of Epistaxis — May be due to the bleeding itself or as a consequence of the packs used to tamponade the bleeding:

- **Severe Bleeding** — seen more commonly with posterior bleeds; transfusion may be needed if there are signs of cardiovascular compromise.

- **Sinusitis and otitis media** — due to obstruction of the sinus ostia and the eustachian tubes by nasal packing.

- **Toxic shock syndrome (TSS)** — due to the rapid growth of toxin-producing staphylococcal organisms precipitated by nasal packing.

- **Hypoxia and hypercarbia** — occur in association with posterior packs. It is postulated that these packs promote bronchoconstriction and increase vascular resistance via the "nasopulmonary reflex". Other contributing factors may include hypoventilation due to the use of sedating agents and aspiration of blood during pack placement.

- **Pressure necrosis of the columella or nasal ala** — from improper padding.

- **Fatal airway obstruction** — precipitated by accidental dislodgment of a posterior pack into the airway.

- **Bradycardia, dysrhythmias and coronary ischemia** — can be precipitated by posterior packing.

ACUTE AIRWAY OBSTRUCTION

I. Signs and Symptoms

- **Labored respirations** (tachypnea, chest retractions, nasal flaring)
- **Stridor** — a high-pitched crowing sound caused by airflow through a partially obstructed <u>upper</u> airway (larynx or trachea). Although it is most commonly heard during inspiration, it may be biphasic or expiratory when the obstruction is more distal (trachea).

  1. Inspiratory → (supraglottic or glottic) — indicates obstruction above or at the larynx, e.g. epiglottitis.

  2. Biphasic → (subglottic) — indicates obstruction below the larynx, e.g. croup.

  3. Expiratory → indicates bronchial or lower tracheal obstruction.

- **Hoarseness**
- **Dysphagia**
- **Coughing**
- **Cyanosis**

> The degree of airflow in the <u>upper</u> airway is dependent upon the diameter of the airway in any given situation: ↓ airway diameter → ↑ resistance to airflow (by a factor of ~ 4)

II. Differential Diagnosis

- **Infections (retropharyngeal abscess, bacterial tracheitis, epiglottitis)**
- **Angioedema (hypersensitivity to irritants, allergens, ACE inhibitors)**
- **Trauma (including burns)**
- **Foreign body aspiration**
- **Vascular anomalies**
- **Neoplasms**
- **Croup**

  1. Most commonly occurs in children 1 to 4 years of age; males are more commonly affected.

  2. Although any type of object may be aspirated, peanuts are the most common offending agent.

  3. The narrowest part of the upper airway is where most airway foreign bodies become lodged:
     a. In adults → vocal cords
     b. In children → cricoid cartilage

4. The presenting signs vary with the location of the foreign body and the degree of obstruction produced:
   a. Aphonia → complete <u>upper</u> airway obstruction
   b. Stridor → incomplete <u>upper</u> airway obstruction
   c. Wheezing → incomplete <u>lower</u> airway obstruction
   d. Coughing → incomplete obstruction at the larynx or distal airways.

   <u>Note</u>: Cough is a presenting symptom in at least 80% of patients.

5. Consider a diagnosis of foreign body aspiration in a previously well child of the appropriate age who has a history of any of the following:
   a. A choking episode
   b. An acute bout of paroxysmal coughing
   c. Sudden onset of wheezing without an associated URI or past history of wheezing
   d. Persistent or recurrent pneumonia

6. The initial approach to the child who has aspirated a FB (example: a penny) and has no airway obstruction is to determine the location of the object. Although this can often be accomplished with plain x-rays or fluoroscopy, diagnostic laryngoscopy or bronchoscopy is sometimes required, especially when the object is small and radiolucent.
   a. PA and lateral CXRs can be used to distinguish a radiopaque FB in the esophagus from one in the trachea. In the <u>esophagus</u>, a flat FB (like a coin) lies in the frontal/coronal plane and appears round in the PA view. A <u>tracheal</u> FB is generally oriented in the sagittal plane and appears round in the <u>lateral</u> view.
   b. The PA and lateral CXRs may also show indirect signs of the presence of an airway foreign body; complete bronchial obstruction produces resorption atelectasis distal to the site of obstruction and pulmonary infiltrates may be seen in the presence of an inflammatory reaction to a foreign body (particularly vegetable matter).
   c. The presence of a radiolucent foreign body that is <u>partially</u> obstructing a mainstem bronchus can be demonstrated on an expiratory film or bilateral decubitus CXRs (in the young uncooperative child). These views accentuate the "ball valve" effect of a partially obstructing foreign body, thereby producing <u>hyperinflation</u> of the obstructed lung (due to air-trapping) and a shift of the mediastinum away from this side. **Review x-rays (expiratory and bilateral decubitus CXRs) that demonstrate air-trapping.**

7. Definitive management of a FB in the airway entails its removal in the operating room (under anesthesia) by laryngoscopy or rigid bronchoscopy.

- **Infections**

Croup and epiglottitis are the most important. You should know these "cold" for the exam. ***Look up the x-rays so that you know how to identify these entities on soft-tissue films.*** Examples can be found online at MedPix (Medical Image Database); look for a link on our website under "resources".

1. Croup (laryngotracheobronchitis)
   a. Clinical picture and epidemiology
      (1) Age group → usually 6 months to 3 yrs. (male predominance)
      (2) Organism → virus (most commonly parainfluenza virus)
      (3) Season → fall and winter (particularly October through December) when the causative viruses are most prevalent
      (4) Site of inflammation/obstruction → glottic and subglottic area
      (5) Prodrome → preceding viral URI of 2 to 3 days duration with a gradually increasing cough
      (6) Onset and progression → insidious (over days)
      (7) General appearance → nontoxic
   b. Signs and symptoms
      (1) Barking cough (worse at night)
      (2) Hoarse voice
      (3) Respiratory distress (tachypnea, dyspnea, retractions and stridor)
      (4) Nasal discharge
      (5) Fever is low-grade or absent
   c. Diagnosis
      (1) In children who present with the classic clinical picture and the characteristic barking, seal-like cough, the diagnosis can be made on clinical grounds alone.
      (2) When the presentation is less typical, x-rays can (when positive), confirm the diagnosis and R/O other causes of airway compromise (epiglottitis, foreign body aspiration, retropharyngeal abscess). These x-rays should be taken in the ED as portable studies.
      (3) Characteristic x-ray findings include:
         (a) PA CXR → subglottic narrowing of the tracheal air column ("steeple sign")
         (b) Soft tissue lateral of the neck → distended hypopharynx, normal epiglottis and normal retropharyngeal space
   d. Treatment
      (1) Cool mist*
      (2) Oxygen prn
      (3) Hydration (PO or IV)
      (4) Racemic epinephrine aerosol (0.5mL of a 2.25% solution diluted in 3mL of saline) — should be administered to patients with resting stridor and respiratory distress that is not relieved by the above measures.

---

*Use is personal preference, not evidence-based.

Note: Although evidence to support the phenomenon of "rebound" is lacking, children sick enough to receive racemic epinephrine should be observed in the ED for 3 - 4 hours following therapy to assure that they do not return to their pretreatment stridorous state once the effect of racemic epinephrine wears off.

    (5) Steroids (dexamethasone 0.15 - 0.6mg/kg IM, IV or PO as a one time dose) is beneficial for outpatient management.

  e. Admission criteria

    (1) Persistent stridor at rest

    (2) Inability to tolerate fluids

    (3) Unreliable social situation

    (4) Incomplete response to racemic epinephrine

    (5) Multiple doses of racemic epinephrine

    (6) Severe croup at presentation (even if responsive to therapeutic measures) particularly in children < 1 year of age due to the smaller diameter of the airway

2. Epiglottitis (supraglottitis) — a true emergency

  a. Clinical picture and epidemiology

    (1) Age group → any age, *including adults*; peak incidences occur in children 2 - 6 years old and adults 20 - 40 years old.

    (2) Organisms → since the introduction of the *H. influenza type B* (HIB) vaccine, *Strep. pneumonia* (and *pyogenes*) and *Staph aureus* have replaced HIB as the most common pathogens in pediatric epiglottitis. [Note: An association between *group A strep.* and varicella zoster virus infection leading to epiglottitis has been known for some time.]

    (3) Season → nonseasonal

    (4) Site of inflammation/obstruction → supraglottic tissues, i.e. the epiglottis, aryepiglottic folds and arytenoids in children; extension to the prevertebral soft tissues, valleculae, base of the tongue and/or soft palate may occur in adults.

    (5) Prodrome → usually none in children; however, adults will often experience a 1 - 2 day URI-like prodrome

    (6) Onset and progression → typically rapid (over hours) although adults infected with an organism other than HIB have a more insidious onset (HIB infection will cause an acute onset of symptoms with a severe clinical course and will most likely necessitate aggressive airway therapy...especially in children.)

    (7) General appearance → toxic

  b. Signs and symptoms

    (1) Patient is usually sitting in a tripod position with chin thrust forward and mouth open.

    (2) Muffled ("hot potato") voice

    (3) Sore throat with dysphagia and drooling

    (4) Respiratory distress (tachypnea, dyspnea and inspiratory stridor)

    (5) Tachycardia out of proportion to fever...or a high fever

    (6) Restlessness

Note: The diagnosis may be missed in some adults who have a more benign clinical presentation, i.e. sore throat and dysphagia without evidence of acute distress...unless you think of the possibility.

c. Diagnosis

(1) Is ideally confirmed in the OR (under controlled conditions) when the swollen cherry-red epiglottis is visualized. This is particularly true in the case of patients in severe respiratory distress; they should <u>not</u> be disturbed for the purpose of x-ray evaluation and attempts to visualize the epiglottis in the ED should be avoided.

(2) In less severe cases, diagnosis may be confirmed with a lateral soft-tissue x-ray of the neck that demonstrates the classic finding of an enlarged "thumbprint-like" epiglottis. The x-ray should be <u>portable</u>; if this is not feasible, someone skilled in airway management must accompany the patient to the x-ray suite with bag-valve-mask, intubation and other invasive airway equipment.

(3) In cooperative patients with <u>mild to moderate</u> symptoms and a <u>negative</u> lateral neck x-ray,[*] careful direct visualization of the epiglottis may be performed to resolve the problem of false negative results on lateral neck x-rays in patients with early epiglottitis. It is unlikely that this procedure will trigger acute airway obstruction in these patients. If direct inspection of the airway is not feasible, CT may be of value but should only be done in patients without airway distress.

d. Treatment

(1) Avoid agitation of the patient; allow him to assume a position of comfort and remain in the company of his family.

(2) Provide supplemental humidified oxygen.

(3) Set up airway stabilization equipment at bedside.

(4) Obtain immediate ENT and anesthesia consultations.

(5) Following airway stabilization by consultants, draw appropriate lab work, start an IV and initiate hydration and antibiotics. Acceptable antibiotics include a second <u>or</u> third generation cephalosporin (cefuroxime, cefotaxime, ceftriaxone) <u>or</u> ampicillin-sulbactam.

(6) Admit to ICU setting.

Note: If *H. flu* type b is isolated, household contacts require prophylaxis with rifampin, particularly if there is an unvaccinated child $\leq$ 4 years old in the contact group.

3. Bacterial tracheitis (membranous laryngotracheobronchitis) — a rare, but life-threatening, bacterial infection of the subglottic region that is characterized by copious tracheal secretions. It is often superimposed upon a viral URI and has features of both croup and epiglottitis (as well as inflammation).

[*]This study has only a 40% sensitivity and 75% specificity for epiglottitis.

a. Clinical picture and epidemiology
   (1) Age group → 3 months to 10 years
   (2) Organism → most commonly *Staph. aureus*; others include:
       (a) *H. influenza*
       (b) *S. pyogenes*
       (c) *Moraxella catarrhalis*
   (3) Season → nonseasonal
   (4) Prodrome → preceding viral URI or croup symptoms of several days duration
   (5) Onset and progress → hours to days; once bacterial superinfection occurs, progression occurs rapidly (over hours).
   (6) General appearance → toxic

b. Signs and symptoms
   (1) Barking cough (present in 50% of cases)
   (2) Respiratory distress (stridor and retractions)
   (3) High fever

c. Diagnosis
   (1) Suspect this diagnosis when a child with symptoms of viral croup becomes acutely more toxic, develops a high fever and has progressive respiratory distress that is unresponsive to usual croup management.
   (2) Direct laryngotracheobronchoscopy confirms the diagnosis. It is performed by ENT in the controlled setting of the OR and reveals pseudomembranes and purulent secretions. Removal of this debris via suctioning helps prevent airway obstruction.

d. Treatment
   (1) Provide supplemental humidified oxygen.
   (2) Obtain immediate ENT and anesthesia consultations.
   (3) Following airway suctioning and stabilization by consultants, obtain appropriate lab work (including Gram stain and culture of trachea), hydrate with IV fluids and administer antibiotics effective against *Staph. aureus*. Acceptable choices include IV nafcillin, methicillin or oxacillin plus ceftriaxone or another third-generation cephalosporin.
   (4) Admit to ICU setting.

ORAL AND PHARYNGEAL INFECTIONS

Infections can occur throughout the mouth and throat, and can range from minor localized infections to deep and spreading infections that may lead to airway compromise and other complications.

I.   **Oral Infections – can occur in and around the teeth as well as in the facial spaces.**

A.   *Masticator Space Abscess*

1.   The masticator space is the area bounded by muscles of mastication (the masseter and internal pterygoid muscles).

2.   Infection is secondary, resulting from extension of an anterior space infection (buccal, sublingual or submandibular spaces) or from an infection around the third molar.

3.   Causative organisms — streptococci and anaerobes

4.   Signs/symptoms include lateral facial swelling with pain, fever and trismus.

5.   Treatment
     a.   IV antibiotics (PCN or clindamycin are the drugs of choice.)
     b.   Emergent ENT consultation
     c.   Admission

B.   *Ludwig's Angina* – a progressive cellulitis of the floor of the mouth. The submandibular, sublingual and submaxillary spaces are involved bilaterally producing massive swelling that can result in airway obstruction (33% of cases). Common precipitants include an abscess of (or trauma to) the posterior mandibular molars.

1.   Causative organisms — these infections are typically caused by a combination of anaerobic (Bacteroides species) and aerobic (*Strep.*, *Staph.*) oral flora.

2.   Signs and symptoms include: dysphagia, odynophagia, dysphonia, trismus, drooling, neck and sublingual pain, massive swelling of the floor of the mouth and anterior neck that is brawny in character, fever and an elevated tongue.

3.   Treatment
     a.   If possible, allow the patient to maintain a sitting position; supine positioning can result in sudden airway obstruction.
     b.   Set up definitive airway management equipment at bedside; the most frequent cause of death in these patients is asphyxiation.
     c.   Obtain immediate ENT consultation.
     d.   Administer parenteral antibiotics (PCN + metronidazole, cefoxitin clindamycin, ampicillin-sulbactam or ticarcillin/clavulanate).
     e.   Admit to ICU.

4. Complications include:
    a. Airway compromise
    b. Extension of infection into the deeper layers of the neck or into the thoracic cavity (mediastinitis, mediastinal abscess).

II. Pharyngeal Space Infections

Review soft tissue films of the neck with a radiologist. Ask him / her to teach you the normal size limits of the following spaces: peripharyngeal, peritonsillar, retropharyngeal and prevertebral. Then look at films that demonstrate infection or abscess formation in these spaces.

A. *Peripharyngeal Abscess* — occurs in the space lateral to the pharynx and medial to the masticator space. This space (which is also referred to as the lateral pharyngeal or pharyngomaxillary space) extends from the base of the skull to the hyoid bone. Common precipitants of abscesses in this region are dental, pharyngeal and tonsillar infections.

1. Causative organisms — these infections are typically caused by a combination of anaerobes and aerobes; the specific organisms isolated reflect the original site of infection.

2. Signs and symptoms include: neck pain, sore throat, dysphagia, odynophagia, <u>unilateral</u> swelling of the neck and angle of the mandible, restricted movement of the neck, torticollis, pharyngitis, bulging of the pharyngeal wall, drooling, cervical adenopathy and fever.

3. Treatment
    a. Emergency airway equipment set up at bedside
    b. Parenteral antibiotics (same as for Ludwig's angina)
    c. Emergent ENT consultation
    d. ICU admission

4. Complications include: airway obstruction, spread of infection into the surrounding spaces, cranial nerve neuropathies (IX-XII), carotid artery erosion and septic thrombosis of the internal jugular vein.

B. *Peritonsillar Abscess* – occurs between the tonsillar capsule and the superior constrictor muscle; it is usually the complication of untreated or partially treated suppurative tonsillitis and is most frequently seen in teenagers and young adults. Typically, the patient gives a history of a sore throat for two or more days that has worsened and localized to one side. If you are unable to visualize the abscess, CT and ultrasound can help identify it.

1. Causative organisms — This is usually a polymicrobial infection caused by a mixture of aerobes and anaerobes. *Group A beta-hemolytic Strep* is the predominant species. Other Strep species, *H. influenza type B*, *Staph*, *Bacteroides* and *Fusobacterium* species are less frequent pathogens.

2. Signs and symptoms:
   a. Sore throat
   b. Dysphagia and odynophagia → drooling
   c. Muffled ("hot potato") voice
   d. Inferior and medial displacement of the involved tonsil
   e. Deviation of the uvula to the opposite side
   f. Ipsilateral ear pain
   g. Trismus
   h. Fever
   i. Tender cervical adenopathy
   j. Foul breath odor

3. Treatment
   a. IV hydration
   b. Parenteral antibiotics (penicillin, ampicillin-sulbactam, clindamycin, cefoxitin or erythromycin)
   c. ENT consultation
   d. Abscess evacuation by needle aspiration or incision and drainage. While usually performed by the ENT consultant, needle aspiration may be performed by the ED physician if trained in the technique; I & D is performed by ENT. Gram stain and culture of aspirated fluid should be ordered.
   e. Discharge with close follow-up or admit as appropriate.
      (1) Following abscess evacuation, many patients have significant relief of their symptoms and may be discharged to home on oral antibiotics (amoxicillin-clavulanate, clindamycin or a second-generation cephalosporin). These patients should be followed up by ENT in 24 hours.
      (2) If the abscess cannot be drained or the patient remains symptomatic, appears toxic or cannot tolerate fluids, he should be admitted to ENT and continued on IV antibiotics.

C. *Retropharyngeal Abscess* — occurs in the space anterior to the prevertebral fascia and posterior to the pharynx and most commonly affects children 6 months to 3 years of age.

1. Causative organisms — *Staph. aureus*, *Group A Strep*. and anaerobes are the most common pathogens.

2. Clinical features include:
   a. Sore throat
   b. Dysphagia → refusal to eat and drooling
   c. Labored respirations and (sometimes) stridor
   d. Muffled voice
   e. Fever
   f. Unilateral bulging of the posterior pharyngeal wall
   g. Swelling of the anterolateral neck

      h. Tender anterior cervical adenopathy
      i. Systemic toxicity
      j. A preference for the supine position with the head and neck held in extension

Note: The presence of chest pain suggests that mediastinal extension has occurred.

3. X-ray evaluation
    a. A soft-tissue lateral film of the neck — is the initial study of choice. Supportive findings include widening of the retropharyngeal space with anterior displacement of the larynx and the presence of air or an air-fluid level in this space.
      (1) The normal width of the retropharyngeal space is less than 1/2 the width of the adjacent vertebral body.
      (2) The film must be taken during <u>inspiration</u> with neck in slight <u>extension</u>: the expiratory phase of respiration and neck flexion → buckling and redundancy of the retropharyngeal tissues → false positive result.
    b. CXR — to R/O mediastinitis
    c. CT or MRI of the neck and mediastinum — confirms the diagnosis and establishes the presence and extent of complications.

4. Treatment
    a. Airway stabilization equipment at bedside
    b. IV hydration
    c. Parenteral antibiotics
      (1) A penicillinase-resistant PCN + metronidazole <u>or</u>
      (2) Clindamycin <u>or</u>
      (3) Cefoxitin <u>or</u>
      (4) Ampicillin/sulbactum
    d. Emergent ENT consultation for I + D
    e. ICU admission

5. Complications — include airway obstruction, aspiration, invasion of contiguous structures (mediastinum, vessels) and sepsis.

D. ***Prevertebral Infection*** — occurs in the space between the prevertebral fascia and the cervical spine; it can be hard to differentiate from retropharyngeal infection except by patient age. It usually results from cervical osteomyelitis, i.e. Staph or TB. Clinical manifestations may include bulging of the pharynx (usually bilateral) and tenderness of the cervical spine on palpation. Lateral neck films revealing retropharyngeal swelling or osteomyelitis of the cervical spine are suggestive. CT, MRI or a cervical myelogram are needed to confirm the diagnosis. These patients require hospital admission, neurosurgical consultation and parenteral antibiotics.

PHARYNGITIS

Pharyngitis is an inflammation or infection of the mucous membranes of the oropharynx. Both noninfectious (trauma, irritant gas) and infectious (viral, bacterial, fungal) agents may be responsible. Patient complaints include dysphagia, sore throat, fever and cervical adenopathy. Airway compromise is a potential complication. In the Emergency Department, the work-up of pharyngitis is primarily aimed at the diagnosis of *group A beta-hemolytic Strep (GABHS)*; appropriate treatment of this infection limits its spread, decreases the incidence of suppurative complications, is effective in preventing rheumatic fever and it accelerates clinical recovery.

I. Trauma — pharyngeal injuries, foreign bodies and burns may present as pharyngitis

---

II. Irritant Inhalant — Many gases and vapors irritate the throat (chlorine, steam, smoke). Assess respiratory effort and oxygenation. The patient may need supplemental oxygen or intubation.

III. Viruses — are the <u>most frequent cause</u> of pharyngitis. Adenovirus, Epstein-Barr virus, influenza virus, parainfluenza virus, enteroviruses and herpes simplex virus are commonly implicated. These infections are usually self-limited and require only symptomatic treatment.

A. *Infectious Mononucleosis* — is caused by the Epstein-Barr virus (human herpes virus 4) and most commonly affects patients 10 - 25 years old. Patients classically present with sore throat, fever, malaise and fatigue. Abdominal pain and/or left shoulder pain (Kehr's sign), particularly if associated with dizziness, nausea and LUQ tenderness, suggests splenic rupture (a serious complication). Exam reveals an exudative pharyngitis and tender cervical adenopathy. <u>Posterior</u> cervical adenopathy is characteristic and helps distinguish infectious mononucleosis from other causes of pharyngitis. Enlargement of the spleen and liver is also common; splenic rupture may occur with minor trauma. Peripheral blood smear reveals a lymphocytosis (> 50%)

---

and an increase in the proportion of atypical lymphocytes (> 10%). A mono-spot test (heterophile antibody) confirms the diagnosis if positive. False negatives do occur, however, particularly in children less than 4 yrs. of age. Treatment is supportive, but steroids are indicated for those who develop complications such as impending airway obstruction, severe hemolytic anemia, thrombocytopenia or neurologic manifestations (e.g. encephalitis, Guillain-Barré syndrome). Patients should also be advised to avoid contact sports for at least a month.

B. *Herpes Simplex Pharyngitis* — most commonly affects young adults and may be the result of a primary infection or reactivation. It is characterized by the presence of grouped vesicles on an erythematous base. These lesions are exquisitely tender and subsequently erode to form superficial ulcers. Treatment in the immunocompromised patient is with acyclovir (which may also benefit immunocompetent patients, but is not yet established).

IV. Bacteria

A. *Diphtheria*

1. Etiology
   a. This is a rare but serious cause of pharyngitis that typically occurs secondary to noncompliance with the DPT immunizations. Spread is primarily by contact with respiratory secretions and the period of incubation is approximately one week.
   b. Morbidity is due to both infectious and toxic reactions.
      (1) Infectious invasion causes enough tissue necrosis to produce a pseudomembrane in the posterior pharynx which can progressively enlarge and lead to airway obstruction.
      (2) *Cornyebacterium diphtheriae* elaborates a powerful exotoxin that can cause widespread organ damage:
         (a) Myocarditis/AV Block/Endocarditis
         (b) Nephritis
         (c) Hepatitis
         (d) Neuritis with both bulbar and peripheral paralysis
            <u>1</u> The most commonly observed paralysis involves the intrinsic and extrinsic muscles of the eyes → ptosis and strabismus.
            <u>2</u> Involvement of the palate produces a change in voice quality and difficulty speaking. (The palate muscles are usually the first to become paralyzed).
            <u>3</u> Limb paralysis and loss of DTRs may also occur.

2. **Clinical Picture**
   The patient presents with acute onset of sore throat, fever and general malaise. He appears toxic and is tachycardic. His voice is hoarse, muffled or even absent. Physical exam reveals an exudative pharyngitis with a white to gray, closely adherent pseudomembrane, marked cervical adenopathy ("bull neck") and fetid breath ("dirty mouse" smell). A serosanguineous nasal discharge may also be present.

3. Lab findings
   a. CBC may show thrombocytopenia.
   b. Gram stain of pharyngeal swab specimen reveals gram-positive rods with clubbing.
   c. Culture on Loeffler's or tellurite media is positive.

4. Treatment
   a. ABC stabilization as indicated.
   b. Definitive treatment is aimed at both the bacteria and the exotoxin and should be initiated as soon as the diagnosis is suspected. Do not wait for a positive culture report:
      (1) Parenteral PCN or erythromycin <u>and</u>
      (2) Diphtheria antitoxin
   c. All patients should be hospitalized with respiratory isolation.
   d. Recommendations for close contacts
      (1) Asymptomatic, <u>immunized</u> contacts should be given a Td booster if more than 5 years have elapsed since their last dose.
      (2) Asymptomatic, <u>partially immunized</u> or <u>unimmunized</u> contacts must receive one dose of IM PCN (7 - 10 days of oral erythromycin may be used in the PCN-allergic patient) and begin the immunization series.

B. *Arcanobacterium (Corynebacterium) Hemolyticum* — produces a pharyngitis that can be clinically indistinguishable from that produced by *group A beta-hemolytic Strep (GABHS)*. It most commonly occurs in patients 10 - 30 years of age; an associated rash (scarlatiniform, urticarial, erythema multiforme) is present in the majority of cases. A membranous pharyngitis resembling that of diphtheria can also occur. The treatment of choice is erythromycin.

C. *Gonorrhea* — should be considered in adolescents and adults who engage in orogenital sex. When it occurs in young children, child sexual abuse should be suspected. Treatment is with ceftriaxone, ciprofloxacin or ofloxacin. If ceftriazone or cipro is used, a regimen that is effective against chlamydia (azithromycin, doxycycline) should also be prescribed since coinfection with this organism may be present. If oxflacin is used, single-dose therapy can be used since this drug is also effective against chlamydia.

D. *Mycoplasma and Chlamydia* — may be common causes of pharyngitis in adults. Treatment is with erythromycin, azithromycin or doxycycline.

E. Group A Beta-Hemolytic Streptococcus (GABHS) – is often seen in late winter, usually in patients under 20 yrs. of age in crowded living conditions. It is rare in children less than 3 yrs. old. Patients classically have fever, tender cervical adenopathy, exudative tonsillitis and no cough (Centor Criteria). Associated complaints of abdominal pain, vomiting and headache are common in children. Accurate diagnosis can only be made by culture. Rapid Strep screens are useful in conjunction with the Centor Criteria. Throat cultures are not routinely recommended. Treatment is with a 10-day course of oral PEN VK or, if compliance is a problem, a single IM dose of benzathine PCN. Erythromycin may be used in the PCN-allergic patient. First and second-generation cephalosporins (e.g. cephalexin, cefadroxil, cefaclor, cefuroxime axetil) and azithromycin are also very effective but are usually reserved for patients with recurrent infections. A single IM dose of dexamethasone (when given in conjunction with antibiotic therapy) has been shown to decrease the duration of symptoms and provide significant pain relief; it should be considered for patients with significant discomfort.

▲ Complications of *GABHS* are both suppurative and nonsuppurative; they include the following:
   a. Pharyngeal space infections (suppurative complication) —Appropriate antibiotic therapy of *GABHS* decreases the incidence of this complication.
   b. Glomerulonephritis (<u>non</u>suppurative complication) — Treatment of *GABHS* is <u>not</u> effective in preventing this complication. It results from prior pharyngeal <u>or</u> cutaneous infection with *GABHS*. Patients present after a latent period of 1.5 - 3 weeks with facial edema, decreased urinary output and dark, tea-colored urine. The most useful lab test for making this diagnosis is the U/A which reveals RBCs, WBCs and casts. Other lab findings include an elevated ESR, a mild normochromic anemia and hyperkalemia.
   c. Rheumatic fever (<u>non</u>suppurative complication) — Treatment of Strep pharyngitis within 9 days of infection prevents this complication. Patients usually present after a latent period of 2.5 - 5 wks. They initially complain of severe migratory joint pain. More than a third go on to develop carditis and valvular damage (mitral valve most commonly involved). Morbidity is most closely associated with this feature. The Jones Criteria (revised), listed below, are a combination of clinical and laboratory features used to establish the diagnosis of rheumatic fever:
      (1) Major - polyarthritis
                  - carditis
                  - chorea
                  - erythema marginatum (evanescent, erythematous, non-pruritic lesions found on the trunk and proximal extremities)
                  - subcutaneous nodules

(2) Minor   - fever
                  - arthralgias
                  - history of rheumatic fever or rheumatic heart disease
                  - laboratory findings: leukocytosis, ↑ESR, ↑CRP,
                                      ELISA pos. for GABHS,
                                      ↑PR interval on ECG

Evidence of a preceding GABH *Strep* infection (positive throat culture, ↑ASO titer, scarlet fever) plus the presence of 2 major (or 1 major and 2 minor criteria) make the diagnosis highly probable. PCN is the treatment of choice. Adjunctive therapy includes ASA or NSAIDs for arthritis and steroids for carditis.

F.   ***Group C and G Streptococci*** — may also cause pharyngitis and can result in the same suppurative complications as GABHS. They have also been linked with the development of scarlet fever and glomerulonephritis (non suppurative complications) but have not been shown to cause rheumatic fever. These infections are clinically indistinguishable from group A infections and should be managed in the same manner.

V.   **Fungi (Candida, Cryptococcus, Histoplasma)** — *can produce pharyngitis in immuno-compromised patients.*

Candida albicans overgrowth occurs most commonly in immunocompromised patients (e.g. HIV, chemotherapy, diabetes, chronic steroid use) and neonates. Physical exam reveals white, removable plaques on an erythematous base. Treatment is with nystatin swish & swallow or systemic fluconazole.

TEMPORAL ARTERITIS

I. Pathology

Temporal arteritis (also known as giant cell arteritis) is a segmental vasculitis involving one or more branches of the carotid artery. Commonly involved branches include the temporal artery, the ophthalmic artery and the posterior ciliary artery.

II. Typical Clinical Presentation

- Woman > 50 years of age (female to male ratio is 4:1)
- Temporal headache (often unilateral) is the most common symptom.
- Jaw claudication
- Polymyalgia rheumatica (a syndrome of aching, pain and stiffness) is present in 50% of patients.
- Constitutional symptoms (fever, night sweats, malaise, anorexia)
- Scalp tenderness
- Tender, thickened (and sometimes pulseless) temporal arteries
- Visual defects/loss (blurred or diminished vision, diplopia)
- Sudden, painless, monocular loss of vision (due to vascular occlusion of the ophthalmic or posterior ciliary artery with infarction of the optic nerve or retina) is the most serious complication; visual loss is usually permanent.

III. Diagnosis

- Clinical picture
- Markedly elevated sed rate (50 - 100mm/hr); elevated acute phase reactants (CRP)
- Mild anemia and a leukocytosis
- Temporal artery biopsy confirms the diagnosis in most cases (sensitivity of 95%); however, given the segmental nature of this disease process, false-negatives do occur. It should be performed within 1 - 2 days of the initiation of treatment since the histologic findings are rapidly reversed with steroid therapy.

IV. Treatment

- High-dose steroids (oral prednisone 60 - 80 mg/day or IV methylprednisolone 250mg Q 6hrs.) as soon as the diagnosis is suspected.
- NSAIDs for pain control.
- Emergent consultation with rheumatology, ophthalmology or neurology.
- Admission or discharge with close follow-up as appropriate. If the patient has an impending vascular complication (or is unable to care for herself), she should be admitted. Patients with less severe symptoms, who are able to care for themselves (and have an identified physician), may be discharged if close follow-up can be arranged for them.

Note: Temporal arteritis is also discussed in the Neurology chapter on p. 919 and in the Eye chapter on p. 1083.

FACIAL INFECTIONS

I. Sinusitis: an infection that is usually precipitated by an acute viral URI

A. *Definition* — An infection of the paranasal sinuses (ethmoid, maxillary, frontal or sphenoid). Maxillary sinusitis, either in isolation or in combination with ethmoid or frontal sinusitis, is the most common. Infection of the sphenoid sinuses is rare.

1. Acute sinusitis — infection < 3 weeks duration

2. Chronic sinusitis — infection > 3 months duration

B. *Pathophysiology* — sinusitis results from occlusion of the sinus ostia and is usually precipitated by a viral URI or allergic rhinitis; ostial obstruction → ideal culture medium in occluded sinus → secondary bacterial infection.

C. *Causative Organisms*

1. Acute sinusitis — nontypeable *H. influenza* and *Strep. pneumoniae* are the most common; others include *Strep. pyogenes*, *Staph. aureus* and *Moraxella (Branhamella) catarrhalis*.

2. Chronic sinusitis — predominantly anaerobes (> 50%)

D. *Signs and Symptoms*

1. Headache or facial pain in a distribution defined by the sinuses involved

2. Percussion tenderness over the involved sinus

3. Swollen erythematous nasal mucosa

4. Purulent yellow-green discharge

5. Low-grade fever

6. Partial or complete opacification of the sinus on transillumination

7. Nasal congestion

E. *Diagnosis* — In most instances, the diagnosis of acute sinusitis can be made on the basis of the history and physical exam findings alone. If the diagnosis is uncertain (or complications are suspected) imaging studies may be indicated. Options include:

1. Plain x-rays (Waters, Caldwell, submentovertex and lateral views)*

    a. Most useful in diagnosing maxillary and frontal sinusitis.

    b. Can confirm sinusitis but can<u>not</u> rule it out (especially ethmoid and sphenoid sinusitis)..

    c. Suggestive findings include sinus opacification, an air-fluid interface and ≥ 6mm of mucosal thickening.

2. CT of the sinuses

    a. Is the most sensitive technique and the "gold standard" for diagnosing sinus disease and its complications.

    b. Suggestive findings include sinus opacification, air-fluid levels, mucosal thickening ≥ 4mm and sinus wall displacement. [See MedPix (Medical Image Database) link on our website under "resources."]

F. *Treatment*

1. Topical decongestants (oxymetazoline or phenylephrine) for a maximum of 3 days to avoid rebound effect.

2. Oral decongestants (pseudoephedrine) for 2 - 4 weeks.

3. Antibiotic therapy — should be reserved for patients with mild to moderate sinusitis who do not respond to symptomatic treatment. For those with severe or persistent symptoms (>1 week) and specific findings of acute sinusitis (nasal discharge, facial pain or tenderness), amoxicillin or trimethoprim/sulfamethoxazole are favored by many as first-line agents. However, in regions with a high percentage of beta-lactamase-producing bacteria, a broad-spectrum agent should be selected: amoxicillin-clavulanate, a second or third generation cephalosporin (e.g. cefuroxime axetil, cefprozil, cefaclor, cefpodoxime, proxetil, loracarbef) or one of the newer macrolides (clarithromycin or azithromycin). Antibiotics should be continued for 10 - 14 days.

*Not recommended for diagnosis of uncomplicated sinusitis.

4. Adjunctive therapy

    a. Analgesics

    b. Mucolytics (e.g. guaifenesin)

    c. Local heat

G. Complications

1. Ethmoid sinusitis can lead to periorbital/orbital cellulitis and abscess formation (especially in children). Physical findings may include:
   a. Redness and swelling of the eyelid
   b. Chemosis
   c. Proptosis
   d. Limitation of extraocular muscle function
   e. Fever

2. Frontal sinusitis may extend anteriorly and posteriorly.
   a. If it extends to the anterior table of the frontal bone, it may produce osteomyelitis of the surrounding bone ("Pott's Puffy Tumor"). These patients present with a doughy-feeling, tender mass above their eye.
   b. If it extends to the posterior table of the frontal bone, it may cause osteomyelitis which can lead to:
      (1) Meningitis
      (2) Epidural abscess
      (3) Subdural empyema
      (4) Brain abscess

3. Sphenoid or ethmoid sinusitis can extend intracranially via the vascular or lymphatic channels of these sinuses, thus producing cavernous sinus thrombosis. Findings include:
   a. Proptosis
   b. Eyelid edema
   c. Dilatation of the episcleral veins
   d. Palsies of cranial nerves III - VI
   e. Venous engorgement of the fundus
   f. Decreased mental status
   g. High fever

Patients demonstrating these complications require admission, parenteral antibiotics and appropriate consultation.

II. Parotitis: an infection of the parotid gland that is caused by a virus (most commonly the mumps virus) or bacteria (usually *Staph. aureus*).

A. *Paramyxovirus ("mumps")*

1. Most commonly occurs in children 5 - 15 years of age in the winter and spring.

2. Incubation period is 12 - 25 days.

3. Characteristic clinical findings:
   a. Tender parotid swelling at the angle of the jaw (frequently bilateral).
   b. Low-grade fever, headache, malaise
   c. Clear saliva from the opening of Stensen's duct

4. Occasionally, the infection may involve:
   a. Gonads (epididymitis, orchitis)
   b. Meninges (meningoencephalitis)
   c. Pancreas (pancreatitis)

5. Treatment
   a. Hydration
   b. Analgesics
   c. Antipyretics

6. Infected individuals are contagious up to 6 days before to 9 days after the onset of parotid swelling.

B. *Suppurative Parotitis*

1. Most commonly occurs in elderly, debilitated or postoperative patients with decreased salivary flow due to drugs, dehydration or irradiation.

2. Causative organism — *Staph. aureus*

3. Characteristic clinical findings
   a. Tender parotid swelling (often unilateral)
   b. Trismus
   c. Purulent discharge from the opening of Stensen's duct
   d. Fever

4. Treatment
   a. An antistaphylococcal antibiotic
   b. Hydration
   c. Local heat
   d. Massage
   e. Sialogogues (sour candy, lemon juice)

III. Mastoiditis: a suppurative infection of the mastoid air cells.

A. *Etiology:* usually a complication of untreated or inadequately treated acute otitis media (especially if it is recurrent).

B. *Causative Organisms* – include *Strep. pneumoniae* (most frequent isolate), *H. influenzae*, *Strep. pyogenes* and *Staph. aureus*).

C. *Signs and Symptoms*

1. Otalgia/Otorrhea + fever

2. Headache/hearing loss

3. Outward and downward displacement of the pinna

4. Posterior auricular (mastoid) tenderness and inflammation

5. Abnormal TM (scarring, erythema, perforation)

D. *Potential Complications of Untreated Mastoiditis*

1. Osteitis

2. Labyrinthitis

3. Meningitis

4. Encephalitis

5. Brain abscess

6. Damage to facial nerve (VII)

E. *Radiographic Evaluation*

1. CT scan of the temporal bone — has replaced plain films; it confirms the diagnosis and identifies the presence of complications.

2. MRI — may be even more useful than CT, especially if intracranial complications are suspected, but is rarely readily available.

F. Treatment

1. Hospitalization

2. Parenteral antibiotics — a third-generation cephalosporin (such as ceftriaxone), ampicillin/sulbactam or a semisynthetic penicillin in combination with chloramphenicol.

3. Immediate ENT consultation regarding the possible need for surgical debridement (myringotomy drainage with tympanostomy tube placement or mastoidectomy).

4. Analgesia

FACIAL FRACTURES

In facial injuries, consider the possibility of concomitant cervical spine injury.

I. Mandibular Injuries

Hallmarks of mandibular dysfunction: limited opening or deviation on opening of the mouth, malocclusion, pain and trismus.

A. *Mandibular Fractures* – The mandible is the second most commonly fractured facial bone (nose is the first). Due to its ringlike structure, the mandible fractures in two or more places in 50% of cases (so don't stop looking after you have found the first fracture). The most common sites of fracture are the condyle, the body and the angle.

1. A dental panoramic view of the maxilla and mandible (Panorex) is the best study for diagnosing mandibular fractures. If Panorex cannot be done, standard x-rays of the mandible (PA, bilateral oblique and Towne's views) should be obtained. However, these films may miss subtle fractures and dental injuries. If a condylar fracture is suspected (but not apparent on standard x-rays) a CT of the condyles should be ordered.

2. Clinical findings
   a. Teeth that are angulated and sometimes avulsed → alveolar Fxs.
   b. Lateral crossbite → unilateral condylar fractures
   c. Displacement of the lower incisors, interruption of arch continuity → symphysis fractures
   d. Ecchymosis or hematoma of the floor of the mouth → highly suspicious for a mandibular fracture
   e. Anesthesia of the lower lip → injury of the inferior alveolar or mental nerve secondary to a mandibular fracture

3. Treatment
   a. Mandibular fractures require consultation with an ENT or oral surgeon for reduction and fixation. The time course involved (immediate or delayed) is determined by the specific injury, the presence of airway compromise and associated injuries.
      (1) Patients with open fractures[*] require antibiotics. Penicillin is the drug of choice. Other alternatives include clindamycin or a first-generation cephalosporin.
      (2) Patients with closed fractures that are nondisplaced may be discharged to home if there is no question of airway compromise. All subcondylar fractures and fractures in edentulous patients are considered "closed" unless accompanied by a laceration.

[*]Any fracture in the tooth-bearing region should be considered "open" because the periodontal ligament communicates with the oral cavity.

    b. Tetanus prophylaxis should be updated as needed.

    c. If discharged, the patient should be placed on a liquid diet and given adequate analgesia.

    d. Admission is required for patients with:

       (1) Airway compromise (early intubation is critical)

       (2) Excessive bleeding

       (3) Severely displaced fractures (impair swallowing)

       (4) Grossly infected fractures

       (5) Comorbid disease/disability (uncontrolled diabetes, elderly)

B. *Mandibular Dislocation* — can result from trauma, yawning or laughing. The jaw is locked open, (mandibular condyle is locked anterior to the articular eminence) and the patient has difficulty talking or swallowing. Bilateral dislocation will present with an anterior open bite; if the dislocation is unilateral, the jaw is displaced toward the unaffected side. *Be able to identify on x-ray.* The treatment is manual reduction with downward pressure applied to the posterior teeth to dislodge the condyle; the chin is then pressed posteriorly so that the condyle returns to the fossa. IV midazolam or diazepam may be required if significant muscle spasm is present. X-ray evaluation to R/O fracture should be obtained prior to manipulation if the dislocation is trauma related. Following reduction, the patient should be placed on a soft diet, advised to avoid opening the mouth widely and referred to an oral surgeon for follow-up. A muscle relaxant + NSAID should also be prescribed.

C. *Temporomandibular Joint (TMJ) Dysfunction* — Patients typically complain of dull, aching unilateral pain in the region of the TMJ that worsens as the day progresses. Referred ear pain is also common. On exam, there is pain on palpation of the TMJ joint and the muscles of mastication (masseter and internal pterygoid muscles). Palpable spasm of these muscles, and a limited ability to open the mouth widely, may also be present. Treatment consists of NSAIDs, a muscle relaxant and referral to a dentist (with a specialty in TMJ disorders) for a bite splint. Warm moist heat to the area, limited jaw movement and a soft diet are also helpful.

II. Midfacial Fractures

This area includes the occlusal teeth up to the lateral canthus of the eye. Check these patients for CSF rhinorrhea with a dexistick reagent strip or send a fluid sample to the lab for glucose analysis.

A. *Isolated Zygomatic Arch Fractures* — If depressed, the cheek may be flattened and opening of the mouth may be painful or limited. These fractures are best visualized on the submental-vertex ("jug-handle") view. Treatment is generally delayed until facial swelling has resolved. Surgical elevation and wiring are indicated for compromised mandibular excursion and unacceptable cosmesis.

B. *Zygomatic-Maxillary Complex ("tripod") Fractures* — generally result from a blow to the cheek and involve fractures at three sites: the zygomatic arch, zygomaticofrontal suture and infraorbital foramen. Fracture of the lateral wall of the maxillary sinus is also invariably present. Clinical findings include flattening of the cheek (if seen early), periorbital swelling and ecchymosis, diplopia, a palpable step-off deformity of the inferior orbital rim and anesthesia of the cheek, upper teeth, lip and gum. On plain films, the best views for demonstrating these fractures are the Waters and submental vertex views. However, coronal CT scanning is replacing plain films in the evaluation of all facial fractures. Treatment consists of controlling bleeding and arranging appropriate consultation. In the absence of eye involvement, patients with these fractures can often be discharged to home with follow-up in 5 - 7 days. Adequate analgesia should be prescribed. Open reduction with wire fixation is required for open/displaced fractures.

C. *Orbital Floor Fractures* — may occur as isolated injuries resulting from blunt ocular trauma ("blowout" fracture) or as a component of a zygomatico-maxillary complex fracture. Orbital fat, bone and extraocular muscles may protrude into the maxillary sinus and become entrapped. Possible clinical findings include diplopia, enophthalmos, upward gaze palsy and hypesthesia of the infraorbital nerve. The best view for visualizing these fractures is the modified Waters view. CT scanning provides more detailed information, but is usually reserved for patients who might require surgery. All of these patients should be referred to ophthalmology for follow-up, and prophylactic antibiotics should be considered for patients with evidence of sinus involvement (subcutaneous emphysema, blood in the maxillary sinus). Persistent enophthalmos and muscle entrapment are indications for surgical repair. [*Be able to identify this fracture on x-ray.*]

Note: Further discussion of blowout fractures can be found in the Eye chapter on pp. 1089 - 1090 and in the Trauma chapter on pp. 487 - 488.

D. Maxillary Fractures

1. Result from massive, direct facial trauma, e.g. high-speed deceleration injuries and may result in airway compromise.

2. They are classified as follows:

    *   Le Fort I (palate-facial disjunction) — a horizontal fracture of the maxilla at the level of the nasal floor.

    *   Le Fort II (pyramidal disjunction) — includes fractures through the maxilla, nasal bones and infraorbital rim.

    *   Le Fort III (craniofacial disjunction) — involves fractures through the zygomaticofrontal suture or zygoma and the frontal bone above the nose.

3. Clinical clues include massive soft-tissue swelling, midfacial mobility, malocclusion and CSF rhinorrhea.

4. Plain films (Waters and lateral views) demonstrate these fractures and are helpful in making the initial diagnosis; however, CT of the facial bones is generally needed to delineate the extent and number of fractures as well as the presence of associated injuries..

5. Treatment includes: airway management, C-spine assessment (including associated neuro deficits), evaluation of the globe and administration of prophylactic antibiotics if the sinuses are involved with possible admission if surgical repair is indicated.

Note: Be able to recognize these fractures on x-ray. Online images of facial fractures can be found at MedPix™ and RadiologyEducation™.com (look for links on our website under "resources".) Also, the third edition of the Harwood-Nuss text has a nice picture on p. 470.

DENTAL EMERGENCIES

I. Neuroanatomy of the Face

Sensory innervation of the face and mouth is via the three branches of the trigeminal nerve (Cranial V): ophthalmic branch, maxillary branch and the mandibular branch. The detailed anatomy of these branches is somewhat complex (especially the maxillary branch). The schematics that follow have been over-simplified to facilitate the learning process. The sensory nerves that are starred (*) are those involved in nerve blocks.

A. Ophthalmic Branch of the Trigeminal Nerve

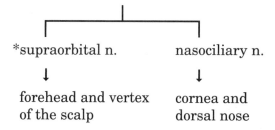

```
                    |
        +-----------+-----------+
        |                       |
  *supraorbital n.        nasociliary n.
        ↓                       ↓
  forehead and vertex     cornea and
  of the scalp            dorsal nose
```

B. Maxillary Branch of the Trigeminal Nerve

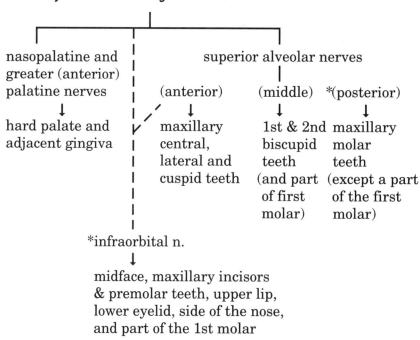

```
                              |
    +-------------------------+---------------------------+
    |                         |                           |
nasopalatine and             :          superior alveolar nerves
greater (anterior)           :                    |
palatine nerves              :        +-----------+-----------+
    ↓                        :    (anterior)  (middle)  *(posterior)
hard palate and              :        ↓          ↓          ↓
adjacent gingiva             :/    maxillary   1st & 2nd  maxillary
                             :     central,    biscupid   molar
                             :     lateral and teeth      teeth
                             :     cuspid teeth (and part (except a part
                             :                  of first   of the first
                             :                  molar)     molar)
                             :
              *infraorbital n.
                     ↓
          midface, maxillary incisors
          & premolar teeth, upper lip,
          lower eyelid, side of the nose,
          and part of the 1st molar
```

C. *Mandibular Branch of the Trigeminal Nerve*

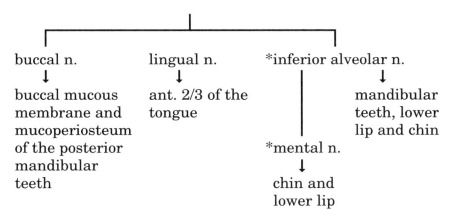

II. Facial and Oral Anesthesia

Intraoral local anesthesia can be achieved with dental syringes and prefilled carpules (1.8mL) of an anesthetic agent (usually Lidocaine or Marcaine). Unless contraindicated, a vasoconstrictor such as epinephrine (1:100,000) is generally combined with the anesthetic agent to prolong its duration of action.

A. *Nerve Blocks*

1. SUPRAORBITAL NERVE BLOCK → anesthesia to ipsilateral forehead/scalp

2. POSTERIOR SUPERIOR ALVEOLAR NERVE BLOCK → anesthesia to ipsilateral maxillary molars (except a portion of the first molar)

3. INFRAORBITAL NERVE BLOCK → anesthesia to the ipsilateral
    *   Midface
    *   Maxillary incisors
    *   Premolars
    *   Lower eyelid
    *   Upper lip
    *   Side of the nose
    *   Portion of the 1st molar

4. INFERIOR ALVEOLAR NERVE BLOCK → anesthesia to ipsilateral mandibular teeth, lower lip and chin

B. *Supraperiosteal Infiltrations*

1. Provide anesthesia to individual teeth.

2. Are used to perform MENTAL NERVE INFILTRATIONS which provide anesthesia to ipsilateral lower lip and chin. Bilateral mental infiltrations are required for midline lip lacerations.

C. Complications of Nerve Blocks

1. Neural injury

2. Vascular injection and spasm

3. Needle misplacement resulting in incomplete anesthesia or inadvertent anesthesia of other facial structures

4. Motor paralysis (if the facial nerve is punctured or injected)

5. Infections in peripharyngeal spaces (especially with INFERIOR ALVEOLAR NERVE BLOCK)

III. Anatomy of a Tooth

The tooth has two main portions: crown and root. Enamel covers the dentin which, in turn, covers the pulp (the neurovascular supply of the tooth). The tooth is embedded in the alveolar bone and held in place by cementum and a periodontal ligament. Sensory innervation of the teeth is via the anterior, middle and POSTERIOR SUPERIOR ALVEOLAR NERVES (maxillary teeth) and the INFERIOR ALVEOLAR NERVE (mandibular teeth).

IV. Dental Emergencies

A. Trauma

1. Tooth Fractures — management is determined by the extent of the fracture and the patient's age
   a. ELLIS I
      (1) Only the enamel is fractured; there is no pain or hot and/or cold sensitivity.
      (2) Treatment is elective (dentist).
   b. ELLIS II
      (1) The enamel is fractured and dentin is exposed; hot and/or cold sensitivity is often present.
      (2) Treatment
         (a) < 12 yrs. of age – apply a dressing of calcium hydroxide paste over the exposed dentin and cover it with aluminum foil or dental dry foil.
         (b) > 12 yrs. of age – a dressing can be placed on the tooth for comfort.
      (3) All patients should receive follow-up by a dentist within 24 hrs. and be advised to avoid temperature extremes in food and drink.

   c. ELLIS III: <u>This is a true dental emergency</u>.
     (1) The enamel is fractured and both dentin and pulp are exposed; a pink tinge or drop of blood on the fracture site is characteristic (indicates pulpal exposure); severe pain is common, but may be absent if the neurovascular supply of the tooth has been disrupted.
     (2) Immediate dental referral is indicated. If a dentist or endodontist is not immediately available, place a piece of moist cotton over the exposed pulp and cover with a piece of tin foil; tetanus immunization should be provided as needed.

2. Alveolar fractures
   a. May be evident (exposed bone) or diagnosed per x-ray (panorex).
   b. May be associated with dental fractures/avulsions/subluxations.
   c. Treatment
     (1) Immediate dental/oral surgery evaluation for reduction and fixation; wire stabilization is accomplished via the dentition.
     (2) Prophylactic antibiotics (PCN or a cephalosporin) and tetanus immunization (if indicated).

3. Avulsed tooth
   a. Permanent tooth
     (1) Holding the tooth by its crown, rinse it gently with saline and immediately replace it in the socket. Do not "brush" the tooth clean as this will remove the periodontal ligament.
     (2) Viability of the tooth decreases with length of time out of the socket.
     (3) Immediate dental referral for stabilization is indicated.
     (4) Prophylactic antibiotics (PCN or erythromycin) should be prescribed and tetanus immunization should be provided (if indicated).
    <u>Note</u>: If a tooth cannot be immediately reimplanted, the best storage and transplant medium is Hank's solution ("Save-A-Tooth"). Viability of the periodontal ligament can be maintained for 4 - 6 hrs. or more in this solution.
   b. Deciduous/primary tooth (children 6 months to 5 years of age) — should <u>not</u> be replaced since alveolar ankylosis may result. These patients should be referred to a pedodontist because space-maintaining procedures/appliances are sometimes required.

4. Intraoral lacerations
   a. Close with absorbable sutures.
   b. Recheck in 24 - 48 hrs.
   c. Although controversial, antibiotic coverage (PCN or erythromycin), is recommended by many, particularly if the wound is extensive or involves significant amounts of crushed tissue.

B. *Hemorrhage* — may be due to one of the following:

1. Trauma

2. Recent dental manipulation (cleaning, extraction, etc.)

3. Gingivitis

4. Blood dyscrasias or coagulopathies

C. *Orofacial Pain*

1. Dental Pain
   a. Tooth eruption in adults
      (1) Usually involves the third molars ("wisdom teeth").
      (2) If the gingivae are inflamed (pericoronitis), instruct the patient to irrigate the area with warm saline or hydrogen peroxide.
      (3) If fluctuance and pus are present (pericoronal abscess), perform a superficial incision and drainage and place the patient on an antibiotic (PEN-VK or clindamycin).
      (4) Refer these patients to an oral surgeon for definitive treatment (extraction).
   b. Dental caries
      (1) Oral analgesia and dental referral are usually all that is needed.
      (2) Suspect an associated periapical abscess if the patient complains of sharp, severe pain on tooth percussion, especially if the tooth is sensitive to hot or cold. A fluctuant swelling requires incision and drainage, an antibiotic and warm saline rinses every two hours. The patient should be seen by a dentist within 24 hours.
   c. Postextraction pain
      (1) Periostitis
         (a) Pain within 24 hours of extraction
         (b) Responds well to oral analgesics
      (2) Alveolar osteitis ("dry socket")
         (a) Is due to loss of clot plus localized osteomyelitis.
         (b) Clinical presentation: history of a pain-free interval of 2 - 4 days postextraction followed by sudden onset of excruciating pain unrelieved by analgesics and a foul breath odor.
         (c) Treatment
            <u>1</u> Anesthetic nerve block
            <u>2</u> Irrigation of the socket
            <u>3</u> Packing with iodoform gauze saturated with a medicated dental paste (such as Bipps or "Sed-a-Dent"), eugenol or Campho-Phenique – placement of the packing provides almost immediate relief.
            <u>4</u> Dental follow-up in 12 - 24 hours
   d. Acute necrotizing ulcerative gingivostomatitis ("Trench mouth")
      (1) ANUG is the only periodontal lesion in which bacteria actually invade <u>non</u>necrotic tissue.
      (2) It is caused by Fusobacteria and spirochetes.

(3) Clinical presentation
    (a) The patient complains of pain, a metallic taste and foul breath which is frequently accompanied by fever, malaise and regional lymphadenopathy.
    (b) Gingivae are swollen and fiery red; the interdental papillae (tissue between the teeth) are swollen, ulcerated (or "punched out") and covered with a grayish pseudomembrane.
(4) Treatment
    (a) Warm saline irrigation + hexadine rinse
    (b) Antibiotic (PCN, erythromycin or clindamycin) for patients with fever and lymphadenopathy — provides dramatic relief within 24 hours.
    (c) Systemic analgesics and topical local anesthetic agents can provide the patient sufficient relief to use warm saline rinses, as well as eat and drink.
    (d) Dental follow-up is required; a potential complication is the destruction of underlying alveolar bone.

2. Other causes of facial pain
- Sinusitis
- Trigeminal neuralgia ("tic-douloureux")
- Herpes zoster
- Ischemic heart disease
- TMJ disease
- Temporal arteritis
- Cluster headache

D. Systemic Diseases with Oral Manifestations

1. Infections
  a. Herpes
  b. Coxsackie virus
  c. Gonococcus
  d. Syphilis

2. Inflammatory states
  a. Systemic Lupus Erythematosus (SLE) — large intraoral ulcerations with necrotic borders.
  b. Reiter's Syndrome (urethritis, arthritis, conjunctivitis, oral ulcers)
  c. Sjogren's Syndrome
    (1) An autoimmune disease characterized by diminished secretion of the lacrimal and salivary glands.
    (2) Symptoms include a gritty sensation of the eyes, dry mouth (xerostomia) and diminished sense of taste.

3. Toxic/metabolic states
   a. Heavy metal poisoning
      (1) Gingival "lead line" in lead poisoning
      (2) Argyria: a blue to bronze discoloration of the oral mucosa in silver poisoning
   b. Gingival hyperplasia
      (1) Diabetes mellitus
      (2) Phenytoin ⌐ not related to toxicity; may be secondary to alter-
      (3) Nifedipine ⌐ ation of calcium metabolism.

4. Granulomatous diseases
   a. Tuberculosis – granulomatous ulcerations of the oral cavity
   b. Wegener's granulomatosis — gingival hyperplasia with petechiae

5. Benign tumors and tumor-like lesions
   a. Pyogenic granuloma
      (1) A proliferation of capillary-rich connective tissue that develops mostly on the lips and gingiva and commonly occurs secondary to trauma
      (2) Particularly common during pregnancy ("pregnancy tumor")
   b. Epidermoid cyst

6. Blood dyscrasias
   a. Acute leukemia: a marked hyperplastic gingivitis (almost covers the teeth) that has a bluish-red discoloration.
   b. Thrombocytopenic purpura
      (1) Petechiae of the oral mucosa
      (2) Spontaneous gingival bleeding

7. HIV/AIDS
   a. Oropharyngeal candidiasis
      (1) Painless curd-like plaques on an erythematous base that are easily removed with a tongue blade
      (2) Frequently one of the earliest manifestations of AIDS
   b. Hairy leukoplakia
      (1) Asymptomatic white patches with hair-like projections; most commonly located on the lateral aspect of the tongue; cannot be removed with a tongue blade
      (2) Believed to be associated with the Epstein-Barr virus (EBV)
      (3) 80% of patients presenting with these lesions go on to develop AIDS within the ensuing 3 years.
   c. Oral Kaposi's sarcoma
      (1) Flat bluish-red lesions with irregular borders; most commonly found on the hard palate, but can be located anywhere in the mouth
      (2) Most common AIDS - related malignancy

Journal References

AM FAM PHYSICIAN, Douglass, A.B., Douglass, J.M., 2003, 67:511-516, "Common Dental Emergencies."

AM FAM PHYSICIAN, Knutson, D., Aring, A., 2004, 69:535-540, "Viral Croup."

AM FAM PHYSICIAN, Sander, R., 2001, 63:927-936, 941-922, "Otitis Externa: A Practical Guide to Treatment and Prevention."

ANN EMER MED., Cooper, R.J., Hoffman J.R., Bartlett, J.G., Besser, R.E., Gonzales, R., Hickner, J.M., Sande, M.A., 2001, 37:711-719, "Principles of Appropriate Antibiotic Use for Acute Pharyngitis in Adults: Background."

ANN INTERN MED, Snow, V., et. al., 2001, 134: (495-497),"Position Paper: Principles of Appropriate Antibiotic Use for Acute Sinusitis in Adults."

ARCH. PEDIATR ADOLESC MED, Heikkinen, Terho, and Olli Ruuskanen, January 1995, "Signs and Symptoms Predicting Acute Otitis Media."

CLINIC INFECT DIS, Bernstein, T., Brilli, R., Jacobs, B., 1998, 27:458-462 "Is Bacterial Tracheitis Changing? A 14-Month Experience in a Pediatric Intensive Care Unit."

CLINIC INFECT DIS, Bisno, A. L., et. al., September 1997, "Diagnosis and Management of Group A Streptococcal Pharyngitis: A Practice Guideline." (in Emer. Med Abstracts, 1998)

DEN TRAUMATOL, Flores, M.T., 2002, 18:287-298, "Traumatic Injuries in the Primary Dentition."

EMERGENCY MEDICINE, Stewart, C., March 2001, "Recognizing the Potential Danger of Supra-glottitis."

EMERGENCY MEDICINE NEWS, Roberts, James R., August, 1995, "The Baffling Clinical Features of Streptococcal Pharyngitis."

EMERGENCY MEDICINE NEWS, Roberts, James R., September 1995, "Pharyngitis: The Value of Laboratory Testing."

EMERGENCY MEDICINE NEWS, Roberts, James R., October 1995, "Acute Pharyngitis: How Effective is Therapy?"

EMERGENCY MEDICINE NEWS, Roberts, James R., November 1995, "Treatment of Strep Throat: Penicillin."

EMERGENCY MEDICINE NEWS, Roberts, James R., December 1995, "Strep Throat: Alternate Therapies and Symptomatic Relief."

EMERGENCY MEDICINE NEWS, Roberts, James R., January 1996, "Symptomatic Treatment of Acute Pharyngitis."

EMERGENCY MEDICINE REPORTS, Bosker, G., 1998, "Antibiotic Selection in Acute Otitis Media: Treatment Guidelines and Management Pathways for Optimizing Clinical Outcomes." (Critical Pathways in Pediatric Emergency Medicine)

EMERGENCY MEDICINE REPORTS, Camp, J.H., and Stewart, C., May 1995, "Dental Trauma: Diagnostic Considerations, Emergency Procedures, and Definitive Management."

EMERGENCY MEDICINE REPORTS, Cohn, Arnold M. and Terry L. Donat, January 23, 1995, "The Challenging Spectrum of Sinusitis and Its Dreaded Complication: Current Diagnostic Strategies, Management Approaches and Therapeutic Guidelines."

EMERGENCY MEDICINE REPORTS, Colucciello, S.A., April 1995, "The Treacherous and Complex Spectrum of Maxillofacial Trauma: Etiologies, Evaluation, and Emergency Stabilization."

EMERGENCY MEDICINE REPORTS, Hals, Gary and Michael Sayre, February 5, 1995, "The Difficult Airway: Access, Intervention and Stabilization Part I: Step-by-Step Techniques for Advanced Clinical Management."

EMERGENCY MEDICINE REPORTS, Hals, Gary and Michael Sayre, February 19, 1996, "The Difficult Airway: Targeting Clinical Applications, Part II: Indications and Contraindications for Intubation and Invasive Management."

EMERGENCY MEDICINE REPORTS, Karras, D. J., May 1996, "Managing Otitis Media in Children."

EMERGENCY MEDICINE REPORTS, Ponder, M., and Cydulka, R. K., December 1996, "Inflammatory Conditions of the Head and Neck."

HOSPITAL PHYSICIAN, Liang, B. C., September 1996, "Neurologic Manifestations of Giant Cell (Temporal) Arteritis."

LANCET, Rovers, M.M., Schilder, A.G., Zielhuis, G.A., Rosenfeld, R.M., 2004, 363:465-473, "Otitis Media."

LANCET INFECT DIS, Rubin Grandis, J., Branstetter, B.F., Yu, V.L., 2004, 4:34-39, "The Changing Face of Malignant (Necrotising) External Otitis: Clinical, Radiological, and Anatomic Correlations."

MAYO CLIN PROCEEDINGS, Swanson, J.A., and Hoecker, J.L., February 1996, "Concise Review for Primary-Care Physicians."

OTOLARYNGOL HEAD NECK SURG, Johnson, R.F., Stewart, M.G., Wright, C.C., 2003, 128:332-343, "An Evidence-Based Review of the Treatment of Peritonsillar Abscess."

PEDIATRIC EMERGENCY MEDICINE REPORTS, Bosker, G., February, 1997, "Otitis Media in Children: Antimicrobial Strategies for Overcoming Barriers to Clinical Cure."

PEDIATR INFECT DIS, Shulman, S. T., et. al., January 1994, "Streptococcal Pharyngitis: The Case for Penicillin Therapy." (in Emer. Med. Abstracts, 1994)

PEDIATR INFECT DIS, McMillan, J. A., April 1993, "Pharyngitis Associated with Herpes Simplex Virus in College Students." (in Emer. Med. Abstracts, 1993)

PEDIATRICS, 2001, 108: 798-808, "Clinical Practice Guideline: Management of Sinusitis."

PEDIATRICS, Craig, F.W., Schunk, J.E., 2003, 111: 1394-1398, "Retropharyngeal Abscess in Children: Clinical Presentation, Utility of Imaging, and Current Management."

PEDIATRICS, McCormick, D.P., Saeed, K.A., Pittman, C., Baldwin, C.D., Friedman, N., Teichgraeber, D.C., Chonmaitree, T., 2003, 112: 982-986, "Bullous Myringitis: A Case-Control Study".

SYMPOSIA MONITOR, Avant, Robert F. and David W. Kennedy, Co-Chairs, September 1990, "First-line Management of Sinusitis: A National Problem?"

Specific Text References

Atlas of Emergency Medicine. Knoop, K. J., et. al., First Edition, (McGraw-Hill, 1997).

CDC Manual for the Surveillance of Vaccine-Preventable Diseases. 1999 Edition.

Ear, Nose and Throat Disorders in Primary Care. Woodson, G. E., (W. B. Saunders Company, 2001).

Fractures and Dislocations - Closed Management. Connolly, J. F., Volume 1, (Philadelphia, Pennsylvania 1995).

Oral and Maxillofacial Surgery. Fonseca, R. J., First Edition, (W. B. Saunders Company, 1997).

Oral and Maxillofacial Surgery. Fonseca, R. J., Second Edition, (W. B. Saunders Company, 2000).

Otolaryngology-Head and Neck Surgery. Cummings, C. W., Third Edition, (Mosby Year Book, 1998).

Web and Other Sources

AGENCY FOR HEALTH CARE POLICY AND RESEARCH, Lau, J., et.al, Evidence Report/ Technology Assessment #9, "Diagnosis and Treatment of Acute Bacterial Rhinosinusitis."

ACEP/ASIM, Vol. 134, No. 6, 2001, "Principles of Appropriate Antibiotic Use for Acute Pharyngitis in Adults: Background." (position paper)

PRESCRIBER'S LETTER, Vol. 9, No. 828, August 28, 2002, "Infectious Diseases."

General Text References, Acep Clinical Policies and LLSA Reading Lists for all chapters located in the back of both volumes.

NOTES

NOTES

GASTROINTESTINAL EMERGENCIES

1. The most common cause(s) of oropharyngeal (transfer) dysphagia is/are:

   (a) Obstructive lesions
   (b) Spasm
   (c) Neuromuscular disorders and inflammatory lesions
   (d) Carcinoma

2. All of the following statements regarding Boerhaave's Syndrome are accurate except:

   (a) It is usually the result of sudden, violent, repeated vomiting.
   (b) It is a partial thickness tear of the esophageal wall.
   (c) Physical findings associated with this entity include subcutaneous emphysema and the presence of a mediastinal crunch (Hamman's sound).
   (d) X-ray findings may include a left pneumothorax, a left pleural effusion, mediastinal emphysema and a widened mediastinum.

3. The most common area for an esophageal foreign body to lodge in an adult is the:

   (a) Aortic arch (T_4)
   (b) Cricopharyngeal muscle (C_6)
   (c) Lower esophageal sphincter/diaphragmatic hiatus (T_{10} - T_{11})
   (d) Tracheal bifurcation (T_6)

4. Which of the following is the most appropriate therapy for a button battery lodged in the esophagus?

   (a) Observation
   (b) Removal with a Foley catheter
   (c) IV glucagon
   (d) Removal via endoscopy

5. What is the most likely diagnosis in patients with abdominal pain that awakens them at night and is relieved by food intake and ingestion of antacids?

   (a) Duodenal ulcer
   (b) Myocardial ischemia
   (c) Gastric ulcer
   (d) Perforated peptic ulcer

6. All of the following statements regarding stress ulcers are true except:

   (a) They are best diagnosed with an upper GI.
   (b) They are more superficial than peptic ulcers.
   (c) They are generally located in the body and fundus of the stomach.
   (d) They are referred to as Cushing's or Curling's ulcers.

7. Factors which have definitely been demonstrated to predispose people to peptic ulcer disease include all of the following except:

    (a) Alcohol ingestion
    (b) Cigarette smoking
    (c) Type O blood
    (d) Use of NSAIDs or ASA

8. Which of the following statements regarding sucralfate is accurate?

    (a) It neutralizes gastric acid.
    (b) It works most effectively at a gastric pH of 4.5.
    (c) It inhibits secretion of mucus.
    (d) It inhibits pepsin, adsorbs bile acids and increases mucosal prostaglandin production.

9. The most common cause of small bowel obstruction is:

    (a) Neoplasms
    (b) Hernias
    (c) Adhesions
    (d) Gallstones

10. All of the following statements regarding volvulus are accurate except:

    (a) Although cecal volvulus can occur at any age, it most commonly affects patients in their twenties and thirties.
    (b) Volvulus is an example of a closed loop obstruction.
    (c) Sigmoid volvulus occurs in patients with a history of chronic, severe constipation; it primarily affects elderly, bedridden patients with significant comorbid disease and psychiatric patients of any age.
    (d) Cecal volvulus occurs more commonly than sigmoid volvulus.

11. The following statements regarding ulcerative colitis are accurate except:

    (a) Inflammation involves all layers of bowel as well as the mesenteric lymph nodes.
    (b) There is a much higher incidence of colon cancer in patients with ulcerative colitis than in the general population.
    (c) It is characterized clinically by bloody stools associated with crampy abdominal pain.
    (d) Complications include intestinal hemorrhage and toxic megacolon.

12. Unlike small bowel obstruction due to other causes, an important therapeutic modality in the treatment of small bowel obstruction due to Crohn's disease is:

    (a) Administration of antibiotics
    (b) NG suction
    (c) Administration of steroids
    (d) IV hydration and correction of electrolyte imbalance

13. All of the following statements regarding pseudomembranous colitis are accurate except:

    (a) It is due to ingestion of broad-spectrum antibiotics (such as the cephalosporins or ampicillin) which alter the gut flora.
    (b) Although they may be delayed, symptoms usually begin within 7 - 10 days following the initiation of a course of antibiotics.
    (c) Diagnosis is confirmed by culturing the stool for Clostridium difficile.
    (d) Effective therapeutic agents include oral metronidazole and oral vancomycin.

14. A patient presents with the complaint of slight hematochezia and intense rectal pain with bowel movements that lingers for several hours and then resolves. The most likely diagnosis is:

    (a) Internal hemorrhoids
    (b) Anal fissure
    (c) Thrombosed external hemorrhoid
    (d) Perirectal abscess

15. A patient presents to the Emergency Department complaining of frothy, foul-smelling diarrhea and abdominal pain. He says he feels bloated and has a lot of gas. Nine days ago he returned from a hiking trip in Colorado where he had been drinking water from streams. The most likely cause of his diarrhea is:

    (a) *Giardia lamblia*
    (b) *Vibrio parahemolyticus*
    (c) *Aeromonas hydrophilia*
    (d) *Vibrio cholera*

16. With the exception of _____, the primary mechanism by which the following bacteria induce illness is by excretion of a toxin.

    (a) *Staphylococcus aureus*
    (b) *Bacillus cereus*
    (c) *Clostridium difficile*
    (d) *Yersinia enterocolitis*

17. An adolescent presents with fever, crampy abdominal pain and watery diarrhea. Physical exam reveals exquisite RLQ tenderness and a wet mount of the stool reveals WBCs. The most likely organism responsible for this presentation is:

    (a) *Yersinia enterocolitica*
    (b) *Shigella*
    (c) *Clostridium perfringens*
    (d) *Vibrio parahemolyticus*

18. The organism most often responsible for Traveler's diarrhea is:

    (a) Salmonella
    (b) Invasive *E. coli*
    (c) *Giardia lamblia*
    (d) *Enterotoxigenic E. coli*

19. Staining of the stool for leukocytes is helpful in uncovering the probable cause of an acute episode of diarrhea as well as determining appropriate therapy, particularly when this information is combined with a detailed history. Leukocytes are typically present with infections induced by all of the following organisms except:

    (a) *Clostridium difficile*
    (b) Viruses
    (c) Invasive *E. coli*
    (d) Salmonella

20. All of the following statements regarding Scombroid fish poisoning are accurate except:

    (a) It is most commonly associated with ingestion of dark-fleshed or red-muscled fish.
    (b) It results from ingestion of toxins with histamine-like properties that form in improperly preserved or refrigerated fish.
    (c) There is no specific effective treatment.
    (d) Symptoms include facial flushing, conjunctival hyperemia, palpitations, nausea, vomiting and diarrhea.

21. The most common cause of post-transfusion hepatitis is:

    (a) Hepatitis A
    (b) Hepatitis B
    (c) Hepatitis C
    (d) Hepatitis D

22. During the "window period" between the disappearance of HB_sAg and the appearance of anti-HB_s, the only marker of Hepatitis B infection that may be present in the serum is:

    (a) HB_eAg
    (b) Anti-HB_e
    (c) Anti-HB_c
    (d) HB_cAg

23. The presence of anti-HB_s in the serum indicates:

    (a) Ongoing viral replication and high infectivity
    (b) Immunity
    (c) The carrier state
    (d) Low infectivity

24. The presence of marked eosinophilia is typical in patients infected with:
    (a) *Necator americanus*
    (b) *Enterobius vermicularis*
    (c) *Giardia lamblia*
    (d) All of the above

25. A 50-year-old male with a history of chronic alcoholism presents with hema-temesis. The bleeding followed an episode of violent and repeated vomiting. It was moderate in quantity and associated with pain on swallowing, but has resolved on its own. The diagnostic study of choice for evaluating this patient is:
    (a) A CXR
    (b) A barium esophagogram
    (c) A CT of the chest
    (d) Endoscopy

26. An 8-year-old patient presents with a foreign body sensation in his throat and relates that he "accidentally swallowed" a quarter a couple of hours prior to presentation. The PA view of the chest reveals the flat surface of the coin. Where is the coin located?
    (a) In the esophagus
    (b) In the trachea
    (c) Unable to tell from the information given

27. All of the following types of viral hepatitis may be associated with the development of a chronic infectious state except:
    (a) Hepatitis B
    (b) Hepatitis C
    (c) Hepatitis delta
    (d) Hepatitis E

28. All of the following statements regarding *Helicobacter pylori* are accurate except:
    (a) It is a gram-negative, spiral-shaped organism that colonizes only gastric mucosa.
    (b) It has been associated with the development of peptic ulcer disease (particularly duodenal ulcers).
    (c) In patients with peptic ulcer disease who are infected with this organism, eradication of the infection effectively eliminates the ulcer diathesis.
    (d) Single-agent therapy with either bismuth or amoxicillin is very effective in eliminating this organism.

29. A 38-year-old woman presents with epigastric pain of several hours duration. She states that it started shortly after eating a meal of fried shrimp and onion rings. She recalls that she has had similar pain in the past, but states that it has never lasted this long. She is moderately obese and has a history of hypercholesterolemia for which she is taking Lopid. Her PMH is otherwise noncontributory and there is no prior history of abdominal surgery. Examination reveals epigastric and RUQ tenderness. She is afebrile and her rectal exam is negative. The most useful <u>initial</u> test for evaluating this patient is:

    (a) A CT scan of the abdomen
    (b) Biliary scintiscanning (HIDA, DISIDA)
    (c) Abdominal ultrasonography
    (d) Plain films of the abdomen

30. The most accurate study for confirming diagnosis of acute cholecystitis is:

    (a) A CT scan of the abdomen
    (b) Biliary scintiscanning (HIDA, DISIDA)
    (c) Abdominal ultrasonography
    (d) Plain films of the abdomen

31. All of the following statements regarding anal canal tumors are accurate except:

    (a) They are defined as tumors which occur proximal to the dentate line.
    (b) Presenting symptoms may include rectal bleeding, decrease in stool caliber, constipation and weight loss.
    (c) They represent 80% of all anorectal tumors.
    (d) They are slow to metastasize and have a low-grade malignant potential.

32. The majority of all acute episodes of diarrhea are caused by:

    (a) Viruses
    (b) Enterotoxin-producing bacteria
    (c) Invasive bacteria
    (d) Parasites

33. Which of the following statements regarding diarrhea in patients with AIDS is false?

    (a) Cytomegalovirus and Cryptosporidium are the two most common causes of diarrhea in these patients.
    (b) Multiple organisms are responsible in up to 25% of cases.
    (c) It is not a self-limited disease in these patients.
    (d) Empiric antibiotics should be administered immediately.

34. Which of the following statements regarding chest pain due to esophageal spasm is least accurate?

    (a) It is frequently triggered by emotional upset.
    (b) It can be precipitated by drinking extremely hot or cold liquids.
    (c) It can produce a dull discomfort, localized pressure or a sensation of severe squeezing pressure across the middle of the chest.
    (d) Pain associated with esophageal spasm can be distinguished from that which occurs in association with myocardial ischemia by evaluating its response to nitroglycerine; pain of esophageal spasm is not relieved by NTG.

35. The finding of _____ on plain abdominal films is strongly suggestive of mesenteric infarction.

    (a) Ileus
    (b) Pneumatosis intestinalis
    (c) Gasless abdomen
    (d) Sentinel loop

36. Work-up of an elderly patient who presents with severe abdominal pain reveals a diagnosis of nonocclusive mesenteric ischemia. In the absence of peritonitis/necrotic bowel, definitive therapy for this patient consists of:

    (a) Systemic heparinization
    (b) Urokinase infusion
    (c) Intra-arterial papaverine infusion
    (d) Exploratory laparotomy

37. In a patient with acute pancreatitis, which of the following lab reports is most likely to be associated with the highest mortality rate according to Ranson's criteria?

    (a) Amylase 800, SGOT(AST) 300, WBCs 3000
    (b) Lipase 1100, SGOT(AST) 350, WBCs 17,000
    (c) LDH 300, SGPT 200, glucose 50
    (d) LDH 400, glucose 400, WBCs 18,000

38. Hepatitis D is caused by:

    (a) An RNA virus
    (b) A defective RNA virus
    (c) A DNA virus
    (d) A defective DNA virus

39. Which of the following lab findings is not consistent with a diagnosis of alcoholic hepatitis?

    (a) AST > ALT
    (b) AST and ALT levels in the thousands
    (c) Prolongation of the PT
    (d) Elevation of bilirubin and alkaline phosphatase levels

40. The toxic metabolite responsible for producing hepatic necrosis in patients who overdose on acetaminophen is:

   (a) APAP-mercapturate and Cysteine
   (b) APAP-sulfate
   (c) APAP-glucuronide
   (d) NAPQI

Answers: 1. c, 2. b, 3. c, 4. d, 5. a, 6. a, 7. a, 8. d, 9. c, 10. d, 11. a, 12. c, 13. c, 14. b, 15. a, 16. d, 17. a, 18. d, 19. b, 20. c, 21. c, 22. c, 23. b, 24. a, 25. d, 26. a, 27. d, 28. d, 29. c, 30. b, 31. d, 32. a, 33. d, 34. d, 35. b, 36. c, 37. d, 38. b, 39. b, 40. d

Use the pre-chapter multiple choice question worksheet (p. xxv) to record and determine the percentage of correct answers for this section.

GASTROINTESTINAL EMERGENCIES

I. Esophageal Disorders

A. Functional Anatomy

1. The esophagus originates in the hypopharynx at the level of the cricoid cartilage (C_6) and terminates in the cardia of the stomach (T_{11}). It is about 25cm (10") long and is divided into three segments:
    a. Upper (cervical) = 4 - 5cm ⎤ helpful in locating FBs and
    b. Middle (thoracic) = 15 - 20cm ⎬ abnormalities of contiguous
    c. Lower (abdominal) = 2 - 3cm ⎦ structures on x-ray

2. Layers of the esophagus
    a. Inner mucosa Esophagitis involves both the inner mucosa and submucosa; if severe and prolonged, esophagitis may result in scarring and stricture formation. Treatment is dilatation. If the cause is eliminated, recurrent stricture is not a problem.
    b. Submucosa Since there is no serosa, perforation of the submucosa extends into surrounding mediastinal structures and leads to a diffuse, malignant, often rapidly progressive and fatal mediastinitis.
    c. Muscle layers If the two muscle layers are split by bougienage or by repeated dilatation, they scar, which leads to stricture formation. Treatment is dilatation, but strictures recur.
      (1) Cricopharyngeal muscle (upper esophageal sphincter) — is located at the level of C_6
      (2) Muscle composition of the esophagus:
        (a) Upper third — striated muscle
        (b) Middle third — smooth and striated muscle
        (c) Distal third (and remaining GI tract) — smooth muscle

3. Blood vessels
    a. Arteries
      (1) Inferior thyroid (cervical)
      (2) Branches of the aorta (thoracic)
      (3) Left gastric and phrenic (abdominal)
    b. Veins
      (1) Inferior thyroid (cervical)
      (2) Azygous (thorax)
      (3) Coronary and short gastric veins (are part of the portal system in the abdomen; portal obstruction, e.g. cirrhosis of the liver, causes submucosal esophageal varices.)

4. Neuromuscular anatomy
   a. Extrinsic nervous system
      (1) Spinal accessory nerve — innervates the cervical esophagus.
      (2) Vagus nerve — innervates the remainder of the esophagus. Stimulation of this parasympathetic nerve during esophageal intubation and endoscopy causes bradycardia.
      (3) Sympathetic fibers from the cervical and thoracic ganglia — also innervate the esophagus. Stimulation causes dysphagia and referred pain to the chest and epigastrium.
   b. Intrinsic nerve supply (Auerbach's and Meissner's plexuses which are contained between the muscle layers of the esophageal wall) is altered in motor disorders (achalasia, diffuse spasm) and destroyed by corrosives and some collagen vascular disorders (scleroderma, those associated with Raynaud's syndrome).

B. Esophageal Bleeding

1. Mild bleeding (< 10% of blood volume) is usually due to capillary bleeding or nonrecurrent arterial bleeding. Causes include injury, infection and inflammation. Volume replacement is not required.

2. Moderate bleeding (10 - 20% of blood volume) is generally the result of an arterial or venous laceration. Causes include Mallory-Weiss tears, FB ingestion and instrumentation. Crystalloid replacement (one liter) is indicated. Transfusion of 1 - 2 units of blood may also be needed.

3. Severe bleeding (20 - 40% of blood volume) is due to laceration of a varix or an artery which cannot retract (one that is bound down in scar tissue). Crystalloid replacement (≥ one liter) and 2 - 4 units of blood are needed.

4. Massive bleeding (> 40% blood volume) is usually due to a ruptured varix, but can also be due to a perforated artery at the base of a peptic ulcer. Initial crystalloid replacement (two liters) and > 4 units of blood are needed.
   a. Endoscopy should be performed in a timely fashion to confirm the source of bleeding (but not prior to, or at the expense of, adequate shock management).
   b. Check for and treat associated coagulation abnormalities.
   c. Specific treatment of a ruptured varix is as follows:
      (1) Immediate therapy is with an infusion of ocreotide or vasopressin:
         (a) Octreotide infusion
            1 Dose is a bolus of 50mcg followed by an infusion of 25 - 50mcg/hr.
            2 This synthetic somatostatin analogue is more effective than vasopressin and has fewer side effects. Vasopressin infusion (20 units in 200mL NS)

      (b) Vasopressin infusion (20 units in 200mL NS)
        <u>1</u> Dose is 0.2 - 0.5 units/min.
        <u>2</u> Simultaneous infusion of nitroglycerine to diminish the side effects associated with vasopressin therapy (e.g. HTN, cardiac and splanchnic ischemia) is advisable.
  (2) Subsequent measures may include one or more of the following:
      (a) Endoscopic variceal sclerotherapy or band ligation — are the preferred methods for controlling variceal bleeding; they also decrease the risk of early rebleeding.
      (b) Insertion of a Sengstaken-Blakemore (or similar type) tube.
      (c) Gelfoam embolization of the left gastric vein.
      <u>Note</u>: Rebleeding is common in patients hospitalized for variceal bleeding (incidence of 42 - 70%) and the mortality rate is $\geq$ 30%.

C. *Dysphagia*

Dysphagia is defined as "difficulty swallowing"; it signifies the presence of <u>organic</u> pathology of the esophagus in nearly all cases. Odynophagia means "<u>pain</u> on swallowing"; it often indicates the presence of an inflammatory or infectious lesion. Globus hystericus is the <u>feeling</u> that there is something stuck in the throat; it is not associated with swallowing and, therefore, is not dysphagia.

1. Oropharyngeal (transfer) dysphagia (difficulty swallowing)
    a. Symptoms occur within the first two seconds of swallowing.
    b. Neuromuscular disorders and painful or mechanically obstructive inflammatory lesions account for most cases. (Difficulty swallowing <u>liquids</u> [particularly cold ones] suggests a neuromuscular disorder.)
      (1) Inflammatory/infectious causes
        (a) Pharyngitis (Strep, Candida, herpes)
        (b) Aphthous ulcers
        (c) Oropharyngeal abscess
        (d) Epiglottitis
      (2) Neuromuscular causes (80% of cases)
        (a) CVA
        (b) Polymyositis and dermatomyositis
        (c) Scleroderma (> 50% c/o dysphagia)
        (d) Myasthenia gravis (reversible with edrophonium)
        (e) Multiple sclerosis, ALS, Parkinson's disease
        (f) Magnesium deficiency
        (g) Lead poisoning
      (3) Infectious/neuromuscular causes
        (a) Poliomyelitis
        (b) Diphtheria
        (c) Botulism
        (d) Rabies
        (e) Tetanus
    c. Cancer of the tongue, pharynx or larynx may also cause oropharyngeal dysphagia.

2. Upper esophageal dysphagia
   a. Difficulty swallowing occurs within the first 2 - 4 seconds and is caused by <u>obstructive</u> lesions in the majority of cases.
      (1) Intrinsic causes of luminal narrowing are esophageal webs (are associated with iron deficiency anemia) and carcinoma.
      (2) Extrinsic compression can be produced by numerous conditions, e.g. thyroid enlargement, Zenker's diverticulum, left atrial enlargement, aortic aneurysm.
   b. Unlike the intermittent and variable dysphagia caused by motility lesions, dysphagia due to obstructive lesions is typically <u>progressive</u> (starts with solid foods and eventually progresses to liquids).

3. Lower esophageal dysphagia (difficulty swallowing)
   a. Symptoms occur 4 - 10 seconds after the bolus is swallowed and are usually worse with solids.
   b. Patients typically complain of a substernal "sticking" sensation and are usually able to accurately pinpoint the location.
   c. Lower esophageal dysphagia is usually due to <u>luminal narrowing</u>. This narrowing can be either constant (e.g. strictures, carcinoma) or intermittent (e.g. spasm).
      (1) Carcinoma is the most common cause of lower esophageal dysphagia. Difficulty swallowing solids occurs initially and progresses to dysphagia with semisolids and, finally with liquids.
      (2) Achalasia is a disorder characterized by marked increase in the resting pressure of the lower esophageal sphincter and absent peristalsis in the body of the esophagus. Dysphagia is the most common presenting complaint. A diagnostic clue is that dysphagia occurs with <u>both</u> solids and liquids.
      (3) Esophageal strictures result from esophageal reflux. There is a history of heartburn before the onset of dysphagia which is worse with solid foods and is constant; reflux-induced spasm without stricture produces intermittent dysphagia.
      (4) "Steakhouse syndrome" is characterized by intense discomfort that develops shortly after swallowing a large piece of meat. It can occur in patients with a normal esophagus but is more commonly associated with one of the following if the problem has occurred repeatedly:
      (a) Carcinoma
      (b) Stricture
      (c) Schatzki's ring (a fibrous, diaphragm-like stricture near the gastroesophageal junction) ... is actually an esophageal web.

d. Lower esophageal dysphagia and chest pain — esophageal reflux disease (GERD) or ischemic heart disease? Chest pain arising from the esophagus may mimic chest pain due to myocardial ischemia because of similar segmental innervation of the heart and esophagus; both may present with ST segment abnormalities on ECG. **The patient's history is by far the most useful aid in differentiating these two entities.**

   (1) A substernal burning sensation (heartburn/pyrosis) is a common complaint in patients with esophageal reflux. However, a dull discomfort, localized pressure or severe squeezing pain across the middle of the chest may be seen when reflux is associated with esophageal spasm.

   (2) Exacerbation of symptoms with stooping, lying or leaning forward suggests reflux. Postural exacerbation of pain is uncommon with ischemic heart disease.

   (3) Water brash (a hypersalivation response) is commonly associated with reflux.

   (4) Radiation of pain into the abdomen occurs more often in patients with reflux than those with coronary artery disease. Radiation into both arms is rarely seen in reflux.

   (5) A feeling of fullness after meals and relief of chest pain with antacids are key points in the history. This history is rarely present in patients with ischemic heart disease.

   (6) Esophageal spasm without reflux may appear clinically similar to myocardial ischemia. Differentiating features include the following:

      (a) Emotional upset frequently triggers spasm.

      (b) Chest pain from esophageal spasm occurs spontaneously and most often at rest.

      (c) Diffuse spasm may be precipitated by swallowing liquids of extreme temperatures (hot or cold).

      (d) Dysphagia that is present during an episode of esophageal spasm usually prevents the patients from swallowing either liquids or solids.

Note: Esophageal spasm and myocardial ischemia are both relieved by nitroglycerine (NTG). Although the latter generally responds more quickly, response to NTG is not useful in distinguishing these clinical entities.

4. Esophagitis
   a. Symptoms may include chest pain, dysphagia, odynophagia or those of reflux. The chest pain is typically constant, acute in onset and unresponsive to treatment with antacids.
   b. Causes include:
      (1) Infections
         (a) Fungal (*Candida albicans*)
         (b) Viral (*herpes simplex*, varicella-zoster, cytomegalovirus)
         (c) Bacterial (mycobacterium)
      (2) Radiation
      (3) Corrosive agents (alkalis, acids)
      (4) Antibiotics (esp. doxycycline & tetracycline), anti-inflammatory agents, potassium chloride and iron sulfate
   c. Treatment — is directed towards the underlying cause.
      (1) Ketoconazole is the drug of choice for esophageal candidiasis.
      (2) Immunocompromised patients with herpes simplex should receive acyclovir.

D. Esophageal Trauma

1. Causes
   a. Swallowing (foreign body, caustic agent)
   b. Instrumental (surgery, bougienage, rigid endoscopy, intubation, etc.)
   c. Chest trauma (open, closed)
   d. Sudden, violent, and usually repeated increase in the intra-abdominal pressure against a weakened esophageal wall. The most common cause is violent and repeated vomiting/retching.
      (1) <u>Mallory-Weiss Syndrome</u>
         (a) A <u>partial thickness</u> tear (mucosa and submucosa) of the <u>right</u> posterolateral aspect of the distal esophagus or gastric cardia associated with dysphagia, odynophagia and upper GI bleeding.
         (b) The <u>prominent symptom</u> is <u>bleeding</u> which is usually mild to moderate and, in most cases, resolves spontaneously.
         (c) Predisposing factors include:
            <u>1</u> Alcoholism
            <u>2</u> Hiatal hernia
            <u>3</u> Gastritis/esophagitis
         (d) The diagnostic study of choice is endoscopy.
      (2) <u>Boerhaave's Syndrome</u>
         (a) A <u>full-thickness</u> tear (perforation) of the <u>left</u> posterolateral aspect of the distal esophagus (an intrinsically weak area) associated with epigastric and retrosternal chest pain that often radiates into the back, neck, left chest or shoulders.
         (b) The <u>prominent symptom</u> is severe, lancinating <u>chest pain</u>.
         (c) Physical findings include: subcutaneous emphysema, mediastinal "crunch" (Hamman's sound) and a <u>left</u> pneumothorax and/or pleural effusion. Epigastric tenderness may also be present.

(d) Chest x-ray: characteristic findings include a left pneumo-thorax, a left pleural effusion, mediastinal emphysema and a widened mediastinum.

(e) An esophagogram using <u>water-soluble</u> oral contrast (Gastrografin) confirms the diagnosis.

(f) Treatment
<u>1</u> Fluid resuscitation
<u>2</u> Broad-spectrum IV antibiotics
<u>3</u> Emergent surgical consultation

(g) This lesion produces the most malignant type of mediastinitis (acid burn and bacterial infection). Morbidity and mortality, due to shock and septicemia, occur very rapidly (< 48 hrs. from the time of perforation). Hence, immediate repair is indicated.

2. Diagnosis of esophageal trauma is confirmed by Gastrografin swallow or endoscopy.

3. Contraindications for insertion of an NG tube:
a. Posterior laryngeal lacerations
b. Esophageal tears
c. Foreign bodies (associated with esophageal wall trauma)
d. Caustic ingestions
e. Near-total obstruction of the esophagus secondary to stricture

E. Esophageal Foreign Body Ingestion

1. FBs tend to lodge or impact at the sites where esophageal narrowing occurs:
a. Cricopharyngeus muscle (C_6) — most common site in kids < 4 yrs.
b. Adjacent to the aortic arch (T_4)
c. Lower esophageal sphincter/diaphragmatic hiatus ($T_{10\text{-}11}$) — most common site in adults
[Note: The majority of esophageal impactions (80%) occur in children and involve true FBs (coins, buttons, marbles, etc.); obstruction occurs less frequently in adults and is usually the result of a food impaction.]

2. Symptoms of a lodged or impacted esophageal FB
a. Patients < 16 yrs. of age
(1) Vomiting
(2) Gagging
(3) Choking (also R/O tracheal FB, especially if it is associated with stridor, wheezing, coughing or other signs of respiratory distress)
(4) Neck or throat pain
(5) Dysphagia
(6) FB sensation in the chest
(7) Refusal to eat

b. Patients >16 yrs. of age
   (1) Anxiety and discomfort
   (2) FB sensation
   (3) Substernal chest pain (sometimes)
   (4) Progressive dysphagia and inability to handle secretions
   (5) Odynophagia
   Note: The patient can usually accurately locate the position of the impacted esophageal foreign body.

3. The following x-rays should be ordered in symptomatic patients: soft tissue films of the neck (AP and lateral) and chest films (PA and lat.)
   a. A flat object (such as a coin) will be oriented in the frontal (coronal) plane if it is located in the esophagus and the PA or AP view will reveal the flat surface of the coin; if it is in the trachea, the coin will be oriented in the sagittal plane (reflecting the angle of the coin required to pass through the vocal cords) and the PA or AP view will reveal the edge of the coin.
   b. An esophageal FB will show on chest x-ray; a tracheal FB may not.
   c. Pull-tabs from aluminum cans are difficult to detect on plain films because they are relatively radiolucent and may overlie the more radiodense vertebral bodies.
   d. Some fish bones are radiolucent and not visible on plain films. This is also true of plastic objects and toothpicks.
   e. X-ray evaluation of asymptomatic patients with suspected or known ingestions should also be considered because many patients are without symptoms; up to one-third of children with esophageal FBs are asymptomatic.
   f. If the FB is not detected by neck and chest films, an esophagogram or endoscopy should be performed.
      (1) Esophagogram — if a perforation is suspected, a water-soluble contrast agent should be selected. If aspiration is a concern, use barium. If both perforation and aspiration are considerations, a nonionic contrast media should be used. Prior to the procedure, an NG tube should be inserted above the obstruction to prevent aspiration of unswallowed liquids which collect there.
      (2) Endoscopy — if readily available, is the diagnostic modality of choice because it can be used to both visualize and remove the FB. Note: Barium should not be used if subsequent endoscopy is anticipated because it may limit or obscure visualization of the FB by the endoscopist.

4. Although objects do occasionally lodge or become impacted in the esophagus (particularly those with sharp edges) the majority will pass spontaneously. In fact, once an object has traversed the gastroesophageal junction, the probability of eventual passage is > 90%. The FB usually arrives at the rectum in 3 - 5 days. As long as the patient is asymptomatic, management in these cases is expectant.

5. A <u>lodged or impacted</u> FB must be dislodged or removed.
    a. Since most esophageal FBs are in the cervical esophagus, removal is usually accomplished with a laryngoscope and Magill forceps or an endoscope.
    b. Food impactions
        (1) A <u>distal</u> esophageal food impaction can occasionally be dislodged with IV Glucagon,* sublingual nitroglycerine or nifedipine.
            (a) IV Glucagon relaxes smooth muscle and decreases lower esophageal sphincter pressure. Following a test dose to rule out hypersensitivity, administer 1mg IV; an additional 2mg may be given if there is no relief in 20 minutes.*
            (b) Sublingual nitroglycerine also works by relaxing smooth muscle. Administer 0.4mg sublingually.
            (c) Nifedipine decreases the amplitude of lower esophageal sphincter contractions and the pressure at this sphincter. Administer 10mg sublingually.
        (2) Gas-forming agents (e.g. E-Z Gas, carbonated beverages) may also be used to dislodge an esophageal food impaction. They work by producing CO_2 which increases intraluminal pressure and pushes the food bolus into the stomach. These agents are avoided in patients with chest pain (possible perforation) or those with symptoms > 24 hours duration.

        <u>Note</u>: The use of a proteolytic enzyme (such as papain) is associated with a 3% incidence of associated esophageal perforation and is no longer recommended.

    c. The practice of removing an impacted, smooth FB (such as a coin) with a Foley or Fogarty catheter requires a co-operative patient, fluoroscopic guidance and an object that has been present for < 24 - 72 hours. This procedure is best avoided; the FB may slip from the esophagus to the trachea and lead to respiratory compromise.
    d. Alkaline disk batteries (button batteries)
        (1) 90% pass through the GI tract in 48 - 72 hours without any untoward effect.
        (2) If the patient is <u>asymptomatic</u> and the battery has already passed into the stomach, expectant management (observation at home) is adequate.
        (3) If a button battery becomes <u>lodged</u>, it usually does so in the esophagus.
        (4) A button battery lodged in the esophagus is associated with severe morbidity and requires <u>emergent</u> endoscopic removal. The corrosive action of these batteries can produce esophageal burns, necrosis and perforation within 4 - 6 hours post-ingestion.
    e. Impacted foreign bodies that cannot be dislodged or removed by direct visualization must be extracted surgically (approximately 1% of all FB ingestions).

*Glucagon frequently causes nausea and vomiting.

6. Sharp or pointed objects, as well as objects longer than 5cm and wider than 2cm, must be removed endoscopically. They should be removed before they pass the pylorus because 15 - 35% will cause perforation, usually in the region of the ileocecal valve.

7. Following the removal of an esophageal FB, the patient should have a complete evaluation of esophageal function (including motility studies) to ensure that there is no underlying pathology which led to the obstruction. This is particularly true of adults with meat impactions; underlying pathology of the esophagus is present up to 97% of the time.

II. Peptic Ulcer Disease (PUD)

A. Pathophysiology

1. Peptic ulcers are mucosal defects that extend beyond the muscularis mucosae. They are most commonly located along the lesser curvature of the stomach or in the first portion of the duodenum.
   a. Gastric ulcers are thought to be due to damage to the gastric mucosal barrier itself; damage to this barrier allows diffusion of hydrogen ions from the lumen to the gastric mucosa and results in ulceration.
   b. Duodenal ulcers are usually associated with hypersecretion of gastric acid (by an enlarged parietal cell mass) and with markedly increased gastric emptying that overwhelms the capacity of the duodenum to neutralize gastric acid and results in damage to the duodenal mucosal barrier.

2. Uncommon sites of peptic ulceration
   a. Distal esophagus
   b. Ectopic gastric mucosa with a Meckel's diverticulum
   c. Margins of surgical anastomoses ("marginal ulcers")

3. A stress ulcer is not the same as a peptic ulcer, i.e., the mucosal lesion of a stress ulcer does not extend through the muscularis mucosae. Stress ulcers are most commonly found in the body and fundus of the stomach and are a common cause of gastric bleeding (hemorrhagic gastritis). When stress ulcers are the result of an acute traumatic insult, CNS tumor or sepsis, they are referred to as Cushing's (gastric) or Curling's (duodenal) ulcers.

4. The pain associated with gastric and duodenal (peptic) ulcers is visceral in nature and, therefore, is vague (not well defined) and is generally felt in the midline. It is typically described as gnawing, aching or burning.

a. Gastric pain is generally perceived at the midline or to the left of the epigastrium.

b. Duodenal bulb pain is usually perceived to the right of the midepigastrium. With posterior penetration, the pain may radiate straight through to the back.

B. Predisposing Factors

- Infection with *Helicobacter pylori*
- Agents such as NSAIDs and ASA that alter the mucosal barrier
- Zollinger-Ellison syndrome
- Cigarette smoking
- Bile salts
- Emotional stress
- Type O blood
- Prolonged use of corticosteroids
- Caffeinated beverages (coffee, soda, tea)
  [Diet and alcohol are not predisposing factors.]

C. Clinical Picture

The patient presents with epigastric pain that may be easily confused with the substernal chest pain of myocardial ischemia. A significant diagnostic clue is the character of the pain — a patient with peptic ulcer disease will describe the pain as a burning sensation; the MI patient generally will not. Ask the patient if there is any relationship between the onset of pain and food intake — the pain of a gastric ulcer usually occurs shortly after eating; duodenal ulcer pain awakens the patient at night, occurs 2 - 3 hours after meals and is relieved (partially or completely) by food; the onset and relief of pain associated with myocardial ischemia usually have no relationship to food intake. (There are reports, however, of anginal pain occurring after eating, presumably due to "portal steal," i.e., increase in portal circulation at the expense of central circulation.)

D. Definitive Diagnosis — is generally not made in the Emergency Department.

1. Peptic ulcers — may be diagnosed with an upper GI or endoscopy. Endoscopic evaluation with biopsy is key to differentiating malignant from benign gastric ulcers and should be suspected in patients > 50 years old as well as those with markers of malignancy.

2. Stress ulcers — are diagnosed with endoscopy.

3. Infection with *Helicobacter pylori* — can be diagnosed noninvasively via serology, the urea breath test or by tests which require endoscopy (rapid urea /CLO test, histology).

E. ***Treatment of Uncomplicated Peptic Ulcer Disease*** — is generally on an outpatient basis and may be initiated from the Emergency Department.

1. Advise patients to avoid substances which exacerbate gastric and duodenal ulcers (smoking, alcohol, NSAIDs, etc.) A bland diet with frequent feedings has not been demonstrated to be effective and is probably unnecessary.

2. Provide pain relief and facilitate ulcer healing with one of the following agents:

   a. Antacids
      (1) Provide pain relief and accelerate healing. They work by neutralizing gastric acid.
      (2) The dose is 30mL at bedtime and at 1 and 3 hours after meals.
      (3) Their major drawback is how frequently they must be taken, which decreases compliance. They may also cause constipation (aluminum salts) or diarrhea (magnesium salts). In addition, antacids decrease the absorption of certain drugs (warfarin, digoxin, several anticonvulsants and some antibiotics).

   b. Histamine (H_2) - Antagonists
      (1) Promote healing by inhibiting gastric acid secretion.
      (2) The major advantage of these drugs is their convenient dosing; they may be taken either once or twice daily.
      (3) The various H_2-antagonists and their dosing schedules are listed below. All of these agents are primarily excreted in the urine; in the presence of renal disease, these dosages should be reduced. They are all equally efficacious but vary in terms of the frequency of adverse effects they produce. Cimetidine is associated with the greatest incidence of adverse effects. The other agents have fewer side effects and fewer or no recognized drug interactions.
         (a) Cimetidine
            • Dose is 800mg PO Q HS or 400mg PO bid
            • Adverse effects include:
               ▲ Interaction with other drugs (warfarin, phenytoin, propranolol, diazepam, chlordiazepoxide, lidocaine, theophylline and tricyclic antidepressants); it <u>inhibits the cytochrome p450 system</u>, thereby <u>increasing</u> the blood levels of these drugs.
               ▲ CNS dysfunction (particularly in the elderly)
               ▲ Painful gynecomastia
               ▲ Reversible impotence (in patients with pathologic hypersecretory disorders such as Zollinger-Ellison syndrome)
               ▲ Thrombocytopenia
         (b) Ranitidine — 300mg PO Q HS or 150mg PO bid
         (c) Famotidine — 40mg PO Q HS or 20mg PO bid
         (d) Nizatidine — 300mg PO Q HS or 150mg PO bid

   c. Proton Pump Inhibitors (PPIs)
      (1) Promote healing by blocking the secretion of gastric acid.
      (2) They <u>inhibit</u> the H^+/K^+ ATPase enzyme system (the "proton pump") of parietal cells, thereby preventing the release of hydrogen ions into the gastric lumen.

(3) They are indicated for the <u>short</u>-term treatment of duodenal and gastric ulcers, and are usually reserved for those that failed to respond to H_2-blockers.

(4) Agents, dosing and drug interactions:

(a) Omeprazole
  - Dose is 20 mg QD
  - Drug interactions → can <u>prolong</u> the elimination of drugs metabolized via oxidation in the liver (e.g., warfarin, diazepam, phenytoin) and some of those metabolized by the cytochrome p450 system (e.g., benzodiazepines, disulfiram, cyclosporine).

(b) Lansoprazole
  - Dose is 15 - 30 mg QD
  - Drug interactions — unlike omeprazole, lansoprazole does not have any significant interaction with drugs metabolized by the cytochrome p450 system.

(c) Pantoprazole
  - A new PPI that is available in IV form
  - Has been shown to ↓ bleeding from peptic ulcers
  - Dose is 80mg Q 8hrs.

d. <u>Misoprostol</u>

(1) A synthetic prostaglandin E_1 analogue that acts in a way similar to the naturally occurring prostaglandins secreted by the gastric mucosa in response to injury. Both promote healing by stimulating local mucus and bicarbonate secretion, enhancing mucosal blood flow and inhibiting gastric acid secretion.

(2) Is only indicated for the <u>prevention</u> of <u>NSAID-induced gastric ulcers</u> in high-risk patients (the elderly, those with concomitant debilitating disease or a history of ulcers).

(3) Can cause spontaneous abortion and is, therefore, contraindicated in pregnant women and women of childbearing age who are not using reliable contraceptive measures.

(4) Dose is 200mcg PO qid with food.

(5) Most common side effects are diarrhea and crampy abdominal pain (both of which are dose-dependent).

e. <u>Sucralfate</u>*

(1) Works <u>locally</u> at the ulcer site where it binds to the base of the ulcer, thereby protecting it from the adverse effect of gastric acid. It also adsorbs bile acids, inhibits pepsin activity and increases mucosal prostaglandin production.

(2) Dose is 1 gm PO qid on an empty stomach. It works best in an acid environment (pH < 3.5). Thus, simultaneous administration of antacids should be avoided.

(3) Adverse reactions (rare) include constipation and dry mouth.

*Drug of choice for erosive esophagitis secondary to "stuck pills" (e.g. doxycycline, colace) that are large in size

f. <u>Bismuth compounds</u> (bismuth subsalicylate / subcitrate)
  (1) Are the most commonly used in triple drug treatment regimens for eradication of *H. pylori*.
  (2) Work by diminishing pepsin activity, increasing mucus secretion and creating a barrier to additional acid damage of ulcerated surfaces. They also augment prostaglandin synthesis, slow hydrogen ion diffusion through the mucosal barrier, and have a bactericidal effect on H. pylori.
g. <u>Eradication of *Helicobacter pylori* (if present)</u>
  (1) *H. pylori* is a gram-negative spiral-shaped organism that colonizes only gastric-type epithelium and is associated with the development of peptic ulcer disease (PUD); it is responsible for about 95% of duodenal ulcers and $\geq$ 70% of gastric ulcers.
  (2) In patients with PUD who are infected with this organism, eradication of the infection effectively eliminates the ulcer diathesis; relapses and recurrences are markedly reduced; — the need for chronic suppressive therapy with H_2-blockers is eliminated.
  (3) Management of patients with suspected or confirmed PUD should, therefore, include a referral for diagnostic testing to determine if infection with *H. pylori* is present.
  (4) Patients with confirmed infections should be started on a regimen that is effective in eradicating this organism. Choose <u>one</u> of the following triple therapy options:
    (a) Bismuth subsalicylate, metronidazole and tetracycline
    (b) Ranitidine bismuth citrate, clarithromycin and tetracycline
    (c) Omeprazole, clarithromycin and amoxicillin

F. Complications of Peptic Ulcer Disease

The most common complications are bleeding (20% of ulcer patients), perforation (7%) and gastric outlet obstruction; they can be the earliest manifestation of ulcer disease in some patients (particularly the elderly).

1. <u>Bleeding</u>
   a. Peptic ulceration is the most common cause of upper GI bleeding.
     (1) Duodenal ulcers (most common) → 29% of upper GI bleeds
     (2) Gastric ulcers → 16% of upper GI bleeds
     (3) Combined, gastric and duodenal ulcers cause 45 - 50% of all upper GI bleeding.
   b. Treatment
     (1) Volume replacement with NS or LR via 2 large-bore IVs
     (2) Oxygen at 6 - 8 L/min.
     (3) NG tube drainage
     (4) Foley catheter placement to monitor volume resuscitation

(5) Lavage
    (a) Can be used to monitor a patient's blood loss and prepare them for endoscopy, but is not helpful in stopping the bleeding or preventing its recurrence.
    (b) To prevent complications, only <u>room-temperature</u> solutions (normal saline or water) should be used and pneumoperitoneum must first be ruled out.

(6) Blood transfusion as required

(7) Administer an H_2-antagonist — These agents (as well as pantoprazole[*]) are effective in promoting healing of the underlying ulcer and have shown to be of some benefit in reducing the rate of rebleeding, surgery and death in patients with gastric ulcers.

(8) Consultation with a gastroenterologist and a general surgeon is prudent in any patient with significant upper GI bleeding.
    (a) If the patient does not respond to the above measures and bleeding persists, early or emergent endoscopic evaluation may be needed for both localization of the bleeding site and treatment. Although arteriography is also useful in locating the bleeding site (if the rate of bleeding is ≥ 0.5mL/min.), it has largely been supplanted by endoscopy which is usually more accurate; it is currently reserved for situations in which endoscopy is unavailable or non-diagnostic.
    (b) Surgical intervention is indicated for patients who fail to respond to medical therapy and endoscopic hemostasis.

2. <u>Perforation</u>
  a. Exposure of the peritoneal cavity to gastric or duodenal contents produces a chemical peritonitis which, in the absence of prompt and adequate treatment, rapidly progresses to bacterial peritonitis.
  b. Sudden onset of abdominal pain with guarding and rebound is characteristic of anterior perforations; back pain is characteristic of posterior perforation of a duodenal ulcer.
  c. Absence of free air on x-ray does not R/O the diagnosis.
    (1) Anterior perforations → Only 60 - 70% demonstrate free air.
    (2) Posterior perforations → No free air will be evident because the posterior duodenum is located retroperitoneally.
  d. Clinical presentation of a posterior, perforated, duodenal ulcer may appear <u>similar</u> to pancreatitis (but the serum lipase will be normal or slightly elevated initially if the perforation is adjacent to the pancreas) or the perforation may actually <u>cause</u> pancreatitis.
  e. Treatment
    (1) IV fluid (NS or LR) and electrolyte replacement
    (2) NG tube drainage
    (3) Broad-spectrum IV antibiotics
    (4) Immediate surgical consultation

---

[*]Pantoprazole is the only proton pump inhibitor available in IV form; this is important in active GI bleeders who may not be able to take a PPI by mouth — the dose is 40mg.

3. Gastric outlet obstruction
   a. When an ulcer heals, it can form a scar that blocks the pyloric outlet. The resulting obstruction can result in gastric dilation, vomiting, dehydration and hypokalemic, hypochloremic, metabolic alkalosis.
   b. Signs and symptoms include:
      (1) Upper abdominal pain and vomiting (most common).
      (2) Early satiety
      (3) Recent weight loss
      (4) A succussion splash (a splashing sound elicited by gently rocking the abdomen)
   c. An upright abdominal x-ray typically reveals a prominently dilated stomach shadow with a large air-fluid level.
   d. Treatment
      (1) Constant NG suctioning
      (2) Fluid replacement and correction of electrolyte abnormalities
      (3) Admission for further evaluation and definitive management

   [Note: Anticholinergic agents are contraindicated because they may aggravate gastric distention by decreasing gastric motility.]

III. Perforated Viscus

A. Gastric and Duodenal Perforations

1. Gastric and duodenal ulcer perforations occur with greater frequency in benign ulcers than in malignant ones.

2. Anterior ulcers perforate into the abdomen and produce severe abdominal pain; posterior duodenal ulcers can perforate into the pancreas producing pancreatitis and pain that radiates straight through the back.

3. Ulcer perforation is rarely associated with significant concomitant hemorrhage.

B. Gallbladder Perforation (rare)

1. Gallstone obstruction of the cystic or common bile duct → gallbladder distention → vascular compromise → gangrene → perforation.
   a. More commonly, gallstones erode through the gallbladder wall, cystic duct or common duct and produce fistulas between the GB and another portion of the GI tract rather than perforate directly into the peritoneal cavity. After such fistula formation, a large gallstone can lodge in the terminal ileum and produce a small bowel obstruction (gallstone ileus). On x-ray, one sees pneumobilia (air in the biliary tree from erosion of the stone into the small bowel) and signs of small bowel obstruction.

b. Gangrene of the gallbladder (with subsequent perforation) can occur in the absence of stone formation (acalculous cholecystitis), especially in diabetics.

2. Patients at risk of gallbladder perforation
   a. The elderly
   b. Diabetics
   c. Those with atherosclerotic cardiovascular disease
   d. Those with a history of gallstones and repeated cholecystitis
   e. Those with a hemolytic disorder (sickle cell disease)

3. Suspect the diagnosis in a patient with the following **clinical picture:** an elderly male with fever who appears ill and has a tender RUQ mass on physical exam. A careful history reveals one or more risk factors. In addition, a nonalcoholic may give a past history of jaundice or pancreatitis, which should suggest common duct stones. Lab studies reveal leukocytosis, possibly an elevated bilirubin and slight elevation of the serum amylase. On abdominal film, a stone may be seen free in the abdomen ...and also check the right diaphragm because subhepatic or subphrenic abscesses can form following a gallbladder perforation and cause restricted movement of the right leaf of the diaphragm.

C. Small Bowel Perforation

1. Causes of jejunal rupture include:
   a. Drugs (enteric-coated potassium tablets)
   b. Infection (e.g. typhoid, TB)
   c. Tumor
   d. Strangulated hernia
   e. Regional enteritis (Crohn's disease)

2. A jejunal perforation causes a chemical peritonitis that is more severe than that caused by an ileal perforation because the pH of the jejunal contents is higher (8) and there are also a greater number of enzymes present in this part of the bowel; ileal perforations are associated with considerable bacterial contamination; these small bowel perforations can rapidly wall off (particularly in patients with Crohn's disease) so that early evaluation may reveal only localized findings.

3. Mortality varies directly with the extent of peritoneal soiling and time delay to diagnosis and treatment.

D. Large Bowel Perforation

1. Causes
   a. Carcinoma
   b. Diverticulitis
   c. Colitis
   d. Foreign body
   e. Diagnostic instrumentation

2. The signs and symptoms of large bowel perforations are largely due to sepsis and, therefore, are usually slower in onset than those produced by small bowel perforations.

3. **Clinical picture** — The patient appears septic and he has a feculent breath odor. His abdomen is distended and he tells you he has been unable to pass stool. When you insert an NG tube and hook it to suction, fecal material is seen in the aspirate. X-ray often demonstrates free air and small bowel obstruction.

E. Treatment for a Known or Suspected Perforated Viscus

1. IV fluid replacement with NS or LR; large volumes (up to 12 L/24 hrs.) may be required due to third spacing.
2. Bladder catheterization (to monitor urine output/volume status)
3. NPO NG tube drainage
4. Broad-spectrum IV antibiotics
5. <u>Immediate</u> surgical consultation (delay in surgical intervention significantly increases mortality)

IV. Other Causes of an Acute Abdomen

A. Appendicitis

1. The most common indication for emergency surgery is appendicitis. It is also the most common surgical emergency seen in pregnancy, and the most common cause of emergent abdominal surgery in the pediatric age group.

2. Although all age groups are affected, the highest incidence is in patients 10 - 30 years of age (particularly males).

3. Pathophysiology
   a. Obstruction of the appendiceal lumen (the <u>primary</u> inciting event) → increased intraluminal pressure and distention → vascular compromise of the appendiceal wall and bacterial invasion.
   b. Causes of appendiceal obstruction include:
      (1) Fecalith (most common)
      (2) Enlarged lymphoid follicles
      (3) Inspissated barium
      (4) Worms
      (5) Granulomatous disease
      (6) Tumors
      (7) Adhesions
      (8) Dietary matter (seeds)

4. Common findings (listed in order of decreasing frequency)
  a. Symptoms
     (1) Abdominal pain
     (2) Anorexia
     (3) Nausea and vomiting
     (4) Fever and chills
     (5) Diarrhea (can be a particularly prominent symptom in very young children and patients with pelvic appendices which often results in misdiagnosis as acute gastroenteritis).
  b. Signs
     (1) Abdominal tenderness
     (2) Percussion or rebound tenderness
     (3) Rectal tenderness
     (4) Cervical motion tenderness (28 - 34%)
     (5) Psoas sign (RLQ pain on passive extension of right hip)
     (6) Obturator sign (RLQ pain on passive internal rotation of the flexed right hip)
     (7) Rosving's sign (RLQ pain on palpation of the LLQ)
     (8) RLQ pain on rectal exam → retrocecal appendicitis

5. **Clinical picture** — Visceral <u>pain</u> is the first symptom to develop; it is dull and vague in character. In the nonpregnant patient, pain usually begins in the periumbilical area and then, over time, moves to the RLQ. Where the pain eventually migrates is determined by the actual location of the appendix; radiation of pain to the flank should make one suspicious of a retrocecal appendicitis. (Remember that kidney stone pain usually comes on suddenly; retrocecal appendiceal pain usually has a gradual onset). In the pregnant patient, the appendix moves laterally and superiorly as the uterus enlarges, so be suspicious of flank or RUQ pain in these patients. <u>If the appendix is located near the uterus, ovary or tubes, there will be pain on cervical motion.</u> (Patients with PID are generally seen later in the course of their illness, have fewer GI symptoms, and have a more elevated sedimentation rate). Anorexia, nausea and vomiting usually begin after the onset of pain. A sudden decrease in pain followed by a dramatic increase suggests perforation.

> Unfortunately, one-third to one-half of patients do not present "classically" (migratory abdominal pain and the typical associated signs and symptoms); the pain can be anywhere. Be particularly suspicious of the very young and the very old patient; their symptoms are frequently vague and clinical presentation is less classic. Delayed diagnosis with resulting perforation and increased morbidity and mortality is common in these age groups.

6. Diagnostic studies — may provide additional information even when the history and physical are classic; they can also be helpful in less typical cases when the diagnosis remains in doubt.

a. Routine studies
   (1) Pregnancy test — should be done in all women of childbearing age to exclude ectopic pregnancy.
   (2) CBC — the white count is usually (but not always) elevated with an increase in the number of PMNs and immature forms.
   (3) UA — pyuria and hematuria may occur if the inflamed appendix lies in close proximity to the ureter — a few WBCs and RBCs in the urine is characteristic in this case.
   (4) Plain abdominal films[*] — a calcified fecalith in the RLQ is very suggestive of appendicitis but is present in only 2 - 22% of cases.

b. Additional studies — may be indicated when the diagnosis remains uncertain and should be chosen in consultation with the evaluating surgeon. Availability and usefulness of these studies may be institution-dependent.
   (1) Abdominal CT — is generally considered the radiographic procedure of choice for diagnosing acute appendicitis in adult males and non-pregnant females. Data suggest that abdominal CT is > 97% sensitive and 98-100% specific for acute appendicitis. (In addition, abdominal CT may unmask other cases of abdominal pain.) Abdominal CT is performed with IV contrast and oral or rectal contrast; presence of peri-appendiceal fat stranding is the most specific radiographic finding for appendicitis.
   (2) Diagnostic laparoscopy — an invasive study that demonstrates a high sensitivity and specificity. It is clearly indicated in equivocal cases of surgical abdominal pain and its use as a diagnostic tool is increasing because laparoscopic appendectomies are now performed more frequently than surgical appendectomies.
   (3) Graded compression ultrasonography — has a sensitivity of ~ 40%, a specificity of ~ 90% and may be especially valuable for evaluating pediatric and pregnant patients. It is noninvasive, without radiation exposure, safe in pregnancy, rapid, inexpensive and rarely requires sedation in kids. Visualization of a noncompressible, immobile appendix > 6mm in diameter is very suggestive of the diagnosis. Furthermore, an alternative definitive diagnosis can be established in up to 50% of patients when appendicitis is absent. The disadvantages of ultrasound are: it is not always available, it's operator-dependent and it has a very poor sensitivity in the presence of perforation.

   Note: Barium enema is not used for the diagnosis of appendicitis. While nonfilling of the appendix and a pressure effect on the cecum do suggest the diagnosis of appendicitis, visualization of a normal appendix does not exclude this diagnosis.

---

[*]An option to be considered only if CT is unavailable.

7. Clinical conditions that mimic appendicitis
   a. Mesenteric adenitis
   b. Yersinia gastroenteritis
   c. PID
   d. Ectopic pregnancy
   e. Ovarian cyst
   f. Pyelonephritis
   g. Crohn's disease
   h. Diverticulitis

8. Treatment for suspected appendicitis
   a. Keep the patient NPO
   b. Establish an IV
   c. Obtain <u>early</u> surgical consultation. (Delay in laparoscopy or surgical intervention → gangrene → perforation → <u>increased</u> morbidity and mortality, particularly in the very young and the very old.)
   d. If a decision to operate is reached, administer prophylactic parenteral antibiotics (they decrease the incidence of postoperative wound infection and, in patients who have perforated, they decrease the incidence of postoperative abscess formation). Acceptable regimens:
      (1) Piperacillin/tazobactam <u>or</u>
      (2) Cefoxitin <u>or</u>
      (3) Cefotetan <u>or</u>
      (4) Ampicillin + gentamicin + metronidazole/clindamycin
   e. Judicious amounts of parenteral narcotic may be administered for pain relief and to facilitate diagnostic evaluation.*

B. Bowel Obstruction

1. Causes
   a. Small bowel obstruction
      (1) Adhesions (most common)
      (2) Hernia (second most common)
      (3) Neoplasms [lymphoma, adenocarcinoma]
      (4) Intussusception (common in children < 2 yrs. old)
      (5) Gallstones [Gallstone ileus]
      (6) Bezoars
      (7) Crohn's disease
      (8) Radiation enteritis
      (9) Foreign bodies
   b. Large bowel obstruction
      (1) Tumor
         (a) Most common cause of large bowel obstruction.
         (b) Remember that tumors on the left side cause obstruction while tumors on the right side present with bleeding.

---

*ACEP clinical policy: Critical issues for the initial evaluation and management of patients presenting with a chief complaint of nontraumatic acute abdominal pain.

(2) Diverticulitis*
(3) Volvulus (sigmoid and cecal)
(4) Fecal impaction
- The elderly
- Narcotic and laxative abusers
- The mentally retarded
- Nursing home patients

2. Pathophysiology
    a. Mechanical obstruction refers to partial or complete compromise of the bowel lumen.
    b. Closed-loop obstruction refers to a segment of bowel that is blocked proximally and distally. It results in rapid increase of intraluminal pressure. Intestinal ischemia, infarction and perforation can ultimately develop. Examples include:
    (1) Volvulus (twisting of a bowel loop on its mesenteric axis)
    (2) Herniation of a bowel loop in the omentum or mesentery or a loop of intestine caught in a hernia sac
    (3) A complete colonic obstruction (such as carcinoma or impaction) in the presence of a competent ileocecal valve causes progressive distention of the involved bowel and creates a form of closed-loop obstruction; if the ileocecal valve is incompetent, decompression can occur by reflux into the ileum.
    c. Peristalsis is initially increased early in the course of bowel obstructions (hyperactive bowel sounds). Passage of stool and flatus often continues in the first few hours following an obstruction. With persistent complete obstruction, the bowel loses its ability to contract rigorously, bowel sounds become infrequent, and the passage of stool/flatus stops.
    d. Strangulation occurs most often in the small bowel and is due to vascular compromise which leads to infarction. In the large bowel, strangulation can occur with a volvulus.

3. Signs and symptoms
    a. Pain
    (1) Crampy, intermittent and poorly-localized pain is typical.
    (2) A change in the quality of the pain (greater intensity, more constant) may indicate that a complication has developed.
    b. Vomiting
    (1) The more proximal the obstruction, the sooner it begins.
    (2) If it is bilious, the obstruction is distal to the pylorus.
    (3) Feculent emesis is associated with distal ileal and large bowel obstruction and, if long-standing, may be due to infarcted bowel.
    c. Abdominal distention — the more distal the obstruction, the more pronounced the distention.
    d. Tympany — may be present on percussion.
    e. Abdominal tenderness
    (1) Mild, diffuse tenderness is typical.
    (2) A tender mass may be palpated with a closed-loop obstruction.
    (3) Severe localized tenderness or rebound tenderness suggests the possibility of gangrenous or perforated bowel.

*One of the most common causes of large bowel obstruction in adults

4. Radiographic studies
   a. Gas patterns in small and large bowel obstructions:
      (1) Colon gas is distinguished from gas in the small bowel by its peripheral location and the presence of haustrations which do not involve the entire transverse diameter of the bowel.
      (2) Small bowel gas is more central in location and one can see valvulae conniventes that involve the entire transverse diameter of the small bowel. They are spaced closer together than the haustrations of the large bowel.
   b. Radiographic signs of small bowel obstruction:
      (1) Dilated loops of small bowel above the point of obstruction
      (2) Air-fluid levels on the upright or decubitus film
      (3) "String of pearls" sign on upright film*
   c. Radiographic signs suggesting a closed-loop obstruction:
      (1) "Coffee bean sign:" a single distended loop of bowel ("sentinel loop") whose lumina are separated by a broad dense band of edematous bowel.
      (2) Pseudotumor: a completely closed loop whose lumen is filled with fluid and looks like a mass.
   d. X-ray signs in volvulus are described below in the section on volvulus.

5. Treatment
   a. IV fluid (NS or LR) and electrolyte replacement — dehydration and hypokalemia are common, particularly in patients with small bowel obstruction who present late.
   b. NG tube placement to decompress the bowel
   c. Broad-spectrum antibiotic coverage
   d. Early surgical consultation

C. Volvulus

1. Volvulus is a closed-loop obstruction that results from the twisting of a mobile segment of bowel on its mesocolon; it is responsible for approximately 10 - 13% of colonic obstructions in the United States.

2. Sigmoid volvulus occurs more commonly (60%); cecal volvulus occurs less frequently (40%).

3. Epidemiology and pathophysiology
   a. Sigmoid volvulus — occurs almost entirely in two-patient populations: elderly, bed-ridden patients with debilitating comorbid diseases and patients of any age with profound neurologic or psychiatric illness. These patients invariably have a history of chronic severe constipation which leads to an elongated (redundant) sigmoid colon.
   b. Cecal volvulus — results from incomplete embryologic fixation of the cecum, ascending colon and terminal ileum to the posterior abdominal wall. Although it occurs in patients of all ages, it is most common in patients in their twenties and thirties.

---

*Small amounts of gas caught between the valvula conivents in a largely fluid-filled, mechanically obstructed bowel.

4. Signs and symptoms of sigmoid and cecal volvulus
   a. Sudden onset of crampy lower abdominal pain
   b. Nausea, vomiting, obstipation
   c. Diffuse abdominal tenderness
   d. Progressive abdominal distention
   e. Tympany

5. X-ray findings — a markedly <u>dilated single loop of colon</u>
   a. Sigmoid volvulus — The loop arises out of the left side of the pelvis and its superior aspect projects upward producing a "bent inner tube-like" appearance.
   b. Cecal volvulus — The loop is usually seen in the mid or upper abdomen toward the left, but may be anywhere given the relative mobility of the cecum. It has a "coffee bean" shape and is often accompanied by distended loops of small bowel.

6. Treatment — initial measures are the same as those for bowel obstruction (IV hydration, NG tube decompression and broad-spectrum antibiotics). Specific measures depend on the type of volvulus present.
   a. Sigmoid volvulus
      (1) Surgical consultation and nonoperative reduction using a rectal tube via the sigmoidoscope or barium enema. Since recurrence is common (90%), this is usually followed by an elective resection if the patient's underlying medical condition can tolerate it.
      (2) If nonoperative management fails or strangulation is suspected, immediate operative reduction is required.
   b. Cecal volvulus — early surgical reduction

D. Mesenteric Vascular Ischemia/Infarction

1. Most commonly affects patients who are > 50 years old and have a history of cardiovascular disease.

2. Mortality rate is 50% overall (but rises to 70% or more once infarction has occurred) and reflects the difficulty in making an early diagnosis as well as the presence of significant underlying disease.

3. Etiology
   a. Acute mesenteric arterial occlusion is responsible for 65 - 75% of cases and is the result of embolization from the heart in most instances. The remaining cases are due to in situ thrombosis and occur in patients with chronic severe atherosclerosis.
   b. Mesenteric venous thrombosis is responsible for 5 - 15% of cases and most commonly occurs in association with a hypercoagulable state (e.g. polycythemia vera, antithrombin III deficiency). Affected patients are usually younger in age and up to 60% of them have a history of peripheral DVT.
   c. Nonocclusive mesenteric ischemia (a multifactorial syndrome where no mechanical occlusive lesion can be identified) accounts for 20% of cases; it is caused by conditions which induce a sustained reduction

in cardiac output (e.g. CHF, recent MI, hypovolemia) or medications that reduce mesenteric blood flow (e.g. digitalis, vasoconstrictors). Elderly, critically ill patients are the most commonly affected.

4. Predisposing factors for...
   a. Arterial occlusion
      (1) Dysrhythmias (particularly atrial fibrillation)
      (2) Atherosclerotic heart disease
      (3) Valvular heart disease
      (4) Recent MI
   b. Venous thrombosis
      (1) History of prior thromboembolic events
      (2) Hypercoagulable states
   c. Nonocclusive ischemia
      (1) Use of diuretics or vasoconstrictive medications
      (2) Hypotension
      (3) CHF

5. Clinical presentation — The patient is typically middle-aged or elderly and presents with <u>severe abdominal pain</u>, fever and tachycardia; sudden onset suggests arterial occlusion while insidious onset suggests venous thrombosis or nonocclusive ischemia. A history of similar, spontaneously-resolving pain episodes following meals ("intestinal ischemia") is not uncommon. Early on, the pain is poorly localized and **out of proportion** to findings on physical exam. Diarrhea is common and is frequently guaiac positive. Grossly bloody stool may also occur. Other commonly associated symptoms are anorexia, nausea and vomiting. Abdominal distention and peritoneal signs are <u>late findings</u> and signal the presence of bowel <u>infarction</u>.

6. Diagnostic studies — With the exception of emergency angiography, the results of these studies are most useful in ruling out other diagnoses and establishing a needed baseline.
   a. CBC — reveals hemoconcentration (increased Hct) and leukocytosis (WBC count is often >15,000).
   b. Serum amylase — is usually moderately elevated (lipase is normal)
   c. Serum phosphate — may be elevated.
   d. D-lactate — is usually significantly elevated.
   e. ABG — often reveals a metabolic acidosis, particularly late in the disease course.
   f. Plain abdominal and upright chest x-rays — are usually the first radiographic studies to be obtained, although they are often normal (especially early on). Findings may include:
      (1) Ileus
      (2) Small bowel obstruction
      (3) Gasless abdomen
      (4) Irregular thickening of the bowel wall ("thumbprinting")*
      (5) Gas in the bowel wall (pneumatosis intestinalis) or portal venous system*

*Although rarely seen, these findings strongly suggest intestinal infarction.

g. Abdominal CT, US and MRI are not the initial studies of choice for emergency diagnosis of bowel ischemia; however, they do provide ancillary data to the plain film evaluation, e.g. bowel wall thickening on abdominal CT suggests mesenteric ischemia.

h. Angiography — is the <u>most important diagnostic tool</u> and should be obtained without delay when this diagnosis is suspected.

7. Management
   a. Initial stabilization measures include:
      (1) IV of NS or LR — to correct volume deficit
      (2) Supplemental oxygen
      (3) NG tube — to decompress stomach and bowel
      (4) Initial labs, type and cross, cultures and x-rays
      (5) Broad-spectrum IV antibiotics
      (6) Correction of precipitating or predisposing causes of ischemia (e.g., CHF, dysrhythmias)
      (7) Immediate surgical consultation
      (8) Infusion of papaverine* (an intra-arterial vasodilator) through the angiographic catheter
   b. Specific treatment measures — depend on the underlying etiology of the ischemia and if peritoneal signs or necrotic bowel are present.
      (1) <u>Nonocclusive</u> mesenteric ischemia — unless peritonitis or necrotic bowel is present, treatment is <u>nonoperative</u>; papaverine alone is considered definitive therapy in these patients.
      (2) Mesenteric <u>venous</u> thrombosis — <u>immediate</u> anticoagulation with heparin is the initial treatment of choice and, in the absence of peritonitis and necrotic bowel, may be the only treatment given.
      (3) Acute mesenteric arterial occlusion (embolic and thrombotic) — is initially treated with papaverine. The need for subsequent surgery is determined by the patient's response, underlying condition and the angiographic findings.
      (4) Immediate surgery is indicated for:
         (a) Patients with peritonitis
         (b) Those requiring a revascularization procedure
         (c) Resection of necrotic bowel

E. Hernias

1. Definitions
   a. Hernia → the protrusion of a structure from its normal position into another through an opening that is either congenital or acquired.
   b. External hernia → protrudes to the outside (e.g. umbilical)
   c. Internal hernia → protrudes within the body (e.g. diaphragmatic)
   d. Incisional hernia → protrudes through a previous incision
   e. Reducible hernia → protruding contents can be pushed back in
   f. Irreducible (incarcerated) hernia
      (1) Protruding contents cannot be moved back into place
      (2) Seen most often when large contents herniate through a small defect
   g. Strangulated hernia → vascular compromise of herniated contents

*Is used to diagnose <u>arterial</u> (not venous) thrombosis.

2. Types
   a. Inguinal hernia
      (1) Direct
         - Protrudes directly through the floor of Hesselbach's triangle
         - Results from relaxation/weakening of the abdominal musculature
         - Increased frequency with age
         - Rarely incarcerates
      (2) Indirect
         - Protrudes through the internal inguinal ring lateral to the inferior epigastric vessels
         - Represents a <u>congenital</u> defect (incomplete closure of processus vaginalis)
         - Most common hernia occurring in both males and females
         - Most common in younger patients
         - Frequently incarcerate, especially in infancy
   b. Femoral hernia
      - Protrudes below the inguinal ligament and the femoral vessels in the femoral canal
      - More common in women
      - Frequently incarcerates
   c. Umbilical hernia
      - Usually presents as a lump
      - Common in newborns
      - Most close spontaneously by two or three years of age
   d. Obturator hernia
      - Protrudes through the obturator foramen into the medial thigh
      - Majority occur in elderly women
      - Patients present with pain and decreased sensation along the medial aspect of the thigh to the knee.

F. Ileitis and Colitis

1. Crohn's disease (terminal ileitis, granulomatous ileocolitis, regional enteritis)
   a. Pathology
      (1) A chronic inflammatory disease that <u>involves all layers</u> of the bowel as well as the mesenteric lymph nodes.
      (2) Any segment of the GI tract from the mouth to the anus may be affected.
      (3) The disease is <u>discontinuous</u> with normal areas of bowel ("<u>skip areas</u>") between one or more involved areas; the ileum is usually involved in the majority of cases.
      (4) The bowel wall is thickened; this leads to narrowing of the lumen which frequently results in obstruction.
      (5) Longitudinal deep ulcerations are characteristic; with progression of the disease, a "cobblestone" appearance of the mucosa results from crisscrossing of these ulcers with intervening normal mucosa.

      (6) Noncaseating granulomas are present in ≥ 50% of specimens and are helpful (but not necessary) in making the diagnosis.

      (7) Perianal complications occur in 90% of cases and may be the initial presenting symptom in many patients.

  b. Epidemiology

      (1) Most commonly seen in the 15 - 40 age group

      (2) Greater incidence in whites than blacks

      (3) Four to eight times more common in Jews than non-Jews

      (4) Family history in 10 - 15% of patients

      (5) Incidence has been increasing over the past 30 years

      (6) Etiology remains undetermined

  c. **Clinical pictures**

      (1) Abdominal pain and diarrhea (inflammation of ileum and/or colon)

        (a) Past history of recurrent abdominal pain, diarrhea and fever for several years.

        (b) Weight loss is common.

      (2) RLQ pain and tenderness (acute inflammation of the terminal ileum only)

        (a) Looks like appendicitis — anorexia, diarrhea, vomiting, fever and leukocytosis.

        (b) Diagnostic clue — occult blood and fecal leukocytes favor regional enteritis.

  d. Extraintestinal manifestations — occur in one-quarter to one-third of cases and may be the presenting and/or dominant manifestation of the disease process in some patients:

      (1) Arthritic (peripheral arthritis, ankylosing spondylitis)

      (2) Vascular (vasculitis, arteritis, thromboembolic disease)

      (3) Hepatobiliary (gallstones, pericholangitis, chronic active hepatitis)

      (4) Dermatologic (erythema nodosum, pyoderma gangrenosum)

      (5) Ophthalmic (uveitis, episcleritis, iritis, conjunctivitis)

      (6) Miscellaneous (growth retardation, hyperoxaluria with renal stones)

  e. Complications

      (1) Perianal (abscess, fissure, fistula, rectovaginal fistula, rectal prolapse)

      (2) Intestinal (obstruction, abscess, fistula, stricture, perforation, hemorrhage)

      (3) Toxic megacolon is an infrequent complication of Crohn's disease and is associated with massive GI bleeding in > 50% of cases.

      (4) Malignancies of both the small and large bowel are three times more frequent in patients with Crohn's disease than in the general population.

  f. Diagnosis

      (1) Previously undiagnosed patients require radiologic, colonoscopic, and histologic confirmation to establish the local and systemic extent of the disease,

      (2) This can be accomplished on an outpatient basis in reliable patients with mild disease.

g. Treatment
   (1) Make a diligent effort to R/O associated small bowel obstruction because early institution of NG suction, IV fluids and steroids may reduce inflammatory edema, restore bowel patency and avoid the need for emergency surgery.
   (2) Fluid and electrolyte replacement prn (especially those patients with a history of anorexia, vomiting and diarrhea).
   (3) Indications for admission — include the presence of:
       (a) Dehydration or metabolic/electrolyte disturbances
       (b) Severe exacerbation of the primary illness
       (c) Acute complications (e.g. obstruction, hemorrhage, peritonitis)
   (4) Outpatient therapy for mild cases
       (a) Bed rest, analgesics, antidiarrheal agent
       (b) Milk products should be avoided; they frequently aggravate diarrhea in these patients in whom the incidence of lactose intolerance is quite high.
       (c) Steroids—Institution of (or change in dose) should be done in conjunction with the patient's primary physician since these agents have many side effects and are ineffective as maintenance therapy.
       (d) Antibiotic therapy with sulfasalazine, especially when combined with a steroid preparation, has been demonstrated to induce symptomatic improvement for patients with active Crohn's colitis.
       (e) Metronidazole
           1 Is useful in treating the perianal and colonic Crohn's disease.
           2 Is used in patients who are unresponsive to or unable to tolerate sulfasalazine.
       (f) Azathioprine and its metabolite 6-mercaptopurine (immunosuppressive agents) are useful:
           1 As steroid-sparing agents (they allow patients to decrease their dose of prednisone)
           2 In patients with refractory disease and contraindications to surgery
           3 In patients with enterocutaneous or enteroenteric fistulas

2. Ulcerative colitis
   a. Pathology
      (1) Ulcerative colitis is a chronic inflammatory and ulcerative disease of the colon and rectum, most often characterized clinically by bloody diarrhea and crampy abdominal pain.
      (2) Inflammation is generally limited to the mucosa and submucosa; the muscular layer and serosa are usually spared.
      (3) Unlike the "skip lesions" of Crohn's disease, mucosal involvement in ulcerative colitis is continuous and uniform; it always begins in the rectum and can remain limited to this area or spread proximally to involve the upper segments of the colon.
      (4) Chronic inflammation leads to the formation of crypt abscesses, epithelial necrosis and mucosal ulceration.

b. Epidemiology — closely approximates that of Crohn's disease.

c. Clinical features (occur intermittently with complete remission between attacks)

    (1) Mild disease — 60% of cases

        (a) < 4 bowel movements/day

        (b) No systemic symptoms

        (c) Few extraintestinal manifestations

    (2) Severe disease (fulminant colitis) — 15% of cases

        (a) > 6 bowel movements/day

        (b) Fever, tachycardia, weight loss, anemia

        (c) Extraintestinal manifestations (essentially the same as those seen with Crohn's disease).

d. Complications

    (1) Hemorrhage — is the most common; however, massive hemorrhage is infrequent (occurs in only 2 - 3% of patients).

    (2) Toxic megacolon (occurs more commonly with ulcerative colitis than with Crohn's disease)

        (a) **Clinical picture** —The patient appears severely ill and has abnormal vital signs (hypotension, tachycardia and fever). The abdomen is distended, tender and tympanitic. Lab studies reveal leukocytosis with anemia, electrolyte imbalance and hypoalbuminemia. Plain film of the abdomen reveals dilatation of the colon with a colonic diameter > 6cm.

        (b) Management

            <u>1</u> NG suction, IV fluids and broad-spectrum antibiotics

            <u>2</u> IV steroids (hydrocortisone or methylprednisolone)

            <u>3</u> Frequent abdominal exams and x-rays with surgery (colectomy) if no improvement in 24 - 48 hrs.

    (3) Perforation (occurs more often during <u>first</u> episodes of colitis)

    (4) Obstruction (due to stricture)

    (5) Perianal fistulas and abscesses (occur less commonly with ulcerative colitis than with Crohn's disease).

    (6) Carcinoma of the colon (the incidence is 10 - 30 times greater in patients with ulcerative colitis than in the general population and correlates with the duration and extent of disease).

e. Diagnosis

    (1) The most sensitive method for establishing the diagnosis of ulcerative colitis and determining the extent of disease is a colonoscopy.

    (2) Diagnosis of toxic megacolon is usually obvious on plain films.

f. Treatment

    (1) Mild to moderate disease

        (a) Sulfasalazine

            <u>1</u> Is the mainstay of therapy.

            <u>2</u> The therapeutic properties of this drug are due to its 5-aminosalicylic acid (5-ASA) component.

            <u>3</u> If sulfasalazine is not well tolerated, a 5-ASA derivative (mesalamine or olsalazine) should be substituted.

   (b) Corticosteroids — may also be needed, either as supplemental therapy or as alternative therapy when sulfasalazine is ineffective.

   (c) 5-ASA and corticosteroid enemas — are useful for patients with ulcerative proctitis and left-sided colitis.

   (d) Supportive therapy (supplemental iron + a lactose-free diet) [Antidiarrheal agents should be avoided; they are usually ineffective and they can precipitate toxic megacolon.]

   (e) Azathioprine, cyclosporine and 6-mercaptopurine are used in patients who do not respond to steroid therapy.

  (2) Severe ulcerative colitis (inpatient therapy)

   (a) IV fluids and correction of electrolyte abnormalities

   (b) NG tube

   (c) IV steroids or ACTH

   (d) Broad-spectrum antibiotics active against coliforms and anaerobes (ampicillin, clindamycin or metronidazole)

   (e) Surgical consult if toxic megacolon suspected

3. Pseudomembranous enterocolitis

 a. An inflammatory bowel disorder characterized by the formation of yellowish exudative pseudomembranous-like plaques that overlie and replace necrotic intestinal mucosa, particularly in the area of the rectosigmoid.

 b. Pathophysiology and epidemiology

  (1) Ingestion of broad-spectrum antibiotics alters the gut flora → proliferation of the cytopathic <u>toxin</u>-producing bacterium, *Clostridium difficile.*

  (2) Most commonly implicated antibiotics:

   (a) Cephalosporins

   (b) Ampicillin

   (c) Clindamycin

   (d) Lincomycin

  (3) Nosocomial transmission among hospitalized patients via hands of health care workers (contaminated with C. difficile toxin) who are caring for them also occurs, even in the absence of antimicrobial therapy.

 c. **Clinical picture** — The patient presents with crampy abdominal pain, fever and watery diarrhea (which may be bloody). Symptoms generally begin 7 - 10 days following the initiation of antibiotics, but may occasionally be delayed several weeks past their discontinuation. The presence of *C. difficile* <u>toxin</u> in the stool <u>confirms</u> the diagnosis. If this assay is not readily available, colonoscopy or sigmoidoscopy can be used to establish a tentative diagnosis.

 d. Treatment

  (1) D/C antibiotics and institute supportive therapy with IV fluids and electrolyte replacement.

  (2) Oral metronidazole is the initial drug of choice for most patients.

  (3) Oral vancomycin is the alternative agent; it is usually reserved for severe cases and those unresponsive to metronidazole.

Note: Antimotility drugs (such as Lomotil) should be avoided; they can worsen symptoms and their use is associated with an increased risk of developing toxic megacolon.

G. Irritable Bowel Syndrome (IBS)

1. Definition — a state of disturbed intestinal motility (without anatomic cause) that is precipitated by psychosocial factors such as stress.

2. Epidemiology
   a. Patients are usually 20 - 40 years old.
   b. Women are affected more often than men (ratio is 2:1).
   c. A familial association is common (? genetic vs. learned behavior).
   d. Psychosocial stressors are often present.

3. **Clinical picture** — The patient is usually a young woman who presents with recurrent episodes of altered bowel function (diarrhea or constipation) with or without associated abdominal pain. The episodes are usually precipitated by stress. The abdominal pain is described as crampy or achy in character and is confined to the lower abdomen. It generally occurs in association with constipation and is relieved by defecation or the passage of gas. Extracolonic symptoms (e.g. bloating, belching, gastroesophageal reflux) are common. Associated anorexia, fever and weight loss are denied. Exam findings are most often nonspecific but may include vague lower abdominal tenderness and a palpable stool-filled sigmoid colon. Lab evaluation is unremarkable.

4. Diagnosis — IBS is a diagnosis of exclusion. Thus, if the history is suggestive and the initial evaluation in the ED is unremarkable, these patients should be referred back to their personal physicians for a more complete work-up (cultures, barium enema, sigmoidoscopy) to R/O an underlying organic disease process, e.g. lactose deficiency, colitis.

5. Treatment modalities
   a. High-fiber, low-fat diet
   b. Bulk-forming agents (psyllium preparation, bran)
   c. Elimination of foods that precipitate or exacerbate symptoms (fatty or fried foods, beans, cabbage, caffeinated drinks)
   d. Drug therapy* — should be reserved for patients who fail to respond to the above measures and may include one or more of the following:
      (1) Antidiarrheal agents
      (2) Antispasmodic (anticholinergic) agents
      (3) Anxiolytics
      (4) Antidepressants

---

*A number of new drugs are currently in phase II and phase III trials, some of which are narcotic receptor modulators and new anticholinergics.

H. Colonic Diverticular Disease

1. Diverticula — are saclike herniations of colonic mucosa through the muscularis that result from colonic muscular dysfunction and a fiber-deficient diet. Increased muscular tone of bowel wall → shortening of the bowel with muscle thickening → saclike protrusions of mucosa through the muscularis at its weakest point (where the intramural blood vessels penetrate it). Though the location of diverticula may vary, most are confined to the sigmoid colon. (LLQ)

2. The frequency of diverticular disease is directly correlated with age, especially if the diet is low in fiber and roughage. As one grows older, there is a 50% probability of developing diverticular disease. However, only a small portion (10 - 20%) of patients with this disease become symptomatic. Massive painless lower GI bleeding in the elderly is one clinical presentation of diverticulosis. (Diverticulosis is one of the most common causes of massive lower GI bleeding.) In most instances, the bleeding stops spontaneously.

3. Painful diverticular disease
   a. Pathophysiology
      (1) Like irritable bowel syndrome (IBS), painful diverticular disease is also associated with a disturbance in intestinal motility and can be precipitated by either stress or eating.
      (2) Food ingestion or emotional stimuli → ↑ intraluminal pressure with stretching of the bowel wall → abdominal pain.
   b. **Clinical picture** — is similar to that seen in IBS, but the patient is older and pain is more localized. The patient is typically more than 40 years of age and presents with LLQ pain accompanied by diarrhea or constipation. He/she relates a history of similar episodes in the past and states that these episodes are usually precipitated by either stress or eating and are relieved by the passage of stool or flatus. On exam, there is tenderness in the LLQ; a tender, mobile, rope-like sigmoid may be palpable, but signs of peritonitis are absent and labs are normal.
   c. Treatment
      (1) High fiber diet
      (2) Bulk laxatives and stool softeners (↓ intraluminal pressure and prevent constipation)
      (3) Anticholinergics for muscle spasm and sedation to alleviate the tension prn
      (4) Local heat application (heating pad)

4. Diverticulitis = diverticulosis + inflammation
   a. Diverticulitis is the most frequent complication of diverticulosis.
   b. Pathophysiology — fecal material in the neck of a diverticulum hardens → fecalith → fecalith erodes the mucosa or compromises its blood supply → ↑ susceptibility to bacterial invasion → inflammation and microperforation of the diverticulum.

c. The **clinical picture** is similar to painful diverticular disease with the following differentiating features:

(1) The stool is positive for occult blood in > 50% of cases but gross bleeding is rare.

(2) Signs and symptoms of peritonitis are often present:

(a) Abdominal tenderness and guarding localized to the left lower quadrant that is associated with mild abdominal distention

(b) Fever and leukocytosis

(c) Anorexia, nausea and vomiting (sometimes)

d. Plain abdominal films — are most useful in excluding the complications of diverticulitis (perforation, obstruction, fistula and abscess formation). Findings may include:

(1) An ileus pattern

(2) Obstruction (Diverticulitis is one of the most common causes of large bowel obstruction in adults)

(3) Free air (peritonitis)

(4) Extraluminal air collection (walled-off abscess)

e. Endoscopy and contrast x-ray studies — while useful in confirming the diagnosis, are relatively <u>contraindicated</u> in the acute phase due to the potential risk of perforation.

f. Abdominal CT — is the preferred study for defining the extent of the disease process (e.g. associated abscess). It is also helpful when the diagnosis is unclear, since it can demonstrate and exclude other abdominal pathophysiology. Furthermore, it is not associated with the risk of perforation.

g. Treatment

(1) IV fluids and broad-spectrum antibiotics providing both aerobic and anaerobic bacterial coverage; a combination of metronidazole and a fluoroquinolone (ciprofloxacin or levofloxacin) are effective and may be given orally or IV.

(2) Keep the patient NPO (to rest the bowel)

(3) NG suction if ileus or intestinal obstruction is present

(4) Surgical consult (15 - 45% require surgery)[*]

(5) Analgesia

(a) Meperidine is beneficial because it interferes with segmental contraction of the colon, but it also causes dysphoria, has a high addictive potential and causes seizures in a non-dose-related manner.

(b) Oral opiates (morphine, codeine) are not recommended for outpatients because they increase the intraluminal pressure within the sigmoid colon; however, short-term use of IV opiates may be used judiciously in hospitalized patients with significant discomfort; morphine and dilaudid (administered parenterally) are now used preferentially by many clinicians.

[*]In patients with diverticular abscess, percutaneous aspiration performed by interventional radiology is an alternative to laparotomy in select patients.

V. Anorectal Disorders

A. Hemorrhoids

1. Definition — Hemorrhoids are dilated venules of the hemorrhoidal plexuses. They are associated with chronic constipation, straining, increased intra-abdominal pressure, pregnancy, increased portal pressure and a low-fiber diet.

2. Types
   a. External hemorrhoids — arise from below the dentate line (which separates the rectum from the anus) and are covered with well-innervated squamous epithelium. They are visible on external inspection.
   b. Internal hemorrhoids — originate from above the dentate line and are covered by relatively insensitive rectal mucosa. Although not normally palpable on exam, they can be visualized with anoscopy at the 2, 5, and 9 o'clock positions.

3. Presentations
   a. Patients with external hemorrhoids most commonly present with painful thrombosis. Exam reveals a tender mass at the external anal orifice.
   b. Patients with internal hemorrhoids usually present with painless bright-red bleeding that occurs in association with defecation. (Hemorrhoids are the most common cause of rectal bleeding). The blood covers the stool or drips into the toilet bowl and is usually small in volume.

4. Treatment
   a. Thrombosed external hemorrhoids
      (1) If pain is tolerable and/or the thrombosis is not acute (> 48 hrs.) warm (40°C/104°F) sitz baths, systemic analgesics, increased dietary fiber, stool softeners or bulk laxatives. Topical agents (e.g., steroids, analgesics, antibiotics) are of limited value and are probably best avoided.
      (2) If pain is severe and the thrombosis is acute (< 48 hrs.) → excision of clots under local anesthesia followed by warm sitz baths 6 - 12 hours post-drainage
   b. Bleeding internal hemorrhoids
      (1) If bleeding is minor and resolves post-defecation → increased dietary fiber and fluids, stool softeners or bulk laxatives and warm sitz baths
      (2) Persistent, refractory bleeding → IV fluid resuscitation (as needed) → rectal packing and surgical therapy
   c. Surgical indications
      (1) Continued bleeding
      (2) Strangulation or incarceration
      (3) Intractable pain or severe itching

B. Fissure-In-Ano (Anal Fissure)

1. Description
    a. Anal fissures are linear tears of the squamous epithelium of the anal canal. Most (90%) are located in the <u>posterior midline</u>; however, in women they are occasionally found in the <u>anterior midline</u>. Lesions found elsewhere should prompt consideration of an underlying disease process (e.g. inflammatory bowel disease, neoplasm, TB) and referral for further evaluation. Chronic fissures may be accompanied by a sentinel pile (a swollen external tag of skin at the base of the fissure) often confused with an external hemorrhoid.
    b. These lesions are the most frequent anorectal disorders affecting infants and children, the most common cause of rectal bleeding in the first year of life and the most common cause of <u>painful</u> rectal bleeding in adults.

2. Etiology — They are usually produced by the passage of a large, hard stool but may also occur with severe diarrhea.

3. **Clinical picture**: The patient has a history of constipation and complains of <u>severe pain with defecation</u> that lingers for several hours before resolving. The pain is often so severe that the patient avoids defecating and is unwilling to let you perform a digital rectal exam. Scant associated hematochezia is common. Inspection of the anus reveals the classic linear ulcer in the posterior midline.

4. Treatment
    a. Instruct the patient to do the following:
        (1) Thoroughly cleanse the anal area following defecation. (This is essential for healing to occur.)
        (2) Take warm (40°C) sitz baths 3 - 4 times/day (relaxes the sphincter).
        (3) Eat a high-fiber diet (prevents stricture formation).
        (4) Use bulk laxatives and stool softeners.
    b. Analgesic/hydrocortisone-containing ointments provide relief and facilitate healing, but may cause constipation.*
    c. If healing does not occur, surgical correction (partial sphincterotomy and excision of the fissure) may be required.

C. Perirectal (Anorectal) Abscesses

1. Perirectal abscesses have a tendency to occur in any of the potential spaces near the anus or rectum (perianal, ischiorectal, deep postanal, supralevator and intersphincteric). Perianal abscesses are the most common. Most abscesses point at the skin, but an ischiorectal abscess may point in an area some distance from the skin; although it can be quite large, a mass may only be felt on digital exam of the perianal area.

---

*Common opiate side effect; consider adding a stool softener.

2. Etiology — Most anorectal abscesses result from obstruction of mucus-producing glands at the base of the anal crypts. Other causes include inflammatory bowel disease, cancer, radiation injury, trauma, TB and lymphogranuloma venereum. The resulting infections are frequently polymicrobial and involve the colonic flora.

3. Fistula formation is a common sequela.

4. **Clinical picture** — As you walk into the room, the patient looks very uncomfortable and may be febrile. He c/o a dull aching pain in his rectum. The pain is worse just prior to and with a bowel movement and then improves but does not resolve. If the abscess points to the skin, it is readily palpable; sometimes there is only a tender erythematous area over the skin with or without fluctuance. Abscesses that point in, away from the skin, can be missed unless a careful rectal exam is performed.

5. Treatment is <u>surgical</u>. Anorectal abscesses require early and extensive drainage. Simple perianal abscesses may be drained in the Emergency Department under local anesthesia; all other perirectal abscesses need to be drained in the OR. Routine use of antibiotics is not warranted; they should be reserved for immunocompromised patients, diabetics, patients with valvular heart disease and those with associated cellulitis.

D. Miscellaneous Anorectal Disorders

1. Fistula-in-ano
   a. This is an abnormal tract between the anal canal and skin that is lined with granulation tissue.
   b. It most commonly occurs as a complication of a perianal or ischio-rectal abscess; it may also be associated with ulcerative colitis, Crohn's disease, TB, radiation and CA of the anus or rectum.
   c. If the tract remains open, there is a persistent, purulent, blood-stained discharge; if the tract becomes blocked (most common), an abscess may be the only physical finding.
   d. Treatment is surgical excision.

2. Rectal prolapse (procidentia)
   a. Types
      (1) Mucosal prolapse (seen primarily in young children and in asso-ciation with internal hemorrhoids)
      (2) Prolapse involving all layers of the rectum
      (3) Intussusception of the upper rectum into the lower rectum with the apex protruding through the anus
   b. Complete rectal prolapse occurs in the very young and the very old (particularly elderly women).
   c. Patients typically complain of a painless anal mass following strain-ing, coughing or defecation.
   d. Treatment
      (1) Reduction can be accomplished in almost all patients, although recurrence (particularly in the elderly) is likely.

(2) In the presence of vascular compromise, emergency reduction is mandatory.
(3) Following reduction, patients should be placed on stool softeners and referred for further evaluation (to uncover any underlying pathology) and potential surgical correction (commonly required in the elderly).

3. Pilonidal sinus (abscess)
   a. Occurs in the <u>midline</u> (at the superior edge of the buttock crease) and is more common in men than women.
   b. The sinus is formed when an ingrowing hair penetrates the skin and induces a foreign body granuloma reaction.
   c. A single opening at the base of the spine with hair protruding is the most common physical finding.
   d. When the sinus becomes plugged and cannot drain → abscess
   e. Treatment is primarily surgical: incision and drainage followed by referral for definitive surgical excision; antibiotics are indicated if there is an associated cellulitis or the patient is immunocompromised.

4. Anorectal tumors:
   a. Classification — based upon their virulence, these tumors have been arranged into two groups with distinct anatomic locations:
   (1) Anal <u>canal</u> neoplasms (occur <u>proximal</u> to the <u>dentate</u> line)
      (a) Represent 80% of anorectal tumors
      (b) Have a <u>high</u>-grade malignant potential and metastasize early; their prognosis is poor.
      (c) Tumors occurring in this region include:
         <u>1</u> Adenocarcinoma (common)
         <u>2</u> Mucoepidermoid carcinoma
         <u>3</u> Malignant melanoma
         <u>4</u> Kaposi's sarcoma
         <u>5</u> Squamous cell carcinoma
         <u>6</u> Basaloid carcinoma
         <u>7</u> Villous adenoma
   (2) Anal <u>margin</u> neoplasms (occur <u>distal</u> to the <u>dentate</u> line)
      (a) Represent 20% of anorectal tumors
      (b) Have a low-grade malignant potential and are slow to metastasize; their prognosis is good.
      (c) Tumors occurring in this region include:
         <u>1</u> Basal cell carcinoma
         <u>2</u> Squamous cell carcinoma
         <u>3</u> Bowen's disease
         <u>4</u> Extramammary Paget's disease
         <u>5</u> Giant solitary trichoepithelioma
   b. Symptoms include: pruritus, rectal bleeding, pain, weight loss, anorexia, constipation, decrease in stool caliber, tenesmus and obstruction.
   c. Management → prompt surgical referral

5. Rectal foreign bodies
   a. Abdominal x-rays should be obtained to ascertain the location, size, shape and number of objects present as well as R/O the presence of free air; multiple views may be needed to make these determinations.
   b. Perforation is the most frequent complication and results from the foreign body itself or attempts to remove it. Mucosal tears can also occur. Therefore, following removal of the foreign body, the patient should be observed for 12 hours and post-removal x-ray studies and sigmoidoscopy should be performed.
   c. If there is clinical or radiographic evidence of free air, the patient should be prepared for surgery and a stat surgical consult should be obtained.

VI. Diarrhea and Food Poisoning

A. *Viral Diarrheal Diseases (The majority of all acute episodes of diarrhea)*

1. Rotavirus and Norwalk virus are the most frequent causes. The peak incidence of infection with these viruses is during the winter months.
   a. Rotavirus infection occurs primarily in children 6 - 24 months of age. These young children typically present with low-grade fever, vomiting and watery diarrhea; they may also have a URI or pneumonia. Symptoms begin after an incubation period of 2 - 3 days and the diarrhea lasts 3 - 10 days. The diagnosis is confirmed with the Rotazyme test. Treatment is supportive.
   b. Norwalk virus typically infects school-aged children and adults. Family outbreaks and epidemics frequently occur. These outbreaks are often associated with the ingestion of contaminated food and water, particularly poorly cooked or raw shellfish. Following an incubation period of 1 - 2 days, patients typically have an abrupt onset of nausea, vomiting, watery diarrhea, abdominal cramps and low-grade fever; there is no upper or lower respiratory tract involvement. Symptoms last for 1 - 2 days. Treatment is supportive.

2. Enteric type adenovirus (intestinal "flu") has been implicated in outbreaks of acute gastroenteritis. Vomiting and watery diarrhea with low-grade fever and general malaise is the usual picture. Like other viral causes of diarrhea described above, this is a self-limited illness treated with supportive measures only.

3. A wet mount of the stool using methylene blue is helpful in distinguishing viral from bacterial diarrhea:
   a. Viral diarrhea → absence of WBCs
   b. Diarrhea due to invasive organisms/bacteria → presence of WBCs
   c. Diarrhea due to enterotoxins → WBCs usually absent (<u>exceptions</u> are *C. difficile* enterocolitis and enterohemorrhagic *E. coli* serotype O157: H7 hemorrhagic colitis where WBCs are usually present)

B. Bacterial Diarrheal Diseases (20% of acute diarrheal cases)

1. Classification
   a. Invasive bacteria act primarily on the large bowel and produce diarrhea by damaging cell membranes and eliciting an inflammatory response → blood and mucus in the stools:
      (1) *Campylobacter*
      (2) *Salmonella*
      (3) *Shigella*
      (4) *Vibrio parahaemolyticus*
      (5) *Vibrio vulnificus*
      (6) *Yersinia enterocolitica*
      (7) *Enteroinvasive E. coli*
      *(8) Enterohemorrhagic *E. coli* serotype O157:H7
      *(9) *Clostridium difficile*
         *Note: These organisms are actually toxin-producing bacteria that induce diarrhea by elaborating a <u>cytopathic</u> toxin that destroys the intestinal wall. They are grouped with the invasive bacteria because the clinical syndrome they produce most closely resembles that produced by these organisms.
   b. Enterotoxin-producing bacteria release a toxin that acts primarily in the small intestine and produces diarrhea by altering water and electrolyte transport in epithelial cells → profuse watery diarrhea:
      (1) <u>*Staph. aureus*</u>
      (2) *Bacillus cereus*
      (3) Ciguatera fish poisoning
      (4) Scombroid fish poisoning
      (5) Enterotoxigenic *E. coli*
      (6) *Clostridium perfringens*
      (7) *Aeromonas hydrophilia*
      (8) *Vibrio cholera*

2. A wet mount or methylene blue stain of the stool for <u>fecal leukocytes</u>:
   a. May be used as a screen for those patients who may benefit from antibiotic therapy:
      (1) Invasive bacterial pathogens producing fever, systemic illness or bloody stools → salmonella, shigella, campylobacter and e.coli 0157:H7
      (2) Pseudomembranous enterocolitis
      (3) Amebiasis
      (4) Inflammatory bowel disease (Crohn's disease and ulcerative colitis)
   b. Typical findings in various infections and conditions producing diarrheal syndromes:

⊕ Fecal leukocytes	⊖ Fecal leukocytes
Campylobacter	Rotavirus
Salmonella	Norwalk virus
Shigella	Enteric type adenovirus
Vibrio parahaemolyticus	*Staph. aureus*

⊕ Fecal leukocytes | ⊖ Fecal leukocytes

⊕ Fecal leukocytes
Vibrio vulnificus
Yersinia
Amebiasis
Enteroinvasive *E. coli*
Enterohemorrhagic *E. coli*
Clostridium difficile
Ulcerative colitis
Crohn's disease

⊖ Fecal leukocytes
Bacillus cereus
Ciguatera fish poisoning
Scombroid fish poisoning
Enterotoxigenic *E. coli*
Clostridium perfringens
Aeromonas hydrophilia
Vibrio cholera
Giardia lamblia

Note: Although treatment based on the presence or absence of fecal leukocytes is not 100% accurate, it is a good place to start, and is one of the few test results for diarrheal illnesses that is immediately available. When this information is combined with a detailed history and an assessment of the overall toxicity of the patient, a reasonable therapeutic plan can be initiated; if available, immunoassay for the neutrophil marker lactoferrin can provide additional evidence of inflammatory diarrhea.

3. Traveler's diarrhea
   a. Definition — Traveler's diarrhea is a syndrome that is acquired by travelers who eat food or water that is fecally contaminated.
   b. The risk of acquiring it is particularly high in people who:
      (1) Travel to developing tropical regions (Mexico, Latin America, southern Asia, Africa) where sanitation is poor.
      (2) Eat food prepared by street vendors.
      (3) Ingest certain unsafe (often contaminated) items such as tap water, ice cubes, unpasteurized dairy products, raw vegetables, unpeeled fruit and raw or undercooked seafood or meat.
   c. Most cases (70 - 75%) are caused by bacteria, of which enterotoxigenic *E. coli* is the most commonly involved pathogen; it is responsible for up to 50% of cases worldwide.
   d. Symptoms often begin abruptly and consist of watery diarrhea and abdominal cramps. Other associated symptoms may be present and vary with the particular etiologic agent involved.
   e. Antibiotic prophylaxis — is not recommended for healthy individuals due to the associated risks (e.g., emergence of resistant organisms, allergic reactions, photosensitivity reactions, etc.). Initiation of treatment at the onset of symptoms is preferred.
   f. Treatment
      (1) Oral rehydration — with Gatorade, caffeine-free soft drinks or diluted fruit juice effectively maintains the fluid and electrolyte balance in the majority of patients.
      (2) Antibiotics — a 3 to 5 day course* of a quinolone (ciprofloxacin, norfloxacin, ofloxacin) or TMP-SMX should be considered for all clinical presentations of Traveler's diarrhea; these agents provide rapid relief of symptoms and decrease the duration of illness.
      (3) Antimotility agents — such as loperamide provide rapid symptomatic relief but should not be continued for more than 2 days and should not be used in patients who are febrile or have blood in the stools because they tend to prolong the duration of the infection.

*Actually, one dose taken at onset of symptoms is usually effective.

(4) Bismuth subsalicylate (Pepto-Bismol®) — an antisecretory agent that is also effective in reducing the number of stools passed and the duration of illness. It works by decreasing the outpouring of fluids by the mucosa of the small intestine. This agent is also effective prophylactically in preventing diarrhea.

4. Specific bacterial infections
   a. *E. coli* — several strains of *E. coli* have been shown to be diarrheagenic, two of which are discussed below. These strains differ in terms of their virulence, epidemiology and clinical characteristics.
      (1) Enterotoxigenic E. coli
         (a) Most common cause of Traveler's diarrhea worldwide.
         (b) Acquired by ingesting fecally-contaminated food and water.
         (c) Causes diarrhea by producing both heat-labile and heat-stable toxins.
         (d) Incubation period of 1 - 4 days.
         (e) Symptoms usually begin suddenly and consist of watery diarrhea associated with abdominal cramping.
         (f) Treatment — most cases will resolve in 2 to 3 days with supportive measures alone. The use of antibiotics and antimotility agents, as described in the section above on Traveler's diarrhea, can shorten the duration of this syndrome.
      (2) Enterohemorrhagic *E. coli* serotype O157:H7 (a common cause of hemorrhagic colitis)
         (a) Most outbreaks are associated with the ingestion of contaminated, undercooked ground beef, seed sprouts or unpasteurized milk; however, person-to-person spread also occurs.
         (b) Most commonly occurs in children, the elderly and patients who are status-post-gastrectomy.
         (c) Incubation period is 4 to 9 days.
         (d) This organism produces Shigella-like toxins (serotoxin) that are <u>cytotoxic</u> to the intestinal vascular endothelium.
         (e) **Clinical picture** — The patient presents with diarrhea, crampy abdominal pain and vomiting. The cramps can be severe enough to masquerade as an acute abdomen. The diarrhea is watery early on, but eventually becomes bloody. Fever is absent or low grade. WBCs are present on the wet mount, but are few in number.
         (f) Diagnosis — fecal testing for Shiga toxin along with cultures for *E.coli* O157:H7.
         (g) Treatment
            1 Antibiotic therapy is <u>not</u> recommended; it has not been shown to decrease the duration of the clinical course and may, in fact, increase the incidence of complications, i.e. hemolytic uremic syndrome.
            2 Most cases resolve in 7 to 10 days with supportive measures alone.

      (h) Complications
         1 Hemolytic uremic syndrome (more common in children)
         2 Thrombotic thrombocytopenic purpura

b. *Shigella* (a common cause of bacterial diarrhea)

  (1) Shigellosis (bacillary dysentery) occurs world-wide but is especially common in countries where adequate sanitary facilities are lacking.

  (2) The causative organism (*Shigella sonnei*, *Shigella flexneri* or *Shigella dysenteriae*) is highly infectious and is primarily spread by fecal-oral transmission; as few as 50 - 100 organisms can cause disease.

  (3) The spectrum of the illness ranges from asymptomatic to severe fulminant disease (especially in infants and the elderly) that can lead to marked dehydration and death.

  (4) **Clinical picture** — The patient frequently presents with fever, crampy abdominal pain and diarrhea 24 - 48 hours after exposure; temperature as high as 104° - 105° may be seen in children. Stools are frequent in number (7 - 12 / day), watery and appear greenish-yellow in color. Bloody mucoid stools (dysentery) occur in approximately one-third of patients and vomiting is not infrequent. A young child without a history of diarrhea who presents with high fever and a febrile convulsion is often thought to have meningitis; a clinical clue is the child who is being held for a lumbar puncture and expels a diarrheal stool.

  (5) Lab studies
    (a) CBC → leukocytosis with a <u>marked left shift</u>; an absolute band count > 800 is suggestive of shigellosis.
    (b) A wet mount of the stool with methylene blue → <u>numerous</u> fecal leukocytes
    (c) Stool cultures → are positive in most cases, particularly if obtained within the first few days of illness.

  (6) Treatment
    (a) Antibiotics decrease the duration of illness and the excretion of shigella organisms in the stool. They are recommended in patients with dysentery, in cases of institutional outbreaks and in the very young and the very old. Their use in patients with mild to moderate illness (without fever and dysentery) remains controversial, in that the infection is usually self-limited (the majority of patients recover in 5 - 7 days).
      1 The quinolones (ciprofloxacin, norfloxacin, ofloxacin) are the drugs of first choice but they are contraindicated in pregnancy and in children < 17 years.
      2 Alternatives include TMP/SMX and ampicillin (<u>not</u> amoxicillin); however, the resistance to these alternative agents is high (15 to 40%).
    (b) Antimotility drugs should be avoided; they can worsen bacterial invasion of the bowel wall.

(7) Complications of Shigellosis
  (a) Dehydration secondary to profuse diarrhea
  (b) Arthralgias
  (c) Reiter's syndrome (nongonococcal urethritis, polyarthritis, conjunctivitis)
  (d) Hemolytic uremic syndrome
  (e) Febrile seizures (common in children < 3 yrs. old)
  (f) Pneumonitis

c. *Salmonella*
  (1) Salmonella is among the most common causes of food-borne illness in the U.S. (Int. Med., Fourth ed., Stein, p. 2140; Wilderness Med., Third ed., Auerbach, p. 1040)
  (2) Many serotypes of salmonella infect animals as well as humans. *Salmonella typhi*, the cause of typhoid fever, is the most virulent serotype, whereas *Salmonella typhimurium* is the most common.
  (3) Most cases of salmonellosis occur in the summer months and result from ingestion of contaminated water or food (especially eggs, egg products and poultry), but person-to-person as well as animal-to-person transmission (pet turtles, iguanas, cats and dogs) also occurs.
  (4) Infection can result in a variety of clinical syndromes, including gastroenteritis, septicemia (enteric fever), typhoid (enteric) fever and asymptomatic carrier state.
  (5) High-risk groups for Salmonella infection include:
    (a) Children (< 5 yrs. old) and the elderly
    (b) Immunosuppressed patients
    (c) Splenectomized patients
    (d) Patients with hemolytic anemias (including Sickle Cell)
    (e) Drug addicts
    (f) Patients who are S/P gastrectomy or taking H_2-blockers (or other agents) which decrease gastric acid secretion.
    (g) Severe atherosclerosis
    (h) Intravascular prosthetic devices
  (6) **Clinical presentations**
    (a) Salmonella gastroenteritis — Patients present with nausea, vomiting, diarrhea, fever, crampy abdominal pain 8 - 48 hrs. following the ingestion of contaminated food. Their stools are watery, foul and brownish-green in color; they contain blood, leukocytes, and mucus. The disease course is generally self-limited with symptoms lasting only a few days.
    (b) Septicemia (Enteric fever) develops in 10 - 15% of patients and is indistinguishable from other causes of sepsis. It is most common in infants, the immunosuppressed and those with hemoglobinopathies. Focal infections generally involve sites adjacent to the bowel (such as the gallbladder) but seeding of the brain and other (more distant) organs may occur.

(c) Typhoid (enteric) fever is characterized by septicemia with a protracted toxic course. Clinical clues to the diagnosis include:

<u>1</u> An incubation period of 1 - 2 weeks caused by S. typhi

<u>2</u> Intractable fever

<u>3</u> Relative bradycardia; *bradycardia despite high fever*

<u>4</u> Absence of diarrhea

<u>5</u> Crampy abdominal pain

<u>6</u> Maculopapular skin lesions ("rose spots")

(d) Asymptomatic carrier state

(7) Lab studies

(a) Stained fecal smear — reveals numerous WBCs and, occasionally, occult blood.

(b) Stool cultures — confirm the diagnosis.

(c) Blood cultures — are reserved for toxic patients; they are the best method for diagnosing Typhoid fever.

(8) Treatment

(a) Salmonella gastroenteritis

<u>1</u> Uncomplicated cases in normal hosts should be treated with fluid replacement alone; these patients do not require antibiotic therapy.

<u>2</u> Patients with serious underlying illness or immunosuppression should receive antimicrobial therapy.[*] A fluoroquinolone (ciprofloxacin, norfloxacin) is the drug of choice. TMP-SMX is also effective.

(b) Septicemia or typhoid fever (enteric fever) — ceftriaxone is the agent of choice for these patients. Alternative agents include ciprofloxacin, chloramphenicol and ampicillin.

(c) Antidiarrheal agents are contraindicated; they prolong the illness and increase the incidence of bacteremia and the carrier state.

d. <u>Campylobacter enteritis</u>

(1) Campylobacter is the most common cause of bacterial diarrhea.

(2) It is transmitted by the ingestion of fecally-contaminated water or food (particularly poultry) or direct contact with feces of infected animals or humans and produces disease by directly invading the colonic epithelium.

(3) The incidence of infection is greater in young children.

(4) Incubation period is 2 - 5 days.

(5) **Clinical presentation** — After a 1 - 2 day prodrome of fever, headache, myalgia and general malaise, the patient develops anorexia, nausea, abdominal cramping and diarrhea. Abdominal tenderness is usually present and may be localized, thus mimicking a "surgical abdomen." The stools are initially loose, and then watery, but often progress to become bloody or melanotic. A wet mount of the stool reveals WBCs and blood.

[*]...although antibiotics may prolong the duration of shedding.

    (6) Lab studies

       (a) Wet mount — shows blood and fecal leukocytes

       (b) Stool culture — confirms the diagnosis

    (7) Treatment

       (a) Antimotility agents should be avoided.

       (b) If the patient is still symptomatic when the culture results return, he should be treated with a fluoroquinolone* (ciprofloxacin, norfloxacin) or erythromycin (reduces diarrhea only if given within 4 days of onset).

    (8) Complications

       (a) Reiter's syndrome

       (b) Hemolytic uremic syndrome

       (c) Guillain-Barré syndrome (a late sequela)

  e. *Yersinia* enterocolitis

    (1) Infection results from ingestion of contaminated food or drink and is most common in childhood.

    (2) **Clinical picture**: The patient presents with fever and diarrhea 2 - 6 day post-exposure that is accompanied by severe cramping abdominal pain. Dysentery (bloody diarrhea) may be present in up to 25% of patients. On physical exam, the abdomen is tender and, if the organism has caused mesenteric adenitis or terminal ileitis (which it sometimes does), you may think the patient has appendicitis. Recent exposure to domestic, farm or wild animals can be a significant diagnostic clue. Postinfectious manifestations (erythema nodosum, polyarthritis) sometimes occur, particularly in adults.

    (3) Clinical presentations

       (a) A child with fever and diarrhea (most common)

       (b) A young adult with fever and severe crampy abdominal pain with little or no vomiting; an historical clue is that the diarrhea was initially profuse and watery and later became bloody.

    (4) Lab studies

       (a) Wet mount of the stool — shows fecal leukocytes and occasionally RBCs.

       (b) Stool culture (special techniques are required) — confirms the diagnosis.

    (5) Treatment

       (a) Mild-moderate infections → supportive therapy

       (b) Severe infections → may be treated with TMP-SMX, a fluoroquinolone (ciprofloxacin, norfloxacin), doxycycline and an aminoglycoside or ceftriaxone.

       (c) Antimotility drugs should be avoided.

  f. *Clostridium perfringens*

    (1) Is a common cause of food poisoning; relatively large outbreaks are typical.

    (2) Food poisoning occurs when food contaminated with the live organism (usually precooked or reheated meat, poultry or gravy) is ingested. In the gut, the organism produces an enterotoxin → diarrhea and abdominal cramps.

---

*Campylobacter infections acquired in southern Asia may be quinolone-resistant.

(3) Incubation period is generally 12 hours (range of 6 - 24 hours).
(4) **Clinical picture**: The patient presents with abdominal cramps and watery diarrhea. Fever, headache and chills may also be present but are not prominent features. No WBCs are seen on the stool wet mount.
(5) Since this is a self-limited disease, only supportive treatment is indicated. Symptoms resolve in 12 - 24 hours.

g. *Clostridium difficile* (pseudomembranous enterocolitis)
(1) Pseudomembranous enterocolitis is a severe form of colitis with a high mortality rate. The disease is unique in that an organism normally present in the colon (*Clostridium difficile*) causes illness only after administration of oral or parenteral antibiotics. The offending antibiotic suppresses normal bowel flora and allows overgrowth of a toxin-producing bacterium, *C. difficile.*
(2) Commonly implicated antibiotics include clindamycin, lincomycin, ampicillin and the cephalosporins.
(3) **Clinical picture** — The typical patient is an adult who presents with fever and crampy abdominal pain associated with diarrhea that is watery and occasionally bloody. If there is a history of current or recent antibiotic usage, the diagnosis becomes suspect. Find out if the patient has been constipated or is taking a constipating drug such as Lomotil or a narcotic; these conditions favor multiplication of the organism and build up of toxin in the colon, thus making the diagnosis more probable. Patients who are on chemotherapy (or recently hospitalized), should also be suspect.
(4) Diagnosis
(a) Wet mount of the stool usually reveals WBCs.
(b) A stool toxin assay is the best way to make the diagnosis.
(c) Endoscopy is the usual means of confirming the diagnosis since pseudomembranous plaques are seen in most patients.
[Note: Stool culture is <u>not</u> diagnostic since the organism is part of the normal bowel flora.]
(5) Treatment
(a) D/C offending antibiotic.
(b) Provide adequate hydration.
(c) Antibiotics are indicated if diarrhea is severe or unrelieved by cessation of previous antibiotics. Metronidazole PO is the initial drug of choice in mild to moderate cases. Vancomycin PO is more effective for severe cases because it is poorly absorbed from the GI tract.[*]
(d) Avoid antidiarrheal agents.
Note: Further discussion of this topic can be found earlier in this chapter in the section on Ileitis and Colitis, p. 269.

h. *Staphylococcus aureus* (the most common cause of food poisoning)
(1) Illness results from the release of preformed enterotoxin following ingestion of protein-rich foods (ham, eggs, mayonnaise) contaminated with the organism.
(2) Large outbreaks are common.

*Because it costs more than metronidazole, vancomycin is not the DOC for mild to moderate cases.

(3) Incubation period is 1 to 6 hours.

(4) **Clinical picture**: The usual scenario is that the patient went to a barbecue or buffet about 6 hours PTA where he had eaten some potato salad or sliced ham that had been sitting at room temperature for several hours. He now presents with profuse vomiting, abdominal cramps and diarrhea.

(5) Treatment — supportive therapy; the disease is self-limited and usually resolves in 6 - 10 hours.

i. *Bacillus cereus*

(1) Two clinical syndromes

  (a) An emetic syndrome (resembles the one that is produced by the Staphylococcal enterotoxin)

    <u>1</u> Begins 1 - 6 hours following the ingestion of contaminated food (usually fried rice).

    <u>2</u> Symptoms include vomiting and crampy abdominal pain.

  (b) A diarrheal syndrome (similar to the one that is produced by C. perfringens)

    <u>1</u> Begins 6 - 24 hours after ingestion of a contaminated meal (usually meat or vegetables).

    <u>2</u> Symptoms include diarrhea and abdominal cramps.

(2) Suspect if $> 10^5$ organisms are isolated from the stool or responsible food item.

(3) Treatment is symptomatic. Recovery occurs within 10 - 24 hours.

j. *Aeromonas hydrophila*

(1) Is usually acquired by drinking untreated water from a well or spring.

(2) Most commonly affects children and the immunocompromised patient.

(3) **Clinical picture**: a patient with a history of AIDS presents with watery stools, abdominal cramps and vomiting. A careful history reveals that he has recently returned from a hiking trip, during which he had been drinking water from a fresh spring.

(4) Diagnosis is confirmed by stool culture.

(5) Treatment

  (a) Supportive measures

  (b) Antibiotic therapy with one of the following agents:

    <u>1</u> A quinolone (ciprofloxacin, norfloxacin, ofloxacin)

    <u>2</u> TMP-SMX

    <u>3</u> Tetracycline

    <u>4</u> An aminoglycoside

    <u>Note</u>: Without antimicrobial therapy, the diarrhea generally persists for 2 weeks or longer.

k. *Vibrio cholera*

(1) This organism is transmitted by the ingestion of contaminated water or seafood (especially raw oysters) which produces an enterotoxin-mediated diarrheal illness (cholera).

(2) A large inoculum of the organism is required to produce disease because of the acid sensitivity of the bacteria.

(3) Copious amounts of watery diarrhea (rice water stools) is the hall-mark of clinical cholera and can lead to significant fluid and elec-trolyte imbalances:

(a) Severe dehydration (loss of isotonic fluid from bowel)

(b) Hyperchloremic acidosis (loss of bicarb in the stool)

(c) Hypokalemia (loss of potassium in the stool)

(4) **Clinical picture**: Following an incubation period of 2 - 6 days, the patient presents with copious watery diarrhea and abdomi-nal distention. Vomiting may also be present. Wet mount of the stool is negative for WBCs.

(5) Treatment

(a) Fluids (oral or IV) — should be the focus of therapy.

(b) Antibiotic therapy with tetracycline for 3 days or single-dose therapy with doxycycline or a fluoroquinolone shortens the duration of illness and the excretion of organisms.

l. *Vibrio parahemolyticus*

(1) Is the most frequent cause of food-borne bacterial enteritis in Japan.

(2) It is an <u>invasive</u> bacteria that produces illness by inducing an inflammatory response in the intestinal mucosa.

(3) It is acquired by ingestion of raw or improperly prepared seafood (especially oysters, clams, shrimp and crabs).

(4) In temperate climates, this infection is usually confined to the summer months.

(5) Symptoms begin after an average incubation period of 12 hours and range from mild gastroenteritis to explosive diarrhea with vomiting, cramps and dysentery. Fever may also be present.

(6) Wet mount of the stool reveals numerous WBCs.

(7) Treatment

(a) Symptomatic therapy is generally all that is needed, as the illness is self-limited and resolves in 2 - 3 days.

(b) Tetracycline or a quinolone may be given for severe infections (dysentery) but their efficacy remains unclear; they do not shorten the clinical course nor do they decrease the duration of shedding of the organism.

m. <u>Scombroid fish poisoning</u>

(1) The most commonly implicated fish is mahi mahi (blue dolphin or dolphin fish) but it is also common with ingestion of tuna, mackerel and other dark-fleshed or red-muscled fish.

(2) Poisoning results from ingestion of <u>heat-stable</u> toxins with <u>his-tamine-like properties</u> produced by bacterial action on <u>dark-meat fish</u>, i.e. high levels of histamine correlate with the mani-festations of the illness. Formation of the toxin is related to impro-per preservation and refrigeration of the fish. [<u>Note</u>: This is <u>not</u> an allergic reaction.]

(3) Clinical features
    (a) Twenty - thirty minutes after ingestion of the fish, the patient presents with signs and symptoms of histamine intoxication:
        <u>1</u> Facial flushing (resembles a sunburn and can extend over the entire upper body)
        <u>2</u> Conjunctival hyperemia
        <u>3</u> Throbbing headache
        <u>4</u> Abdominal cramps
        <u>5</u> Nausea, vomiting and diarrhea
        <u>6</u> Palpitations
        <u>7</u> Bronchospasm or hypotension (with severe toxicity)
    (b) Historical clue — At time of ingestion, the patient noticed a sharp, metallic, bitter or peppery taste to the fish.
(4) Treatment is parenteral antihistamine therapy with diphenhydramine 50mg IM or IV; if this is ineffective, then cimetidine 300mg IV or ranitidine 50mg IV should be given. Additional therapy may be required:
    (a) Prochlorperazine (for nausea and vomiting)
    (b) Albuterol + steroids (for bronchospasm)
    (c) Epinephrine (for anaphylactoid reaction)

n. <u>Ciguatera fish poisoning</u>
(1) The most common cause of nonbacterial fish-associated food poisoning in the U.S.
(2) Results from ingestion of <u>ciguatoxin</u>, a tasteless, odorless, <u>heat-stable neurotoxin</u> that accumulates in the flesh of certain carnivorous tropical and semitropical coral-reef fish when a particular dinoflagellate (Gambierdiscus toxicus) is present in their food chain during the late spring and summer months. The most commonly affected species are grouper, snapper, barracuda, king fish and jack. Since the toxin accumulates in the flesh of these fish, the bigger and older the fish, the more likely that it carries the toxin.
(3) The incubation period is usually 2 - 6 hours but ranges from 15 minutes to 24 hours.
(4) The illness generally begins with vomiting and diarrhea and is followed by neuromuscular and neurosensory manifestations such as myalgias, weakness, paresthesias, <u>reversal of hot and cold sensation</u> (pathognomonic), burning sensation in hands and feet, and a feeling that the teeth are loose. GI symptoms usually resolve within 24 - 48 hours, but neurosensory symptoms may persist for months and are exacerbated by the ingestion of alcohol.
(5) Treatment
    (a) Supportive measures (IV fluids, antiemetics, analgesics)
    (b) Mannitol (20% solution) 1gm/kg (up to 50gms) IV over one hour — has recently been shown to decrease the neurologic and neurosensory manifestations of this illness and should be considered for those patients with moderate to severe symptoms who present during the acute phase (days 1 - 5).

      (c) Absolute abstinence from alcohol, seafood and nuts until all symptoms have resolved; continued abstinence is recommended for 3 - 6 months after exposure.

   5. Empiric antibiotic therapy
     a. Should be limited to the patients who are significantly ill or toxic in appearance that are believed (based on clinical grounds) to have an invasive or infectious diarrhea.
     b. Early administration of antibiotics to these patients decreases the intensity and duration of symptoms, prevents systemic and suppurative sequelae and reduces spread of the infection.
     c. Unless contraindications exist, e.g., pregnancy, children <17 years, the fluoroquinolones are the agents of choice; they are effective against all of the common bacterial causes of infectious diarrhea and have few side effects. Acceptable regimens include:
       (1) Ciprofloxacin 500 mg PO bid for 3 - 5 days or
       (2) Norfloxacin 400mg PO bid for 3 - 5 days.

C. Parasitic Gastrointestinal Infections *

   1. Entamoeba histolytica
     a. Transmission is via asymptomatic carriers who pass cysts via the fecal-oral route or through anal-oral sexual practices.
     b. Symptoms, if they occur, are produced by trophozoites (the reproductive form of this parasite); however, the majority of patients (> 80%) are asymptomatic carriers.
     c. Prevalence is greatest among:
       (1) Patients with AIDS
       (2) Male homosexuals
       (3) Institutionalized persons
       (4) Native Americans living on reservations
       (5) Travelers returning from underdeveloped countries (especially tropical Africa, Asia or Latin America--where it is endemic)
     d. Clinical features
       (1) Intestinal
         (a) Abdominal cramps, intermittent diarrhea (which may contain blood-streaked mucus) and flatulence → colitis or
         (b) Profuse bloody diarrhea, fever and severe abdominal cramps → amebic dysentery
       (2) Extraintestinal → abscess formation
         (a) Liver (most common)
         (b) Lung
         (c) Heart
         (d) Kidney
         (e) Brain
     e. Diagnosis of intestinal amebiasis
       (1) Is based on the finding of trophozoites or cysts in the stool; since fecal shedding of cysts is irregular, several specimens may need to be examined to make the diagnosis.

*All patients with GI symptoms lasting > 7 days should be tested for parasites.

(2) Sigmoidoscopy with rectal biopsy can be helpful when the stool examination is negative.

(3) Serologic tests are sensitive and specific in patients with symptomatic infection and may provide additional information.

(4) Eosinophilia is absent.

f. The diagnosis of amebic liver abscess (extraintestinal amebiasis) is based on the combination of:

(1) A compatible clinical syndrome

(2) A positive serology and

(3) Imaging studies (radioisotope liver scanning, US or CT)

[Note: Examination of the stool in patients with extraintestinal amebiasis is rarely helpful since organisms are found in less than 20% of these patients.]

g. Treatment

(1) Asymptomatic carriers → Iodoquinol (eradicates the cyst stage)

(2) Mild-moderate intestinal illness → Metronidazole (or tetracycline) plus iodoquinol or paromomycin

(3) Severe illness → Emetine (or dehydroemetine) plus iodoquinol — Chloroquine may be added to this regimen in the presence of live parasites.

2. Giardia lamblia (the most common intestinal parasite in the US)

a. Giardiasis is transmitted by cysts via the fecal-oral route.

(1) Most infections are associated with the ingestion of contaminated water, particularly water from remote streams and wells. For this reason, Giardiasis is often referred to as "backpackers diarrhea."

(2) Beavers play a role in the spread of this disease by contaminating streams with cysts.

(3) Venereal transmission among homosexuals (by direct fecal-oral contamination) is also common.

b. Symptoms, if they occur, are produced by trophozoites and begin after an incubation period of 1 - 3 weeks; most patients, however, are asymptomatic.

c. Prevalence is highest among:

(1) Homosexual men

(2) Immunocompromised patients

(3) Institutionalized persons

(4) Native Americans living on reservations

(5) Children attending day care centers

(6) Travelers returning from underdeveloped countries (especially Russia) or a backpacking trip to Colorado

(7) Patients with decreased gastric acidity

d. **Clinical picture**: The patient has recently returned from a backpacking trip in Colorado (or from travel to Russia) and presents with abdominal pain and feeling bloated and gaseous. He also c/o post-prandial abdominal cramping, an urgency to defecate and has diarrhea that is frothy and foul-smelling. A stool specimen sent to the lab may be negative for ova and parasites because the cysts are only passed sporadically. If this is negative, an Entero-Test (string test) or duodenal aspiration can be done to look for trophozoites.

   e. Diagnosis

      (1) Is based on the finding of trophozoites or cysts in the stools — (several stools may need to be examined to make the diagnosis; symptoms may precede cyst excretion by more than a week) — or ELISA testing for fecal Giardia antigen (most cost-effective).

      (2) A string test or duodenal aspiration may need to be performed in asymptomatic patients and those with chronic symptoms.

      (3) Eosinophilia is absent.

   f. Treatment — should be provided for all patients whether or not they are symptomatic. Effective agents include:

      (1) Metronidazole (drug of choice)

      (2) Furazolidone (though less effective than metronidazole is available as a suspension and, for this reason, is often the preferred agent in children).

   g. Patients with recurrent or refractory giardiasis should be tested for immunoglobulin A deficiency.

3. <u>Cryptosporidium</u> (most common cause of chronic diarrhea in patients with AIDS)

   a. Transmitted by <u>cysts</u> from human or animal sources via the fecal-oral route.

   b. Symptoms, if they occur, are produced by trophozoites after an incubation period of 1 - 2 weeks; some patients are asymptomatic.

   c. People at high risk include:

      (1) Immunocompromised patients (especially those with AIDS)

      (2) Homosexual men

      (3) Animal handlers

      (4) Children attending day care centers

      (5) Travelers returning from Russia

   d. Clinical features

      (1) Patients present with profuse watery diarrhea, abdominal cramping, anorexia, nausea and flatulence.

      (2) In <u>immunocompetent</u> patients, these symptoms may persist for 1 - 3 weeks and result in significant dehydration, but they are generally self-limited.

      (3) In <u>immunocompromised</u> patients, malabsorption and significant weight loss occurs as well; symptoms may persist for months to years, producing significant discomfort and morbidity.

   e. Diagnosis

      (1) Is made by examining stool for oocysts using an acid-fast stain or enzyme immunoassay testing for cryptosporidium (> 95% sensitive)

      (2) Fecal blood and leukocytes are usually absent.

      (3) Eosinophilia is absent.

  f. Treatment
   (1) Immunocompetent patients
    (a) Rehydration and symptomatic therapy.
    (b) Nitazoxanide may hasten recovery.
   (2) Immunodeficient patients — are resistant to treatment.
    (a) When possible, therapy should be directed toward correcting the underlying immunodeficiency.
    (b) Nitazoxanide or paromomycin plus azithromycin — may lessen symptoms in these patients, but is not curative.
    (c) In AIDS patients, antiretroviral therapy with AZT (azidothymidine) is probably the best treatment since it directly increases host immunity by suppressing HIV replication.

4. Isospora belli
 a. Transmitted by <u>cysts</u> via the fecal-oral route.
 b. Symptoms, when present, begin after an incubation period of 1 - 2 weeks and last for 2 - 6 weeks; some immunocompetent patients are asymptomatic, whereas immunocompromised patients tend to have a severe protracted course.
 c. Usually an opportunistic infection, it is seen most commonly in patients with AIDS (especially in developing countries).
 d. **Clinical picture**: The patient is a 30-year-old Haitian male with a history of AIDS who presents with profuse watery diarrhea, abdominal cramps, nausea and vomiting. He also c/o weight loss and has signs of malabsorption. Examination of the stool reveals oocysts.
 e. Diagnosis
  (1) Is usually made by identifying oocysts in the stool, performing acid-fast staining of a stool specimen or by identifying intracellular forms on biopsy of the small bowel.
  (2) Leukocytosis with moderate eosinophilia is common and further supports the diagnosis.
 f. Treatment
  (1) TMP-SMX — is the drug of choice; prolonged therapy is required in AIDS patients.
  (2) Pyrimethamine, nitrofurantoin or furazolidone — may be used in patients allergic to sulfa.

5. Necator Americanus (hookworm)
 a. Infection occurs when the hookworm larvae penetrate through intact skin on contact with feces-contaminated soil.
 b. Most commonly occurs in warmer climates (tropics, southeastern USA) where people walk around barefoot and sanitation is poor.
 c. After penetrating the skin, the larvae enter the bloodstream, ascend the trachea, descend the esophagus to differentiate into adult worms and migrate to the upper intestine where they attach to the mucosal wall and feed on host blood.
 d. Clinical features
  (1) Patients may present with intermittent diarrhea, epigastric discomfort, weakness, low-grade fever, cough, rash and weight loss.
  (2) Hypochromic microcytic anemia may develop in those children who are heavily infected.

e. Diagnosis
(1) Is made by identifying ova in the stool.
(2) The presence of hypochromic microcytic anemia and marked eosinophilia further support the diagnosis.
f. Treatment — mebendazole, albendazole or pyrantel pamoate (plus an iron supplement).

6. Enterobiasis (pinworm)
a. Transmission is via ingestion of Enterobius vermicularis eggs.
b. Once ingested, eggs develop into adult worms in the large bowel; then the gravid females migrate to the anus at night to deposit their eggs.
c. Outbreaks often occur in schools, day care centers and other institutional settings.
d. Clinical features
(1) Patients most commonly c/o pruritus ani, particularly at night.
(2) Secondary skin changes and bacterial infection may also be present.
(3) Other associated problems may include insomnia, enuresis, UTIs and vaginitis.
e. Diagnosis
(1) Is made by identifying either adult worms migrating in the perineal area or eggs on a cellophane tape swab of the anus.
(2) Eosinophilia is absent.
f. Treatment — is a single dose of mebendazole (Vermox) or pyrantel pamoate (Antiminth) that is repeated again after two weeks. All family members should be treated.

D. Diarrhea in the Patient with AIDS

1. Patients who are HIV positive are more susceptible to the typical enteric organisms and to many opportunistic organisms as well. In addition, it is believed that HIV itself may produce an enteropathy.
a. Cytomegalovirus (CMV) and Cryptosporidium are the two most common causes of diarrhea in these patients. *Mycobacterium avium* is another important cause.
b. Multiple organisms are responsible in some patients (up to 25%).
2. Unlike diarrheal illness in the immunocompetent patient, diarrheal illness in the AIDS patient is not a self-limiting disease. Due to decreased immunity and poor baseline nutritional status of these patients, diarrheal illness can have devastating consequences which require a more aggressive approach to the work-up and treatment.
a. Initial evaluation should include stool cultures/stains, blood cultures and proctosigmoidoscopy (if colitis or proctocolitis are present.)
b. Empiric antimicrobials should not be administered.

VII. Cholecystitis

A. *Cholecystitis is an acute inflammation of the gallbladder that is more common in women than in men. In most cases, it is associated with an obstruction at the neck of the gallbladder or within the cystic duct due to gallstones. About 20 million people in the USA have gallstones (30% of people > 40 years of age).*

B. *Risk Factors — are the same as those for cholelithiasis and include:*

1. Female gender

2. Increasing parity

3. Advancing age

4. Obesity

5. Rapid weight loss

6. Drugs (hypolipidemic agents, estrogen therapy)

7. Family tendency

8. Cystic fibrosis

9. Presence of chronic hemolysis

C. *Variations and Complication of Cholecystitis*

1. Acalculous cholecystitis (5% of cases)
   a. Occurs in post-partum/post-op patients and those with burns or other major trauma, vascular disease, diabetes, sepsis and CHF.
   b. Is more common in the elderly.
   c. Gangrene and perforation are relatively frequent in contrast to calculous cholecystitis.

2. Calculous cholecystitis is the most frequent cause of acute pancreatitis → a gallstone passes into the common bile duct and may occlude the pancreatic duct at the sphincter of Oddi.

3. Ascending cholangitis
   a. Occurs when stones passing through the common bile duct cause a purulent infection within the bile ducts that extends into the liver.
   b. Clinical features: fever and chills, abdominal pain and jaundice (Charcot's triad). In severe cases, mental confusion and shock may also be present (Reynold's pentad).
   c. This is a surgical emergency with a high mortality rate.

4. Emphysematous cholecystitis (rare) → infection with gas-forming bacteria (*E. coli*, *Clostridium perfringens*, *Klebsiella* and/or anaerobic strep).

5. Empyema of the gallbladder (an advanced stage of cholecystitis) → bacterial invasion of the gallbladder wall leads to gross suppuration.

6. Gallstone ileus (uncommon)
   a. Mechanism: a large gallstone erodes into the duodenum, lodges in the terminal ileum and produces intestinal obstruction.
   b. Most commonly seen in elderly women with multiple underlying medical problems and a history of gallstones.
   c. X-ray findings include: pneumobilia (air in the biliary tree . . . be able to identify), evidence of mechanical small bowel obstruction and a stone in the GI tract.

D. Clinical Features

1. History
   a. Family history of GB disease (common)
   b. Fatty food intolerance (common)
   c. Nausea (common)
   d. Bile-stained vomitus (variable since vomiting may not be present)
   e. Abdominal pain — most common presenting complaint, often precipitated by ingestion of a fatty or heavy meal. Initially, the pain is visceral in nature and felt in the midline. With prolonged obstruction of the cystic duct, somatic fibers become involved and the pain localizes to the RUQ.
      (1) Distention of the GB (due to obstruction of the cystic duct by a gallstone) → epigastric pain
      (2) Prolonged obstruction of the cystic duct → increased intragallbladder pressure → chemical and/or bacterial inflammation of the GB wall → RUQ pain (which may radiate to the interscapular area, right scapula or shoulder)

2. Physical exam
   a. Tachycardia and fever
   b. Tenderness in the RUQ or epigastrium
   c. Murphy's sign: ↑ pain and transient arrest of inspiration when direct pressure is applied to the RUQ while the patient is taking a deep breath.

3. Diagnostic studies
   a. Lab abnormalities
      (1) Mild leukocytosis with a left shift
      (2) Bilirubin and alkaline phosphatase (may be normal).
         (a) Mildly elevated → cholecystitis alone
         (b) Highly elevated → common duct stone
      (3) Significantly elevated serum amylase or lipase → pancreatitis due to a common duct stone
   b. Radiologic abnormalities
      (1) Plain films of the abdomen are usually negative or demonstrate nonspecific findings. Positive findings, when present, include:
         (a) Radiopaque gallstones (10 - 15%)
         (b) Sentinel loop in the RUQ

        (c) Air or an air-fluid level in the gallbladder → emphysematous cholecystitis

        (d) Air in the biliary tree → biliary enteric fistula

    (2) Ultrasonography — is the most useful <u>initial test</u> for imaging the gallbladder in the emergency setting; it is rapid, noninvasive and can identify the following:

        (a) Thickness of the GB wall (5mm or greater is diagnostic of cholecystitis)

        (b) Gallstones

        (c) Common duct stones

        (d) Dilated common duct

        (e) Pericholecystic fluid

        (f) Other sources of RUQ pain (pathology of the liver, pancreas and kidneys)

    (3) Biliary Scintiscanning (HIDA, DISIDA) — is the most <u>accurate test</u> for establishing the diagnosis of cholecystitis.

        (a) Is indicated if no stones are seen on ultrasound or there was equivocal thickness of the GB wall.

        (b) If the isotope does not pass into the gallbladder within 1 hr. of ingestion, the cystic duct is presumed to be obstructed.

    (4) CT scanning — rarely offers any advantage over ultrasound.

E. Treatment

1. Patients with acute cholecystitis (fever, leukocytosis, significant abdominal tenderness and vomiting) and/or its complications (pancreatitis, ascending cholangitis, jaundice) should be admitted.

2. Initial therapy should consist of:
   a. IV fluids
   b. Antiemetics and NG tube suction (if persistent vomiting is present)
   c. Surgical consultation
   d. Pain relief (meperidine is the preferred agent)
   e. Broad-spectrum IV antibiotics
      (1) A second- or third-generation cephalosporin is adequate in most cases.
      (2) Triple antibiotic therapy (ampicillin, an aminoglycoside <u>and</u> clindamycin or metronidazole) is indicated in the presence of sepsis.

3. Definitive therapy is cholecystectomy at the earliest convenient time (usually within 72 hours).

VIII. Hepatitis

A. *Viral Hepatitis*

1. <u>Sequence of events</u>: Hepatic enzymes begin to elevate prior to the prodromal phase → prodromal symptoms (usually constitutional) for 1 - 2
   weeks → icteric phase (when present) may be preceded by pruritus and
   dark urine followed by jaundice and, possibly, RUQ pain with hepatomegaly or splenomegaly [<u>Note</u>: Most patients do not develop jaundice]
   → recovery phase (symptoms resolve and hepatic enzymes normalize).
   In most cases, there is complete recovery in 3 - 4 months.

2. <u>Hepatitis A</u> (formerly known as infectious hepatitis)
   a. Is caused by an RNA virus (HAV) and is spread by the fecal-oral route
      directly via person-to-person contact or indirectly through the inges-
      tion of <u>contaminated</u> water or food (particularly raw or under-cooked
      shellfish).
   b. The illness is generally mild with a 15 - 50 day incubation period.
   c. Fecal shedding of the virus is maximal late in the incubation period
      and early in the prodromal phase.
   d. There is <u>no carrier state</u> and it does <u>not</u> cause chronic liver disease.
   e. Serologic marker is anti-HAV:
      (1) Anti-HAV IgM — indicates acute infection
      (2) Anti-HAV IgG — indicates prior infection and confers immunity

3. <u>Hepatitis B</u> (formerly known as serum hepatitis)
   a. Is caused by a DNA virus (HBV) and is spread primarily by the per-
      cutaneous route but may also be transmitted by intimate contact via
      blood, semen or saliva.
   b. The illness is usually more severe and protracted when compared to
      that produced by Hepatitis A and has a 45 - 160 day incubation period
      (mean = 120 days); fulminant hepatic failure develops in 1% of cases
      (rapidly rising bilirubin levels, coagulopathy and encephalopathy) —
      80% of comatose patients will die.
   c. Chronic hepatitis or a chronic carrier state develops in 90% of infec-
      ted neonates and 10% of infected adults. These chronic carriers are
      all at increased risk for developing hepatocellular cancer; those with
      circulating virus continue to be a source of possible transmission.
   d. Serologic markers in hepatitis B infection
      (1) Hepatitis B surface antigen (HB_sAg) — Represents the outer pro-
          tein coat of the virus. In the vast majority of cases (>90%), it is
          detectable in the serum prior to elevation of hepatic enzymes and
          the appearance of clinical symptoms; it lasts about 6 months.
          Its presence <u>implies active hepatitis or the carrier state</u> but not
          necessarily infectivity.
      (2) Antibody to HB_sAg (anti-HB_s) appears in the serum 2 - 6 months
          after the disappearance of HB_sAg; it is a sign of previous infection
          or vaccination and <u>indicates immunity</u>. [<u>Note</u>: Chronic carriers
          usually have persistent HB_sAg in their serum and, therefore, do
          <u>not</u> develop anti-HB_s.]

(3) Hepatitis B core antigen (HB_cAg) — (the core of the virus) is only present in hepatocytes, not in the serum. Its presence, in conjunction with a negative anti-HB_s, is suggestive of early infection.

(4) Antibody to HB_cAg (anti-HB_c) is present in the serum approximately 2 weeks following the appearance of HB_sAg. It may be the only marker of recent infection during the "window period" between the disappearance of HB_sAg and the appearance of anti-HB_s. The presence of IgM anti-HB_c in high titer indicates acute infection and high infectivity, whereas the presence of IgG anti-HB_c in association with anti-HB_s implies remote infection.

(5) Hepatitis B epsilon antigen (HB_eAg) is found in serum containing Hb_sAg. Its presence indicates ongoing viral replication and high infectivity. The antigen disappears in those patients who recover from Hepatitis B, but persists in those who develop chronic hepatitis.

(6) Antibody to HB_eAg (anti-HB_e) appears during the acute phase of Hepatitis B and implies that the patient is not likely to be infective. Anti-HB_e persists several months after the disappearance of HB_eAg.

Sound confusing? Well, it is, especially since the presence of active infection does not necessarily correlate with infectivity, i.e. how likely the patient is to transmit the disease. Here's one way of evaluating the serologic results:

No infectivity	Low infectivity	+ infectivity	High infectivity
+ anti-HB_s	+ anti-HB_e	+ HB_sAg	+ HB_eAg

Note: Only 2 serologic markers (HB_sAg and IgM anti-HB_c) are actually needed to establish the diagnosis of infection with Hepatitis B and determine its chronicity; HB_sAg confirms that infection is present, while IgM anti-HB_c implies that it is acute.

   e. The CDC believes that successful hepatitis B vaccination (i.e., that which is documented by anti-hepatitis B surface antibodies $\geq$ 10 IU at anytime during a patient's life) confers lifetime protection. Therefore, do not test the source of (or recipient of) a blood exposure (e.g. needle stick) if the patient has been successfully immunized. Otherwise, perform routine testing (including anti-hepatitis B surface antibodies).

4. Hepatitis C
   a. Is caused by an RNA virus (HCV) and seems to spread in a fashion similar to Hepatitis B.
   b. It is the most common cause of viral hepatitis in the USA.
      (1) Prior to 1992, most cases occurred in association with the transfusion of blood/blood products; thus, hepatitis C was referred to as "post-transfusion hepatitis". Since the introduction of a marker in 1992 to screen blood for hepatitis C (anti-HCV), the number of transfusion-related cases of hepatitis C has been decreasing.

(2) Currently, IV and intranasal drug abuse accounts for a growing number of new infections with hepatitis C.

c. The incubation period is 15 - 160 days (mean = 50 days) and the illness produced is similar to (but milder than) that caused by hepatitis B.

d. Chronic hepatitis develops in 50 - 85% of these patients, many of whom go on to develop cirrhosis. The delayed development of hepatocellular CA in these cirrhotics is not uncommon.

e. Anti-HCV is the serologic marker for hepatitis C; it is detectable in the serum 1 to 6 months following the onset of symptoms; anti-HCV indicates the presence of chronic infection and potential infectivity.

5. Hepatitis E
   a. Is caused by an RNA virus (HEV); incubation period is 15 - 60 days.
   b. Resembles Hepatitis A in its mode of transmission and the clinical course, but is associated with a higher incidence of fulminant liver failure and mortality, particularly in pregnant females.
   c. Chronic infection does not occur.
   d. A serologic marker has not yet been identified.

6. Hepatitis delta (HDV)
   a. Is a "defective" RNA-containing virus that can only occur in patients who are currently infected with HBV. Infection may occur concomitantly with an acute HBV infection or as a superinfection in patients with chronic hepatitis B.
   b. Acute concomitant infection has a better prognosis than superinfection; the illness is generally self-limited.
   c. Superinfection is associated with a high mortality rate (relative to acute HBV infection) and the frequent development of chronic HDV hepatitis with subsequent cirrhosis.
   d. The serologic marker is anti-HDV.

7. Lab findings
   a. Serum aminotransferases are elevated; aspartate (AST) is 10 - 100 times normal and alanine transferase (ALT) is usually higher than the AST.
   b. Bilirubin (total and direct) — is elevated.
   c. PT — is usually normal; prolongation points to a more complicated course and a poorer prognosis.

8. Prevention and prophylaxis
   a. Immune globulin (IG), formerly known as gamma globulin or serum immune globulin, is 80 - 90% effective in preventing infection with HAV if administered within 14 days of exposure.
   b. Hepatitis A vaccine should be recommended for travelers to endemic areas. It becomes effective 20 days post-administration.
   c. Hepatitis B immune globulin (HBIG) and Hepatitis B vaccine have both been demonstrated to prevent Hepatitis B; HBIG confers passive immunity while the vaccine confers active immunity. For maximum effectiveness, HBIG must be administered within 7 days of exposure; the sooner the better.

d. There is no vaccine available for hepatitis C; postexposure prophylaxis with immune globulin is not recommended; results with interferon are inconclusive.

   (1) For potential exposures, the CDC recommends determining the serostatus of the source case; however, the average incidence of anti-HCV seroconversion after unintentional needle stick or other sharp exposure from an HCV positive source is only 1.8% (range of 0 - 7%)

   (2) The exposed worker should have baseline hepatitis C antibody tests (EIAs) and LFTs (including AST and ALT) which should be repeated in 6 months.

e. There is no specific vaccine for Hepatitis delta. The best preventive measure is vaccination for Hepatitis B as infection with Hepatitis delta cannot occur in the absence of infection with Hepatitis B.

f. There is no vaccine available for Hepatitis E and the immune globulin that is produced in the USA is <u>not</u> protective against HEV (it does not contain anti-HEV titers).

g. Detailed recommendations for clinical practice regarding post-exposure hepatitis prophylaxis can be found in <u>Rosen's Text</u>, Fourth ed., Table 116-3, p. 1986 or Fifth ed., Table 85-3, p. 1255.

9. Indications for admission include:

   a. Refractory vomiting

   b. Fluid or electrolyte imbalance

   c. Prolonged PT (> 3 - 5 secs. when compared with the control)

   d. Bilirubin > 20 - 30 mg/dL

   e. Hypoglycemia

   f. Immunosuppression

   g. Severe underlying disease

   h. Early signs of encephalopathy (e.g. agitation, altered mental status)

   i. Age > 45 - 50 years

B. Toxic Hepatitis

1. Hepatotoxins that can produce morphologic changes in the liver and resemble those of acute viral hepatitis:

   a. <u>Halothane</u>

      (1) Produces toxicity via a toxic metabolite and a hypersensitivity reaction.

      (2) Most cases (75%) occur in patients who have been exposed to the anesthetic in the past.

      (3) Is more common in adults (particularly females) and the obese.

      (4) Postoperative fever, rash and eosinophilia may be present.

      (5) Onset is abrupt; usually occurs a couple of days post exposure.

      (6) Mortality rate is 20 - 40% in severe icteric cases.

   b. <u>Methyldopa</u>

      (1) Produces injury via a toxic metabolite and a hypersensitivity reaction.

(2) Mild transient elevation of transaminase levels is seen in about 5% of patients treated with this drug and < 1% actually develop acute hepatitis.

(3) Development of a rash, arthralgias and lymphadenopathy may precede the onset of jaundice.

(4) Clinical improvement occurs when the drug is discontinued, but cases of chronic hepatitis and cirrhosis have been described.

  c. Isoniazid (INH)

(1) Produces toxicity via a toxic metabolite.

(2) Incidence of developing toxic hepatitis is age-related; it is rare in patients < 20 years old but approaches 3% in those over 50.

(3) Susceptibility is potentiated by alcoholism and by the concurrent use of rifampin or pyrazinamide.

  d. Phenytoin

2. Hepatotoxins that produce cholestatic changes in the liver with clinical manifestations of malaise, anorexia, nausea and vomiting:

  a. Anabolic steroids

  b. Oral contraceptives

  c. Chlorpropamide

  d. Chlorpromazine

  e. Erythromycin estolate

  f. Haloperidol

  g. Verapamil

  h. Phenobarbital

3. Hepatotoxins that can produce massive hepatic necrosis:

  a. Acetaminophen

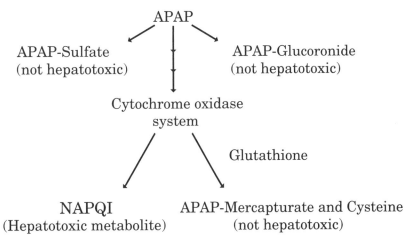

[Mechanism of toxicity]

APAP

APAP-Sulfate (not hepatotoxic)   APAP-Glucoronide (not hepatotoxic)

Cytochrome oxidase system

Glutathione

NAPQI (Hepatotoxic metabolite)   APAP-Mercapturate and Cysteine (not hepatotoxic)

↑ dose of APAP → saturation of the sulfate and glucuronide pathways + depletion of glutathione → build up of toxic metabolite (NAPQI)

  b. Carbon tetrachloride

  c. Yellow phosphorus

  d. Mushrooms (e.g. amanita phalloides)

IX. Alcoholic Liver Disease

A. Syndromes

1. Hepatic steatosis (fatty liver)
   a. Consumption of even moderate amounts of alcohol can lead to deposition of fat within hepatocytes.
   b. The most common clinical finding is nontender hepatomegaly associated with mild elevation of serum transaminase.
   c. Resolves in 4 - 6 weeks with abstinence from alcohol.

2. Alcoholic hepatitis
   a. Clinical severity ranges from a mild illness to acute liver failure, depending on the degree of hepatocellular necrosis and intrahepatic inflammation.
   b. Patients classically present with generalized weakness, anorexia, nausea, abdominal discomfort and weight loss. They may also note that their urine is dark in color.
   c. Examination usually reveals a low-grade temperature, jaundice and a tender, enlarged liver.
   d. Lab findings:
      (1) CBC → macrocytic anemia, leukocytosis, thrombocytopenia
      (2) Bilirubin and alkaline phosphatase levels are increased
      (3) AST/ALT levels 2 - 10 times normal with the AST > ALT
      (4) Prolonged prothrombin time (prolongation above normal range that is > 8 secs. is a poor prognostic sign)

3. Alcoholic (Laennec's) cirrhosis
   a. An irreversible disease that produces permanent histologic changes in the liver (hepatocytic nodules and fibrous tissue) which disrupt normal hepatic blood flow and result in portosystemic shunting with concomitant portal hypertension.
   b. Patients typically present with chronic fatigue and anorexia; however, some remain relatively asymptomatic and do not present until they develop a complication (hepatic encephalopathy, GI bleed).
   c. Classic clinical findings include jaundice, spider angiomata, palmar erythema, gynecomastia, muscle wasting, Dupuytren's contracture, ascites and pedal edema.
   d. Lab findings:
      (1) CBC → anemia, leukopenia, thrombocytopenia
      (2) AST/ALT levels are minimally elevated
      (3) Prolonged PT*
      (4) Elevated bilirubin* and alkaline phosphatase levels
      (5) Hypoalbuminemia
      (6) Hyponatremia
      (7) Hypokalemia

* useful predictor(s) of severity of liver disease

B. Complications

1. Bleeding esophageal varices
   a. 30 - 33% of all cirrhotics die from this complication.
   b. Clinical picture: hemorrhagic shock with <u>massive</u> hematemesis.
   c. Emergency endoscopy should be performed ASAP to confirm the diagnosis, R/O other sources of bleeding and to provide therapy.

   <u>Note</u>: Further discussion of this topic can be found earlier in this chapter in the section on Esophageal Disorders, pp. 244 - 245.

2. Portosystemic encephalopathy
   a. Is due to accumulation of toxic substances in the blood.
   b. Occurs in cirrhotics with extensive portosystemic shunting when the diseased liver is no longer able to perform its metabolic function of detoxifying wastes adequately.
   c. Precipitating factors include:
      (1) Azotemia (GI bleeding, high protein diet)
      (2) Injudicious use of medications (sedatives, analgesics and tranquilizers)
      (3) Hypokalemic metabolic alkalosis
      (4) Infection
      (5) Hypoxemia
      (6) Hypoglycemia
      (7) Dehydration
   d. Clinical features include an altered LOC, fetor hepaticus and asterixis ("liver flap" — best demonstrated with the dorsiflexed wrist) along with other signs and symptoms of chronic liver disease; the serum ammonia level is usually elevated.
   e. Management
      (1) General supportive measures
      (2) Correction/elimination of precipitating factors
      (3) Administration of lactulose and/or neomycin (to eliminate NH_3)
      (4) Protein restricted diet

3. Hepatorenal syndrome
   a. A syndrome of acquired renal failure of unknown cause that occurs in decompensated cirrhotics.
   b. Pathogenesis: vasoconstriction + shunting of blood away from renal cortex → ↓ glomerular filtration rate → ↓ renal output → azotemia.
   c. The prognosis is dismal; the mortality rate is nearly 100%.

4. Spontaneous bacterial peritonitis (SBP)
   a. Occurs in up to 33% of patients with liver disease + ascites.
   b. This diagnosis should be suspected in patients with liver disease who present with fever, abdominal tenderness, worsening ascites and decreasing hepatic function.
   c. Evaluation of ascitic fluid (obtained via paracentesis) confirms the diagnosis.
      (1) A granulocyte count > 500 mm^3 is very suggestive.
      (2) A positive culture is diagnostic.

   d. *E. coli* and Strep species are the most common bacterial isolates.

   e. Treatment is with IV antibiotics (e.g. a third generation cephalosporin).

   f. Mortality rate ranges from 30 - 100%.

X. Pancreatitis

A. Etiology

1. Acute pancreatitis is most often due to ethanol ingestion or biliary tract disease (gallstones). Other causes include abdominal trauma, surgery, endoscopic retrograde cholangiopancreatography (ERCP), drugs (thiazides, furosemide, azathioprine, tetracycline, sulfonamides), penetrating peptic ulcer, hyperlipidemia, hypercalcemia, infections (mumps, viral hepatitis, infectious mononucleosis, mycoplasma) and pregnancy.

2. Chronic pancreatitis is the result of repeated episodes of acute pancreatitis and is usually due to chronic alcoholism of long duration (75% of cases in USA). Other causes include severe protein-calorie malnutrition, hyperthyroidism and pancreas divisum.

B. Clinical Picture: Patients classically present following ingestion of a fatty meal or after binge drinking and complain of epigastric pain, nausea and vomiting. The epigastric pain is <u>constant</u> in nature with radiation directly into the back and it is often eased when the patient leans forward. Exam may reveal epigastric tenderness with guarding, tachycardia (due to fever, hypovolemia and pain), tachypnea (due to pulmonary involvement), a low-grade fever and hypoactive bowel sounds. Because of the retroperitoneal location of the pancreas, however, rebound is generally absent. Grey Turner's sign (bluish discoloration in the left flank) and Cullen's sign (bluish discoloration around the umbilicus) indicate the presence of retroperitoneal hemorrhage and point to the diagnosis of hemorrhagic pancreatitis; unfortunately, these signs are not usually present. Serum amylase and lipase levels are typically elevated in acute pancreatitis; however, the degree of elevation does not correlate with the severity of the disease. Very high levels are usually seen when biliary tract disease (gallstones) is the underlying cause. On the other hand, patients with chronic pancreatitis do not usually have elevation of pancreatic enzymes since their pancreas is "burned out". Endoscopic retrograde cholangiopancreatography (ERCP) is the most reliable diagnostic tool since it readily demonstrates pancreatic ductal abnormalities.

C. Labs

1. Serum amylase
   a. Rises shortly after the onset of symptoms and returns to baseline levels within 1 to 4 days.
   b. Elevation 1.5 times the upper limit of normal is indicative of acute pancreatitis (specificity > 98%).
   c. Since other organs (fallopian tubes, salivary glands, ovaries) release this enzyme, elevation may be due to another disease.
   d. Its sensitivity is decreased in patients with alcohol-related pancreatitis (serum lipase is a better test in these cases) and in patients with chronic pancreatitis who have an acute exacerbation (levels may be normal or only mildly elevated in these patients).
   e. Isoamylase determinations increase specificity slightly, but are less sensitive, more time-consuming and are not readily available.

2. Amylase-creatinine clearance ratio
   a. When serum amylase is normal, send a urine specimen for amylase + creatinine levels to determine the amylase-creatinine ratio:

   $$\frac{\text{amylase clearance}}{\text{creatinine clearance}}\ \% = \frac{\text{urine amy.}}{\text{serum amy.}} \times \frac{\text{serum creatinine}}{\text{urine creatinine}} \times 100$$

   b. Interpretation of results
      (1) A ratio ≤ 3 is "normal" and should distinguish the hyperamylasemia of nonpancreatic disorders (ectopic pregnancy, parotitis).
      (2) A ratio ≥ 5 implies acute pancreatitis (although it may be elevated in patients with burns or DKA who have altered renal tubular function).
   c. While this test seems to be more sensitive and specific than the serum amylase, false positives and negatives do occur.

3. Serum lipase
   a. Unlike serum amylase (which is released by several organs) serum lipase is found primarily in the pancreas.
   b. It is as sensitive as serum amylase, but has the advantage of being more specific; specificity is almost 100%.
   c. Assays are readily available, reliable and inexpensive.

4. Other labs which should be assessed include:
   a. Glucose — to R/O hyperglycemia
   b. Calcium — to R/O hypocalcemia (most common lab abnormality)
   c. WBC — leukocytosis is common
   d. Hct — to R/O ↓ Hct (suggestive of hemorrhagic pancreatitis)
   e. ABG — to R/O ↓ pO_2 (suggestive of severe disease or development of a complication such as ARDS)
   f. BUN and creatinine — usually elevated due to hypovolemia
   g. SGOT(AST) and LDH — significant elevation suggests severe disease

D. Plain x-rays — are most helpful in excluding other diagnoses. Radiographic findings associated with pancreatitis include:

1. Abdominal films
   a. Scattered calcifications in the area of the pancreas are suggestive of <u>chronic</u> pancreatitis.
   b. Evidence of ileus + air-trapping in the small bowel adjacent to the pancreas → sentinel loop (suggests acute pancreatitis)
   c. Distended colon + collapse of the distal colon → colon-cutoff sign

2. CXR
   a. Left pleural effusion or elevated left hemidiaphragm
   b. Findings consistent with ARDS may be seen in patients with severe disease.

E. Management

1. Severe pancreatitis requires aggressive fluid resuscitation with NS or LR because profound shock may result from sequestration of large volumes of fluid in the retroperitoneum (third-spacing).

2. NG suctioning is indicated for severe cases to prevent vomiting, reduce abdominal distention and decrease stimulation of the pancreas.

3. Antiemetics and analgesics prn; meperidine is preferred to morphine (which may induce spasm of the sphincter of Oddi)

4. Surgical consultation for patients with severe pancreatitis.

F. Poor Prognostic Signs (Ranson's Criteria)

1. <u>On admission</u>
   a. Age > 55 years
   b. Leukocytosis >16,000/mm^3
   c. Hyperglycemia > 200 mg/dL
   d. SGOT (AST) > 250 SF units
   e. LDH > 350 IU/L

2. <u>48 hours later</u>
   a. Calcium < 8 mg/dL
   b. PO_2 < 60 mmHg (suggests ARDS)
   c. >10% fall in Hct (suggests hemorrhagic pancreatitis)
   d. > 5 mg/dL rise in BUN
   e. Base deficit > 4 mEq/L
   f. Sequestration > 4 L of fluid
   [Adapted from Ranson THC: Am J of Gastroenterol 77:663, 1982]

Mortality correlates <u>directly</u> with the number of poor prognostic signs present; the greater the number, the greater the mortality.

G. Complications

1. Pleural effusions (usually left-sided)

2. ARDS — is due to deactivation of surfactant (most common cause of death due to acute pancreatitis)

3. Pancreatic phlegmon → pseudocyst

4. Pancreatic abscess → sepsis

5. Hemorrhage (intrapancreatic or intraperitoneal) → shock

6. Pancreatic ascites

7. Third spacing of fluids → hypovolemia → ATN

8. DIC

GASTROINTESTINAL

Journal References

AMERICAN JOURNAL OF ROENT, Sivit, C. J., et. al., October 2000, "Imaging Evaluation of Suspected Appendicitis in a Pediatric Population: Effectiveness of Sonography Versus CT."

AMERICAN JOURNAL OF SURGERY, Chase, C. W., December 1996, "Serum Amylase and Lipase in the Evaluation of Acute Abdominal Pain."

AMERICAN JOURNAL OF SURGERY, Horton, May 2000, "A Prospective Trial of Computed Tomography and Ultrasonography for Diagnosing Appendicitis in the Atypical Patient."

AMERICAN JOURNAL OF SURGERY, Horwitz, J. R., Gursoy, M., Jaksic, T., Lally, K. P., February 1997, "Importance of Diarrhea as a Presenting Symptom of Appendicitis in Very Young Children."

ANNALS OF EMERGENCY MEDICINE, Gallagher, E.J., Lukens, T.W., Colucciello, S.A., et. al., 2000, #36 "Clinical Policy: Crital Issues for the Initial Evaluation and Management of Patients Presenting with a Chief Complaint of Nontraumatic Acute Adbominal Pain".

ANNALS OF EMERGENCY MEDICINE, Mikulich, V.J., Schriger, D.L., "The Management of Occupational Exposures to Blood and Body Fluids: Revised Guidelines on New Methods of Implementation."

AUDIO-DIGEST: EMERGENCY MEDICINE, Birnbaumer, D., August 1996, "Abdominal Pain in the Emergency Department."

AUDIO-DIGEST: EMERGENCY MEDICINE, Gerberding, J., February 1998, "AIDS Exposure."

AUDIO-DIGEST: EMERGENCY MEDICINE, Moran, G. J., January 1998, "Abdominal Infections."

AUDIO-DIGEST: EMERGENCY MEDICINE, Parrillo, S. J., January 1997, "Gastrointestinal (GI) Emergencies: Board Review."

AUDIO-DIGEST: GASTROENTEROLOGY, Boyer, T.D., May 1995, "Viral Hepatitis."

AUDIO-DIGEST: INTERNAL MED., May 3, 1995, "Infection Connections: Peptic Ulcer/Bad Food."

CLINICAL INFECTIOUS DISEASES, Gill, C.J., Lau, J., Gorbach, S.L., et al., 2003, 37(3), "Diagnostic Accuracy of Stool Assays for Inflammatory Bacteria Gastroenteritis in Developed and Resource-Poor Countries."

CLINICAL PHARMACY REVIEW, Mattson, C., 1995, "Treatment of Acid Peptic Disorders."

ED LEGAL LETTER, Salkin, M. S., December 1996, "Appendicitis: Avoiding Failure to Diagnose."

EMERGENCY MEDICINE, Johnson, D. A., February 1996, "New Dimensions in Helicobacter Pylori Infection."

EMERGENCY MEDICINE NEWS, Roberts, James R., January 1995, "Myths and Misconceptions about NSAID Gastropathy, Part II."

EMERGENCY MEDICINE REPORTS, Castellone, J. A. and Powers, R. D., September 1997, "Ischemic Bowel Syndromes: A Comprehensive, State-of-the-Art Approach to Emergency Diagnosis and Management."

EMERGENCY MEDICINE REPORTS, Seamens, C. M. and Schwartz, G., June 1998, "Food-Borne Illness: Differential Diagnosis and Targeted Management."

EMERG MED CLIN NORTH AM, Hunter, D., August 1996, "Gastrointestinal Emergencies, Part I."

FORESIGHT, Domeier, R. M., July 1996, "Acute Appendicitis."

HOSPITAL PHYSICIAN, Chey, W. D., February 1997, "Diagnosis of Helicobacter Pylori."

JOURNAL OF CLINICAL MICROBIOLOGY, Savola, K.L., Baron, E.J., Tomkins, L.S. et al, "Fecal Leukocyte Stain Has Diagnostic Value for Outpatients But Not Inpatients."

N ENGL J MED, Rao, P. M., et. al., January 1998, "Effect of Computed Tomography of the Appendix on Treatment of Patients and Use of Hospital Resources." (in Emer. Med. Abstracts, 1998)

MAYO CLINIC PROCEEDINGS, Gross, Jr., J.B., April 1998, "Clinician's Guide to Hepatitis C".

MAYO CLINIC PROCEEDINGS, Roberts, L. R., and Kamath, P. S., October 1996, "Pathophysiology and Treatment of Variceal Hemorrhage."

P & T UNIV OF WI SCHOOL OF PHARMACY, Laine, L., and Bloom, B., April 1997, "Helicobacter Pylori and Peptic Ulcer Disease: Selection of Antimicrobial Therapy."

Specific Text References

Atlas of Clinical Gastroenterology. Misiewicz, Bartram, Cotton, Mee, Price and Thompson (Glaxo/Roche, N.C., 1985)

Emergency Medicine Clinics of North America. Munter, D. W., Gastrointestinal Emergencies, Part I (Saunders, Philadelphia, 1996)

Emergency Medicine Clinics of North America. Munter, D. W., Gastrointestinal Emergencies, Part II (Saunders, Philadelphia, 1996)

Slieisenger & Fordtrans "Gastrointestinal and Liver Disease". Feldman, M., Slieisenger, M., Scharschmidt, B., 6th Edition, (W. B. Saunders, Philadelphia, 1998).

Textbook of Gastroenterology. Yamada, T., Alpers, D. H., et. al., Third Edition, (Lippincott Williams & Wilkins, Philadelphia, 1999)

Web and Other Sources

1997 SCIENTIFIC ASSEMBLY: AMERICAN COLLEGE OF EMERGENCY MEDICINE, Coppola, M., October 1997, "Current Management of Peptic Ulcer Disease."

EMEDICINE (www.emedicine.com), Santacroce, L., "Helicobacer Pylori Infection."

General Text References, Acep Clinical Policies and LLSA Reading Lists for all chapters located in the back of both volumes.

NOTES

PULMONARY EMERGENCIES

1. The most common cause of community acquired bacterial pneumonia is:

   (a) *Group A strep*
   (b) *Hemophilus influenza*
   (c) *Strep pneumoniae*
   (d) *Klebsiella pneumoniae*

2. An adequate sputum specimen is characterized by:

   (a) > 5 epithelial cells, few PMNs and many bacterial forms
   (b) > 5 epithelial cells, > 25 PMNs and a predominant bacterial form
   (c) < 5 epithelial cells, few PMNs and many bacterial forms
   (d) < 5 epithelial cells, > 25 PMNs and a predominant bacterial form

3. A sputum gram stain revealing encapsulated gram-positive lancet-shaped diplococci is most consistent with:

   (a) *Staph. aureus*
   (b) *Hemophilus influenza*
   (c) *Mycoplasma pneumonia*
   (d) *Strep. pneumoniae*

4. Although abscess formation is not frequent, it can be seen in association with each of the following causes of pneumonia except:

   (a) *Klebsiella pneumoniae*
   (b) *Chlamydia pneumoniae*
   (c) *Pseudomonas aeruginosae*
   (d) *Staph. aureus*

5. The antiviral agent used to treat infants and children with severe RSV (Respiratory Syncytial Virus) pneumonia or bronchiolitis is:

   (a) Rimantadine
   (b) Ribavirin
   (c) Adenosine Arabinoside
   (d) Amantadine

6. A 55-yr.-old male smoker presents in August with signs of an atypical pneumonia, relative bradycardia and gastrointestinal complaints. He is on no medications. The most probable cause of this patient's pneumonia is:

   (a) *Mycoplasma pneumoniae*
   (b) *Pasteurella (Francisella) tularensis*
   (c) *Legionella pneumophiliae*
   (d) *Coxiella burnetii*

7. All of the following statements regarding *Klebsiella* pneumonia are true except:

    (a) Sputum gram stain reveals encapsulated gram-positive organisms which occur in pairs.
    (b) The sputum is thick and brown in color, resembling currant jelly.
    (c) Alcoholics, diabetics and patients with COPD are most commonly afflicted.
    (d) CXR commonly reveals a necrotizing RUL infiltrate.

8. Which of the following statements regarding the TB skin test is most accurate?

    (a) It is positive in 100% of the patients with TB meningitis.
    (b) A positive reaction indicates the presence of infection with Mycobacterium tuberculosis but not necessarily the presence of active disease.
    (c) It is always positive in patients infected with M. tuberculosis.
    (d) Criteria for interpreting the test as positive are the same for all patients regardless of background/concurrent illnesses.

9. INH therapy for TB is associated with the multiple complications listed below. Which one of these complications can be prevented or minimized by the simultaneous administration of pyridoxine?

    (a) Phenytoin toxicity
    (b) Hepatitis
    (c) Hypersensitivity reaction
    (d) Peripheral neuritis

10. On which of the following views of the chest is a small pleural effusion most likely to be detected?

    (a) Supine
    (b) PA
    (c) Lateral decubitus
    (d) Lateral

11. All of the following are appropriate in the acute treatment of aspiration pneumonia except:

    (a) Administration of steroids and prophylactic antibiotics
    (b) Administration of supplemental oxygen
    (c) Bronchoscopy to remove large particles
    (d) Use of CPAP

12. The severity of pulmonary injury resulting from aspiration of foreign material is determined by all of the following factors except:

    (a) The presence of bacterial contamination
    (b) The pH and volume of the aspirate
    (c) The presence of particulate matter
    (d) The position of the patient at the time of aspiration

13. A small pneumothorax in a hypotensive patient may be detected on a _____ chest film.

    (a) Inspiratory
    (b) Expiratory
    (c) Lordotic
    (d) Supine

14. Signs and symptoms of a tension pneumothorax may include all of the following except:

    (a) JVD, cyanosis and dyspnea
    (b) Hypertension
    (c) Hyperresonance to percussion and absence of BS on the affected side
    (d) Deviation of the trachea to the contralateral side

15. Which modality assesses the degree of airflow obstruction in the asthmatic patient?

    (a) ABGs
    (b) PFTs (PEFR or FEV_1)
    (c) Pulse oximetry
    (d) CXR

16. The initial treatment of choice for the asthmatic patient is:

    (a) Corticosteroids
    (b) Atropine
    (c) Inhaled beta-adrenergic agents
    (d) Subcutaneous beta-adrenergic agents

17. All of the following are accurate indicators of a severe asthmatic attack except:

    (a) The presence of wheezing
    (b) The use of accessory muscles
    (c) The presence of diaphoresis and cyanosis
    (d) The presence of a pulsus paradoxus > 12mmHg

18. All of the following statements regarding the use of beta-adrenergic ago-
    nists in the treatment of asthma are accurate except:

    (a) Their primary effect is on the large central airways.
    (b) They promote bronchodilation by increasing cyclic AMP.
    (c) Their onset of action is < 5 minutes.
    (d) Agents with beta$_2$-selectivity are preferred.

19. Which of the following statements is true regarding the role of steroids in
    the treatment of PCP pneumonia?

    (a) They have no role.
    (b) They are beneficial as adjunctive therapy in patients with moderate
        to severe PCP pneumonia.
    (c) They are beneficial as adjunctive therapy in patients with mild PCP
        pneumonia.
    (d) They should be used as a primary therapeutic modality in all patients
        with PCP pneumonia.

20. Frequent metabolic derangements in near-drowning victims include all of
    the following except:

    (a) Hypoxemia
    (b) Acidosis
    (c) Serum electrolyte abnormalities
    (d) Hypercapnia

21. All of the following are causes of noncardiogenic pulmonary edema except:

    (a) Fat embolus
    (b) Fluid overload
    (c) Drug overdose
    (d) Multiple trauma

22. All of the following statements regarding noncardiogenic pulmonary edema
    are true except:

    (a) The heart size is small or normal
    (b) PAWP is elevated
    (c) CXR shows bilateral pulmonary infiltrates
    (d) Lung compliance is reduced

23. Pneumonia is most commonly acquired via _____.

    (a) Hematogenous spread from another site
    (b) Direct introduction of organisms into the pleura or lungs
    (c) Aspiration of oropharyngeal secretions
    (d) None of the above

24. All of the following statements regarding pneumococcal pneumonia are accurate except:

 (a) Patients usually give a history of a single shaking chill followed by the development of a cough productive of rust-colored sputum.
 (b) The WBC count is usually < 12,000.
 (c) A pleural effusion may be present in up to 25% of patients.
 (d) PCN is still the treatment of choice.

25. The serotype of *H. influenza* that is responsible for 95% of human infections is:

 (a) *Type a*
 (b) *Type b*
 (c) *Type c*
 (d) *Type d*

26. Atypical pneumonias are characterized by all of the following except:

 (a) Abrupt onset
 (b) Moderate fever
 (c) Presence of constitutional symptoms
 (d) Nonproductive cough

27. A pet shop employee presents with severe headache, malaise, myalgias and cough. Exam reveals a fever of 104° F, hepatosplenomegaly and a relative bradycardia. Lab evaluation reveals patchy perihilar infiltrates on CXR, elevated LFTs and proteinuria. The organism most likely responsible for this patient's pneumonia is:

 (a) *Coxiella burnetii*
 (b) *Francisella tularensis*
 (c) *Hantavirus*
 (d) *Chlamydia psittaci*

28. The agent of choice for the treatment of the patient described in the question above is:

 (a) Tetracycline
 (b) PCN
 (c) Chloramphenicol
 (d) Ribavirin

29. All of the following statements regarding near-drowning are accurate except:

    (a) Salt water drowning is more common than fresh water drowning.
    (b) Males are more commonly affected than females, regardless of age.
    (c) Children < 5 years old and teenagers are most commonly affected.
    (d) The final common pathway in both "wet" and "dry" drownings is profound hypoxemia.

30. ARDS most commonly occurs in association with:

    (a) Aspiration
    (b) Trauma
    (c) Sepsis
    (d) Massive blood transfusions

Answers: 1. c, 2. d, 3. d 4. b, 5. b, 6. c, 7. a, 8. b, 9. d, 10. c, 11. a, 12. d, 13. d, 14. b, 15. b, 16. c, 17. a, 18. a, 19. b, 20. c, 21. b, 22. b, 23. c, 24. b, 25. b, 26. a, 27. d, 28. a, 29. a, 30. c

Use the pre-chapter multiple choice question worksheet (p. xxv) to record and determine the percentage of correct answers for this section.

PULMONARY EMERGENCIES

I. Pneumonia

A. Bacterial Pneumonia (most common cause of a focal infiltrate)

1. Epidemiology
    a. Accounts for up to 10% of hospital admissions in the U.S.
    b. Most pneumonias are the result of a single species of bacteria:
        (1) *Strep pneumoniae* (60 - 90% of the time)
        (2) *Hemophilus influenza*
        (3) *Pseudomonas aeruginosa*
        (4) *Klebsiella pneumoniae*
        (5) *Staphylococcus aureus*
        (6) *Escherichia coli*
        (7) *Group A streptococci*
        (8) *Moraxella catarrhalis*
    c. Mechanisms of infection
        (1) Aspiration of oropharyngeal secretions is the primary mechanism of acquisition.
            (a) 50% of normal healthy individuals aspirate in their sleep.
            (b) In the presence of an altered mental status, an abnormal swallowing mechanism and/or GI disease, the frequency of aspiration is much greater.
        (2) Other mechanisms include hematogenous spread from another site and direct introduction of organisms into the pleura or lungs, both of which are uncommon.
    d. Predisposing factors
        (1) Impaired cough and gag reflex
            • Altered mental status
            • Seizures
            • Syncope
            • CVA
        (2) Impaired mucociliary transport
            • Smoking
            • Viral or mycoplasmal infection
            • COPD
        (3) Chronic underlying disease
            • Hepatic/renal failure
            • Diabetes mellitus (DM)
            • CHF
        (4) Impaired immunity
            • AIDS
            • Chemotherapy
            • Alcoholism
            • Cystic fibrosis

- Malnutrition
- Sickle cell disease/splenectomy
- Congenital immune deficiencies

(5) Underlying lung pathology
- Bronchial obstruction (FB, tumor)
- Pulmonary embolus/contusion
- Atelectasis

(6) Chest wall dysfunction
- Neuropathies/myopathies
- Postoperative pain
- Chest trauma

(7) Mechanical bypass of normal defense mechanisms
- ET tube
- NG tube
- Chest tube
- Bronchoscopy

(8) Altered upper respiratory tract flora
- Recent antibiotic therapy/hospitalization

e. Defense mechanisms
(1) Cough and gag reflex prevents gross aspiration.
(2) Tracheobronchial tree cilia remove particles > 5μm.
(3) Alveolar macrophages remove particles < 5μm.
(4) Surfactant, complement IgG and IgA limit bacterial growth.

2. Diagnostic studies
a. White blood cell count (a normal count does not R/O pathology)
(1) In a young normally healthy patient, a markedly elevated WBC count (> 15,000) is highly suggestive of bacterial pneumonia.
(2) In an elderly or debilitated patient, WBCs may be normal or decreased (even if there is an associated sepsis); the only clue may be a left shift.
(3) A very high or very low WBC count is associated with increased mortality.

b. Chest x-ray
(1) Certain patterns suggest a specific organism:
(a) *S. pneumoniae* (most common cause of lobar pneumonia)
<u>1</u> Singular lobar infiltrate in the LLL, RLL or RML
<u>2</u> Small pleural effusion
<u>3</u> Abscess formation
(b) *Group A strep*
<u>1</u> Patchy, multilobar infiltrates (usually lower)
<u>2</u> Large pleural effusion
(c) *H. influenza*
<u>1</u> Patchy (frequently basilar) infiltrates
<u>2</u> Occasional pleural effusion
(d) *Klebsiella pneumoniae*
<u>1</u> Upper lobe infiltrates
<u>2</u> Bulging fissure
<u>3</u> Abscess formation

      (e) *Staph. aureus*
         <u>1</u> Patchy, multicentric infiltrates
         <u>2</u> Abscess formation
         <u>3</u> Empysema
         <u>4</u> Pneumothorax
      (f) *Pseudomonas aeruginosa*
         <u>1</u> Patchy, mid or lower lobe infiltrates
         <u>2</u> Abscess formation
      (g) *E. coli* — patchy, bilateral lower lobe infiltrates
    (2) When infiltrates (patchy or lobar) are identified, always scan the films for other associated findings:
      (a) Pneumothorax
      (b) Pleural effusion
      (c) Abscess formation
    (3) Leukopenic or dehydrated patients may have normal-appearing x-rays.
    (4) Conditions that simulate pneumonitis on x-ray:
      (a) Pulmonary infarction
      (b) Pulmonary edema
      (c) Metastatic CA
      (d) Pleural thickening
      (e) Parenchymal scarring
      (f) Atelectasis

c. Pulse oximetry/arterial blood gases
    (1) In patients with pneumonia, the lungs are adequately perfused but poorly ventilated; the result is hypoxia.
    (2) If the saturation on pulse oximetry is < 95%, obtain an ABG to determine the actual pO_2 with pCO_2 levels.
    (3) If the pO_2 is < 60mmHg on room air, the patient should probably be hospitalized.

d. Sputum analysis (Consider primarily for high-risk patients who are hospitalized)*
    (1) Obtaining an adequate specimen is important in high-risk patients who will be hospitalized. Specimen collection is facilitated by heated saline nebulization, postural drainage or both. However, samples are not usually clinically useful unless they are obtained via an invasive method (e.g. bronchoscopy, tracheal suctioning). Fiberoptic bronchoscopy is the standard invasive procedure of choice for seriously ill or immunocompromised patients.
    (2) Gross exam findings (may suggest a particular organism)
      (a) Bloody or rusty → pneumococcus
      (b) Thick "currant jelly"
         <u>1</u> *Klebsiella*
         <u>2</u> Type 3 pneumococcus
      (c) Foul-smelling → anaerobic infection
      (d) Green color
         <u>1</u> *Pseudomonas*
         <u>2</u> *H. flu*
         <u>3</u> *S. pneumoniae*

*ACEP Clinical Policy on community-acquired pneumonia in adults

(3) Microscopic exam findings of a gram-stained specimen[*]
    (a) > 5 squamous epithelial cells is a contaminated specimen.
    (b) < 5 squamous epithelial cells + > 25 PMNs is an <u>adequate</u> specimen. ⎤
    (c) A predominate bacterial form suggests infection; sensitivity is 40 - 60%. ⎦ order sputum culture
(4) Smears for AFB should be done in patients at risk for TB (immigrants, patients with AIDS, IV drug abusers).

  e. Blood cultures should only be ordered in patients who are seriously ill as well as those with presumed bacteremia, comorbid disease, immunosuppression or rigors. "Routine" cultures on patients with pneumonia are discouraged due to a low yield of clinically useful data.

  f. Pleural fluid aspiration, although not generally an ED procedure, is helpful in ruling out empyema and, in the case of a large pleural effusion, drainage can reduce respiratory embarrassment as well. With smaller effusions, determination of the fluid pH is helpful in determining treatment: pH > 7.3 → antibiotics; pH < 7.3 → drainage.

3. Pneumococcal pneumonia
  a. Microbiology
    (1) Caused by *S. pneumoniae*, a gram-positive lancet-shaped, encapsulated diplococcus.
    (2) At least 83 serotypes have been isolated:
      (a) Types 1,3,4,6,7,8,12,14,18,19 = adult disease
      (b) Types 1,6,14,19 = children's disease
  b. *S. pneumoniae* is the most common cause of community-acquired bacterial pneumonia and the number one cause of bacterial pneumonia in HIV-infected patients.
    (1) Occurs 1 in 500 persons annually.
    (2) Peak incidence is in winter/early spring.
    (3) Mortality rate is < 5% if treated, but up to 30% if left untreated.
  c. **Clinical picture**
    The patient appears acutely ill and he can usually tell you exactly when he became very ill (abrupt onset). The presence of tachypnea and tachycardia is coupled with sharp chest pain associated with marked splinting on the affected side. There is a history of a <u>single</u> acute <u>shaking chill</u> followed by a cough productive of a rust-colored sputum. Flank or back pain, anorexia and vomiting are additional symptoms. On physical exam, the skin may be cyanotic or jaundiced, auscultation reveals crackles in the involved region and there are signs of pulmonary consolidation (bronchial breath sounds, egophony, increased tactile and vocal fremitus). If you listen carefully, you may also pick up a pleural friction rub.
  d. Associated lab findings
    (1) WBCs 12,000 - 25,000 but may be higher; a low count suggests severe sepsis.

---

[*] Sputum gram stain results are helpful in making therapeutic decisions in only about one-third of patients.

(2) Chest x-ray
   (a) Single lobar infiltrate (patchy in infants and the elderly)
   (b) Bulging fissures are occasionally present.
   (c) Pleural effusion (25%)
(3) Gram stain reveals a single predominate gram-positive organism in pairs or chains. Sputum culture is positive in 50% and blood cultures are positive in 30% of cases.

e. Treatment (See algorithm next page)
   (1) Despite the prevalence of increasingly resistant strains (up to 40%), penicillin is still a drug of choice.
   (2) Macrolides or doxycycline are preferred for uncomplicated infections in outpatients. Fluoroquinolones are no longer recommended for emperic outpatient therapy in otherwise healthy patients; they are reserved for outpatients with comorbidities (COPD, diabetes, renal failure, CHF or malignancies) and for those who have recently received antibiotics for another infection.
   (3) For those patients requiring IV therapy, one of the following protocols is recommended:
      (a) Cefotaxime or ceftriaxone ± a macrolide* or
      (b) Monotherapy with an extended spectrum fluoroquinolone
   (4) For inpatients with one of the following conditions requiring general medical admission:
      (a) Suspected aspiration with infection → amoxicillin-clavulanate or clindamycin
      (b) Recent antibiotic therapy for another condition → azithromycin or clarithromycin plus a beta-lactam or a respiratory fluoroquinolone alone -- the regimen selected will depend on the nature of the recent antibiotic therapy.
   (5) For ICU patients in whom:
      (a) Pseudomonas infection is not an issue → a beta-lactam + an advanced macrolide (azithromycin, clarithromycin) or a respiratory fluoroquinolone
      (b) Pseudomonas infection is not an issue, but the patient has a beta-lactam allergy → a respiratory fluoroquinolone (with or without clindamycin)
      (c) Pseudomonas infection is an issue →
         1 An antipseudomonal agent (piperacillin, imipenem, meropenem, cefepime, or piperacillin-tazobactam) + ciprofloxacin or
         2 An antipseudomonal agent + an aminoglycoside + a respiratory fluoroquinolone or a macrolide
      (d) Pseudomonas infection is an issue but the patient has a beta-lactam allergy →
         1 Aztreonam + levofloxacin or
         2 Aztreonam + moxifloxacin or gatifloxacin (with or without an aminoglycoside)

* Preferred regimen by the CDC

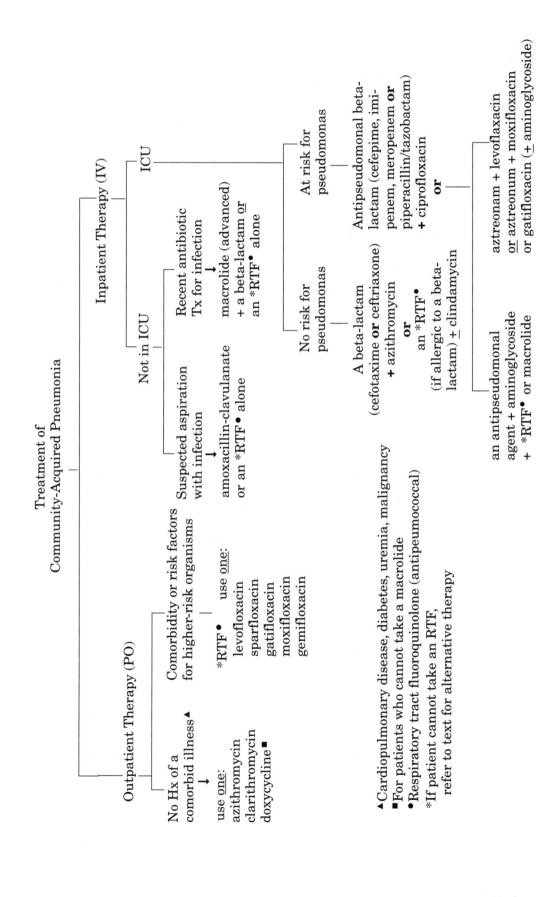

Treatment of
Community-Acquired Pneumonia

Outpatient Therapy (PO)

No Hx of a
comorbid illness ▲

use one:
azithromycin
clarithromycin
doxycycline ■

Comorbidity or risk factors
for higher-risk organisms

*RTF●   use one:
levofloxacin
sparfloxacin
gatifloxacin
moxifloxacin
gemifloxacin

Inpatient Therapy (IV)

Not in ICU

Suspected aspiration
with infection

amoxacillin-clavulanate
or an *RTF● alone

Recent antibiotic
Tx for infection

macrolide (advanced)
+ a beta-lactam or
an *RTF● alone

ICU

No risk for
pseudomonas

A beta-lactam
(cefotaxime or ceftriaxone)
+ azithromycin
or
an *RTF●
(if allergic to a beta-
lactam) + clindamycin

At risk for
pseudomonas

Antipseudomonal beta-
lactam (cefepime, imi-
penem, meropenem **or**
piperacillin/tazobactam)
+ ciprofloxacin
or

an antipseudomonal
agent + aminoglycoside
+ *RTF● or macrolide

aztreonam + levoflaxacin
or aztreonum + moxifloxacin
or gatifloxacin (± aminoglycoside)

▲ Cardiopulmonary disease, diabetes, uremia, malignancy
■ For patients who cannot take a macrolide
● Respiratory tract fluoroquinolone (antipeumococcal)
*If patient cannot take an RTF,
refer to text for alternative therapy

    f. Complications of *S. pneumoniae*
      (1) Sepsis
      (2) Meningitis
      (3) Endocarditis/pericarditis
      (4) CHF
      (5) Empyema (< 20%)
      (6) Peritonitis
      (7) Septic arthritis

    g. *S. pneumoniae* types 1 and 3 carry a poor prognosis as do patients with any of the following:
      (1) Multilobular involvement
      (2) Leukopenia(< 5000 WBCs) / bacteremia
      (3) Jaundice
      (4) Sickle cell anemia
      (5) COPD
      (6) CHF
      (7) Diabetes
      (8) Alcoholism
      (9) Splenectomy

4. Hemophilus pneumonia
    a. Microbiology
      (1) Caused by *H. influenza*, a gram-negative pleomorphic rod that exists in both encapsulated and unencapsulated forms.
      (2) Both forms cause pneumonia, but only the encapsulated form produces bacteremia on a regular basis.
      (3) The capsular forms are separated into 6 serotypes (a-f); type "b" causes 95% of all human infections.

    b. Epidemiology
      (1) The second most common cause of community-acquired bacterial pneumonia (in adults).
      (2) Is especially common among patients with COPD and AIDS.

    c. **Clinical picture** (peak incidence is in the winter/early spring) The patient is elderly, debilitated and may be diabetic, alcoholic or both. If he has COPD, ask if his cough and sputum production have been getting worse. He complains of fever, SOB and pleuritic-type chest pain. When you listen to breath sounds, there are rales but no signs of consolidation.

    d. Associated lab findings
      (1) Chest x-ray reveals patchy alveolar infiltrates and, occasionally, a pleural effusion.
      (2) The organism is frequently overlooked on gram stain.

    e. Treatment
      (1) Effective agents include:
        (a) Amoxicillin-clavulanate
        (b) Cephalosporins (second-or-third-generation)
        (c) Azithromycin (the preferred macrolide)
        (d) TMP-SMX
        (e) Tetracycline or doxycycline
        (f) Fluoroquinolones (levofloxacin, sparfloxacin)

(2) When patients require IV therapy, a second-or-third-generation cephalosporin (cefuroxime, ceftriaxone) should be used.
    f. Complications
       (1) Sepsis
       (2) Meningitis
       (3) Empyema
       (4) Arthritis

5. Klebsiella pneumonia
    a. Microbiology
       (1) Caused by *K. pneumoniae* - - a short, plump, encapsulated gram-negative bacillus that occurs in pairs.
       (2) On a poor-quality gram stain, *Klebsiella* is easily confused with pneumococcus.
    b. Most commonly occurs in:
       (1) Alcoholics
       (2) Diabetics
       (3) Patients with COPD
    c. **Clinical picture**
      Sudden onset of cough followed by multiple shaking chills and shortness of breath. The patient (usually a middle-aged or older male) complains of pleuritic-type chest pain and is noted to be cyanotic. Signs of pulmonary consolidation are present on physical exam.
    d. Associated lab findings
       (1) Leukocytosis (75% of cases)
       (2) Chest x-ray
         (a) Necrotizing RUL infiltrate or abscess formation with an air-fluid level
         (b) Perihilar and patchy infiltrates are occasionally seen.
         (c) Bulging minor fissure (35%)
       (3) Gross sputum exam: dark brown, tenacious and occasionally blood-stained; it resembles currant jelly.
    e. Treatment
       (1) Attentive airway management since the sputum is frequently so thick that clearance is difficult.
       (2) IV cephalosporin (ceftriaxone, cefuroxime or cefotaxime) plus an aminoglycoside (gentamicin, tobramycin or amikacin) are the initial agents of choice. Alternative agents include aztreonam and imipenem.
    f. Complications
       (1) Empyema within 24 - 48 hrs. (20%)
       (2) Sepsis
       (3) Pneumothorax

6. Other gram-negative pneumonias (occur rarely)
    a. Organisms
       (1) *E. coli*
       (2) *Pseudomonas*
       (3) *Enterobacter*
       (4) *Serratia*

  b. Usually occur in the immunosuppressed and debilitated patient.
  c. Treatment: carbenicillin or ticarcillin <u>plus</u> an aminoglycoside.

7. Staphylococcal pneumonia
    a. Organism: Large gram-positive cocci in pairs and clusters.
    b. Etiology
        (1) 1% of all bacterial pneumonias
        (2) Peak incidence is during measle and flu epidemics.
        (3) Affects IV drug abusers, nursing home patients, the debilitated
             and patients recovering from influenza infection.
    c. **Clinical picture**
        The patient presents with fever, multiple chills and pleuritic chest
        pain. He had the flu which was followed by the insidious onset of a
        cough productive of purulent sputum. Coarse rhonchi and rales are
        heard on exam of the chest; there are rarely signs of consolidation.
    d. Associated lab findings
        (1) WBC usually > 15,000
        (2) Chest x-ray
            (a) A patchy infiltrate that is initially multicentric or peripheral
                 (since it results from hematogenous spread) ultimately pro-
                 gresses to lobar consolidation and abscess formation.
            (b) Empyema is common.
            (c) A pleural effusion may also occur.
        (3) Blood cultures are usually negative unless the pulmonary involve-
             ment is metastatic.
    e. Treatment:
        (1) IV oxacillin or nafcillin are the antibiotics of choice.
        (2) IV vancomycin is the alternative agent; it is usually reserved for
             patients who are allergic to (or resistant to) PCN.

8. Group A streptococcal pneumonia (rare)
    a. Organism: gram-positive cocci in pairs or chains
    b. **Clinical picture**
        There is sudden onset of fever, chills and productive cough. The spu-
        tum is usually bloody and purulent; chest exam reveals fine rales
        without signs of consolidation.
    c. Chest x-ray: multilobular bronchial infiltrates with a large pleural
        effusion.
    d. Treatment: — Due to the high mortality associated with this rapidly
        progressive pneumonitis, patients generally require admission for
        IV antibiotics:
        (1) Aqueous PCN is the drug of choice;
        (2) A cephalosporin (ceftriaxone) or erythromycin are alternative
             agents.

9. Patient Assessment and Risk Stratification: The Pneumonia Specific Severity Index (PSI)*
   a. There are five severity classes based on mortality rate:
   - Classes I, II, & III → < 1% mortality
   - Class IV → 10% mortality
   - Class V → 27% mortality
   b. Patients in Class I are < age 50 with:
   - No comorbid conditions
   - Normal (or near-normal) vital signs
   - Normal mental status exam
   c. Patients in Classes II-V are determined by a point system:
   (1) Age in years (-10 for women) ____
   (2) Nursing home patient   +10
   (3) Coexisting illness
   - Neoplastic   +30
   - Liver   +20
   - CHF   +10
   - CVA/TIA   +10
   - Kidney   +10
   (4) Physical exam
   - Altered mental status   +20
   - RR > 30/min.   +20
   - Systolic BP < 90mmHg   +20
   - Temp < 30° C or 40°C   +15
   - Pulse > 125/min.   +10
   (5) Lab and x-ray
   - Arterial pH < 7.35   +30
   - BUN < 130   +20
   - Na^+ < 130   +20
   - Glucose > 250   +10
   - Hematocrit < 30   +10
   - pO_2 < 60% / O_2 sat. < 90   +10
   - Bilateral pleural effusion +10
   (6) Classification based on scoring
   - Class I (< 51 points)
   - Class II & III (51 - 70 & 71 - 90)
   - Class IV (91 - 130)
   - Class V (> 130)
   (7) Disposition (based on the IDSA** Guidelines)
   - In general, home care is recommended for patients in Classes I, II or III. However, admission is recommended in all patients with pre-existing conditions that compromise the safety of home care or those with mitigating factors (e.g. inabiliy to take oral meds, frailty, social/psych problems, unstable living situation, homelessness, etc.)

* ACEP Clinical Policy for the Management and Risk Stratisfication of Community Acquired Pneumonia in Adults in the Emergency Department. ANN EMERG MED 2001; 38:107-113
** Infectious Disease Society of America (Guidelines published in 2003)

B. Atypical Pneumonia

1. General characteristics
   a. Insidious onset of headache, myalgias, moderate fever and nonproductive cough
   b. Many WBCs but <u>no</u> predominant organism on Gram stain
   c. WBC normal or only moderately elevated
   d. Interstitial infiltrates (usually bilateral)
   e. Protracted clinical course

2. Mycoplasma pneumonia
   a. Epidemiology
      (1) Most common cause of atypical "walking" pneumonia
      (2) Accounts for 10 - 20% of community-acquired pneumonia
      (3) Most commonly affects children ≥ 3 yrs. old and adults < 40 yrs. old (but is often underdiagnosed in older adults)
      (4) Incubation period is 1 - 3 weeks
   b. Clinical signs and symptoms are variable.
      (1) Most patients have fever, chills, headache, malaise, sore throat, a dry cough and pleuritic chest pain. Other symptoms include:
         (a) URI (50%)
         (b) Earache (33%)
         (c) Anorexia, nausea, vomiting and diarrhea in the first week (12 - 14%)
      (2) Most patients have segmental rales and rhonchi on physical exam. Other findings include:
         (a) Conjunctivitis
         (b) Pharyngitis
         (c) Bullous myringitis (3 - 10%)
   c. Complications — are more common than previously thought and may include:
      (1) Aseptic meningitis or encephalitis
      (2) Hemolytic anemia
      (3) Glomerulonephritis
      (4) Guillain-Barré syndrome
      (5) Congestive heart failure, chest pain and other cardiac abnormalities, e.g. pericarditis, myocarditis, AV block
      (6) Splenomegaly
      (7) Erythema multiforme
   d. Associated lab findings
      (1) WBC is usually normal or moderately elevated.
      (2) CXR
         (a) One or more segmental infiltrates, dense consolidation or a generalized interstitial pattern may be present.
         (b) Segmental (or patchy) infiltrates are usually in the lower lobes and appear as streaks radiating from the hilum.
         (c) Interstitial pneumonia characterized by a reticulonodular pattern is often associated with deterioration of pulmonary function and can progress to respiratory failure.
         (d) Small pleural effusions are present in 20% of patients.

(3) Cold agglutinin titers are elevated in up to 60% of these patients and are supportive of the diagnosis but are neither sensitive nor specific.

(4) A fourfold increase in complement-fixing antibody titers is diagnostic; an initial titer > 1:64 is very suggestive.

e. Treatment:

(1) Erythromycin or one of the advanced macrolides (clarithromycin or azithromycin) are the drugs of choice.

(2) Tetracycline or doxycycline are the alternative agents.

<u>Note</u>: The hallmark of this disease is the disparity between the patient's clinically benign appearance and the extensive radiographic findings.

3. Viral pneumonia . . . is a common cause of CAP; underlying bacterial pneumonia should be considered in patients ill enough to require admission.

a. Types of infecting viruses

(1) <u>Respiratory syncytial virus (RSV)</u>

(a) The most common cause of pneumonia in children < 6 mos. old and those 3 - 5 yrs. old; the elderly and the immunocompromised are also at risk for RSV infection, as are hospitalized patients (and staff).

(b) Seen most commonly in the winter months.

(c) Clinical findings

<u>1</u> Fever, cough and coryza

<u>2</u> Chest x-ray: hyperexpansion of the lungs and patchy bronchial infiltrates.

<u>3</u> RSV antigen detection tests are unreliable in adults and not recommended.

(d) Treatment is primarily supportive. If admission is required, specific therapy may be indicated.

<u>1</u> Infants should receive at least one course of beta-adrenergic therapy during the first 24 hours (albuterol 0.1 - 0.15mg/kg/dose, up to 5mg hourly for the first few doses, then Q 4 - 6 hrs.).

<u>2</u> Aerosolized ribavirin may be used to treat infants and children with severe RSV infection as well as those with underlying cardiopulmonary pathology.

(2) <u>Parainfluenza</u>

(a) The second most common cause of pneumonia in children

(b) Also causes croup and bronchitis.

(3) <u>Adenoviruses</u>

(a) Target populations: children and military recruits

(b) Clinical findings: fever, cough, rhinitis, conjunctivitis and pharyngitis

(c) Chest x-ray: lower lobe infiltrates

(4) <u>Varicella - zoster virus</u>

(a) Occurs primarily in adults and is especially severe in pregnant patients.

(b) The illness begins with a rash which is followed within a week by fever and cough associated with tachypnea and dyspnea. 20 - 40% of patients will also develop cyanosis, hemoptysis and pleuritic chest pain.

(c) Sputum analysis may reveal multinucleated giant cells.

(d) CXR usually reveals an interstitial pneumonia; however, micronodular and lobar patterns may also occur.

(e) This is a serious adult illness and requires admission. Administration of intravenous acyclovir is indicated.

(5) Influenza viruses (most common cause of viral pneumonia in adults)

(a) Occurs between November and April (usually type A).

(b) The usual syndrome has a 1 - 5 day incubation period followed two weeks later by fever, headache and a nonproductive cough.

   1 80% will have an associated bacterial pneumonia.

   2 Up to 40% of patients with a normal chest film will have rales, rhonchi and wheezing on exam.

(c) Pure influenza pneumonia (no associated bacterial infection) is much more deadly. The elderly, pregnant patients and those with heart disease (especially mitral stenosis) are at risk.

   1 Sudden weakness is followed by dyspnea, cyanosis and ARDS.

   2 CXR: bilateral interstitial infiltrates (as well as treatment).

(d) Rapid Antigen Detection Assay is recommended for epidemiologic reasons.

(e) Treatment is primarily supportive. Amantadine (or rimantadine) is helpful in the treatment and prophylaxis of patients with influenza A if it is started within 48 hours of symptom onset.

(6) Cytomegalovirus (CMV)

(a) CMV pneumonia is a complication of transplant recipients and patients with advanced AIDS.

(b) CMV can be either a true pathogen or a coexistent organism:

   1 In transplant recipients, CMV is a true pathogen. It generally produces pneumonia within 1 - 3 months following transplantation and is the most common cause of death in recipients of bone marrow transplants.

   2 In AIDS patients, CMV is often found in association with other pathogens and may represent a coexistent organism rather than a true pathogen. Thus, a definitive diagnosis of CMV pneumonitis in these patients requires all of the following:

      a A compatible clinical picture (fever, hypoxia and infiltrates on CXR)

      b Positive cultures for CMV

      c Absence of other pathogenic organisms

(c) CXR most often reveals bilateral interstitial (or reticulonodular) infiltrates which begin in the periphery of the lower lobes and spread centrally and superiorly.

       (d) Treatment

         <u>1</u> IV ganciclovir or foscarnet

         <u>2</u> Immunoglobulin — is combined with the above regimen in bone marrow recipients (who are particularly susceptible to CMV infection).

   (7) <u>Hantavirus</u>

       (a) Infection results from inhalation of aerosols which contain material contaminated with rodent urine and feces.

       (b) Residents of the southwestern United States (New Mexico, Arizona, Colorado, Utah) are most commonly affected.

       (c) Patients initially have a prodrome of fever, myalgia and malaise that progresses over several days and evolves into a syndrome of severe respiratory distress and shock.

       (d) CXR reveals bilateral interstitial infiltrates (most prominent in the dependent lobes).

       (e) Treatment is supportive care and IV ribavirin (which is still experimental).

4. Chlamydial pneumonia (6% of community-acquired pneumonia)

   a. Organism: Chlamydia pneumoniae (the TWAR agent) is an obligate intracellular, gram-negative organism.

   b. Epidemiology

     (1) *C. pneumoniae* is a common cause of atypical pneumonia in young adults.

     (2) Spread is from person-to-person by droplet transmission.

     (3) Outbreaks generally occur as a cluster of cases in enclosed populations (boarding schools, army barracks, prisons).

   c. **Clinical picture** — The patient is usually a young adult who complains of a dry cough and low-grade fever that was preceded by a sore throat. Other complaints may include: laryngitis/hoarseness (present in one-third of patients), mild headache, myalgias and diarrhea. Exam reveals rales or rhonchi (and sometimes wheezing) on auscultation of the lungs and a nonexudative pharyngitis.

   d. Lab findings

     (1) WBC count is usually normal.

     (2) CXR typically reveals a subsegmental pneumonitis.

     (3) Nasopharyngeal culture or serology confirms the diagnosis.

   e. Treatment

     (1) Tetracycline, doxycycline or erythromycin are the agents of choice; a three-week course of therapy is recommended.

     (2) Azithromycin or clarithromycin (and quinolones)are also effective.

5. Psittacosis

   a. Organism: *Chlamydia psittaci* — an obligate intracellular, gram-negative organism harbored in avian species and transmitted by inhalation of infected dust or droplets.

   b. Owners of pet birds (particularly parrots), pet-shop employees, poultry workers and veterinarians are most commonly affected.

  c. Signs and symptoms include:
    (1) Hyperpyrexia (up to 105°)
    (2) Severe headache (often the major complaint)
    (3) Cough (which is occasionally associated with hemoptysis)
    (4) Hepatosplenomegaly
    (5) A flu-like syndrome consisting of malaise, myalgias and a URI
    (6) Relative bradycardia
  d. Associated lab findings
    (1) Leukopenia (25%)
    (2) Proteinuria
    (3) Abnormal liver profile (high enzymes)
    (4) Patchy perihilar or lower lung field infiltrates on CXR
    (5) Elevated complement fixation antibody titer
      (a) A fourfold rise (1:32) is diagnostic.
      (b) A 1:16 titer is presumptive evidence.
      (c) False positives occur in patients with Brucellosis and Q Fever.
  e. Treatment
    (1) Tetracycline is the drug of choice; a three-week course is recommended.
    (2) Erythromycin is the alternative agent.
  f. Complications are multiple and severe without antibiotic therapy; they include: hepatitis, myocarditis, endocarditis and meningitis.

6. Q Fever pneumonia
  a. The organism is *Coxiella burnetii*, an obligate intracellular rickettsia. It is highly infectious and can survive in dried soil or excrement up to 18 months and in tap water or milk for up to 42 months.
  b. Humans usually become infected by inhaling dust contaminated with excreta, placenta and uterine excretions of infected sheep, goats, cattle and parturient cats.
  c. Slaughterhouse workers, dairy farmers (and those who work closely with animals, especially farm livestock) are most commonly affected.
  d. **Clinical picture** — The patient looks ill, is diaphoretic and febrile. The usual history is sudden onset of shaking chills, high fever, myalgias, severe headache and a nonproductive cough. Chest findings are frequently minimal (fine rales) or absent. Hepatomegaly, if present, is a clinical clue.
  e. Associated lab findings
    (1) Abnormal liver function studies (85%)
    (2) Proteinuria (62%)
    (3) Sterile pyuria (12%)
    (4) Rounded segmental densities in the lower lobes or lobar consolidation on CXR.
    (5) Serologic studies are the diagnostic test of choice.
  f. Early antibiotic therapy helps promote a quick response and prevents relapse or chronic Q Fever.
    (1) Tetracycline 500mg qid <u>or</u>
    (2) Doxycycline 100mg bid <u>or</u>
    (3) Chloramphenicol 500mg qid

g. Complications associated with a prolonged illness:
   (1) Relapse despite antibiotic therapy
   (2) Endocarditis
   (3) Hepatitis
   (4) Meningitis

7. Tularemia
   a. Organism: *Francisella tularensis* — a gram-negative, nonmotile, pleomorphic coccobacillus that is harbored principally in hard ticks and wild rabbits.
   b. Epidemiology
      (1) Transmission is usually via direct contact with tissues or body fluids of infected animals, exposure to an infected tick or inhalation of contaminated dust or water aerosol.
      (2) Hunters, trappers, butchers, cooks and campers are most commonly affected.
   c. Clinical forms of tularemia include:
      (1) Ulceroglandular (most common) — characterized by an indurated skin lesion at the site of inoculation and regional lymphadenopathy
      (2) Typhoidal — characterized by fever, chills, weight loss and hepatosplenomegaly
      (3) Glandular
      (4) Oculoglandular
      (5) Oropharyngeal
   d. Tularemia pneumonia — is usually acquired via inhalation of contaminated aerosol or from bacteremia, but may also arise as a complication of either the ulceroglandular or typhoidal forms.
   e. **Clinical picture** of tularemia pneumonia — The patient (often a male) presents with high fever (104°- 106°), shaking chills and cough (usually nonproductive). Other symptoms include chest pain, shortness of breath and hemoptysis. Exam of the chest is often normal but may reveal rales, consolidation or a pleural rub. Hepatosplenomegaly and a maculopapular rash may also be present. CXR usually reveals bilateral, patchy, poorly-defined or ovoid infiltrates as well as hilar lymphadenopathy and pleural effusion.
   f. Serologic studies (ELISA) confirm the diagnosis:
      (1) A fourfold rise between acute + convalescent titers is diagnostic.
      (2) A single convalescent titer $\geq$ 1:160 is very suggestive.
   g. Treatment*
      (1) Streptomycin is the drug of choice.
      (2) Gentamicin or kanamycin are alternative agents.
      (3) Tetracycline or chloramphenicol are also effective, but are associated with a high rate of relapse and should be reserved for patients who cannot tolerate any of the above agents.
   h. Complications
      (1) Mortality rate is 5 - 30% without antibiotic therapy, < 1% with antibiotic therapy.
      (2) Prolonged course (up to several months) may occur.

*A live, attenuated vaccine has been developed for high-risk lab personnel.

II. Legionnaire's Disease

A. Pathophysiology

1. The most common causative organism is *Legionella pneumophila*, a gram-negative facultative intracellular bacillus that lives in natural and man-made water systems; it is implicated in as many as 6% of CAP cases.

2. Transmission occurs via inhalation of contaminated aqueous aerosols from equipment such as cooling towers, evaporative condensers and shower heads. Person to person spread has not been documented.

3. The illness occurs seasonally (summer and fall) and has an incubation period of 2 - 10 days.

4. Populations at risk
   a. Patients (particularly men) > 50
   b. Cigarette smokers
   c. Patients with a significant underlying disease (alcoholism, diabetes mellitus, COPD)
   d. Immunosuppressed patients (especially those with transplants)
   e. Patients who live or work near construction or excavation sites
   f. Recent travel (especially to spas) or changes in plumbing.

B. Clinical Signs and Symptoms

1. General systemic manifestations (rigors, high fever, headache, malaise, myalgias and weakness)

2. Pulmonary symptoms
   a. Cough — initially dry, but often becomes productive of purulent sputum and is occasionally accompanied by hemoptysis
   b. Dyspnea
   c. Pleuritic chest pain (33%)

3. Gastrointestinal symptoms
   a. Watery diarrhea (50%)
   b. Nausea, vomiting and abdominal pain

4. Neurologic signs
   a. Altered LOC
   b. Gait disturbance
   c. Seizures

5. Clinical clues within the past history:
   a. Failure to respond to β-lactam drugs (PCN, cephalosporins) or aminoglycosides for a recent infection.
   b. Onset of symptoms within 10 days of hospital discharge.

6. Exam findings
   a. Toxic appearance
   b. Disorientation and confusion
   c. Diffuse inspiratory rales progressing to signs of consolidation
   d. Relative bradycardia (50%)

C. Associated Lab Findings

1. WBC count is 10,000 - 20,000 with a left shift

2. ↑ Sed rate

3. Abnormal chemistries
   a. ↑ Liver function tests
   b. ↓ Sodium (< 130mEq/L) and phosphate
      Note: Hyponatremia is seen more commonly with legionella than any other cause of pneumonia.

4. Proteinuria and microscopic hematuria

5. Gram stain: PMNs but no predominant organism

6. CXR
   a. Unilateral patchy alveolar infiltrate (usually in the lower lobes) → progressing to lobar consolidation
   b. Pleural effusions (16 - 33%)
   c. Cavitary lesions (immunosuppressed patients)

D. Diagnostic Studies

1. Preferred diagnostic tests are the urinary antigen assay and culture of aspiratory secretions in selective media.

2. Direct immunofluorescent antibody (DFA) staining of sputum, pleural fluid or lung biopsy has the advantage of providing prompt results but has a sensitivity of only 50%.

3. Indirect immunofluorescent antibody (IFA) test is the most readily available serologic study; however, seroconversion takes 3 - 6 weeks.
   a. A fourfold rise in titer to a minimum of 1:128 from the acute to convalescent phase is diagnostic.
   b. A single convalescent titer > 1:256 is very suggestive of a recent infection.

E. Antimicrobial Therapy*

1. The advanced macrolides (especially azithromycin) are preferred by many for treatment of community-acquired pneumonia.

2. Alternative agents include:
   a. TMP-SMX + rifampin
   b. Quinolones (ciprofloxacin, ofloxacin or perfloxacin)
      Note: Cipro is the drug of choice for transplant patients.

*Mortality rate is up to 75% without early appropriate antimicrobial therapy and < 10 % with therapy.

III. Pneumocystis Carinii Pneumonia (PCP)

A. *Pathophysiology*

1. The causative organism is *Pneumocystis carinii*, an <u>opportunistic</u> pathogen whose classification remains unsettled; although it was previously considered a protozoan, current data suggest that it is probably a fungus. However, its susceptibility to antifungal agents is poor, while the antiparasitic agents (such as pentamidine and atovaquone) are effective.

2. Most cases result from <u>reactivation</u> of latent infection acquired early in life via the respiratory route.

3. This infection is seen almost exclusively in patients who are <u>immunosuppressed</u>:
   a. Patients with AIDS
   b. Patients receiving immunosuppressive therapy for cancer (especially corticosteroids) or organ transplantation
   c. Premature and malnourished infants
   d. Children with primary immunodeficiency disease

4. PCP is the <u>most common</u> opportunistic infection seen in HIV patients and is the leading cause of death in these patients.
   a. 80% of patients will acquire PCP at some time during their illness.
   b. It is the initial opportunistic infection in $\geq 60\%$ of those who are not receiving prophylactic therapy.
   c. In adults, infection generally does not occur until the CD4 lymphocyte count is < 200 cells/mm^3 but may occur with higher counts in the pediatric population.

B. *Clinical Signs and Symptoms*

1. Signs and symptoms develop in a slow and insidious fashion in AIDS patients; most have been symptomatic for two to three weeks at the time of diagnosis. Abrupt onset of signs and symptoms with rapid progression occurs more commonly with oncology patients.

2. Patients usually present with dyspnea, nonproductive cough and fever. Decreased exercise tolerance is also common. Other more variable complaints include weight loss, night sweats, chest pain, fatigue and chills.

3. Typical physical findings are cyanosis with tachypnea, tachycardia and a moderately elevated temperature. Hairy leukoplakia and oral candidiasis are signs of immunosuppression.

4. Lung auscultation is often normal, although rales or rhonchi may be heard in one-third of patients.

5. Extrapulmonary infection also occurs, most commonly in the lymph nodes.

C. Associated Laboratory Findings

1. ABGs — are frequently abnormal. Findings include:
   a. ↓ pO_2
   b. ↓ pCO_2
   c. ↑ alveolar-arterial oxygen gradient
   d. Low oxygen saturation or desaturation with 10 mins. of exercise
   e. Respiratory alkalosis

2. CXR
   a. May be normal in up to 20 to 30% of patients. This is more common early in the disease process.
   b. Classically demonstrates bilateral diffuse interstitial or alveolar infiltrates beginning in the perihilar region and extending in a "bat-wing" pattern.
   c. Atypical apical infiltrates and spontaneous pneumothoraces (10%) may also be seen. These findings are more common in patients who receive aerosol pentamidine prophylaxis. [Note: PCP is the most common cause of pneumothorax in patients with AIDS.]

3. ↑ LDH — the greater the elevation, the worse the prognosis.

4. WBC — may be low as a result of underlying disease or drug therapy; a marker of immunosuppression is a total lymphocyte count < 1000/mm^3.

5. Diffusing capacity for carbon monoxide is abnormal (a sensitive but nonspecific test).

6. Gallium scan is abnormal (a sensitive but nonspecific test).

7. A high-resolution CT scan that reveals patchy nodular densities suggests the diagnosis.

8. Pulmonary function tests are abnormal.

D. Diagnosis — examination of <u>induced</u> sputum* by direct or indirect immuno-fluorescent staining using monoclonal antibodies is the initial diagnostic procedure of choice and has a sensitivity of > 75%. However, fiberoptic bronchoscopy (bronchoalveolar lavage, brush biopsy, transbronchial biopsy) is almost always done to confirm the diagnosis; bronchoalveolar lavage, when performed as a <u>first</u>-line test, has a sensitivity of 86 - 97% and is the mainstay of the diagnosis. TB studies should also be performed since TB can present in a clinically similar fashion in immunocompromised patients (especially early).

---

* Obtained by using a high-flow nebulizer filled with 3% NS; 30 - 45 minutes are spent encouraging the patient to cough.

E. Treatment

1. Oxygen

2. Antibiotics — The two most commonly used drugs for moderate to severe PCP are trimethoprim-sulfamethoxazole (TMP-SMX) and pentamidine isethionate. Each is 50 - 80% effective. Unfortunately, AIDS victims have a particularly high incidence of adverse side effects to these drugs and often require a change from one medication to the other. Combination therapy with these two drugs is <u>not</u> recommended; it is associated with an increased incidence of side effects and <u>no</u> improvement in efficacy.

   a. <u>TMP - SMX</u>
      (1) Is the initial drug of choice in patients who can tolerate sulfa drugs. It has the advantage of providing coverage for some bacterial pneumonias and is well tolerated in non-AIDS patients.
      (2) Dosage is 15 - 20mg/kg/day TMP and 75 - 100mg/kg/day SMX IV or PO divided in four doses × 14 - 21 days.
      (3) Adverse reactions include nausea/vomiting, fever, rash, elevated liver enzymes and neutropenia.

   b. <u>IV Pentamidine</u>
      (1) May be used as an alternative drug for patients with a history of severe allergy/adverse reactions to sulfonamides.
      (2) Dosage is 4mg/kg/day IV over an hour × 14 - 21 days. BP must be carefully monitored during infusion because hypotension is a common side effect.
      (3) Adverse reactions include hypotension, syncope, tachycardia, facial flushing, pruritus, renal toxicity, elevated liver enzymes, hypoglycemia, rash, thrombocytopenia, neutropenia, pancreatitis and hallucinations.

   c. Alternative treatment regimens for patients who cannot tolerate the above agents include:
      (1) Oral TMP (15 - 20mg/kg/day in four divided doses) <u>plus</u> dapsone (100mg/day) — for mild to moderate PCP
      (2) Clindamycin (600mg PO tid or Q 6 hrs. IV) in combination with oral primaquine (15 - 30mg primaquine base/day) — for mild to moderate PCP
      (3) Atovaquone (750mg PO bid)
      (4) Trimetrexate (45mg/m^2/day IV) <u>plus</u> folinic acid (20mg/m^2 PO or IV Q 6 hrs) — for severe PCP
      (5) Aerosolized pentamidine (600mg/day) — for mild PCP

3. Steroids — are beneficial as adjunctive therapy in patients with moderate to <u>severe</u> PCP. They limit oxygen deterioration, decrease mortality and respiratory failure and accelerate recovery.

   a. Administer them to all children and to adult patients with a pO$_2$ < 70mmHg or a P(A-a)O$_2$ gradient > 35mmHg.
   b. Initiate therapy immediately (before the antibiotic is given) since hypoxemia may worsen.

c. Dosage
   (1) Prednisone is administered in a starting dose of 40mg bid × 5 days followed by 40mg qd × 5 days followed by 20 mg qd × 11 days.
   (2) Methylprednisolone may be substituted for prednisone at 75% of the above dosages if IV therapy is preferred.

4. Disposition — Hospitalization is indicated for most patients, especially children and those with a prior history of PCP since the mortality rate increases with subsequent episodes. Patients with mild disease and favorable respiratory parameters can be treated on an outpatient basis if close follow-up can be assured.

F. Prophylaxis

1. Is recommended for the following patients:
   a. Those with a prior episode of PCP pneumonia (the recurrence rate is 60% in AIDS patients).
   b. HIV-infected patients with a CD4 count < 200 cells/mL, unexplained fever (> 100°F) for ≥ 2 weeks or a history of oral candidiasis.
   c. Those undergoing intensive immunosuppressive therapy.

2. Prophylactic therapy is stopped if the CD4 count is > 200 cells/mL in patients on HAART (Highly Active Retroviral Therapy) for 3 - 6 months.

3. Regimens include:
   a. TMP - SMX (1 double strength tablet 3 × per week) or
   b. Dapsone* (50mg qd) or
   c. Aerosolized pentamidine (300mg every four weeks).

IV. Tuberculosis (TB)

A. Epidemiology

1. TB causes more deaths worldwide than any other single infectious agent; one-third of the world's population is infected with *M. tuberculosis*

2. The incidence of TB in the U.S. had been declining for decades, but this trend reversed itself in the mid-1980s; From 1985 - 1992 the number of cases of TB increased dramatically and in epidemic proportions. The incidence of multidrug-resistant strains of TB also increased, due in large part to noncompliance with drug therapy. Since 1993, however, the incidence has been steadily declining with an all-time low reached in 2000.

3. Circumstances that contributed to the resurgence in the mid 1980s included the HIV epidemic, congregate living in nursing homes, prisons and shelters, immigration, a decline in the ability of cities and states to maintain TB control programs and other social factors such as substance abuse, poverty and homelessness. Of these factors, the HIV epidemic is probably the single most significant influence. Comprehensive strengthening of control activities has reduced the rate of transmission.

*Contraindicated in patients with G6PD deficiency

4. TB is an AIDS-defining opportunistic infection and is the <u>only</u> opportunistic infection in patients with AIDS that is transmitted by the respiratory route to <u>both</u> immunocompromised and immunocompetent hosts.

B. Pathophysiology

1. The causative organism is *Mycobacterium tuberculosis*, a weakly gram-positive obligate aerobic rod with acid-fast staining properties that multiplies once every 12 - 24 hours (very slowly).

2. Transmission almost always occurs via aerosolized droplets produced by coughing, sneezing, talking or breathing. Infection develops when these contaminated droplets are inhaled and reach the alveoli.

3. Once in the alveoli, tubercle bacilli are phagocytized (but not killed) by alveolar macrophages and proliferate within these cells to form a primary focus of infection (primary TB) usually in the lower lobes. Organisms may also spread from this initial site of infection through the lymphatics to regional lymph nodes and to distant organs via the bloodstream. This bacillemia is usually <u>asymptomatic,</u> but it produces metastatic foci throughout the body which may become active later in life. These foci are preferentially established in areas of high oxygen tension such as the apical and posterior segments of the upper lobes of the lung, the kidneys, bones and brain.

4. Most infected patients mount an effective immune response and have no further infectious sequelae. T lymphocytes reach sufficient numbers to control the infection 2 - 10 weeks (average 6 - 8 weeks) following exposure. The tuberculin skin test becomes positive at this time, indicating that cell-mediated immunity has developed. Immunocompromised patients, however, may be unable to mount an adequate immune response. In these individuals, a rapidly progressive primary infection resulting in early death can evolve.

5. After a period of dormancy, some infected patients go on to develop active disease. This generally occurs when the patient's immune response is altered in some manner.
    a. The lifetime risk of reactivation in the general population is 10% but is much greater in patients with impaired cellular immunity.
    b. Conditions associated with an increased rate of conversion to active disease include:
        (1) AIDS — rate of progression is 7 - 10%/year
        (2) Immunosuppressive therapy (including steroids)
        (3) Renal failure/hemodialysis
        (4) Diabetes
        (5) Malnutrition/alcoholism
        (6) Malignant disease
        (7) Post-gastrectomy and post-intestinal bypass states
        (8) Transplant recipients

C. Clinical Signs and Symptoms

1. Pulmonary TB (inactive [dormant] *foci*)
   a. Is <u>asymptomatic</u> in ≥ 90% of patients and can only be identified by the development of a positive TB skin test ... and possibly a Ghon complex on chest x-ray.
   b. A pneumonitis may also occur (usually in the lower lobes).

2. Reactivation TB (endogenous reactivation of dormant *foci*)
   a. Is the most common clinical form of TB and is seen most often in the elderly.
   b. Symptoms include low-grade fever, night sweats, malaise, weight loss and productive cough (most common symptom).
   c. Signs of chronic wasting are present in most patients.
   d. Sites of involvement include the apical and posterior segments of the upper lungs, kidneys, bones/joints and brain.
      (1) Pulmonary involvement is present in > 80% of patients.
      (2) Extrapulmonary involvement is present in 15% of the general population but is greater in patients with HIV.

3. Pulmonary TB (active *foci*)
   a. Clinical onsets
      (1) Insidious: patients (usually debilitated) present with a chronic cough (most common symptom) and constitutional symptoms of reactivation such as malaise, weight loss and fever. As the cough progresses over time, it becomes productive of mucopurulent sputum and is often associated with hemoptysis. Patients may also complain of a dull ache or tightness in the chest.
      (2) Abrupt: some patients present with acute onset of fever, chills, cough (most common symptom) and myalgias mimicking an episode of acute bronchitis or pneumonia. Unless TB is considered in the differential Dx and smears of sputum for acid-fast bacilli are obtained, these patients may be misdiagnosed as having bacterial pneumonia.
   b. Chest exam — is often unremarkable, but may reveal rales or consolidation in the presence of extensive pulmonary involvement.

4. Extrapulmonary TB — can result from primary infection or reactivation and may involve almost any organ in the body. It may also take a disseminated form (miliary TB). The signs and symptoms produced are determined by the structures that are affected.
   a. TB meningitis (most rapidly progressive form of TB)
      (1) Results from seeding during the primary infection or from rupture of a subependymal lesion (Rich foci) into the subarachnoid space.
      (2) Clinical onsets
         (a) Insidious: patients often present with a nonspecific febrile illness of 1 - 6 weeks duration followed by intermittent headache, confusion, personality changes, stiff neck, diplopia, photophobia, cranial nerve palsies, ↓ LOC and seizures.
         (b) Fulminant: some patients, particularly children, may present acutely with fever and delirium in association with a severe headache and stiff neck.

      (3) Associated lab findings
         (a) Positive TB skin test (75%)
         (b) CSF analysis (acid-fast stain not usually positive)
           <u>1</u> ↑Pressure and protein
           <u>2</u> ↓Glucose
           <u>3</u> ↑WBC count of 100 - 1000/mL (predominantly lymphs)

b. Pleural TB
   (1) Results from rupture of a parenchymal focus into the pleural space
   (2) The associated pleural effusion is <u>exudative</u> in nature with lab evaluation revealing:
      (a) ↑ Protein
      (b) Low pH
      (c) Normal or low glucose
      (d) WBC count of 1000 - 5000/mL (mostly monos)
      (e) An acid-fast smear that is often negative
   (3) Pleural biopsy is helpful in making the diagnosis.

c. Genitourinary TB
   (1) Patients usually present with urinary symptoms (dysuria, frequency) hematuria or flank pain. Constitutional symptoms may also be present.
   (2) Urinalysis reveals
      (a) Pyuria with<u>out</u> bacteriuria
      (b) Low pH

d. Miliary (disseminated) TB
   (1) A multisystemic process resulting from a progressive primary infection (immunocompromised patients) or from secondary bloodstream seeding during recrudescence of previously dormant foci.
   (2) Symptoms are usually nonspecific and may include fever, anorexia, weight loss and weakness. Depending on the sites of involvement, more specific symptoms (dyspnea, cough, headache) may also be present.
   (3) Physical findings may include:
      (a) Fever
      (b) Pulmonary findings
      (c) Hepatomegaly
      (d) Lymphadenopathy
      (e) Splenomegaly
      (f) Tubercles of the retina[*] (the only specific finding)
   (4) Associated lab findings
      (a) Anemia and WBC abnormalities (leukopenia, leukemoid reactions, agranulocytosis)
      (b) Hyponatremia
      (c) Negative TB skin test 25 - 50% of the time (especially in the elderly and immunocompromised)
      (d) CXR - typically reveals small nodular densities that are uniformly distributed throughout both lung fields. A pleural effusion may also be present.

*Circumscribed, spheroid, granulomatous lesions with 3 distinct zones

5. TB and HIV
    a. TB is an AIDS-defining illness and generally produces disease at an earlier stage of HIV infection than other opportunistic infections.
    b. The incidence of TB in HIV-infected patients approaches 60% and currently represents the greatest health care risk to the general public from the HIV epidemic.
    c. Co-infection with TB and HIV results in:
        (1) A greater incidence of extrapulmonary disease
        (2) More atypical clinical findings
        (3) An increased incidence of tuberculin <u>non</u>reactivity and negative acid-fast bacilli smears
        (4) A greater frequency of unusual and atypical CXRs
        (5) Decreased cavitary disease
        (6) More antibiotic resistance
        (7) Higher relapse and mortality rates
        (8) A larger number of adverse drug reactions and multidrug-resistant TB (especially to Rifampin and Isoniazid)

D. **Diagnosis** — TB must be considered in the differential diagnosis of any patient who presents with respiratory complaints or extrapulmonary symptoms, particularly if the patient is a member of a high risk group (patients with AIDS, immigrants, IV drug abusers, residents/employees of long-term care facilities). Tests used to establish the diagnosis include the TB skin test, CXR and microbiological studies for acid-fast bacilli (AFB).

1. TB skin test
    a. Is the standard test for detecting <u>infection</u> with *M.tuberculosis*.
    b. Involves intradermal administration of purified protein derivative (PPD) and is read 48 - 72 hours following administration.
    c. A positive reaction indicates the presence of infection but not necessarily the presence of active disease (must be confirmed by culture).
    d. Criteria for interpreting the test as <u>true-positive</u> vary with patient background as follows:
        (1) ≥ 5mm induration is positive in patients with:
            • Known or suspected HIV infection
            • An abnormal CXR
            • Close contact with a person with active TB
        (2) ≥ 10mm induration is positive in:
            • Residents/employees of long-term care facilities
            • IV drug abusers
            • Immigrants from an area with a high incidence of TB
            • Certain high-risk minority groups (Hispanics, African-Americans, Native Americans)
        (3) ≥ 15mm induration is positive in all others
    e. A <u>negative</u> test does <u>not</u> exclude the diagnosis since some patients (particularly those who are immunocompromised) are anergic.

f. A <u>false-positive</u> test may be due to infection with *M. avium* or *M. kansasii* (nontuberculous mycobacterium). Clues to this diagnosis include the following:
   (1) No history of risk factors for TB
   (2) A negative skin test (or a reaction smaller than a true-positive)
   (3) History of COPD

2. CXR findings suggestive of TB
   a. Primary TB
      (1) Small parenchymal infiltrates located in any area of the lung and unilateral hilar adenopathy.
      (2) These lesions may subsequently calcify to form a Ghon complex.
      (3) Inflammatory infiltrates of the lower lobes with associated hilar adenopathy are seen in patients with progressive primary infections and clinically evident disease. [<u>Note</u>: Hilar adenopathy is the radiologic hallmark of primary TB in children.]
   b. Reactivation/pulmonary TB
      (1) Is typically an <u>upper</u> lobe process. Nodular densities are most often seen in the apical (Simon's foci) or posterior segments of the upper lobe but may also be found in the upper segment of the lower lobe.
      (2) Associated cavitation may or may not be present.
   c. Miliary (disseminated) TB
      (1) CXR may initially be normal but classically reveals small nodules (1-3mm) scattered throughout both lung fields in a miliary pattern.
      (2) A pleural effusion (frequently unilateral) may also be present.
   d. Findings in HIV-infected patients
      (1) The CXR is often <u>atypical</u> and may even be normal.
      (2) Upper lobe cavitary lesions are rare while hilar or mediastinal adenopathy and lower lobe infiltrates are more common.
      (3) A diffuse interstitial pattern that is easily mistaken for PCP may also be seen.

3. Microbiological studies
   a. Staining of sputum for AFB
      (1) Is done with Ziehl-Neelsen or fluorescent (fluorochrome) staining (which is more sensitive) and provides a rapid <u>presumptive</u> diagnosis of TB; the number of bacilli seen correlates with the degree of infectivity.
      (2) Positive smears have a specificity of 98%.
      (3) Smear results should be confirmed by culture.
   b. Culture of sputum or tissue for AFB
      (1) Is more sensitive than staining and is the "gold standard" for confirming the diagnosis of TB.
      (2) Although traditional cultures take 3 - 6 weeks, new radiometric techniques can confirm the diagnosis in as few as 5 days; DNA probes, reverse transcription and polymerase chain reaction (PCR) tests allow for identification of TB in a matter of hours but, due to technical problems, have not received approval for routine clinical use.

E. TB Therapy

1. As soon as the diagnosis is suspected, have the patient wear a mask and place him in an isolation room.

2. Due to the emergence of multidrug-resistant strains of TB, it is now recommended that initial therapy for TB include four drugs until susceptibility tests are available.

3. The initial drug regimen of choice is isoniazid (INH),* rifampin (RIF), pyrazinamide (PZA) and streptomycin (SM) or ethambutol (EMB); in the absence of drug resistance, isoniazid and rifampin taken for nine months is curative.

4. Side effects associated with these drugs are as follows:
   a. Isoniazid (INH)
      (1) Multiple neurologic entities, including peripheral neuritis — pyridoxine/vitamin B_6 is administered with INH to prevent INH-induced neuropathy.
      (2) Hepatitis
      (3) Hypersensitivity reactions
      (4) Drug-induced interactions with ketoconazole and fluconazole
   b. Rifampin (RIF)
      (1) Hepatitis
      (2) Thrombocytopenia
      (3) Drug interactions with Coumadin, oral contraceptives, digitalis derivatives, methadone, dapsone, cyclosporin, corticosteroids, oral hypoglycemic agents, ketoconazole and fluconazole → decreased blood levels and effectiveness
      (4) Orange-colored tears, saliva and urine
   c. Pyrazinamide (PZA)
      (1) Hyperuricemia
      (2) Hepatitis
      (3) Arthralgias
      (4) Rash
   d. Ethambutol (EMB)
      (1) Optic neuritis
      (2) Rash
   e. Streptomycin (SM)
      (1) Vestibular nerve damage
      (2) Nephrotoxicity

5. Prior to initiating therapy with these agents, baseline studies should be obtained:
   a. LFTs, BUN/creatinine and CBC with platelet count → all patients
   b. Visual acuity (+ red-green color perception) → if treating with EMB
   c. Serum uric acid → for treatment with PZA

---

*Preventive drug therapy also includes INH (i.e. those with a positive PPD).

V. Pleural Effusion: an abnormally large collection of fluid within the pleural space, reflecting the presence of an underlying intrathoracic or extrathoracic disease process.

A. *Pathophysiology*

1. Transudates: excessive hydrostatic pressure (CHF) or insufficient oncotic pressure (↓ serum protein) → low protein plasma infiltrates.

2. Exudates: lymphatic blockage due to malignancy or pleural capillary damage due to infectious disease → high protein plasma infiltrates.

B. *Clinical Signs and Symptoms*

1. Pleuritic pain is common with infection. Other associated symptoms include fever, cough and SOB.

2. Physical exam findings
   a. Splinting ± a pleural friction rub = pleurisy.
   b. Dullness to percussion + ↓ BS + ↓ tactile fremitus = pleural fluid.
   c. Bronchial breath sounds + egophony = atelectasis.
   d. Normal breath sounds + distended neck veins + left parasternal lift + accentuated P_2 on cardiac exam = massive pulmonary embolism.

C. *Diagnostic Workup*

1. CXR — Small effusions are most easily detected on a <u>lateral decubitus</u> film with the affected side down; accumulations of 5 - 50mL of fluid can be detected with this view. Small effusions can be missed entirely on supine films, and are generally not apparent on PA and lateral films until 200mL or more of fluid are present.
   a. Early signs of small effusion
      (1) PA view → faint obscuring of the costophrenic angle
      (2) Lat. view → blunting or loss of the costophrenic angle
      (3) Lateral decubitus view → fluid layers out
   b. Signs of a moderate effusion
      (1) Ground-glass appearance of lung fields
      (2) No air bronchograms
   c. Sign of a large effusion → opacification (partial or complete)
   d. Pleural fluid in a fissure → a "phantom" or "pseudotumor"

2. Thoracentesis — the definitive procedure
   a. Contraindications
      (1) Uncooperative patient
      (2) Coughing or hiccups
      (3) Local skin infection
      (4) Coagulopathies
      (5) Anticoagulant therapy
   b. Technique
      (1) The posterior entry is the primary approach. Insert the needle immediately above the rib to avoid the neurovascular bundle.
      (2) Loculated effusions may require ultrasound or CT-guided needle aspiration.
      (3) Withdrawing fluid
         (a) If an exudate is suspected, remove as much fluid as possible to a maximum 1 - 1.5 liters; removal of a greater amount of fluid increases the probability that reexpansion pulmonary edema will develop.
         (b) If a transudate is suspected, remove only a small amount of fluid for analysis.
      (4) Following the procedure, obtain a CXR to rule out an iatrogenic pneumothorax.
   c. Pleural fluid studies
      (1) CBC with differential
      (2) Serum protein, LDH, amylase and glucose (< 40mg/dl → empyema)
      (3) Cytology studies
      (4) Gram stain and AFB smear
      (5) Cultures for aerobes, anaerobes, mycobacteria and fungi
      (6) pH (< 7.0 suggests empyema; < 6.0 suggests esophageal rupture)
   d. Order serum protein and LDH levels, too, because the criteria for classifying pleural fluid as an exudate or transudate includes the protein and LDH pleural fluid to serum ratios.
   e. Diagnostic criteria
      (1) In the past, a protein concentration > 3gm/dL and a SG > 1.015 were used to classify a pleural effusion as an exudate but these criteria were found to be too inaccurate.
      (2) Current criteria:
         • Pleural fluid protein/serum protein > 0.5
         • Pleural fluid LDH > 200 IU/ml
         • Pleural fluid LDH/serum LDH > 0.6
         • Pleural fluid cholesterol ≥ 60mg/dl
         If one or more of these four criteria are present, the fluid is probably an exudate. If none of the criteria are present, the fluid is probably a transudate. (The only exception to this rule is the patient with CHF who is taking diuretics; in this case, pleural fluid values are unreliable indicators because protein is removed from the pleural space more slowly during diuresis).

f. Differential diagnosis
(1) Transudates
(a) CHF — most common cause of effusions
(b) Constrictive pericarditis
(c) SVC obstruction
(d) Hypoalbuminemia
(e) Nephrotic syndrome
(f) Cirrhosis
(g) Peritoneal dialysis
(2) Exudates:
(a) Infections
  • Bacterial pneumonia ———— 2nd and 3rd most
  • TB (usually primary) ———— common causes
(b) Malignancy ———————— of effusions
(c) Connective tissue and hypersensitivity disorders
  • Rheumatoid arthritis
  • Systemic lupus erythematosus
  • Dressler's syndrome
  • Drug-induced
(d) Pancreatitis
(e) Subphrenic abscess
(f) Abdominal surgery
(g) Uremia
(h) Esophageal rupture
(i) Pulmonary emboli and infarction (along with pneumonia and malignancy, are the most common causes of pleural exudates)
(j) Hemothorax
(k) Chylothorax
(l) ARDS

VI. Aspiration Pneumonia

A. Pathophysiology

1. Aspiration pneumonia is an inflammation of lung parenchyma precipitated by foreign material entering the tracheobronchial tree.

2. The <u>initial</u> pathologic changes (first few minutes) produced by fluid aspiration are <u>nonspecific</u> and <u>independent</u> of the type of fluid aspirated. These changes include collapse and expansion of individual alveoli, reflex airway closure and interstitial edema → ventilation-perfusion mismatching and hypoxia.

3. Final extent and severity of pulmonary injury, however, are determined by the specific substance aspirated and are dependent on three factors:
   • The pH and volume of the aspirate
   • The presence of particulate matter (such as food)
   • Bacterial contamination
      *In <u>Community-Acquired</u> aspiration pneumonia, streptococcal species are the most common aerobic isolates.
      *The most commonly isolated aerobes from <u>nosocomial</u> aspiration pneumonia are gram-negative bacilli and Staph. aureus.

4. The pH and specific content of the aspirate affect the pathologic changes produced as follows:

   $$\boxed{pH > 2.5}$$

   a. The additional injury produced by neutral fluids is determined by the volume and content.
   b. The larger the volume of aspirate, the greater the mortality and morbidity.
   c. Aspiration of lipid material → a chronic granulomatous reaction → lipoid pneumonia
   d. Aspiration of fluid containing food particles → a persistent inflammatory reaction which progresses within 6 hours to hemorrhagic pneumonitis → a granulomatous reaction resembling TB
   e. Aspiration of charcoal → bronchiolitis obliterans

   $$\boxed{pH < 2.5}^{*}$$

   a. Aspiration of fluid with a pH < 2.5 produces pulmonary changes resembling those of a chemical burn.
   b. Aspiration of as little as 0.3mL/kg in kids or 20 - 25 mL in adults → immediate reflex airway closure, destruction of surfactant-producing alveoli, alveolar collapse and irreversible damage to pulmonary capillaries. Sequelae include pulmonary hemorrhage, bronchial epithelial degeneration and pulmonary edema.
   c. Secondary bacterial infection eventually results.
      (1) Anaerobes predominate in community-acquired aspirations.
      (2) A mixture of gram-negative aerobes and anaerobes are typically isolated in hospital-acquired aspirations.

5. Foreign body aspiration
   a. The leading cause of accidental home death in children < 6 yrs. old.
   b. Complete obstruction causes death by asphyxiation in 4 - 6 minutes.
   c. Peripheral aspiration causes pneumonitis and lung abscess.

* Usually due to esophageal rupture

B. Risk Factors

1. Depression of the cough or gag reflex (general anesthesia, chronic illness, drug overdose, use of sedative medications)

2. NG Tubes

3. Esophageal strictures, dysmotility and reflux

4. Esophageal obturator airway (EOA)

5. Tracheostomies

6. Poor oral hygiene

C. Clinical Signs and Symptoms

1. Aspiration of fluid and oropharyngeal bacteria can be silent and actually occurs to some extent in normal individuals during sleep. Pathologic aspirations, however, such as those occurring during a substance abuse stupor or in a comatose state when the normal protective airway reflexes are decreased or lost, tend to produce a more devastating clinical picture:
   a. Sudden onset of coughing or choking
   b. Tachypnea, tachycardia and cyanosis
   c. Wheezing, rales or rhonchi
   d. Large amounts of frothy, bloody sputum
   e. Hypotension

2. Most patients (> 90%) develop signs and symptoms within one hour of the event.

3. Patients who have aspirated a FB (and have incomplete obstruction) present with choking, a spasmodic cough and wheezing. Examination of the chest may reveal asymmetric chest wall movement, decreased BS, wheezing and hyperresonance to percussion on the involved side.

D. Lab Findings

1. ABGs
   a. The usual finding is hypoxia with respiratory alkalosis.
   b. Severe aspiration → respiratory failure with a combined respiratory and metabolic acidosis.
2. CXR
   a. Radiographic findings are often delayed.
      (1) Atelectasis is the initial finding and may be seen as early as one hour post-aspiration.
      (2) Infiltrates develop 6 - 12 hours later and most frequently involve the RLL (if aspiration occurred in the upright position).
   b. FB aspiration → an end-expiratory PA film demonstrates a hyperexpanded lung on the involved side (usually the right side since the right mainstem bronchus has less of an acute angle than the left).

E. Treatment

1. Place the patient in the left lateral decubitus position with head down.

2. Suction the mouth and trachea and determine the pH of the aspirate.

3. Provide supplemental oxygen.
    a. High-flow O_2 by nasal cannula or face mask may be sufficient for some patients.
    b. Those who are hypercarbic (or remain hypoxic) despite these measures should be intubated and mechanically ventilated.
    c. If the patient has an altered level of consciousness and a decreased gag reflex, immediate endotracheal intubation is needed. Oxygenation with PEEP (peak end-expiratory pressure) will lower the mortality rate if it is begun within six hours of aspiration.

4. Initiate intermittent positive pressure ventilation (IPPV) with either CPAP or PEEP.
    a. IPPV has been demonstrated to improve survival and decrease hypoxia if initiated within 6 hours of aspiration.
    b. IPPV → ↑functional residual capacity + ↓atelectasis and interstitial edema → ↓ventilation-perfusion mismatching.

5. Correct hypovolemia (due to fluid loss into the interstitium and alveoli) with adequate volume replacement; use a crystalloid solution.
    a. The rate of administration should be guided by changes in the BP, pulse, urine output and CVP.
    b. Patients with CHF may require Swan-Ganz monitoring of IV fluids.

6. Bronchoscopy is useful in removing large particles and clearing the large airways. Bronchial irrigation with saline solution, however, should be avoided; it has no beneficial effect and may be harmful.

7. Antibiotics should be reserved for elderly and chronically ill patients as well as those who develop clinical evidence of infection (fever, purulent sputum, leukocytosis). Bacterial aspiration pneumonia occurs over a period of several days in > 60% of cases of chemical aspiration. Antibiotic therapy is based on the origin of the infection.
    a. <u>Community-acquired</u> aspiration pneumonia → empiric treatment is with a third or fourth generation cephalosporin **or** a fluoroquinolone (with anti-pneumococcal coverage) **or** a beta-lactam with a beta-lactamase inhibitor and a macrolide.
    b. <u>Nosocomial</u> aspiration pneumonia → empiric treatment is with piperacillin/clavulanate **or** a fluoroquinolone (with antipneumococcal coverage) **and** clindamycin [Note: if an abscess is present, clindamycin has excellent penetration.]

8. Supportive care measures include:
    a. Humidified oxygen
    b. Bronchodilators
    c. Chest physiotherapy

F. Complications of Aspiration Pneumonia
- Acute respiratory failure
- Hypovolemic shock
- Pneumonia, empyema and lung abscess
- Pulmonary fibrosis

G. Mortality Rate . . . varies with the pH and contamination of the aspirate:
40 - 70% if the pH is < 2.5, almost 100% if the pH is < 1.8 or the aspirate is grossly contaminated, i.e. Boerhaave's syndrome.

H. Prevention of Aspiration in the Emergency Department

1. Any patient with a depressed or absent gag reflex should be intubated[*] using a high-volume, low-pressure, cuffed ET tube.

2. When gastric lavage is indicated in the obtunded or comatose patient: intubate first, then place the patient in Trendelenburg on his left side prior to lavage.

3. Do not remove an esophageal obturator airway (EOA) until the patient has been intubated and adequate suction is available.

4. Increase the gastric pH.
   a. Nonparticulate antacids (such as 0.3M sodium citrate) neutralize gastric acidity and have been shown to reduce morbidity and mortality if administered before aspiration occurs.
   b. H_2-receptor blockers (such as cimetidine) have been demonstrated to raise the pH of gastric contents acutely in trauma patients and may play a role in the prevention of pulmonary injury.

5. Administering metoclopramide to accelerate gastric emptying may also be helpful

VII. Lung Abscess

A. Etiology

1. A lung abscess is a cavitation of the lung parenchyma resulting from local suppuration and central necrosis. It is often precipitated by aspiration of oropharyngeal secretions.

2. Predisposing factors (lead to suppression of cough/gag reflexes)
   a. Factors which suppress the cough/gag reflex (ETOH, CVA, seizures)
   b. Esophageal motility disorders, strictures and CA

[*]Rapid sequence intubation is the best way to decrease aspiration risk when intubating.

c. Pulmonary disorders
(1) Pneumonia
(2) Embolic phenomena
- Pulmonary embolus with cystic infarction
- Septic emboli
(3) Vasculitis
(4) Infected cysts
d. Periodontal disease (anaerobic lung abscess)

3. Organisms — Most lung abscesses are <u>polymicrobial</u> and involve either strictly anaerobes or a mixture of anaerobic organisms:
a. Anaerobic
(1) *Fusobacterium*
(2) *Bacteroides*
(3) *Streptococci* (microaerophilic and anaerobic)
b. Aerobic
(1) *Staph. aureus* (often follows influenza in a flu epidemic)
(2) *Strep. pneumoniae*
(3) *Alpha streptococci*
(4) *Pseudomonas*
(5) *Klebsiella pneumoniae*
(6) *E. coli*
(7) *Proteus*
c. Other organisms
(1) *Mycobacterium*
(2) *Histoplasma*
(3) *Coccidioides*
(4) Lung flukes and *Entamoeba histolytica*

B. *Clinical signs and symptoms are coincident with the development of cavitation (1 - 2 wks. after aspiration).*

1. History
a. Systemic signs & symptoms: weakness, fever, weight loss
b. Pulmonary signs & symptoms: dyspnea, chest pain and a cough productive of a fetid and bloody sputum

2. Physical exam
a. Poor dentition, gingivitis and foul-smelling breath
b. Signs of localized consolidation or cavitation on auscultation
c. Hemoptysis

C. Lab Findings

1. CBC: ↑WBCs with a left shift and anemia.

2. Chest x-ray: cavitation with an air/fluid level.
   a. Most common sites are the posterior segment of the RUL and superior segment of the LLL and RLL.
   b. Findings that suggest empyema rather than abscess
      (1) An air/fluid level at the site of a previous pleural effusion
      (2) A cavity with an air/fluid level that tapers at the pleural border
      (3) An air/fluid level that crosses a fissure
      (4) An air/fluid level that extends to the lateral chest wall
   c. Signs of impending hemoptysis
      (1) Emptying and refilling of cavity on serial x-rays
      (2) Varying lucency and height of air/fluid level
      (3) Variable parenchymal densities (blood clots) within the cavity

3. Sputum analysis
   a. Gram stains are of some use in the diagnosis of aerobic infections.
   b. Due to oropharyngeal contamination, only transtracheal or transthoracic specimens are reliable for anaerobic C+S.

D. Treatment

1. Antibiotic therapy
   a. Clindamycin is currently the antibiotic of choice for uncomplicated lung abscess. It is given IV until the patient remains afebrile for a period of 5 days and then is continued orally for 6 - 8 weeks.
   b. Alternative agents include PCN (when PCN resistance is not a problem), metronidazole or cefoxitin.

2. Indications for surgery
   a. Life-threatening hemoptysis
   b. Bronchopleural fistula
   c. Tumor or empyema
   d. A residual cavity

E. Late Complications

- Chronic lung abscess
- Empyema
- Bronchopleural fistula
- Brain abscess

VIII. Empyema — a collection of pus in the pleural space or fissures

A. Etiology

1. Mechanism of formation
   - Hematogenous/lymphatic spread from pneumonia
   - Infection from a chest tube, thoracentesis or thoracotomy
   - Esophageal perforation and mediastinitis
   - Rupture of a mediastinal lymph node
   - Aspiration pneumonia
   - Direct extension from retropharyngeal or subdiaphragmatic abscesses or from vertebral osteomyelitis.

2. Causative organisms — *M. tuberculosis*, *staph.*, *pseudomonas*, gram-negatives and anaerobes

B. Clinical Signs and Symptoms

1. Acute illness: fever and chills with pleuritic chest pain and SOB.

2. Subacute illness (more common): weight loss and fatigue.

3. Physical exam: decreased BS, dullness on percussion and decreased excursion of the involved hemithorax.

C. Diagnostic Work-Up includes the following:

1. Chest x-ray: air-fluid level in the pleural space or loculated fluid

2. Thoracentesis (confirms the diagnosis)

D. Definitive Therapy

1. Pleural drainage via tube thoracostomy, image-directed catheterization, thoracoscopic drainage or thoracotomy with open drainage and decortication.

2. High-dose, broad spectrum IV antibiotics (usually clindamycin and a third-generation cephalosporin) are given for 2 weeks or longer.

E. Complications

1. Empyema necessitans (dissection into the subcutaneous tissues or through the chest wall)

2. Bronchopleural fistula

3. Permanent loss of lung tissue

___

IX. Hemoptysis

A. Definitions

1. Hemoptysis — is coughing up blood originating from the pulmonary parenchyma or the tracheobronchial tree. Most often, it is not life-threatening. However, when hemoptysis is massive, it can produce airway obstruction as well as hemorrhagic shock and requires urgent intervention.

2. Massive hemoptysis — is defined as:
   a. A single expectoration > 50mL or 600mL blood/24 hrs.
   b. Necessitating transfusion to maintain a stable hematocrit.

B. Causes — vary with the age of the patient

1. Infection/inflammation — most common etiology of hemoptysis
   - Bronchitis (especially chronic) - most common cause
   - Pneumonia (esp. *Klebsiella*, *Staph* or influenza virus)
   - Parasites (ascariasis, schistosomiasis)
   - Endocarditis
   - Bronchiectasis
   - Tuberculosis ———— most common causes
   - Lung abscess ———— of <u>massive</u> hemoptysis

2. Neoplasms (esp. bronchogenic Ca)

3. Cardiovascular disorders
   - Mitral stenosis
   - CHF
   - Pulmonary hypertension (primary) or embolism/infarction
   - AV malformation/fistula
   - Congenital heart disease
   - Thoracic aortic aneurysm
   - Pulmonary embolism

4. Trauma

5. Immunologic disorders
   - Goodpasture's syndrome
   - Vasculitis

6. Other
   - Cystic fibrosis
   - Blood dyscrasias
   - Drugs (ASA, TPA, ETOH etc.)
   - Coagulopathies

7. Idiopathic (~ 5 - 15% of cases)

8. Iatrogenic
   - Swan - Ganz catheter → rupture of pulmonary artery
   - Central line (internal jugular) → fistula to trachea

___

C. **Hemoptysis Versus Hematemesis** — Hemoptysis needs to be distinguished from hematemesis or blood swallowed from epistaxis. The color, quality and pH of the sample are helpful in making this distinction. "True" hemoptysis is:

- Initiated and accompanied by vigorous coughing
- Generally bright red and foamy and does not contain particles of food
- Alkaline

D. **Signs and Symptoms** — are determined in large part by the underlying cause. For example, <u>patients with</u>:

1. <u>Bacterial pneumonia</u> — have only small amounts of blood in their sputum, and complain of a productive cough and fever. Exam may reveal rales or rhonchi and signs of consolidation.

2. <u>CHF</u> — often have only small amounts of blood in their sputum, and complain of shortness of breath. Exam may reveal rales, an S_3 gallop, JVD, hepatomegaly, ascites or peripheral edema.

3. <u>Bronchogenic carcinoma</u> — generally have a chronic cough and complain of weight loss. Exam may reveal signs of consolidation and clubbing.

4. <u>TB</u> — may be massive hemoptysis. These patients are often cachectic and have a chronic cough. Exam may reveal post-tussive rales.

E. **Laboratory Evaluation** — The severity and suspected etiology of the hemoptysis determine the extent of the evaluation performed in the ED setting.

1. CXR — should be obtained in all patients and may reveal signs of underlying pulmonary or cardiovascular disease; 50% are normal.

2. CBC — Establishes a baseline hematocrit.

3. PT (INR)/PTT and platelet count — are useful in patients who are on anticoagulants to rule out blood dyscrasias.

4. ABGs — are indicated in patients with respiratory distress or massive hemoptysis.

5. Type and cross — should be obtained in all patients with massive hemoptysis.

6. Sputum — should be sent for Gram and acid-fast stains, culture (for bacteria, fungi and mycobacteria) and cytologic examination.

7. Bronchoscopy — is useful both diagnostically and therapeutically. It should be obtained on an emergent basis in patients with massive hemoptysis.

8. Selective arteriography — can be used to localize and embolize the site of bleeding in patients with massive hemoptysis and is particularly useful when the site is peripheral to the bronchoscope's field of view.

9. High-resolution chest CT — is usually reserved for patients in whom the CXR is normal and bronchoscopy is unrevealing.

F. *Treatment* — is determined by the volume of hemoptysis and the underlying condition:

1. <u>Minimal</u> hemoptysis — In these patients, treatment is aimed at correcting the underlying problem. For example, patients with pneumonia should receive antibiotics. Specific therapy for the hemoptysis itself is generally unnecessary.

2. <u>Massive</u> hemoptysis — Initial therapy is aimed at maintaining the airway, stabilizing the patient and terminating the bleeding.
   a. Place the patient in Trendelenburg with the bleeding side down (to protect the uninvolved lung and maximize gas exchange).
   b. Suction and provide supplemental oxygen.
   c. Establish two large-bore IVs and replace blood loss rapidly.
   d. Obtain immediate consultation with a pulmonologist and a thoracic surgeon.
   e. Intubate via bronchoscopy.

   Once the patient is stabilized and bleeding has been controlled, further evaluation and treatment of the underlying pathology can be undertaken.

X. Pneumothorax

A. *Spontaneous Pneumothorax* — a collection of air in the pleural space (in the absence of trauma) that is divided into primary and secondary forms.

1. Primary (idiopathic) spontaneous pneumothorax
   a. Occurs in <u>healthy</u> individuals who <u>lack</u> evidence of underlying pulmonary pathology; however, most of them are smokers. There may also be a recent history of vigorous exercise.
   b. Results from rupture of a subpleural bleb (often apical) or a weak pleural segment → air leaking into the pleural space → pulmonary collapse.
   c. Causative factors are not always present, but may include:
      • Atmospheric pressure changes (scuba diving, fighter pilots)
      • Performance of the Valsalva maneuver in association with abuse of marijuana/cocaine or injection into the central venous system (the "pocket shot") by IV drug users
      • Marfan's syndrome
      • Cigarette smoking

d. Incidence is greatest in <u>young</u> adults 20 - 40 years of age.
e. More common in males than females (male-to-female ratio is 5:1); tall, thin males who smoke are most commonly affected.
f. Onset is usually during rest or sleep.
g. Recurrence rate is 20 - 50% over the following 2 - 5 years.

2. Secondary spontaneous pneumothorax
a. Occurs in individuals <u>with</u> underlying lung pathology which damages the alveolar/pleural barrier or causes an increase in the intra-bronchial pressures.
b. Associated medical conditions include:
(1) Airway disease
- COPD (most common cause)
- Chronic bronchitis ⎤
- Asthma ⎦ (also common)
- Cystic fibrosis
(2) Infection
- Pneumonia — particularly PCP in patients with AIDS
- TB
(3) Neoplasms
(4) Interstitial lung disease
- Collagen vascular disease
- Pneumoconioses
- Sarcoidosis
- Idiopathic pulmonary fibrosis
(5) Other
- Toxic drugs - especially aerosolized pentamidine
- Chemical and radiation pneumonitis
- Smoking
- Endometriosis ("catamenial" pneumothorax)
c. Individuals > 40-years-old are most commonly affected.

3. Iatrogenic pneumothorax — a pneumothorax that occurs in association with the performance of procedures such as:
- Subclavian vein catheterization and CPR (most common causes in ED)
- Positive pressure ventilation cases
- Intercostal nerve block
- Percutaneous lung biopsy
- Thoracentesis
- Bronchoscopy

B. Clinical Picture

The patient presents with sudden onset of pleuritic chest pain and dyspnea. Mild tachycardia and tachypnea may also be present. Your first thought might be "PE," especially if the patient is a middle-aged female with risk factors for thromboembolic disease. The chest pain is usually anterior, but may radiate into the neck, back or ipsilateral shoulder. An associated cough and subcutaneous emphysema of the neck and chest are occasionally present.

Classic physical findings are: decreased breath sounds, decreased tactile fremitus and hyperresonance to percussion on the affected side. However, these signs may be subtle or absent in patients with COPD or small pneumothoraces. On ECG, ST segment changes and T-wave inversion may be found, thus mimicking cardiac ischemia.

C. Chest X-ray — confirms the diagnosis

1. Findings on a standard PA chest film (taken in inspiration) include:
    a. A fine line (the edge of the collapsed lung) running parallel to the chest wall but separated from it by a space.
    b. Absence of lung markings along the lung periphery in the space beyond this line.

2. If the standard CXR does <u>not</u> reveal a suspected pneumothorax, a <u>supine</u> film may be helpful (especially in the hypotensive* patient). In this position, a pneumothorax will collect along the costophrenic sulcus (rather than along the apex of the lung in an upright position), thus making a small pneumothorax more apparent. Chest x-rays taken in full expiration have not been shown to enhance detection of pneumothorax.

3. Radiologic findings that may be confused with pneumothorax:
    a. Skin folds
    b. Tubing outlines
    c. Clothing
    d. Bullae or cysts

D. Treatment Options — include observation, simple catheter aspiration and tube thoracostomy. The approach selected is determined by the size of the pneumothorax, the degree of symptomatology, the presence of underlying pulmonary pathology, the reliability of the patient and whether the patient has had prior pneumothoraces. All patients should be placed on supplemental O_2 because it hastens resolution of the pneumothorax.

1. Observation (inpatient or outpatient)
    a. Is acceptable if the pneumothorax is small (< 15 - 20%) and the patient is healthy, reliable and minimally symptomatic.
    b. When this option is chosen, serial CXRs must be performed to R/O progressive accumulation of air within the pleural cavity.
    c. One approach is to observe the patient in the ED for 6 hours and then repeat the CXR. If the CXR remains unchanged, the patient may then be discharged to home with instructions to return for a repeat CXR in 24 hours (or sooner if symptoms progress).
    d. Reabsorption occurs at a rate of 1.25% of the volume of intrapleural air per day and is hastened by the administration of 100% oxygen.

*Upright films are not advisable in these patients

2. Simple catheter aspiration
   a. Reduces a large or moderate pneumothorax to a small one which can then be left to resorb on its own.
   b. It is appropriate for mildly to moderately symptomatic patients with primary spontaneous or needle-induced pneumothoraces.
   c. A CXR should be performed immediately following the aspiration (and again 6 hours later) to verify that aspiration was successful and that reaccumulation has not occurred.

3. Tube thoracostomy
   a. Is the therapeutic "gold standard."
   b. It is considered to be mandatory in the presence of:
      - Significant underlying pulmonary pathology
      - An expanding pneumothorax
      - A pneumothorax > 25%
      - Bilateral or tension pneumothorax
      - Trauma
      - Significant dyspnea
      - Detectable pleural fluid
      - Positive pressure ventilation
      - Previous contralateral pneumothorax

E. **Tension Pneumothorax** — a life-threatening complication

1. Evolution of a tension pneumothorax
   Air enters the pleural space on inspiration but cannot escape on expiration (ball-valve effect) → progressive accumulation of air within the pleural cavity and total collapse of the affected lung → a shift of mediastinal structures to the opposite hemithorax → compression of the contralateral lung and impairment of venous return → decrease in the cardiac output and the development of signs of shock.

2. Clinical recognition and management
   The patient is hypotensive, cyanotic and in severe respiratory distress. Air hunger develops and the respiratory rate increases. He becomes agitated, restless and displays decreasing mental activity. The trachea is deviated to the contralateral side and there is hyperresonance to percussion and absent BS on the involved side. JVD may be present. When the diagnosis is made, or even suspected, the positive intrapleural pressure must be released immediately. Do not wait for x-ray confirmation. Insert a large bore needle (14 gauge) anteriorly in the involved hemithorax through the second or third intercostal space midclavicular line. This allows time for a tube thoracostomy to be performed.

XI. Asthma

A. Definition and Epidemiology

1. Asthma is a chronic, nonprogressive lung disorder characterized by:
   - Increased airway responsiveness (an exaggerated bronchoconstrictor response) to a variety of stimuli
   - Airway inflammation
   - Reversible airway obstruction

2. It can occur at any age, but is more common in children and adolescents; 50% of patients develop asthma before age 10.

3. The prevalence of asthma is increasing.

4. Asthma-related morbidity and mortality rates have been climbing over the last twenty years.

5. The most common predictors of fatal asthma seem to be a past history of intubation/mechanical ventilation and underuse of steroid therapy.

B. Etiology

1. In the past, asthma was classified as either intrinsic (not IgE-mediated) or extrinsic/allergic (atopic or IgE-mediated). These distinctions, however, no longer reflect our current understanding of this disorder.

2. Asthma today is viewed as a state of bronchial hyperreactivity with multiple potential "triggers". An immunologic reaction mediated by IgE is only one such "trigger" and it can occur in both atopic and non-atopic individuals.

3. Triggers that can initiate an asthmatic response include:
   - Allergens
   - Viral respiratory infections (may be the most common cause)
   - Sinusitis
   - Exercise
   - Inhaled irritants
   - Strong odors
   - Medications (NSAIDs, ASA, beta-blockers) and food additives (MSG, sulfites, some dyes)
   - Gastroesophageal reflux
   - Cold exposure and changes in humidity
   - Strong emotions (via vagal efferent pathways)
   - Endocrine factors (menses, pregnancy, thyroid disease)

C. *Pathogenesis*

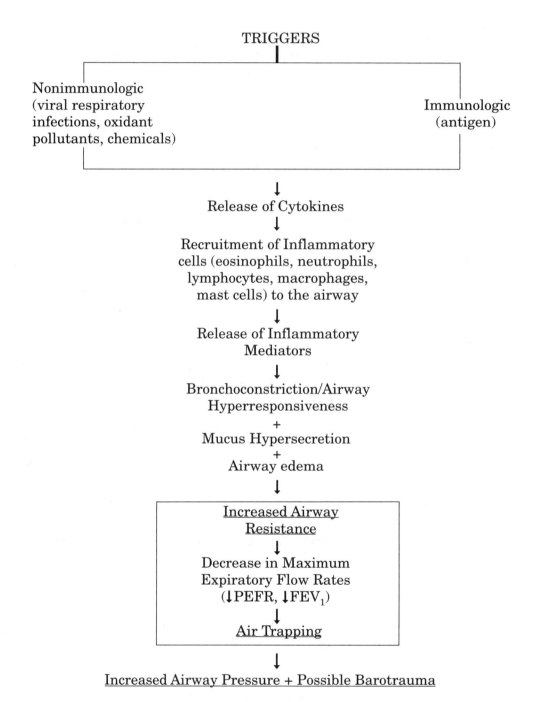

TRIGGERS

Nonimmunologic (viral respiratory infections, oxidant pollutants, chemicals)

Immunologic (antigen)

↓

Release of Cytokines

↓

Recruitment of Inflammatory cells (eosinophils, neutrophils, lymphocytes, macrophages, mast cells) to the airway

↓

Release of Inflammatory Mediators

↓

Bronchoconstriction/Airway Hyperresponsiveness
+
Mucus Hypersecretion
+
Airway edema

↓

Increased Airway Resistance

↓

Decrease in Maximum Expiratory Flow Rates (↓PEFR, ↓FEV$_1$)

↓

Air Trapping

↓

Increased Airway Pressure + Possible Barotrauma

D. Clinical Manifestations

1. Symptoms ... usually awaken the patient at night
   a. Cough — may be dry or productive of sputum
   b. Dyspnea
   c. Wheezing
   d. Chest tightness

2. Typical exam findings
   a. Tachypnea
   b. Tachycardia
   c. Wheezing — although the most common manifestation of asthma, wheezing is <u>not</u> an accurate indicator of the severity of an attack; it may be absent in patients with severe obstruction.
   d. Cough — may be the only finding in patients with cough-variant asthma.
   e. Prolonged expiratory phase
   f. Hyperresonance to percussion

3. Findings suggestive of severe airway obstruction
   a. Dyspnea so severe the patient is only able to speak a few words at a time and poor air movement on auscultation of the lungs.
   b. Use of accessory muscles (sternocleidomastoid, scalenus) — reflects diaphragmatic fatigue
   c. Heart rate > 120
   d. Respiratory rate > 30
   e. Pulsus paradoxus $\geq$ 12mmHg (defined as $\geq$ 12mmHg drop in systolic BP during inspiration) — implies that the FEV_1 is less than one half the normal predicted FEV_1 for that patient and reflects the degree of airway obstruction, air-trapping and ventilatory effort.
   f. Silent chest — indicates that airflow is dramatically reduced and is no longer adequate to promote wheezing.
   g. Diaphoresis
   h. Inability to recline on the stretcher
   i. Paradoxical respirations — herald impending respiratory failure.
   j. Cyanosis — late finding appearing just prior to respiratory arrest.
   k. Altered mental status (confusion, agitation, somnolence) may indicate hypercapnia and often reflects impending respiratory failure.

<u>Note</u>: Asthma indices (e.g. the Fischl scoring system) which incorporate subjective and objective data about an asthmatic attack have <u>not</u> been found to be reliable in assessing the severity of an attack on presentation or in predicting outcome in adults.

E. Differential Diagnosis

- CHF (cardiac asthma) — distinguishing features include older age, bibasilar rales, an S_3 gallop, pink frothy sputum and JVD; β-naturetic hormone assays may be useful in distinguishing the two.

- Upper airway obstruction (CA, laryngeal edema, FB inhalation) — remember that these patients usually have stridor (<u>not</u> wheezing); a patient with wheezing usually has <u>lower</u> airway obstruction. If in doubt, listen to <u>tracheal</u> breath sounds; any abnormality here is indicative of upper airway obstruction.
- Carcinoid tumors — are typically associated with postprandial flushing and GI upset.
- Chronic bronchitis or COPD with acute exacerbation — these patients are generally older, have a smoking history (along with a chronic productive cough) and no true symptom-free intervals.
- Eosinophilic pneumonias and invasive worm infestations.
- Endobronchial conditions (CA, FB aspiration, bronchial stenosis) — wheezing is unilateral.
- Drugs (beta-blockers, ACE-inhibitors)
- Allergic or anaphylactic reactions — urticaria, angioedema, hypotension and/or GI symptoms are clinical clues.
- Chemical irritants, insecticides and anticholinergics — a clue here is a history of exposure in an otherwise normal individual.
- Pulmonary embolus — most of these patients have one or more risk factors for DVT/PE. Order spiral CT with contrast if suspected (V/Q scans may be indeterminant in patients with acute asthma); angiography is indicated if the CT is negative but clinical suspicion is high.
- Noncardiogenic pulmonary edema (ARDS, CNS)

F. Laboratory Evaluation

1. Pulmonary function tests (PEFR or FEV_1)[*]
   a. Should be measured before and after each treatment with an adrenergic agent.
   b. The PEFR is the easiest test to perform in the ED since it is done at the bedside with a portable peak expiratory flow meter (e.g. Wright peak flow meter).
   c. These studies provide an <u>objective measure</u> of the degree of airflow obstruction present; they are useful in assessing the severity of an attack, the response to treatment and the need for close follow-up or admission.
   d. Indicators of <u>severe</u> bronchospasm and probable hospital admission:
      - PEFR < 100L/min or FEV_1 < 1L prior to treatment
      - PEFR or FEV_1 < 50% baseline/predicted (adults)
      - Failure of PEFR to improve by $\geq$ 10% following <u>initial</u> treatment
      - PEFR < 300L/min. or FEV_1 < 2.1 L following aggressive treatment

2. CBC
   a. Adds little to the overall assessment of the patient and is not routinely warranted; fever is a clear indication.
   b. Mild eosinophilia is frequently present, reflecting the asthmatic condition.

[*]Although recommended to gauge treatment efficacy and severity of the exacerbation, PEFR and FEV_1 have not proven beneficial or predictive based on multiple studies. However, they are useful in documenting a trend and serve as a comparison to baseline.

  c. The WBC count is often elevated, from the stress of an asthma at-
     tack or chronic steroid use, but it may also be elevated in the setting
     of pneumonia.

3. Sputum
   a. Eosinophils are typically present and can make the sputum appear
      purulent in the absence of infection.
   b. Other findings may include:
      (1) Charcot-Leyden crystals = crystallized eosinophilic granules
      (2) Curschmann's spirals = spiral casts of the airways formed from
          mucus and epithelial cells
      (3) Creola bodies = clusters of columnar epithelial cells

4. Pulse oximetry
   a. Should be used to assess and follow the adequacy of oxygenation; how-
      ever, a near-normal pulse oximetry may be present in a patient with
      pending respiratory failure due to hypercapnia (the reason is that
      increased minute ventilation and adequate oxygenation can produce
      a near-normal pulse-ox reading); bedside capnometry may be a better
      way to monitor these patients.
   b. Oxygen saturation ≤ 90% indicates a severe asthmatic attack and
      significant hypoxemia; an ABG should be obtained.

5. ABGs
   a. Do not measure pulmonary function per se, but rather the ability to
      exchange oxygen and carbon dioxide.
      • PFTs measure how well a patient is doing.
      • ABGs measure how poorly a patient is doing.
   b. The real value of ABGs lies in the assessment of respiratory failure,
      i.e. detecting the presence of hypercapnia and acidosis.
      (1) They are indicated in patients with signs of impending respira-
          tory failure:
          (a) Fatigue or exhaustion
          (b) An altered sensorium
          (c) Worsening or failure to improve after adequate treatment
          (d) SaO_2 ≤ 90%
      (2) Severity of respiratory failure: ABG results
          (a) Mild respiratory failure: ↑pH ↓pCO_2 nl or ↓pO_2 (R. alk.)
          (b) Moderate respiratory failure: nl pH nl pCO_2 ↓pO_2
          (c) Severe respiratory failure: ↓pH nl or ↑pCO_2 ↓pO_2 (R. acid.)
      (3) ABG values consistent with severe asthma include:
          (a) pO_2 < 60mmHg
          (b) pCO_2 > 45mmHg
          (c) pH < 7.35

6. CXR
   a. May reveal evidence of hyperinflation (increased AP diameter and/or
      flattening of the diaphragms), increased bronchial markings and/or
      atelectasis but is generally nondiagnostic.

b. It is most useful in ruling out the complications of asthma and conditions which mimic it.

c. CXR is not obtained routinely, but is indicated in patients who:
(1) Are febrile
(2) Have focal physical findings suggestive of pneumonia or barotrauma (pneumothorax, pneumomediastinum)
(3) Fail to respond to aggressive treatment
(4) Present with their <u>first</u> episode of wheezing

7. ECG
a. Unless ischemia is suspected, routine ECGs are generally not helpful diagnostically.
b. A right ventricular strain pattern is seen in 30 - 40% of patients.

8. Theophylline level — should be checked in patients taking this agent.

G. Treatment

1. Pharmacologic agents and their mechanism of action
a. Beta$_2$ adrenergic agonists
(1) Promote bronchodilation by <u>increasing cyclic AMP</u>.
(2) They may also modulate mediator release from mast cells and basophils as well as promote mucociliary clearance.
(3) Their primary effect is on the <u>small</u> peripheral airways.
(4) Onset of action is <u>less</u> than 5 minutes.
b. Anticholinergic agents
(1) Promote bronchodilation by inhibiting vagally-mediated bronchoconstriction, i.e. they competitively antagonize acetylcholine (the transmitter released by the vagus nerve) at the post-ganglionic parasympathetic effector cell junction → <u>decrease</u> in <u>cyclic GMP</u> → bronchodilation.
(2) Their primary effect is on the <u>large</u> central airways.
(3) Onset of action is <u>delayed</u> up to 30 mins. and peaks in 1 - 2 hrs.
c. Corticosteroids
(1) Are believed to produce their effects by:
(a) <u>Increasing</u> the responsiveness of beta-adrenergic receptors in airway smooth muscle
(b) <u>Limiting</u> recruitment and activation of inflammatory cells
(c) <u>Interfering</u> with arachidonic acid metabolism and the synthesis of leukotrienes and prostaglandins.
(2) Onset of action is <u>gradual</u> with initial improvement occurring 3 hours following administration and peaking in 6 - 12 hours. Early administration (within one hour) results in fewer hospital admissions and a lower rate of relapse after ED discharge.
d. Antileukotrienes . . . . are being used more frequently in managing chronic asthma.

2. ED management (applies to adults; Tx of children is on pp. 649 - 652 in the Pediatric chapter)
   a. Administer oxygen to all asthmatics; many are hypoxic and treatment with beta-adrenergic agents may initially worsen hypoxia by exacerbating ventilation-perfusion mismatching. Verify the adequacy of arterial oxygen saturation by pulse oximetry and use continuous capnometry (if available) to assess adequacy of ventilation.
   b. Beta-adrenergic agonists — because of their <u>rapid</u> onset of action (< 5 minutes) and effectiveness in promoting bronchodilation, treatment should be <u>initiated</u> with these agents. Aerosolized therapy is preferred over parenteral therapy; it has more rapid onset of action, provides comparable or superior bronchodilation, produces fewer side effects and avoids the need for painful injections. The oral route is <u>not</u> appropriate in the acute setting.
      (1) Inhaled agents: administer one of the following using a handheld nebulizer:
         (a) Albuterol (Proventil®, Ventolin®) 0.5% solution — is the preferred agent due to its beta$_2$-specificity and fewer side effects.
            <u>1</u> The dose is 2.5mg in 2 - 3mL NS Q 20 - 30 mins. up to 3 doses, then hourly.
            <u>2</u> Continuous nebulization in a dose of 15mg/hr. (for 2 hrs.) has been shown to be safe and effective in adults with severe bronchospasm; it should be considered for those patients who present with a PEFR < 200L/min. or an FEV$_1$ < 50% of predicted.
         (b) Metaproterenol sulfate (Alupent®, Metaprel®) 5% solution
            <u>1</u> The dose is 15mg in 2 - 3mL NS Q 20 - 30 mins. up to 3 doses, then hourly.
            <u>2</u> This agent has some alpha- and beta$_1$ - adrenergic effects which limit its usefulness.
      <u>Note</u>: Although numerous studies have demonstrated that delivery of beta agonists (using a metered-dose inhaler with a spacing device) can achieve bronchodilation equivalent to that achieved by nebulization, this method requires more patient effort and is <u>not</u> recommended for patients with severe obstruction.
      (2) Injectable (SQ) meds — should be reserved for those patients who are too sick to provide an effective inspiratory effort; alternative medications include:
         (a) Epinephrine 1:1000 solution
            <u>1</u> The dose is 0.3mg Q 20 - 30 mins. up to 3 doses.
            <u>2</u> It has both alpha and beta effects but beta predominate.
         (b) Terbutaline 1mg/mL
            <u>1</u> The dose is 0.25mg Q 20 - 30 mins. up to 3 doses.
            <u>2</u> This agent is more beta$_2$ - selective than epinephrine and has a longer duration of action.
      <u>Note</u>: These agents should be strongly considered in patients with severe asthma who have an inadequate ventilatory effort with inhaled agents; in these cases, cardiovascular disease is <u>not</u> a contraindication. In life-threatening situations, Epi can be life saving.

   c. Anticholinergic agents
     (1) For all patients who present with exacerbation of acute asthma, anticholinergics and beta-agonist therapy should be used <u>together</u> in the initial management of an acute attack. The efficacy of anticholinergic therapy increases proportionately with the severity of the attack, but some benefit is gained even in less severe attacks.
     (2) When used in combination with beta-adrenergic agonists, effects are additive and a small incremental benefit may be derived; although their effects are delayed in onset, they provide a synergistic reduction in bronchospasm and a more prolonged effect. Addition of anticholinergics to beta-agonists (and glucocorticoid) therapy decreases the rate of hospitalization and improves pulmonary function in the first 90 minutes.
     (3) Nebulized Ipratropium bromide (Atrovent) 500mcg in 2mL NS Q 3 - 4 hours is the agent of choice; it may be added to the nebulizer along with the standard dose of beta-agonist being administered. If ipratropium is being used as a first-line agent, the dose may be repeated with the first three beta-agonist inhalation treatments. This agent is an atropine derivative but has limited systemic absorption and produces far fewer side effects than atropine.
     (4) Ipratropium is also effective in reversing bronchospasm secondary to beta-blocking agents.
   d. Corticosteroids — treat the inflammatory component of asthma and should be administered <u>early</u>; they reduce the rate of relapse and the rate of hospital admission. Underuse of these agents is believed to be an important cause of fatal asthma.
     (1) They should be administered to the following patients:
       (a) Those who show minimal or no improvement following <u>initial</u> sympathomimetic therapy
       (b) Those who are currently taking (or have recently discontinued) a steroid preparation
       (c) Those with signs of severe obstruction, e.g. tachycardia >120, pulsus paradoxus $\geq$ 12mmHg, PEFR or FEV_1 < 40% baseline
       (d) Those with a history of asthma-associated respiratory failure
       (e) Those whose attack has been prolonged (these patients are more likely to have significant bronchial wall edema and mucus impaction)
       (f) Those who relapse (return to the ER for the same asthmatic attack)
     (2) The oral and intravenous routes are equally effective.
     (3) Use one of the following agents:
       (a) Methylprednisolone 60 - 125mg IV... is the parenteral drug of choice.
       (b) Hydrocortisone 200 - 500mg IV
       (c) Methylprednisolone 60mg PO
       (d) Prednisone 1 - 2mg/kg PO

(4) Patients who receive steroids in the ER and are subsequently discharged should be continued on oral steroids (methylprednisolone or prednisone 1mg/kg/day) at home for a minimum of 3 - 5 days and a maximum of 14 days. Prolonged therapy with a gradually tapered dose is recommended for patients taking maintenance doses more than 10 days.

(5) Aerosolized corticosteroids are potentially irritating (can stimulate cough or bronchospasm) and, therefore, should not be used during an acute attack.

e. Other points to consider in the treatment of asthma:

(1) Evaluate for evidence of dehydration and administer replacement fluids (PO or IV) prn.

(2) Do not administer sedatives, narcotics or tranquilizers.

(3) Avoid the use of IV isoproterenol; it is highly dysrhythmogenic and carries a risk of myocardial injury resulting from ischemia or infarction.

(4) Magnesium sulfate should be administered only in severe, nonresponding acute asthma when intubation/mechanical ventilation is being considered. The dose is 2 - 3gm (over 10 mins.) and should be given while continuing inhalation therapy.

(5) Administration of helium should be considered for patients with severe asthma. It decreases the work of breathing and, therefore, buys you time for the meds you've already given to work (which may save you from intubating — a real problem in some asthmatics).

(6) Check serum electrolytes in adult patients who require repeated use of beta-agonists (> 3 doses) since they can cause hypokalemia, hypomagnesemia and hypophosphatemia.

(7) Reserve antibiotics for patients with evidence of infection (fever, infiltrate on CXR, PMNs on sputum exam, evidence of sinusitis); respiratory tract infections that trigger exacerbations of asthma are usually viral in etiology.

f. Noninvasive Positive Pressure Ventilation (NPPV)

(1) May be used in patients with respiratory failure (or impending failure) who are not responsive to therapy but who have normal mentation and facial anatomy.

(2) Nasal BiPAP is the modality of choice for patients who are able to cooperate.

(a) Start with an inspiratory pressure of 8cm-H_2O and expiratory pressure of 3cm-H_2O.

(b) Increase settings based on pulse-ox and ABG results.

(c) Patients who fail to improve over 30-60 minutes require intubation.

g. Intubation with assisted ventilation:

(1) Mechanical ventilation in these patients can produce excessively high airway pressures and is associated with considerable morbidity and mortality.

(2) The initial goal of mechanical ventilation in these patients is not necessarily to restore the pCO_2 to normal; the respiratory rate and tidal volume required to do this can produce excessive peak inflation pressures → alveolar gas trapping and overdistention → high risk of barotrauma.

(3) These patients should be intentionally hypoventilated (a technique referred to as "controlled mechanical hypoventilation" or "permissive hypocapnia"). This technique increases the amount of time available for expiration and thereby minimizes air trapping. Suggested initial ventilator settings are: tidal volume 6 - 8mL/kg, respiratory rate 8 - 10 and an inspiratory flow rate of 60L/min. The moderate hypercapnia that may occur with these ventilator settings is well tolerated and less dangerous than persistently high airway pressures.

(4) Volume-cycled ventilators with high peak pressure and flow rates should be used initially to deliver an adequate tidal volume; if PIP exceeds $50cmH_2O$, switch to pressure-controlled ventilation with a decelerating "ramp" wave form.

(5) Criteria for intubation:
  (a) ABG triad of progressive hypoxemia, hypercapnia and acidosis or
  (b) Persistent hypercapnia in spite of therapy or
  (c) Persistently poor or worsening PFTs or
  (d) Clinical signs of respiratory failure (cyanosis, apnea) or
  (e) Change in mental status (confusion, somnolence) or
  (f) Exhaustion/obtundation (patient looks at you but can't speak)

(6) Adjuncts to intubation/mechanical ventilation:
  (a) Lidocaine — should be used in the asthmatic prior to induction and paralysis in order to minimize exacerbation of bronchospasm.
  (b) Ketamine — can be used to provide sedation for intubation (or as an induction agent for rapid sequence intubation) and has the benefit of inducing bronchodilation; avoid in patients with hypertension and those at risk for CAD (may ↑ P + BP).
  (c) Succinylcholine — is the paralytic of choice. Pancuronium is useful when muscle paralysis is required to facilitate ventilation; it does not cause histamine release.
  (d) Benzodiazepines — may be used when sedation is needed; it will minimize emergence of hallucinations if ketamine was used; opiates induce histamine release and should be avoided.
  (e) Helium — should be considered for mechanically ventilated asthmatics with significant respiratory acidosis and markedly elevated airway pressures; it lowers airway resistance and decreases the work of breathing. A helium-oxygen mixture of 80:20 or 70:30 (preferred) should be used.

h. Asthma in pregnancy:
  (1) The incidence of asthma rises in pregnancy.
  (2) Respiratory alkalosis (pCO_2 of 30 - 35) is a normal finding in pregnancy. Do not be concerned about respiratory compromise unless the pCO_2 is > 35.

(3) Management of asthma in pregnant patients is similar to that in nonpregnant patients. The goal of treatment is to ensure adequate oxygenation for both mother and fetus while avoiding (whenever possible) any drugs that may pose a risk to the fetus.

    (a) All patients should receive supplemental oxygen (maternal hypoxia → impaired fetal oxygenation → fetal complications)

    (b) Inhaled beta-agonists are the first-line drugs of choice. If parenteral therapy is required, terbutaline is preferred over epinephrine; the use of subcutaneous epinephrine early in pregnancy is associated with an increased incidence of congenital malformations and, in late pregnancy, is associated with premature labor... and should be avoided.

    (c) Corticosteroids are also safe in pregnancy and should be administered in all but the mildest exacerbations.

    (d) Anticholinergic agents and theophylline may also be used. The clearance of theophylline in the third trimester, however, is reduced; serum levels must be carefully monitored.

Note: Asthma medications which are appropriate for administration during pregnancy are also safe for use during lactation.

XII. Chronic Obstructive Pulmonary Disease (COPD)*

A. Pathophysiology

1. COPD is often referred to as a single disease but is actually a triad of three distinct disease processes:

    a. Chronic bronchitis — characterized by airway hypersecretion and inflammation that cause a chronic productive cough for an extended period of time.

    b. Emphysema — characterized by irreversible enlargement of the air spaces distal to the bronchioles.

    c. Asthma — characterized by airway hyperreactivity and inflammation. In most COPD patients, these three entities coexist but, the contribution each makes to pulmonary dysfunction varies from individual to individual. However, some COPD patients present with predominately emphysema (pink puffers) or chronic bronchitis (blue bloaters).

2. Evolution

    a. COPD begins in the early twenties and is only detected by pulmonary function testing (end-tidal volume determination). Early pathologic changes are completely silent.

    b. As the disease progresses, signs and symptoms appear with a full-blown clinical picture evolving in the fifties and sixties.

*Fourth most common cause of death

c. Chronic bronchitis ensues with a typical history of chronic, recurrent production of excessive mucus.

d. Repeated inflammation leads to increased resistance or decreased caliber of the small bronchi and bronchioles. As alveolar hypoventilation subsequently occurs, hypoxemia and hypercarbia result. Ventilation-perfusion mismatching occurs (thus promoting hypoxemia), while increased physiologic dead space ventilation leads to alveolar hypoventilation, hypercarbia and further hypoxemia.

e. In addition to obstruction of the peripheral airways, destruction and coalescence of the alveolar cell structure (particularly in dominantly emphysematous disease) results in reduction of the total "matched" alveolar-capillary surface area for diffusion of gases (oxygen cannot get in, CO_2 cannot get out).

f. Later on, chronic and progressive airflow obstruction can lead to right-sided cardiac strain that results in pulmonary hypertension (loud P_2 on auscultation) and cor pulmonale.

B. Predisposing Factors

1. Tobacco smoking (most important factor)

2. Exposure to second-hand smoke

3. Environmental pollution

4. Industrial or occupational exposure

5. Alpha$_1$ - antitrypsin deficiency

6. Cystic fibrosis

7. Recurrent pulmonary infections

C. Causes of Acute Decompensation

1. Superimposed respiratory infection (acute bronchitis, pneumonia)*

2. Changes in ambient temperature, humidity or air pollution levels

3. Noxious environmental exposures

4. Spontaneous pneumothorax

5. Pulmonary embolus

6. Noncompliance with (or underdosing of) medications

7. Inappropriate treatment (beta-blockers, sedatives)

8. Acute CHF

9. Continued cigarette smoking

* The most common precipitating factor of acute COPD exacerbation. Influenza and pneumococcal vaccination recommended.

D. **Clinical Signs and Symptoms...** in combined disease

1. Dyspnea is the most common complaint, followed by cough (occasionally with hemoptysis), chest tightness and fatigue. A history of morning headache may be due to a rising $PaCO_2$ (hypercapnia).

2. Physical findings
   a. Tachypnea
   b. Prolonged expiratory phase
   c. Increased AP chest diameter ("barrel chested")
   d. Decreased breath sounds
   e. Wheezing, rales and rhonchi
   f. Lip-pursing, accessory muscle use, cyanosis and diaphoresis
   g. Pulsus paradoxus
   h. Distant heart sounds, a loud P_2 and right-sided CHF

E. **Clinical Signs and Symptoms...** when emphysema or bronchitis predominate

1. <u>Emphysema</u> (pink puffer)
   a. Dyspneic
   b. Thin, anxious, alert appearance
   c. ↑ AP chest diameter (overinflation)
   d. Tachypneic and hypotensive
   e. Uses accessory muscles to breathe
   f. ↓ BS, faint end-expiratory rhonchi and hyperresonance on percussion

2. <u>Chronic bronchitis</u> (blue bloater)
   a. Productive "wet" cough
   b. Stocky build, polycythemic and cyanotic
   c. Normal chest diameter
   d. Little air-hunger
   e. Subxiphoid or retrosternal heave → right ventricular hypertrophy
   f. Signs of CHF (JVD, S_3 or S_4 gallop, murmur of tricuspid insufficiency, scattered rales and rhonchi, edema)

F. **Lab Findings**

1. Chest x-ray
   a. Is most useful in ruling out other disease processes/complications (pneumonia, pneumothorax, atelectasis, effusions, CA, CHF): > 15% of acutely decompensated COPD patients will have treatable findings.
   b. Signs of overinflation are common (60% of patients):
      (1) ↑ AP diameter
      (2) ↑ retrosternal airspace
      (3) ↑ parenchymal lucency
      (4) Low and flattened diaphragm
      (5) Long and narrow cardiac silhouette (unless chronic bronchitis predominates the clinical picture, in which case, an enlarged right ventricle will be seen on the lateral film)
   c. Bullae may also be seen.

2. ABGs — provide critical information regarding the seriousness and acuteness of airway compromise in the COPD patient.
   a. PaO_2 — is generally low
      (1) Hypoxemia is common in these patients and worsens as the disease progresses as well as with acute exacerbations.
      (2) It is due to ventilation-perfusion mismatching and can usually be corrected by increasing the amount of oxygen being inspired.
   b. $PaCO_2$
      (1) Reflects the adequacy of ventilation.
      (2) Normocarbia may be present early on, but hypercarbia develops with disease progression and may worsen with acute exacerbations.
      (3) A rapid rise in the $PaCO_2$ produces a decrease in the pH whereas, with a more gradual rise, the kidneys are able to compensate by retaining bicarbonate which normalizes the pH. Therefore, it follows that:
         • An ↑$PaCO_2$ + a normal pH + an ↑ bicarbonate level suggests <u>chronic</u> CO_2 retention, while
         • An ↑$PaCO_2$ + a ↓pH + an ↑ bicarbonate level points to <u>acute</u> respiratory failure superimposed on chronic respiratory insufficiency.

3. Pulmonary function tests
   a. Are more useful in patients with asthmatic bronchitis than COPD in evaluating the degree of airway obstruction present and in monitoring the response to treatment.
   b. Either the forced expiratory volume in one second (FEV_1) or the peak expiratory flow rate (PEFR) may be used; both provide a measurable index of airway obstruction.
   c. Because bronchospasm is <u>not</u> the major component of lung dysfunction in COPD patients, the response to treatment is less than that of asthmatics.
   d. Lung volume measurements in COPD patients reveal an increase in the amount of dead space (DS) and a decrease in the vital capacity (VC) so that there is ↑DS and an accompanying ↓VC; clinical signs develop when the VC drops 50%.

4. ECG — detects ischemic disease or dysrhythmias associated with COPD (especially multifocal atrial tachycardia and atrial fibrillation -- both are common and should be assumed to be secondary to CHF) and may also demonstrate evidence of COPD or cor pulmonale. Findings may include:
   a. P pulmonale (peaked P waves in II, III and AVF) → very suggestive of COPD
   b. Low voltage, right axis deviation and poor R wave progression → also very suggestive of COPD
   c. Criteria for right ventricular hypertrophy → very suggestive of cor pulmonale

[Note: Troponin elevation is relatively common in COPD patients with acute exacerbations and is not usually associated with a co-diagnosis of ACS.]

G. Treatment* — is directed toward improving oxygenation and respiratory function

    1. Oxygen... is the <u>most important</u> therapy.

        a. COPD patients who chronically <u>retain</u> CO_2 depend on their hypoxic respiratory drive to breathe. Raising the pO_2 too quickly in these patients depresses the respiratory center and shuts off this drive. Concern over suppressing this drive must be balanced against the need to increase the pO_2 to a satisfactory level.

        b. To minimize the risk, initiate treatment using <u>low</u> concentrations of oxygen and a <u>controlled</u> delivery system such as a Venturi mask. Start with an FIO_2 of 24 - 28% and increase it as needed. The goal is to raise the pO_2 to > 60% and the saturation to > 90%.

        c. Continuous pulse oximetry (supplemented with ABGs when there is concern that the pCO_2 is rising) should be used to monitor response to treatment and guide adjustments in the FIO_2; continuous capnometry can also be useful.

        d. Assurance of adequate oxygenation should take precedence over concern about suppressing the hypoxic respiratory drive; if a high concentration of oxygen is needed, it should be administered.

    <u>Note</u>: There is less risk of oxygen-induced apnea if the patient is <u>tachypneic</u> (rather than <u>bradypneic</u>)... and if the respiratory rate <u>is</u> slow in the COPD patient with an acute exacerbation, and he doesn't respond to low concentrations of oxygen, he needs <u>more</u> oxygen no matter what.

    2. Beta-adrenergic agonists — produce the <u>most rapid</u> response and they should be used for <u>initial</u> therapy. The newer beta$_2$-selective agents are best in that they produce fewer side effects.

        a. Inhaled agents — If the patient can cooperate and provide the necessary inspiratory effort, aerosolized therapy (via a hand-held nebulizer) is preferred; it is associated with equal or superior bronchodilation and less systemic toxicity than parenteral therapy. Delivery via a meter-dosed inhaler with a spacer device may be as effective but requires more patient effort. The usual agents are:

            (1) Albuterol 0.5% solution, 2.5mg in 2 - 3mL NS Q 20 - 30 mins. prn up to 3 doses, then hourly.

            (2) Metaproterenol sulfate 5% solution, 15mg in 2 - 3mL NS Q 20 - 30 mins. prn up to 3 doses, then hourly.

        b. Injectable (SQ) meds — are reserved for patients who are moving little or no air and are, therefore, unable to cooperate with aerosolized therapy. Available agents include:

            (1) Epinephrine 1:1000 solution, 0.3mg Q 20 - 30 mins. prn up to 2 - 3 doses.

            (2) Terbutaline 1 mg/mL solution, 0.25mg Q 20 - 30 mins. prn up to 2 - 3 doses.

    <u>Note</u>: If signs of drug toxicity develop (e.g. increasing tachycardia, ventricular ectopy) the dosing interval should be <u>prolonged</u>.

---

* Beta-adrenergics, anticholinergics and methylxanthines should be used with extreme caution in COPD patients > 40 yrs. old as well as those with coronary artery disease or hypertension.

3. Nebulized anticholinergic agents
   a. Should be used in conjunction with beta-agonists as first-line therapy in COPD patients with an acute exacerbation.
   b. Unlike the beta-agonists (which have their primary effect on the small peripheral airways) these agents preferentially dilate the <u>larger</u> central airways.
   c. They are as effective as, and in some cases even more effective than, the beta-agonists in improving pulmonary function; however, they have a slower onset of action (5 - 15 mins.) and take a <u>longer</u> time to peak (1 - 2 hrs.).
   d. These agents are synergistic with beta-agonists and should, therefore, be administered at the same time.
   e. Ipratropium bromide (Atrovent) is the agent of choice; it has limited systemic absorption and produces far fewer side effects than atropine.
      (1) The dose is 500mcg in 2mL NS Q 3 - 4 hrs.
      (2) It should be added to the nebulizer along with the standard dose of the beta-agonist being administered.

4. Methylxanthines (aminophylline, theophylline)
   a. Although these agents have a role in the chronic outpatient management of COPD (particularly in patients with nocturnal dyspnea), their role in the treatment of acute exacerbations remains unsettled.
   b. They are weak bronchodilators, but this may not be their most important effect. They also function to stimulate the respiratory drive, enhance diaphragmatic contractility and improve mucociliary clearance.
   c. These agents should be administered to those patients who are not responding well to optimal treatment with beta-adrenergic agonists and ipratropium. Studies have demonstrated synergistic activity when all three agents are used (beta-agonist, anticholinergic + theophylline therapy).
   d. A stat serum theophylline level should be obtained in patients who have been taking this medication (8 - 12mg/mL is appropriate). The patient may be placed on a maintenance drip until the level is back.
   e. Dosage guidelines for IV aminophylline:
      (1) Loading dose is 5mg/kg (ideal body wt.) over 10 - 15 minutes.
      (2) Maintenance dose is based on ideal body weight and associated conditions:
         (a) Adult smokers < 50 yrs. → 0.9 mg/kg/hr.
         (b) Adult nonsmokers < 50 yrs. → 0.5mg/kg/hr.
         (c) Adults > 50 yrs → 0.4 mg/kg/hr.
         (d) Patients with CHF/liver disease → 0.25 - 0.35 mg/kg/hr.
   f. Aminophylline also promotes diuresis and has an inotropic effect. Subsequent potassium depletion may lead to cardiac dysrhythmias.
      (1) Since CO_2 retention causes additional potassium wasting and hypochloremic alkalosis, supplemental KCL should be given if the serum potassium is below normal.
      (2) In addition to the inotropic effects of aminophylline, COPD patients also have a high incidence of cardiac disease. Therefore, cardiac monitoring is indicated during therapy.

5. Steroids
   a. Their use in COPD is less compelling than their use in asthma (although they do help reduce the relapse rate).
   b. They should be administered to all acutely ill patients and especially:
      (1) Those who are steroid-dependent
      (2) Those who have an allergic component to their COPD
      (3) Those who are not responding well to oxygen, beta-adrenergic, anticholinergic and methylxanthine therapy
   c. These agents work by decreasing inflammation and increasing responsiveness to beta-agonists and theophylline.
   d. The preferred agent for severe exacerbations is methylprednisolone in a dose of 80 - 125mg IV. Mineralocorticoids (e.g. hydrocortisone) should be avoided; they promote sodium retention and potassium excretion.
   e. Patients who receive steroids in the ED and are subsequently discharged should be continued on oral steroids at home. Start with a dose of 60 - 180mg/day (i.e. between one and three times the maximum adrenal physiologic secretion rate) and taper over one week or as tolerated.
   f. Patients who are in less severe distress (and will be discharged) may be given oral steroids only; a two-week prednisone taper regimen is recommended.

6. Antibiotics — should be administered to patients with signs or symptoms of an associated respiratory infection ($\uparrow$ in sputum volume, change in sputum character or color).
   a. If signs of pneumonia are present, a sputum culture should be ordered (although specimens are not very useful unless obtained by invasive means). These patients often require hospitalization.
   b. The most commonly implicated organisms include Strep. pneumoniae, Hemophilus influenza and Moraxella catarrhalis.
   c. If the patient has acute bronchitis, empiric oral antibiotic therapy aids resolution of COPD exacerbations (which makes a sputum gram stain superfluous).

H. Complications of COPD that require additional therapy:

1. Respiratory decompensation → intubation may be needed (Beware of ventilator complications, especially tension pneumothorax)

2. Cor pulmonale → phlebotomy may be needed to keep Hct < 55%.

3. Multifocal atrial tachycardia → correct any lyte imbalance before attempting drug therapy with verapamil or metoprolol.

4. Pulmonary embolus

5. Pneumothorax

6. $\downarrow PO_4$ (Phosphate)

XIII. Near-Drowning

A. Definition of Terms

1. <u>Drowning</u>: Death from suffocation after submersion

2. <u>Near-Drowning</u>: Temporary or permanent survival after suffocation by submersion

3. <u>Immersion syndrome</u>: Sudden death after submersion in very cold water (presumed to be due to vagally-mediated asystole or V-Fib)

4. <u>Post-immersion syndrome</u> (secondary drowning): Delayed deterioration of a patient who is initially relatively asymptomatic; deterioration is generally due to respiratory insufficiency and may be delayed several hours to several days. This is the major complication of near-drowning

B. Epidemiology

1. Drowning is the third most common cause of accidental death in the U.S., claiming 8000 - 9000 lives/year with brain injury being the major cause of death from drowning.

2. Freshwater drowning (particularly in swimming pools) is more common than saltwater drowning.

3. Age distribution is bimodal, with peaks occurring in children < 5 years old (consider child abuse) and teenagers.

4. Males predominate in every age group.

5. Contributing factors
   a. Drugs (particularly ETOH)
   b. Inadequate swimming skills
   c. Exhaustion
   d. Hyperventilation prior to underwater swimming
   e. Trauma
      • Accidental (C-spine injuries, head injuries)
      • Nonaccidental (child abuse)
   f. Underlying illnesses
      • Hypoglycemia
      • Seizures
      • MI
      • Cardiac dysrhythmias
      • Depression/suicide attempt
   g. Lack of supervision
   h. Hypothermia

C. Pathophysiology

   1. Sequence of events (are essentially the same for freshwater and saltwater submersion)

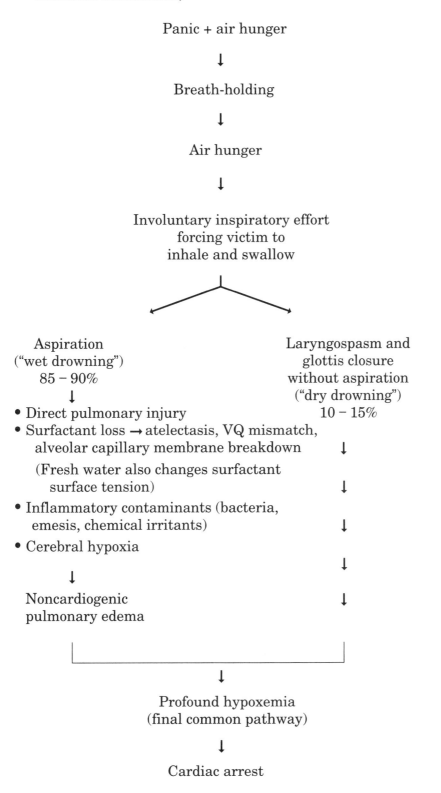

Panic + air hunger

↓

Breath-holding

↓

Air hunger

↓

Involuntary inspiratory effort
forcing victim to
inhale and swallow

Aspiration
("wet drowning")
85 – 90%
↓
• Direct pulmonary injury
• Surfactant loss → atelectasis, VQ mismatch,
  alveolar capillary membrane breakdown

  (Fresh water also changes surfactant
   surface tension)

• Inflammatory contaminants (bacteria,
  emesis, chemical irritants)

• Cerebral hypoxia

↓

Noncardiogenic
pulmonary edema

Laryngospasm and
glottis closure
without aspiration
("dry drowning")
10 – 15%

↓

↓

↓

↓

↓

↓

Profound hypoxemia
(final common pathway)

↓

Cardiac arrest

2. Other pathophysiologic characteristics of near-drowning:
   a. Metabolic acidosis (lactic acidosis type A) develops in many patients and is due to hypoxemia (anaerobic metabolism) and poor perfusion.
      (1) It is usually well tolerated in children and may be reversed with adequate ventilation and oxygenation.
      (2) It is less well tolerated in adults.
         (a) In addition to ventilation and oxygenation, small doses of $NaHCO_3$ may be considered for refractory acidosis.
         (b) Lactic acidosis persists if severe hypoxemia is not corrected.
   b. Most victims do not aspirate enough fluid to cause life-threatening changes in blood volume or serum electrolyte concentrations.
   c. Renal failure occurs infrequently in near-drowning.
      (1) Acute tubular necrosis may develop secondary to hypoxemia.
      (2) In freshwater near-drowning, acute renal failure may result from hemolysis and hemoglobinuria.
   d. Cerebral edema may develop (usually within 6 - 12 hours) from generalized neuronal death. Cerebral edema → ↑ intracranial pressure → ↓ cerebral perfusion pressure and ↓ cerebral blood flow → further ischemic neurologic injury.

D. *Important Points About Prehospital Care*

1. Ineffective and potentially dangerous procedures:
   a. In-water CPR
   b. Attempts to remove fluid from the lungs via postural drainage or the Heimlich maneuver

2. Initial assessment and stabilization
   a. Always start CPR in the pulseless, apneic victim even if there is only a remote possibility of success.
   b. Airway maintenance and supplemental oxygen are of primary importance. An IV should also be started if possible.
   c. Immobilize the C-spine and look for signs of spinal injury:
      (1) Paradoxical respirations
      (2) Unexplained hypotension
      (3) Bradycardia
      (4) Flaccidity
      (5) Priapism
   d. Prevent onset or worsening of hypothermia — Remove wet clothes, dry the patient and wrap in dry blankets.

3. Transport <u>all</u> drowning victims to the hospital.

E. Emergency Department Assessment and Stabilization

1. Evaluate airway patency, adequacy of C-spine immobilization and mental status; naloxone + glucose are indicated if there is an altered LOC.

2. Assess respiratory status, looking for signs of pulmonary insufficiency:
   a. Tachypnea
   b. Dyspnea
   c. Use of accessory muscles
   d. Wheezing, rales or rhonchi

3. Provide supplemental oxygen.
   a. Always use 100% oxygen.
   b. Intubation is indicated if the pO_2 is < 60 in adults or < 80 in children (while on high-flow oxygen).
   c. If the patient has signs of pulmonary insufficiency, use CPAP (if awake) or PEEP (if comatose). Indications include:
      (1) A very high respiratory rate (> 50/min.)
      (2) A PaO_2 < 60 with an FIO_2 < 50%
      (3) A $PaCO_2$ > 35mmHg
      (4) A PaO_2: FIO_2 ratio < 300
   d. Persistent hypoxemia may be due to aspiration of particulate matter which may require active suctioning or bronchoscopy.

4. Treat bronchospasm → aerosolized albuterol 0.5% solution: 2.5mg in 2 - 3mL NS Q 20 - 30 mins. prn.

5. Establish an IV of NS or LR (if not started in the field) and place patient on a cardiac monitor and pulse oximeter.

6. Correct shock (if present) with fluid boluses; if this is unsuccessful, use an inotrope (dobutamine, dopamine).

7. Maintain C-spine immobilization until all seven cervical and first thoracic vertebra have been cleared by cervical spine films (three views).

8. Decompress the stomach with an NG tube.

9. Place Foley catheter to follow urine output.

10. Conduct a thorough search for associated injuries.

11. Assess the patient's temperature to R/O hypothermia (which is not uncommon and alters the therapeutic approach).
    a. Use a rectal thermometer that is specially calibrated to record <u>low</u> temps; most clinical thermometers only read down to 34.4°C (95°F).
       (1) Patients who have been submerged in <u>icy</u> cold water ($\leq$ 5 - 10° C) for longer than forty minutes have been known to survive and have a good neurologic outcome.
       (2) Cold water slows the metabolic rate and shunts blood to the brain, heart and lungs (diving reflex).
    b. Institute appropriate rewarming measures for hypothermia.
    c. Extracorporeal membrane oxygenation (if available) is indicated for patients with severe hypothermia and/or hypoxia.
    d. Continue resuscitation efforts until a near-normal core temperature (95° F) is attained.

12. Obtain baseline lab studies.
    a. C-spine films should be done if there is any suspicion of possible cervical injury.
    b. ABGs
    c. Chest x-ray (50% of patients with abnormal films will require intubation) -- typically, one of three patterns are seen:
       (1) Normal (although this does not necessarily mean there is no lung pathology)
       (2) Perihilar pulmonary edema
       (3) Generalized pulmonary edema
    d. CBC + U/A
    e. Glucose, Lytes, PT (INR) / PTT
    f. Blood alcohol level and drug screen
    g. ECG

13. Do <u>not</u> administer prophylactic antibiotics or steroids; neither have been shown to change the course of aspiration pneumonia in near-drowning victims.

F. Predicting Outcome

1. The most <u>reliable</u> predictors of outcome are the duration of submersion and resuscitation.
   a. Good prognostic indicators include:
      (1) <u>Short</u> submersion time
      (2) BLS and/or ALS at the scene
      (3) Favorable response to <u>initial</u> resuscitative efforts (return of spontaneous respiration)
      (4) Alert on admission
      (5) Older child ($\geq$ 3 yrs. old) or adult
      (6) Water temperature $\leq$ 5 - 10° C
   b. Bad prognostic indicators include:
      (1) Submersion duration > 25 mins.
      (2) Cardiac arrest requiring > 25 mins. ALS
      (3) Ongoing CPR in the ED
      (4) Fixed, dilated pupils in the ED
      (5) pH < 7.1
      (6) Age < 3 yrs. old
      (7) Glasgow Coma Score < 5 in the ED

2. Classification of near-drowning victims based on the neurologic examination within one hour of rescue is also highly predictive of outcome:
   a. Patients who are <u>awake</u> and alert almost always survive intact.
   b. Patients who are <u>blunted</u> (obtunded to stuporous) but arousable and have a purposeful response to painful stimuli, usually recover without neurologic sequelae.

    c. Patients who are <u>comatose</u> and have an abnormal response to pain and abnormal respirations have a more variable outcome; although some will survive intact if appropriate care is provided, many will die or survive with anoxic encephalopathy. These patients were generally submerged for a prolonged period of time.

3. Pulmonary injury and hypoxia are the primary pathophysiologic determinants of outcome.

G. Disposition

1. Asymptomatic patients should be observed for 6 hours. If they remain asymptomatic, are oxygenating normally on room air and have a normal CXR, they may be discharged. Adequate follow-up must be available.

2. Hypoxemic and/or symptomatic patients should be hospitalized.

H. Postimmersion Syndrome — Risk Factors:

- Severe transient hypoxia
- History of unconsciousness in the water
- Presence of symptoms such as dyspnea, coughing and tachypnea
- Underlying cardiopulmonary disease

XIV. Adult Respiratory Distress Syndrome (ARDS)

A. Etiology

1. ARDS is a <u>permeability</u> pulmonary edema (unrelated to high-pressure or cardiogenic pulmonary edema) that leads to:
    a. Severe hypoxemia unresponsive to increased concentrations of inspired oxygen (<u>clinical hallmark</u>)
    b. Intrapulmonary shunting
    c. Reduced lung compliance (< 50mL/cm H_2O)
    d. Irreversible parenchymal lung damage (pulmonary fibrosis)

2. Conditions that may precipitate ARDS:
- Shock states (especially septic shock)
- Substance abuse (opiates, methadone, ethchlorvynol, ASA)
- Toxic inhalation (smoke, corrosives, paraquat, oxygen)
- Liquid aspiration (gastric contents, fresh or saltwater)
- Pneumonia (bacterial or viral)
- Emboli (pulmonary, fat, air, amniotic fluid)
- Hematologic disorders (DIC, TTP)

- Major trauma (burns, pulmonary contusion, multiple injuries)
- Multiple transfusions
- Re-expansion of a collapsed lung
- Eclampsia
- High altitude
- Pancreatitis
- Acute neurologic crisis (head injury, SAH, CVA, brain tumor)
- Cancer therapy (tumor lysis, radiation)

<u>Note</u>: Sepsis (especially gram-negative sepsis) is the most common cause of ARDS, aspiration is the second most common cause; together they account for > 50% of cases.

B. Pathophysiology

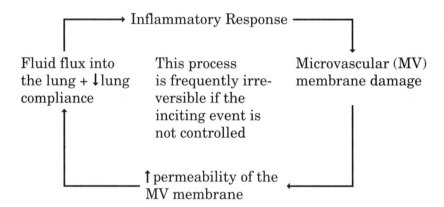

1. The inflammatory response results from activation of enzyme systems (which is caused by the inciting event) and involves a variety of biochemical mediators that typify an inflammatory response.

2. In many disorders associated with permeability pulmonary edema, the activation of enzyme cascades leads to microvascular membrane damage and increased permeability of the microvascular membrane. There are primarily two enzyme cascades that are activated:
   a. The complement system is triggered by:
      (1) Antigen-antibody complexes (the classic pathway)
      (2) Endotoxins
      (3) Exposure to cell surfaces by bacteria or fungi
      (4) Complex polysaccharides
   b. The coagulation pathways are activated when collagen in exposed basement membrane is exposed to plasma. This causes activation of Hageman factor (Factor XII) which, in turn, activates components of the coagulation system, the fibrinolytic system and the kinin generation system.

3. In addition, metabolism of arachidonic acid through major biochemical pathways leads to the release of a variety of mediators (including a host of leukotrienes and prostaglandins) which contribute to further endothelial and alveolar injury.

4. The neutropenic patient may also develop permeability pulmonary edema. Injury to the pulmonary endothelium in this patient results from one of the following:
    a. Direct effects of bacterial endotoxin and complement
    b. Oxygen toxicity
    c. Release of prostaglandins and leukotrienes from alveolar macrophages

5. Once the microvascular membrane is damaged and its permeability is increased, it is no longer an effective barrier to protein flux. Any subsequent increase in hydrostatic pressure will then accelerate fluid flux into the lung. This is why measurement of pulmonary hydrostatic pressure via pulmonary artery wedge pressure (PAWP) monitoring has major therapeutic implications in the management of these patients.

6. To complicate this process, the mechanical properties of the lung are also adversely affected: surfactant is reduced or inactivated → destabilization of lung units (alveoli) → stiff lung (which requires greater pressure to inflate it) → ↓ lung compliance.

7. A patient is said to have ARDS when he has permeability pulmonary edema associated with reduced lung compliance and severe hypoxemia that is refractory to supplemental oxygen.

C. Diagnosis

1. 2 - 24 hours after the inciting event, the patient develops tachypnea and shortness of breath. Fine scattered rales may also be present.

2. Characteristic findings
    a. $PaO_2 <$ 75mmHg when the FIO_2 is ≥ 0.5 ($PaO_2 : FIO_2 < 200$)
    b. Decreased lung compliance (airway resistance is high when the patient is on a mechanical ventilator)
    c. Chest x-ray: <u>diffuse</u> bilateral interstitial and alveolar infiltrates with a <u>normal</u>-sized heart (non-cardiogenic pulmonary edema).
    d. Low to normal capillary wedge pressure

3. A radiologic "pearl" that is helpful in distinguishing ARDS from CHF is the following:
    a. Pulmonary edema + a small heart → ARDS
    b. Pulmonary edema + a large heart → CHF

4. If the diagnosis is uncertain, pulmonary fluid analysis may be helpful; edema fluid protein concentration <u>greater</u> than 70% of the plasma protein concentration supports the diagnosis of ARDS. This is an inhospital procedure that is frequently performed by a critical care specialist.

D. Treatment — is primarily supportive

1. Definitive therapy is directed toward the underlying cause.

2. Supportive therapy involves maintenance of acceptable oxygenation and hemodynamic competence.

   a. The patient with moderate to severe edema should be intubated and put on a mechanical ventilator.

      (1) Incremental oxygen supplementation can be tried first but is frequently ineffective in improving the pO_2.

      (2) The use of positive-end expiratory pressure (PEEP) can improve oxygenation deficits and should be instituted if administration of supplemental oxygen does not improve the pO_2.

         (a) PEEP stabilizes fluid-filled alveoli that are susceptible to collapse and, therefore, increases the number of alveolar units that can participate in gas exchange during ventilation with PEEP. The use of PEEP also allows reduction of the FIO_2 to safer levels ($FIO_2 \leq 0.5$).

         (b) As the level of PEEP is increased, observe the patient carefully for adverse effects.

            <u>1</u> ↓ Venous return → ↓cardiac output and oxygen delivery

            <u>2</u> Pulmonary barotrauma (pneumothorax, pneumomediastinum)

         (c) Optimal PEEP ranges between 0 and 15mmHg.

   b. Swan-Ganz catheterization should be done to monitor hemodynamic competence (as well as confirm the diagnosis):

      (1) Cardiac output

      (2) Arterial and mixed venous oxygen tensions

      (3) Pulmonary artery pressures (including PAWP)

         (a) PAWP should be maintained as low as possible while still maintaining peripheral perfusion.

         (b) When the PAWP is elevated, judicious use of diuretics may be required; vasodilators can increase pulmonary shunting and should be avoided if possible.

   c. IV fluids may be needed to maintain cardiac output and peripheral perfusion, particularly since a decreased venous return may be precipitated by sudden increases of PEEP. However, measurement of PAWP before and after a fluid challenge should always be done to monitor the response.

3. Steroids are <u>not</u> effective in either reversing respiratory failure or in improving survival, and have been shown to increase the incidence of subsequent infections; they should <u>not</u> be administered.

E. Outcome

1. Mortality rate ranges from 40 - 70% and may be declining even though the incidence of ARDS is rising due to higher initial survival rates following emergency care.
   a. 15% of patients die of respiratory failure.
   b. The majority die of multisystem organ failure.

2. Sepsis is the most common cause of fatal ARDS.

XV. Severe Acute Respiratory Syndrome (SARS)

A. ***Background*** — First recognized in southern China in 2002, SARS is a highly communicable infectious disease transmitted by respiratory droplets. As of July 2003, 8000 cases have been reported in 32 countries.

B. ***Pathogenesis*** — The infecting agent is a microbiologically unique Cornavirus and is the <u>first</u> cornavirus known to cause serious disease in humans. It has an incubation period of 2 - 10 days followed by onset of fever and <u>lower</u> respiratory tract symptoms associated with hypoxia; upper respiratory tract symptoms are uncommon and suggest another diagnosis.

C. ***Clinical Diagnosis*** — The CDC criteria are fever >100.4°F (> 38°C) plus one or more of the following:

1. Rapidly progressive respiratory compromise characterized by cough, dyspnea and hypoxia (the classic clinical picture).

2. Travel within 10 days of symptom onset to an area with known community transmission of SARS (especially China and the Asia-Pacific region).

3. Close contact with a person known to have (or suspected of having) SARS within 10 days of symptom onset.

D. ***Laboratory Diagnosis***

1. Presumptive

   a. Combination of thrombocytopenia and lymphocytopenia (which may be absolute) is highly suggestive...especially if the patient also has a cough.

   b. An early finding on chest x-ray is hazy opacities with a ground-glass appearance (much easier to see on high-resolution CT); focal areas of consolidation (especially in the periphery) appear next with progression to extensive bilateral consolidation over 24 - 48 hrs.

   2. Confirmed
      a. Detection of antibody to SARS-CoV (coronavirus) in specimens obtained during acute illness or > 21 days after illness onset <u>or</u>
      b. Detection of SARS-CoV RNA by RT-PCR confirmed by a second PCR assay, using a second aliquot of the specimen and a different set of PCR primers <u>or</u>
      c. Isolation of SARS-CoV

   E. **Management** — is supportive, with most cases resolving spontaneously; antibiotics, steroids and anti-virals have not yet been studied in well-designed clinical trials.

Journal References

ACAD EMER MED, Gibbs, M., Camargo, C., Rowe, B., Silverman., R. 2000; 7: 800-815, "State of the Art: Therapeutic Controversies in Severe Acute Asthma."

AM J EMER MED, Bullard, M.J., et. al., March 1996, "Early Corticosteroid Use in Acute Exacerbations of Chronic Airflow Obstruction." (in Emer. Med. Abstracts, 1996).

AM J MED, Marrie, T. J., et. al., 1996, Vol. 101 (508), "Ambulatory Patients with CAP: The Frequency of Atypical Agents & Clinical Course."

AM J RESPIR & CRIT CARE MED, Georgopoulos, D., et. al., 1996, "Effects of Breathing Route Temperature and Volume of Inspired Gas and Airway Anesthesia on the Response of Respiratory Output to Varying Inspiratory Flow."

AM J RESPIR & CRIT CARE MED, Monso, E., et. al., 1995 "Bacterial Infection in Chronic Obstructive Pulmonary Disease: A Study of Stable and Exacerbated Outpatients Using the Protected Specimen Brush."

AM SURG, Chendrasekhar, A., May 1996, "Are Routine Blood Cultures Effective in the Evaluation of Patients Clinically Diagnosed to Have Nosocomial Pneumonia?"

ANN EMERG MED, Chen, S.Y., Su, C.P., MA, M.H., January 2004, Vol. 43 (1-5), "Predictive Model of Diagnosing Probable Cases of Severe Acute Respiratory Syndrome in Febrile Patients with Exposure Risk."

ANN EMERG MED, Karas, Jr., S., July 2001, Vol. 38 (107-113), "Clinical Policy for the Management and Risk Stratification of Community-Acquired Pneumonia in Adults in the Emergency Department."

ANN EMERG MED, Smith, D., May 2003, Vol. 41(5):706, "Intravenous Epinephrine in Life-Threatening Asthma."

ANN EMERG MED, Su, C.P., Chiang, W.C., MA, M.H., et.al., January 2004, Vol. 43 (34-42), "Valida-tion of a Novel Severe Acute Respiratory Syndrome Scoring System."

ANN EMERG MED, Wang, T.L., Jang, T.N., Huang, C.H., January 2004, Vol. 43 (17-22), "Establishing a Clinical Decision Rule of Severe Acute Respiratory Syndrome at the Emergency Department."

ANNUAL REV MED, Demling, R. H., 1995, "The Modern Version of Adult Respiratory Distress Syndrome."

BRIT MED J, Harries, M., 2003; 327: 1336-1339, "Near Drowning".

CHEST, Marik, P., Kaplan, D., 2003, 124: 328-336, "Aspiration Pneumonia and Dysphagia n the Elderly."

CLIN INFECT DISEASES, Bartlett, J. G., Breiman, R. F., Mandell, L. A., File, Jr., T. M., April 1998, Vol. 26, No. 4, "Community-Acquired Pneumonia in Adults: Guidelines for Management by the Infectious Disease Society of America."

CLIN INFECT DISEASES, Birnbaumer, D. M., October 1998, "Resistant Pneumococcus: The Magnitude of the Problem."

CLIN INFECT DISEASES, Mandell, L., Bartlett, J., Dowell, S., et. al., 2003, 37: 1405-1433, "Update of Practice Guidelines for the Management of Community Acquired Pneumonia in Immunocompetent Adults."

CRIT CARE MED, Garber, B. G., Hebert, P.C., Yelle, J. D., Hodder, R. V., McGowan, J., 1996, "Adult Respiratory Distress Syndrome: A Systemic Overview of Incidence and Risk Factors."

CRITICAL PATHWAYS IN EMERGENCY MEDICINE, Mathey, David and Robin Hemphill, October 12, 1998, "Community-Acquired Pneumonia: Patient Risk Stratification and Prediction Rule for Optimizing Clinical Outcome."

EMERGENCY MEDICINE & ACUTE CARE ESSAYS, Bukata, W. R., July 1998, "Community-Acquired Pneumonia Treatment Guidelines."

EMERGENCY MEDICINE & ACUTE CARE ESSAYS, Bukata, W. R., December 2001, Vol. 25, No. 12, "ATS Pneumonia Guideline Update, 2001."

EMERGENCY MEDICAL ABSTRACTS, Doern, G. V., et. al., October 1998, "Prevalence of Anti-microbial Resistance Among Respiratory Tract Isolates of Streptococcus Pneumoniae in North America: 1997 Results From the Sentry Antimicrobial Surveillance Program."

EMERGENCY MEDICAL ABSTRACTS, Lanes, S. F., et. al., August 1998, "The Effect of Adding Ipratropium Bromide to Salbutamol in the Treatment of Acute Asthma: A Pooled Analysis of Three Trials."

EMERGENCY MEDICAL ABSTRACTS, Plotnick, L. H., et. al., October 10, 1998, "Should Inhaled Anticholinergics Be Added to Beta-2 Agonists for Treating Acute Children and Adolescent Asthma."

EMERGENCY MEDICINE AUSTRALASIA, Harvey, M.G., June 2004: Vol. 16(3):212, "Elevation of Cardiac Troponins in Exacerbation of Chronic Obstructive Pulmonary Disease."

EMERGENCY MEDICINE: ACUTE MEDICINE FOR THE PRIMARY CARE PHYSICIAN, Silverman, Robert, March 1999, "Acute Asthma in Adults."

EMERGENCY MEDICINE REPORTS, Bosker, G., April 22, 2002, Vol. 23, No. 9, "Community-Acquired Pneumonia (CAP) Antibiotic Selection and Management Update - Part I: Evaluation, Risk Stratification and Current Antimicrobial Treatment Guidelines for Hospital-Based Management of CAP: Outcome-Effective Strategies Based on Year 2002 NCCLS Breakpoints and Recent Clinical Studies."

EMERGENCY MEDICINE REPORTS, Bosker, G., May 6, 2002, Vol. 23, No. 10, "Community-Acquired Pneumonia (CAP) Antibiotic Selection and Management Update - Part II: Evaluation, Risk Stratification and Current Antimicrobial Treatment Guidelines for Hospital-Based Management of CAP: Outcome-Effective Strategies Based on New National Committee on Clinical Laboratory Standards (NCCLS) Breakpoints and Recent Clinical Studies."

EMERGENCY MEDICINE REPORTS, Cullison, B., Emerman, C., May 21, 2001, Vol. 22, No. 11, "The Clinical Challenge of Acute Asthma: Diagnosis, Disposition, and Outcome-Effective Management: Year 2001 Update."

EMERGENCY MEDICINE REPORTS, Emerman, C. L., Bosker, G., Miller, L. A., October 12, 1998, "Outpatient and In-Hospital Management of Community-Acquired Pneumonia: Prediction Rules for Patient Disposition and Outcome-Effective Antibiotic Selection."

EMERGENCY MEDICINE REPORTS, Emerman, C. L., Bosker, G., Miller, L. A., November 22, 1999, Vol. 20, No. 24, "Community Acquired Pneumonia (CAP) Update Year 2000: Current Antibiotic Guidelines and Outcome Effective Management: Part I."

JAMA, Sin, D., McAlister, F., Man, P., Anthonisen, N. 2003, 290: 2301-2312, "Contemporary Management of COPD."

INTENSIVE CARE MED, Johanson W., 2003, 23: 23-29, "Nosocomial Pneumonia."

N ENGL J MED, Droston C., Gunther, S., Preiser W., et.al., 2003, Vol. 348: 1967-1976, "Identification of a Novel Coronavirus in Patients With Severe Acute Respiratory Syndrome."

N ENGL J MED, Ksiazek, T.G. and the SARS Working Group, et.al., 2003, Vol. 348: 1953-1966, "A Novel Coronavirus Associated With Severe Acute Respiratory Syndrome."

N ENGL J MED, Small, P., Fujiwara, P., 2001, Vol. 345: 189-200, "Management of Tubercu-losis in the United States."

N ENGL J MED, Nicolaou, S. Al-Nakshabandi, N.A., Muller, N.L., 2003, Vol. 348: 2006, "Radiologic Manifestations of Severe Acute Respiratory Syndrome."

N ENGL J MED, Tsang, K.W., Ho, P.L., Ooi, G.C. et.al., 2003, Vol. 348: 1977-1985, "A Cluster of Cases of Severe Acute Respiratory Syndrome in Hong Kong."

THORAX, Lordan J., Gascoigne, A., Corris, P., 2003, Vol. 58: 814-819, "Assessment and Management of Massive Hemoptysis"

Specific Text Chapter References

Moran, G. J., Talan, D. A., "Tuberculosis." In Harwood-Nuss, A. L., Linden, C. H., Luten, R. C. (eds.) THE CLINICAL PRACTICE OF EMERGENCY MEDICINE, 2nd ed., (Lippencott-Raven: Philadelphia, 1996)

Specific Text References

Clinical Infections Disease, Stamm, W. E., Root, R. K., et. al., (Oxford Univ. Press, Oxford, England, 1999).

Fishman's Pulmonary Diseases and Disorders, Fishman, A. P., Elias, J. A., et. al., 3rd. ed., (McGraw-Hill, New York, 1998).

Respiratory Disease in the Immunosuppressed Host, Shelhamer, J., Pizzo, P. A., Parrillo, J. E., Masur, H., (J. B. Lippincott Co, Philedeliphia, 1999).

Web and Other Sources

ACEP, Pollack, C., File, Jr., T. M., 2001, "Respiratory Tract Infections: New Management Approaches." (video CME Series) (monograph)

EMER MED & ACUTE CARE ESSAYS, Emergency Medical Abstracts, May 2003, Vol. 27, No. 5, "SARS Update."

IDSA GUIDELINES, Mandell, L.A., et.al., December 2003: 37, "Update of Practice Guidelines for the Management of Community-Acquired Pneumonia in Immunocompetent Adults."

General Text References, Acep Clinical Policies and LLSA Reading Lists *for all chapters located in the back of both volumes.*

NOTES

ORTHOPEDIC EMERGENCIES

1. All the following statements regarding anterior shoulder dislocations are true except:

    (a) Subcoracoid dislocations are the most common type.
    (b) Associated neurovascular injury is nonexistent.
    (c) A Hill-Sachs deformity occurs in up to 50% of anterior dislocations.
    (d) Treatment consists of reduction and immobilization in a shoulder immobilizer.

2. Which of the following statements regarding posterior shoulder dislocations is accurate?

    (a) They are best visualized with an axillary or scapular "Y" view.
    (b) They are often associated with damage to the axillary nerve.
    (c) They are the most frequent type of shoulder dislocation.
    (d) They are often associated with fracture of the anterior glenoid rim.

3. Which of the following is not a component of the rotator cuff?

    (a) Subscapularis
    (b) Supraspinatus
    (c) Infraspinatus
    (d) Teres major

4. All of the following statements regarding the rotator cuff are true except:

    (a) It permits abduction and controls internal and external rotation of the shoulder.
    (b) The tendinous insertions of the rotator cuff are on the greater and lesser tuberosities of the humerus.
    (c) It may be torn in association with anterior shoulder dislocations.
    (d) All tears require surgical correction.

5. All of the following statements regarding humeral fractures are accurate except:

    (a) Humeral shaft fractures are frequently associated with radial nerve injuries.
    (b) Proximal humeral fractures are classified according to the Neer classification system.
    (c) Fracture through the surgical neck of the humerus is associated with avascular necrosis of the humeral head.
    (d) Management of proximal humeral fractures is determined primarily by the amount of displacement present.

6. All of the following statements regarding supracondylar extension fractures are true except:

    (a) They generally result from a fall on the outstretched arm.
    (b) They are more common in adults than in children.
    (c) They are associated with the development of Volkmann's ischemic contracture.
    (d) Associated median nerve injury may occur with this injury.

7. A distal radial shaft fracture associated with a distal radioulnar dislocation is referred to as a:

(a) Galeazzi fracture
(b) Monteggia fracture
(c) Nightstick fracture
(d) Maisonneuve fracture

8. All the following statements regarding the ulnar nerve are accurate except:

(a) It passes through Guyon's canal.
(b) Loss of function results in a "claw hand" deformity.
(c) It innervates the interosseous muscles.
(d) It is frequently injured in association with anterior elbow dislocations.

9. Empiric antibiotic coverage from human bite cellulitis associated with involvement of the MCP joint (clenched fist injuries) should be designed to cover all of the following pathogens except:

(a) Anaerobic strep
(b) *Staph aureus*
(c) *Eikenella corrodens*
(d) *Pasteurella multocida*

10. The carpal bone most frequently injured in a fall on the outstretched hand is the:

(a) Lunate
(b) Trapezoid
(c) Scaphoid
(d) Triquetrum

11. The incidence of avascular necrosis in association with scaphoid fractures is highest in fractures of the:

(a) Tubercle of the scaphoid
(b) Distal scaphoid
(c) Waist (middle third) of the scaphoid
(d) Proximal scaphoid

12. Which of the following injuries is most frequently associated with the development of acute carpal tunnel syndrome?

(a) Perilunate dislocation
(b) Lunate dislocation
(c) Scapholunate dislocation
(d) None of the above

13. All but one of the injuries listed below may be sustained in a fall on the outstretched arm. Which of them occurs via a different mechanism?
    (a) Rotator cuff tear
    (b) Proximal humeral fracture
    (c) Radial head subluxation
    (d) Supracondylar fracture

14. The primary cause of death in patients with pelvic fractures is:
    (a) Blood loss
    (b) Associated injuries
    (c) Ruptured diaphragm
    (d) Sepsis

15. All of the following statements regarding posterior hip dislocations are true except:
    (a) They represent 80 - 90% of all hip dislocations.
    (b) Avascular necrosis is a late complication of this injury.
    (c) The limb appears abducted, externally rotated and flexed.
    (d) The mechanism of injury is a direct force applied to the flexed knee.

16. All of the following are signs of pelvic fracture except:
    (a) Destot's sign
    (b) Earle's sign
    (c) McMurray's sign
    (d) Roux's sign

17. Which of the following are stabilizers of the lateral aspect of the knee?
    (a) Vastus lateralis and rectus femoris muscles
    (b) Semimembranous muscle and medial collateral ligament
    (c) Iliotibial band and biceps femoris muscle
    (d) Cruciate ligaments

18. All of the following statements regarding knee dislocations are accurate except:
    (a) The incidence of associated popliteal artery injury is 30 - 40%.
    (b) Findings of a warm foot and palpable pulses rule out the presence of injury to the popliteal artery.
    (c) Findings of paresthesia along the dorsal aspect of the foot and foot drop signal the presence of associated peroneal nerve injury.
    (d) Arteriography is indicated for all patients with this injury.

19. Which of the following is not an early or reliable sign of anterior compartment syndrome?
    (a) Pain with active dorsiflexion of the foot
    (b) Sensory loss in the first web space of the foot
    (c) Absence of peripheral pulses of the foot
    (d) Pain with passive plantar flexion of the foot

20. Which of the following findings is consistent with a third degree sprain of the ankle?

    (a) Moderate swelling
    (b) Able to bear weight
    (c) Positive stress test
    (d) Moderate functional loss

21. All of the following statements regarding calcaneal fractures are true except:

    (a) They have a 10% incidence of associated lumbar fractures.
    (b) They are generally the result of a compression injury (fall).
    (c) They are the second most frequently fractured tarsal bone.
    (d) A Bohler's angle < 20% is consistent with a depressed fracture of the body of the calcaneus.

22. The joint separating the hindfoot from the midfoot is referred to as:

    (a) Charcot's joint
    (b) Chopart's joint
    (c) Lisfranc's joint
    (d) Bohler's joint

23. All of the following statements regarding lunate fractures are accurate except:

    (a) Patients present with pain over the middorsum of the wrist that is increased by axial compression of the third metacarpal.
    (b) Plain x-ray films are usually diagnostic.
    (c) They result from a fall on the outstretched hand.
    (d) Avascular necrosis of the proximal segment is a serious complication.

24. A 28 year-old athlete presents with knee pain. He states that he was playing football about two hours ago and received a direct blow to the lateral aspect of his knee. X-ray of the knee is negative for fracture; exam reveals a hemarthrosis. Ligamentous evaluation reveals instability (joint opening of 5mm) with valgus stress in 30° of flexion. Other tests of stability, including valgus stress in extension, are negative. This athlete most likely has:

    (a) Rupture of the anterior cruciate ligament
    (b) Rupture of the medial collateral ligament
    (c) Rupture of the medial collateral ligament as well as potential injury to the anterior cruciate ligament and posterior capsule
    (d) Rupture of the lateral collateral ligament

25. A 60-year-old woman presents with the complaint of knee pain for 1 day. There is no history of trauma or similar pain in the past. Exam reveals a tender, warm, erythematous knee. Joint aspiration demonstrates cloudy fluid with 10,000 WBCs (> 75% PMNs), normal glucose and rhomboid-shaped crystals that are positively birefringent under polarized light. The most likely diagnosis is:

   (a) Osteoarthritis
   (b) Rheumatoid arthritis
   (c) Gout
   (d) Pseudogout

26. A 40-year-old patient presents with low back pain plus bowel and bladder incontinence. Exam reveals loss of sensation in the "saddle" distribution and loss of anal tone. The most appropriate management of this case is:

   (a) Bedrest for 2 days with appropriate analgesia and muscle relaxants plus orthopedic follow-up in 2 days.
   (b) Bedrest for 2 weeks with appropriate analgesia and muscle relaxants plus orthopedic follow-up in 2 weeks.
   (c) Immediate neurosurgical consultation for acute disc decompression.
   (d) Bedrest for 2 days with appropriate analgesia and muscle relaxants plus neurosurgical follow-up in 2 days.

27. A 62-year-old woman presents with severe shoulder and proximal arm pain following a fall. X-ray reveals a proximal humeral fracture; the lesser tuberosity is displaced from the remainder of the humerus by > 1cm. This type of proximal humeral fracture would most accurately be classified as a Neer:

   (a) One-part fracture
   (b) Two-part fracture
   (c) Three-part fracture
   (d) The Neer classification system does not pertain to this type of fracture.

28. Which of the injuries listed below commonly occurs in association with the particular type of humeral fracture described in the preceding question (#27)?

   (a) Clavicular fracture
   (b) Posterior shoulder dislocation
   (c) Anterior and posterior shoulder dislocations
   (d) Anterior shoulder dislocation

29. All the following statements regarding compartment syndrome are accurate except:

   (a) It can be caused by crush injuries, fractures or constrictive dressings or casts.
   (b) The most commonly affected compartments are the anterior compartment of the lower leg and the volar compartment of the forearm.
   (c) Normal compartment pressure is 10 - 20mmHg.
   (d) Initial management consists of removal of constricting dressings/casts (if present).

30. Which of the following is an absolute contraindication to reimplantation of an amputated digit?
    (a) Single-digit amputation other than the thumb
    (b) Serious underlying systemic illness
    (c) Severely damaged or contaminated part
    (d) Unstable patient with other life-threatening injuries

31. While awaiting a decision from the vascular surgeon regarding reimplantation what is the best method of preserving an amputated part?
    (a) Place it in a container of 10% providine iodine solution and store this container in ice water.
    (b) Irrigate it with normal saline or Ringer's lactate to remove gross contamination, wrap it in sterile gauze moistened with normal saline, place it in a sterile, water-tight container and store this container in ice water.
    (c) Irrigate it with normal saline or Ringer's lactate to remove gross contamination, wrap it in sterile gauze moistened with normal saline and then place it on ice.
    (d) Irrigate it with 10% providine iodine solution to remove gross contamination, wrap it in sterile gauze moistened with normal saline and place it between two ice packs.

32. All of the following statements regarding scapular fractures are accurate except:
    (a) They typically occur in association with high-energy trauma.
    (b) Associated injuries, some of which may be life-or limb-threatening, occur in up to 98% of these patients.
    (c) The most common associated injuries are ipsilateral lung injuries, rib fractures and clavicle fractures.
    (d) Most scapular fractures require orthopedic referral for open reduction and internal fixation.

33. The most commonly injured major ligament of the knee is the _____.
    (a) Medial collateral ligament
    (b) Lateral collateral ligament
    (c) Anterior cruciate ligament
    (d) Posterior cruciate

34. A 48-year-old man presents with knee pain following a fall. Exam reveals a significant hemarthrosis which you aspirate to make him more comfortable. The finding of fat globules in the aspirate is very suggestive of:
    (a) A tear in the anterior cruciate ligament
    (b) A peripheral meniscus tear
    (c) A fracture
    (d) None of the above

35. Innervation of the intrinsic muscles of the hand is provided by:

    (a) The median and ulnar nerves
    (b) The ulnar and radial nerves
    (c) The median and radial nerves
    (d) The median, ulnar and radial nerves

36. Apley's and McMurray's tests are helpful in making the diagnosis of:

    (a) Chondromalacia patellae
    (b) Meniscal tears
    (c) A torn anterior cruciate ligament
    (d) A torn posterior cruciate ligament

Answers: 1. b, 2. a, 3. d, 4. d, 5. c, 6. b, 7. a, 8. d, 9. d, 10. c,
           11. d, 12. b, 13. c, 14. a, 15. c, 16. c, 17. c, 18. b, 19. c,
           20. c, 21. c, 22. b, 23. b, 24. b, 25. d, 26. c, 27. b, 28. b,
           29. c, 30. d, 31. b, 32. d, 33. c, 34. c, 35. a, 36. b

Use the pre-chapter multiple choice question worksheet (p. xxv) to record and determine the percentage of correct answers for this section.

ORTHOPEDIC EMERGENCIES

I. **General Principles of Fracture and Dislocation Management**

A. *Classification and Definitions*

    1. Direct Trauma (direct force over the fracture site)
        a. "Tapping" (nightstick) fracture
            (1) Linear fracture with two fragments
            (2) Little or no soft tissue injury
        b. Crush fracture
            (1) Comminuted or transverse fracture
            (2) Extensive soft tissue injury
        c. Penetrating fracture (often seen with missile wounds)
            (1) High-velocity injuries: fragmentation of bone → bone fragments act as secondary missiles → results in cavitation and extensive soft tissue injury.
            (2) Low-velocity injuries: mild fragmentation of bone.

    2. Indirect Trauma (forces acting at a distance from the fracture site)
        a. Traction (tension) fracture: bone is pulled apart → transverse fracture.
        b. Angulation fracture: bending along the long axis of the bone → transverse fracture with concave surface often splintered.
        c. Compression fracture: compression on the long axis of the bone → axial loading → "T" or "Y" fractures.
        d. Spiral fracture: results from rotational stress (torque).
            (1) A pure rotational injury is rare.
            (2) When associated with an axial load → oblique fracture.

    3. Incomplete fractures (torus and greenstick): only one cortex is interrupted; these fractures occur almost exclusively in children (due to their greater bone elasticity).
        a. Torus (buckle) fracture: characterized by a bulging (buckling) of one cortex; results from compressive forces and usually involves the metaphyseal region.
        b. Greenstick fracture: characterized by a break in one cortex (convex side) and a bending (bowing) of the other cortex (concave side); this results from an angular force applied to a long bone.

    4. Complete fracture: involves both cortices.

    5. Closed (simple) fracture: there is no communication with the external environment; the overlying skin and soft tissue are intact.

6. Open (compound) fracture: there is communication with the external environment through a break in the overlying skin and soft tissue; these fractures are at high risk for infection (osteomyelitis) and are considered an orthopedic emergency. Management includes:

   a. Early emergency department administration of IV antibiotics (a first-generation cephalosporin ± an aminoglycoside)
   b. Tetanus prophylaxis
   c. Wound irrigation + debridement (usually accomplished in the OR)

7. Pathologic fracture: results from bone weakness secondary to an underlying disease process (cysts, tumors, osteogenesis imperfecta, scurvy, rickets, Paget's disease, etc.); should be suspected when trivial trauma results in a fracture.

8. Stress fracture ("march or fatigue fracture"): results from bone fatigue secondary to repeated or cyclical stress; often occurs in association with a sudden increase in the level of training; usually located in the lower extremities (metatarsals, navicular, distal tibia/fibula, femoral neck); plain x-rays may be negative for two or more weeks.

9. Dislocation: complete disruption of the articular surface.

10. Subluxation: incomplete disruption of the articular surface.

B. _**Salter-Harris Classification of Epiphyseal Fractures**_: (aids in determining prognosis — the higher the number, the poorer the prognosis)

1. 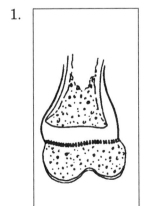 Type I: fracture through the epiphyseal plate (physis) resulting in separation of the epiphysis; good prognosis.

2.

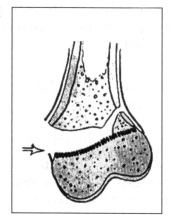

Type II: fracture of the metaphysis with extension through the epiphyseal plate (most common type); seen most frequently in children > 10 yrs. old; a metaphyseal fragment called a "Thurston-Holland Sign" is present; good prognosis.

3.

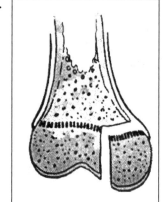

Type III: fracture of the epiphysis with extension into the epiphyseal plate (a totally intra-articular fracture); open reduction is often necessary.

4.

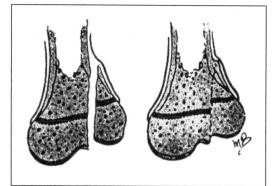

Type IV: fracture through the metaphysis, epiphysis and epiphyseal plate (also a completely intra-articular fracture); open reduction is usually necessary and perfect reduction is essential; growth disturbance is common.

5.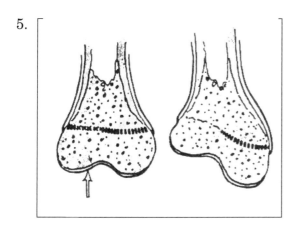

Type V: crush fracture of the epiphyseal plate (opposite of Type I): most commonly seen in knee and ankle; **x-rays may look normal**; poor prognosis, as the blood supply to the epiphyseal plate is interrupted.

C. Complications of Fractures

1. Immediate complications
   a. Hemorrhage (can be extensive with pelvic fractures)
   b. Vascular injuries
      - Anterior shoulder dislocation → R/O axillary artery injury
      - Extension supracondylar fracture → R/O brachial artery injury
      - Post. elbow dislocation → R/O brachial artery injury
      - Knee dislocation → R/O popliteal artery injury
   c. Nerve injuries
      - Anterior shoulder dislocation → R/O axillary and musculo-cutaneous nerve injury
      - Humeral shaft injury → R/O radial nerve injury
      - Extension supracondylar fracture → R/O median, radial and ulnar nerve injury
      - Medial epicondylar fracture → R/O ulnar nerve injury
      - Post. elbow dislocation → R/O ulnar and median nerve injury
      - Olecranon fracture → R/O ulnar nerve injury
      - Acetabular fracture → R/O sciatic nerve injury
      - Posterior hip dislocation → R/O sciatic nerve injury
      - Anterior hip dislocation → R/O femoral nerve injury
      - Knee dislocation → R/O peroneal and tibial nerve injury
      - Lateral tibial plateau fracture → R/O peroneal nerve injury
   d. Associated soft tissue /visceral injuries

2. Intermediate complications
   a. Compartment syndrome
   b. Fat embolism (usually originates from a long bone)

3. Long-term complications
   a. Reflex sympathetic dystrophy
   b. Volkmann's ischemic contracture
   c. Nonunion
   d. Avascular necrosis (femoral head, <u>proximal</u> scaphoid, capitate and talus fractures are particularly predisposed to this complication)
   e. Angulation deformities, overgrowth or shortening
   f. Infection
   g. Joint stiffness
   h. Post-traumatic ossification or arthritis

II. Upper Extremity Trauma

A. Shoulder Dislocations and Ligamentous Tears

1. <u>Sternoclavicular joint injuries</u>
   a. Classification
      (1) First-degree (= sprain) → partial tear of the sternoclavicular and costoclavicular ligaments without associated clavicular subluxation.
      (2) Second-degree (= subluxation) → complete tear of the sternoclavicular ligament plus partial tear of the costoclavicular ligament with subluxation of the clavicle from the manubrium.
      (3) Third-degree (= dislocation) → complete tear of both the sternoclavicular and costoclavicular ligaments with dislocation of the clavicle from the manubrium. The clavicle can dislocate either anteriorly (most common) or posteriorly (uncommon, but a true orthopedic emergency).
   b. Mechanism of injury
      (1) Direct force over sternoclavicular joint → posterior dislocation
      (2) Fall onto the shoulder* → anterior or posterior dislocation
   c. Signs and symptoms
      (1) Tenderness and swelling over the sternoclavicular joint
      (2) Pain with movement of the ipsilateral extremity and with lateral compression of the shoulders.
      (3) With third-degree injuries, the medial clavicle is displaced (anteriorly or posteriorly) relative to the manubrium.
      (4) Shortness of breath, dysphagia or choking (in patients with posterior dislocations associated with compression of mediastinal structures)
   d. X-rays — Dislocations are best demonstrated with tomograms or CT.
   e. Treatment
      (1) First-degree → arm sling for 3 to 4 days and analgesics
      (2) Second-degree → figure-of-eight clavicular strap or arm sling, analgesics and orthopedic follow-up.

*Large amount of force involved, often necessitating trauma work-up and consideration of possible intra-thoracic injuries.

(3) Third-degree → <u>immediate orthopedic</u> consultation and rapid reduction . . .
   (a) Establish an IV and administer analgesia; posterior dislocations often require general anesthesia in the operating room.
   (b) Place the patient in the supine position with a rolled sheet between the shoulders.
   (c) Extend, abduct and apply traction to the ipsilateral arm while an assistant pushes (anterior dislocation) or pulls with a towel clip (posterior dislocation) the clavicle into its normal position.
   (d) Apply a figure-of-eight clavicular strap or arm sling and refer for orthopedic follow-up.
   <u>Note</u>: Life-threatening injuries to adjacent structures (pneumothorax and compression or laceration of the esophagus, trachea or great vessels) occur in up to 25% of <u>posterior</u> dislocations and must be promptly attended.

2. <u>Acromioclavicular separation</u>
   a. Classification
      (1) First degree/Type I (= sprain) → partial tear of the acromioclavicular (AC) ligament without subluxation of the clavicle; the coracoclavicular ligament is intact.
      (2) Second degree/Type II (= subluxation) → complete tear of AC ligament with subluxation of the clavicle; the coracoclavicular ligament is stretched or incompletely torn.
      (3) Third degree/Type III (= dislocation) → complete tears of <u>both</u> the AC and coracoclavicular ligaments with dislocation of the clavicle.
      (4) Fourth degree/Types IV-VI (= displacement) → significant displacement of the distal clavicle posteriorly (Type IV), superiorly (Type V) or inferiorly (Type VI) as well as associated injury/interposition of the deltoid or trapezius muscle.
   b. Mechanism of injury
      (1) Fall on the shoulder with the arm <u>adducted</u> (most common)
      (2) Fall on the outstretched arm
   c. Signs and symptoms
      (1) Tenderness and swelling over the AC joint
      (2) Pain with movement of the affected extremity
      (3) With Type III injuries, the distal clavicle is displaced upward relative to the acromion when compared to the opposite shoulder. (<u>Note</u>: This is best visualized when the patient is examined in the sitting or standing position with the affected arm hanging at his side)
   d. X-ray evaluation
      (1) Obtain AP views of both clavicles (on the same cassette)
      (2) Stress views (taken with 10 lbs. of weight suspended from each wrist) are <u>no longer routinely</u> recommended because they:
         (a) Are associated with increased cost, radiation exposure and patient discomfort
         (b) Provide little additional information and can be misleading

(c) Do <u>not</u> usually alter the course of treatment since most acromioclavicular separations are managed conservatively (non-operatively) and most third-degree injuries are clinically obvious.

(3) Findings — depend on the degree of separation.
  (a) First degree → AC joint is radiographically normal even with stress view.
  (b) Second degree → due to upward displacement of the clavicle, the distance between the acromion and the inferior aspect of the distal aspect of the clavicle is increased by ≤ one-half the width of the clavicle (or ≤ 1cm) on the AP view. The distance seen between the clavicle and the coracoid process is normal.
  (c) Third degree → the distance between the acromion and the distal aspect of the clavicle is increased by > one-half the width of the clavicle (or > 1cm) on the AP view. The distance between the distal clavicle and the coracoid process is also increased.

  e. Treatment
    (1) Type I → sling for 1 - 2 weeks and analgesics, followed by early range of motion exercises.
    (2) Type II → sling until acute pain has subsided, analgesics and orthopedic referral for further evaluation and rehabilitation.
    (3) Type III → is controversial (immobilization versus surgical fixation); immobilize in a sling, provide analgesics and arrange prompt orthopedic referral (within 72 hours).
    (4) Types IV-VI → will likely require surgical fixation as definitive treatment; acute management is the same as Type III.

3. <u>Shoulder dislocation</u> (most common dislocation seen in the ED)
  a. X-ray series
    (1) Standard views should always be ordered (AP shoulder + transcapular lateral or "Y" view)
      (a) In anterior dislocations, the AP view detects the most important associated fracture--the humeral neck; fracture of the lesser tuberosity suggests a posterior shoulder dislocation.
      (b) In posterior dislocations, the Y or axillary view is diagnostic.
    (2) An axillary lateral view is ideal for differentiating anterior from posterior dislocations and it often reveals an impression fracture of the humeral head, but it may be difficult to obtain.
    (3) A modified axillary view (called the West Point view) allows visualization of the anterior glenoid rim; avulsion fractures in this area (that are associated with anterior dislocations) are not infrequent.
  b. Anterior (95 - 97% of all shoulder dislocations)
    (1) Mechanism of injury: abduction, extension and external rotation
    (2) Types of anterior dislocations (where the humeral head is)
      (a) Subcoracoid (most common)
      (b) Subglenoid (head of the humerus is anterior and inferior to the glenoid fossa)

    (c) Subclavicular ——┐
                        ├─ (very rare)
    (d) Intrathoracic ——┘

(3) Examination of the shoulder reveals prominence of the acromion process and flattening of the normal contour of the shoulder. The affected arm is held in slight <u>ab</u>duction + <u>external</u> rotation; the patient is unable to place his palm on the uninjured shoulder.

(4) A clinical clue is resistance to <u>internal</u> rotation and <u>ad</u>duction.

(5) Complications/associated injuries

    (a) Recurrence — is the most common complication and is age-related; the younger the patient the greater the likelihood of recurrence.

    (b) Bony injuries

        1 <u>Hill-Sachs deformity</u>

           <u>a</u> A compression fracture or "groove" of the posterolateral aspect of the humeral head [<u>Rosen's Text</u>, Fourth ed., p. 727, Fig. 44-28 and Fifth ed., p. 594, Fig. 46-27].

           <u>b</u> Results from impaction of the humeral head on the anterior glenoid rim as it dislocates (or reduces).

           <u>c</u> Occurs in up to 50% of anterior dislocations and is particularly common in patients with recurrent dislocation; the humeral head is damaged by the sharp anterior rim of the glenord, creating a lesion called the "hatchet sign" which is apparent on the reduction film.

        2 Avulsion of the greater tuberosity (more common in patients > 45 years old and in those with subglenoid dislocations).

        <u>3</u> Fracture of the anterior glenoid lip (Bankart's fracture)

    (c) Nerve injuries

        <u>1</u> May occur when the shoulder is dislocated or reduced; therefore, it is important to check and document sensation both pre-and post-reduction.

        <u>2</u> Most injuries are neuropraxias and recover well over time.

        <u>3</u> Axillary nerve injury (most common) — exam reveals sensory loss over the lateral aspect of the shoulder and weakness in shoulder <u>ab</u>duction (deltoid muscle).

        <u>4</u> Musculocutaneous nerve injury — exam reveals weakness of forearm flexors and supinators as well as sensory loss along dorsum of forearm.

        <u>5</u> Brachial plexus injuries (require <u>a</u>traumatic reduction)

    (d) Rotator cuff tears (higher incidence in patients > 40 yrs. old)

    (e) Axillary artery injury is rare but should be suspected in an elderly patient with a weak/absent radial pulse or an expanding hematoma.

c. Posterior (2 - 4% of all shoulder injuries)

    (1) Mechanism of injury

        (a) Convulsive seizure or electric shock

        (b) Fall on a forward-flexed, <u>ad</u>ducted and internally-rotated arm

        (c) Significant direct blow to the anterior shoulder

(2) The most commonly <u>missed</u> major dislocation of the body, it is often misdiagnosed as "bursitis" or "adhesive capsulitis;" x-ray diagnosis can be made with an axillary lateral or transscapular lateral "Y" view; an axillary lateral view is an excellent technique for visualization of a posterior dislocation, but it is not usually possible to take because the patient cannot abduct his shoulder. (Be able to identify.) [See <u>Rosen's Text,</u> Fifth ed., p. 597, Fig. 40-34]

(3) Types of posterior dislocation
    (a) Subacromial (98%)
    (b) Subglenoid
    (c) Subspinous

(4) Examination of the shoulder reveals anterior flatness, posterior fullness and prominence of the coracoid process. The affected arm is <u>internally</u> rotated and is usually held in <u>adduction</u>.

(5) A clinical clue is inability to <u>ab</u>duct or externally rotate the arm.

(6) Complications/associated injuries
    (a) Associated fractures of the posterior rim of the glenoid fossa, anteromedial aspect of the humeral head (reversed Hill-Sachs deformity) and lesser tuberosity. In fact, in the presence of an isolated lesser tuberosity fracture, a posterior shoulder dislocation should always be ruled out.
    (b) Recurrence (incidence of 30%)
    (c) Neurovascular complications are <u>un</u>common.

d. Treatment of shoulder dislocations is with reduction using traction, scapular manipulation or leverage and requires conscious sedation with a short-acting narcotic for sedation/pain control (e.g. fentanyl) and a benzodiazepine for sedation and muscle relaxation (e.g. midazolam). Closed reduction can usually be accomplished in the ED.

(1) Reduction techniques for anterior dislocations:*
    (a) Stimson or hanging-weight
    (b) Scapular manipulation
    (c) Traction - countertraction
    (d) External rotation (Hennipen technique)
    (e) Milch forward elevation

(2) Reduction technique for posterior dislocations: axial traction is applied in-line with the humerus and then the humeral head is pushed forward. If this is unsuccessful, reduction may need to be accomplished under general anesthesia. Orthopedic consultation should <u>precede</u> any reduction attempt, as this injury is rare and the rate of complications (fractures) is high.

(3) Shoulder dislocations with an associated fracture should be referred to an orthopedic surgeon for reduction (closed or open).

(4) Following reduction:
    (a) Recheck and document neurovascular exam.
    (b) Order post-reduction films to confirm reduction and <small>R/O</small> any associated injuries; humeral <u>neck</u> fractures are a known complication of anterior shoulder relocation, the result of which is often avascular-necrosis of the humeral <u>head</u>.

*The Kocher maneuver (a leverage technique) and the Hippocratic technique are associated with many complications and should <u>not</u> be used.

(c) Place patient in a shoulder immobilizer or Velpeau's dressing. The length of immobilization will vary from 1 - 4 weeks, depending on the patient's age; the <u>older</u> the patient, the sooner <u>mobilization</u> should be started to avoid stiffness.

(d) Refer for orthopedic follow-up.

4. <u>Rotator cuff tears</u>
   a. The rotator cuff is made up of tendinous insertions of the following muscles that attach to the greater and lesser tuberosities of the humerus:
      (1) Subscapularis ⎤
      (2) Supraspinatus ⎥ permit <u>ab</u>duction and
      (3) Infraspinatus ⎥ control internal/external
      (4) Teres <u>minor</u> ⎦ rotation of the shoulder
      <u>Note</u>: Supraspinatus injuries (tears) are the most frequent.

   b. Mechanisms of injury
      (1) Acute tears - usually occur in association with:
         (a) Forceful <u>ab</u>duction of the arm against significant resistance, (such as a fall on the outstretched arm)
         (b) A fall on the shoulder
         (c) Heavy lifting
      (2) Chronic tears (90% of all lesions) - result from subacromial impingement and decreased blood supply to the tendons, both of which accompany advancing age; these tears can be insidious in onset and can occur in the absence of trauma, particularly in the elderly.

   c. **Clinical picture** — the patient is typically a male in his forties or older who presents with:
      (1) Pain over the anterior aspect of the shoulder that is abrupt in onset and tearing in quality with acute tears; in chronic tears, the pain is more gradual in onset and is typically described as being worse at night.
      (2) Weak and painful <u>ab</u>duction or, if the tear is large or complete, inability to <u>initiate</u> abduction; a positive "drop-arm test" (inability to hold the arm in 90° abduction) is present with significant tears.
      (3) Tenderness on palpation over the insertion site of the supraspinatus on the greater tuberosity

   d. X-rays — may be normal or show degenerative changes and, in the presence of a complete tear, may demonstrate superior displacement of the humeral head (best seen on an external rotation view).

   e. Treatment
      (1) Initial treatment for patients with acute tears consists of sling immobilization, analgesia with NSAIDS and early orthopedic referral. Complete tears require early surgical repair (< 3 weeks) in young, active individuals but are handled more conservatively with the elderly, sedentary patient.

(2) Patients with chronic tears should be immobilized in a sling, given analgesics and referred to an orthopedic surgeon for shoulder rehabilitation exercises and possible corticosteroid injection. Patients who fail to respond to these measures may eventually require surgical repair.

B. Scapular Fractures

1. Result from <u>high-energy</u> trauma, particularly those involving the body or spine of the scapula.

2. Due to the significant force required to produce these fractures, <u>associated injuries</u> are frequent and sometimes life- or limb-threatening; they occur in up to 98% of these patients and include the following:
   a. Rib fractures*
   b. Ipsilateral lung injuries*
      (1) Pneumothorax
      (2) Hemothorax
      (3) Pulmonary contusion
   c. Injuries to the shoulder girdle complex
      (1) Clavicle fractures*
      (2) Shoulder dislocations with associated rotator cuff tears
   d. Neurovascular injuries (rare)
      (1) Brachial plexus injuries
      (2) Axillary artery or nerve injuries
      (3) Subclavian artery injury
      (4) Suprascapular nerve injury
   e. Vertebral compression fractures

3. Mechanism of injury
   a. Direct blow to the scapula
   b. Trauma to the shoulder
   c. Fall on the outstretched arm

4. Classification of these fractures is based on their anatomic location; fractures of the body, neck and glenoid are the most common.

5. **Clinical picture** — the patient is frequently a male who was involved in a high speed MVA or had a significant fall. He presents with the affected arm and shoulder <u>ad</u>ducted against his body and complains of pain over the back of the shoulder. When you examine him, his shoulder pain is increased with <u>ab</u>duction of the arm.

6. X-rays
   a. Routine shoulder x-rays — demonstrate most scapular fractures.
   b. Axillary lateral view — is helpful in evaluating fractures involving the glenoid fossa, acromion and coracoid process.
   c. CXR — R/O associated pulmonary injury.

*The most commonly associated injuries

7. Treatment
    a. Once any associated injuries have been ruled out, most scapular fractures can be managed with sling immobilization (for two weeks or more) and analgesia, followed by early range-of-motion exercises.
    b. Orthopedic referral for open reduction and internal fixation (ORIF) is usually reserved for severely displaced or angulated fractures.

C. Humeral Fractures

1. <u>Proximal Humeral fractures</u> (most commonly seen in the elderly)
    a. Mechanisms of injury
        (1) Fall on the outstretched arm (most common)
        (2) Direct blow to the lateral aspect of the arm.
    b. **Clinical picture** — the patient is usually an elderly, osteoporotic woman who presents with severe upper arm and shoulder pain following a fall; she is likely to be holding the arm in adduction.
    c. Neer classification system [See <u>Tintinalli's Text,</u> Fifth ed., p. 1790, Fig. 263-10 or Sixth ed., p.1700, Fig. 271-8] — is an anatomical classification system for proximal humeral fractures.
        (1) It classifies proximal humeral fractures according to the amount of <u>displacement</u>* of four segments:
            (a) Anatomic neck
            (b) Surgical neck
            (c) Greater tuberosity
            (d) Lesser tuberosity
        (2) Major categories:
            (a) <u>One-part</u> (= minimally displaced) <u>fractures</u> — demonstrate no displacement (as defined below).* These fractures account for 80 to 85% of all proximal humeral fractures.
            (b) <u>Two-part fractures</u> — demonstrate displacement of only one fragment.
            (c) <u>Three-part fractures</u> — demonstrate the displacement of two individual fragments from the remaining proximal humerus.
            (d) <u>Four-part fractures</u> — demonstrate displacement of all four segments.
    d. Treatment — In general, the amount of displacement determines how these fractures are managed. AP, lateral and axillary (if possible) views are essential to make an accurate diagnosis.
        (1) One-part fractures → immobilization with shoulder immobilizer, sling and swath or a Velpeau's dressing, analgesics and referral for orthopedic follow-up.
        (2) Two-, three- and four-part fractures → immobilize as above and obtain emergent orthopedic referral. Many of these fractures will require surgical repair. Four-part fractures may require the insertion of a prosthesis.

*Displacement refers to fragment separation > 1cm or angulation > 45°.

e. Complications and associated injuries
(1) Adhesive capsulitis ("frozen shoulder") — is the most common complication and can be minimized or prevented by early mobilization exercises.
(2) Associated neurovascular injuries (brachial plexus, axillary nerve and axillary artery) should be ruled out in all proximal humeral fractures, particularly surgical neck fractures (as well as fracture-dislocations.)
(3) <u>Posterior</u> shoulder dislocations frequently accompany fractures of the <u>lesser</u> tuberosity due to intense contraction of the subscapularis muscle which inserts at this location; anterior and posterior dislocations occur in association with three-and four-part fractures.
(4) Avascular necrosis of the humeral head — frequently complicates anatomical neck fractures, four-part fractures and fractures of articular surfaces.

2. <u>Humeral Shaft fractures</u>
a. Mechanisms of injury
(1) Direct blow (most common)
(2) Fall on an outstretched arm or elbow
(3) Pathologic fractures (particularly from metastatic breast cancer) are also common
b. The fracture usually involves the <u>middle</u> third of the humeral shaft.
c. Associated injuries
(1) Most common associated injury is damage to the <u>radial nerve</u> → wrist drop (inability to extend the wrist, fingers and thumb) and loss of sensation in the first dorsal web space.
(a) Nerve damage occurring at the time of injury is often due to <u>neuropraxia</u> and resolves spontaneously in most cases.
(b) Nerve palsy occurring after manipulation or immobilization is generally due to nerve entrapment and requires <u>immediate</u> surgical exploration.
(2) Ulnar and median nerve injury may also occur but are much less common.
(3) Brachial artery injury
d. Treatment
(1) Most of these fractures are managed <u>non</u>operatively with one of the following:
(a) A coaptation ("sugar-tong") splint plus sling and swathe — for <u>non</u>displaced fractures
(b) A hanging cast — for displaced or angulated fractures
(2) Operative management is usually reserved for patients with neurovascular compromise, soft-tissue interposition, pathologic fractures or transverse fractures.
e. Complications
(1) Delayed union — is common and may necessitate prolonged immobilization.
(2) Adhesive capsulitis (stiff/frozen shoulder) — may be prevented by early initiation of circumduction exercises.

D. Elbow Injuries

1. Fractures
    a. Radiographic findings helpful in diagnosing occult elbow fractures that may be detected on the lateral x-ray view of the elbow:
        (1) Fat pad signs
            (a) <u>Posterior fat pad sign</u> — is never seen on a normal x-ray. Its presence indicates distension of the joint capsule by effusion (hemarthrosis) and probable fracture.
            (b) <u>Anterior fat pad sign</u> — not as useful diagnostically as the posterior fat pad sign since a small one is present on many normal x-rays. However, superior and anterior displacement of this fat pad suggests a probable fracture.
        (2) Anterior humeral line — a line drawn along the anterior surface of the humerus and extending through the elbow — is helpful in detecting subtle supracondylar fractures; this line normally transects the middle of the capitellum but, with supracondylar <u>extension</u> fractures, transects the anterior third of the capitellum or passes completely anterior to it.
    b. <u>Supracondylar fractures</u>
        (1) More common in children < 15 years old.
        (2) Two types
            (a) Supracondylar <u>extension</u> fractures
                <u>1</u> Most common type
                <u>2</u> Generally results from a fall on the outstretched arm with the elbow in extension or hyperextension.
                <u>3</u> The <u>distal</u> humeral fragment is displaced <u>posteriorly</u>, thus placing the sharp fracture fragments anteriorly, potentially injuring the brachial artery and median nerve, producing weakness of the flexor muscles of the hand + loss of two-point discrimination of the fingertips (especially the index and middle fingertips). Radial and ulnar nerve injury can also occur. Deficits that occur at the time of injury are usually neuropraxias, which resolve over time.
                <u>4</u> These fractures may result in a compartment syndrome of the forearm (Volkmann's ischemia) which, if not treated promptly, will result in Volkmann's ischemic contracture. (See p. 439 in this chapter for further discussion of this topic.)
                <u>5</u> Treatment
                    <u>a</u> Obtain emergent orthopedic consultation.
                    <u>b</u> <u>Nondisplaced</u> fractures should be immobilized in a posterior splint (axilla to palm) with the elbow flexed 90°. Patients may be discharged to home if close neurovascular observation and early orthopedic follow-up can be assured. Parents should be advised to return immediately if pain is unmanageable with OTC medications or the child becomes unable to extend all the fingers of the affected extremity.

  <u>c</u> Displaced fractures require <u>prompt</u> reduction, followed by percutaneous pin fixation or internal fixation by an orthopedic surgeon; however, if vascular compromise threatening the viability of the extremity is present, the ED physician may make one attempt at reducing the fracture. Patients with these fractures should be hospitalized, as delayed swelling leading to neurovascular compromise is common.

(b) Supracondylar <u>flexion</u> fractures

 <u>1</u> Usually result from a direct blow to the posterior aspect of the flexed elbow.

 <u>2</u> The <u>distal</u> humeral fragment is displaced <u>anteriorly</u>.

 <u>3</u> These fractures are frequently open, but associated vascular injuries are uncommon.

 <u>4</u> Ulnar nerve injury is the most commonly associated complication.

 <u>5</u> Treatment

  <u>a</u> <u>Non</u>displaced fractures are treated with splint immobilization and early orthopedic follow-up.

  <u>b</u> Displaced fractures require emergent orthopedic consultation for reduction and percutaneous pinning; open reduction is often required for completely displaced fractures.

c. <u>Olecranon fractures</u>

(1) Mechanism of injury

(a) Direct blow to the point of the elbow

(b) Fall on the outstretched hand with the elbow in flexion

(2) Exam reveals swelling and tenderness over the olecranon and inability to extend the elbow against gravity or resistance due to inadequacy of the triceps mechanism.

(3) Associated injury of the <u>ulnar nerve</u> (paresthesias and numbness in the ulnar nerve distribution or weakness of the interossei muscles) is common; it is usually secondary to ulnar nerve contusion and resolves spontaneously over time.

(4) Treatment

(a) Nondisplaced fractures → elbow immobilization in 30° flexion.

(b) Fractures with > 2mm displacement → emergent orthopedic referral for surgical repair (open reduction with int. fixation).

d. <u>Condylar fractures</u>

(1) The distal humerus is composed of the medial and lateral condyles, each of which has an <u>articular</u> and <u>non</u>articular surface.

(a) Articular surfaces

 <u>1</u> Trochlea (on the medial condyle)

 <u>2</u> Capitellum (on the lateral condyle)

(b) <u>Non</u>articular surfaces

 <u>1</u> Medial epicondyle

 <u>2</u> Lateral epicondyle

(2) Condylar fractures usually involve <u>both</u> the articular surface (trochlea, capitellum) and the nonarticular surface (epicondyle) of the distal humerus.

      (3) Fractures of the lateral condyle are more common than those of the medial condyle.

      (4) Treatment

         (a) Nondisplaced or minimally displaced fractures → immobilization in 90° elbow flexion with forearm supination (lateral condylar fracture) or pronation (medial condylar fracture) and orthopedic referral

         (b) Fractures with > 3mm displacement → surgical fixation

  e. <u>Articular surface fractures</u> (trochlea and capitellum)

      (1) Mechanism of injury

         (a) Trochlea and capitellum fractures usually occur in association with posterior elbow dislocations.

         (b) Capitellum fractures can also result from a fall on the outstretched hand.

      (2) Treatment

         (a) Nondisplaced fractures — splint immobilization

         (b) Displaced fractures (even if minimal) — emergent orthopedic consultation and surgical repair

  f. <u>Epicondylar fractures</u>

      (1) Most commonly seen in children

      (2) Medial epicondylar fractures

         (a) Avulsion fractures of the medial epicondyle most often occur in association with posterior elbow dislocations in children and adolescents, but can also occur as a result of repeated valgus stress of the elbow in adolescents ("little leaguer's elbow") as well as from a direct blow.

         (b) These patients must be evaluated for <u>ulnar nerve</u> injury (present in 60% of patients).

         (c) Treatment

            <u>1</u> Nondisplaced (or minimally displaced) fractures → immobilization

            <u>2</u> Displaced fractures → orthopedic referral and surgical reduction if fragment displaced > 3 to 5mm or if they are intra-articular

      (3) Lateral epicondylar fractures

         (a) Are rare and generally result from a direct blow.

         (b) These fractures are generally nondisplaced and are treated with immobilization.

2. Dislocations

  a. <u>Posterior elbow</u> dislocations

      (1) Are the most common type of elbow dislocations.

      (2) Mechanism of injury: fall on the extended (or hyperextended) and <u>ab</u>ducted arm.

      (3) Physical findings: marked swelling with 45° flexion of the joint and posterior prominence of the olecranon.

      (4) Best demonstrated on the lateral x-ray of the elbow [<u>Tintinalli's Text,</u> Fifth ed., p.1764, Fig. 261-1 or Sixth ed., p. 1685, Fig. 270-1]

(5) Associated injuries
    (a) Fractures about the elbow (occur in 30 to 60% of cases)
    (b) Injuries to the ulnar and median nerves (common)
    (c) Brachial artery injury (occurs in up to 8% of cases — should be suspect when a large opening between the tip of the olecranon and the distal humerus is palpated on exam or seen on x-ray)

(6) Treatment — is reduction, which should be accomplished by the orthopedic surgeon without delay. If vascular compromise is present or orthopedic assistance is not available in a timely fashion, reduction* should be accomplished by the emergency physician. Neurovascular status should be assessed prior to and following reduction.
    (a) Provide conscious sedation.
    (b) Apply traction distally at the wrist while an assistant immobilizes the humerus.
    (c) While maintaining traction at the wrist, flex the elbow and apply posterior pressure to the distal humerus.
    (d) A "clunk" will be heard or felt as the elbow is reduced and the articular surfaces mesh.
    (e) Move the elbow through its full range of motion to check stability and then reassess the neurovascular status.
    (f) Immobilize the elbow in a long-arm posterior splint in 120° of flexion (full flexion) and obtain post-reduction films.
    (g) Observe (preferably in the hospital) for the development of delayed vascular compromise.

b. Anterior elbow dislocations (uncommon)
    (1) Mechanism of injury: a blow to the olecranon with the elbow in flexion.
    (2) Physical findings: the forearm is elongated and supinated while the elbow is generally held in full extension.
    (3) Associated injuries
        (a) There is a much higher incidence of vascular impairment than with posterior dislocations.
        (b) Associated avulsion of the triceps mechanism is common.
    (4) Treatment* — Once the neurovascular status has been assessed and conscious sedation provided, an assistant immobilizes the humerus while the physician applies in-line traction to the wrist (with one hand) and downward and backward pressure to the proximal forearm (with the other hand).

c. A severe disruption of the elbow joint with any type of dislocation may be accompanied by injury to the brachial artery and should be suspected when a wide opening (olecranon to distal humerus) is palpated or seen on a lateral x-ray. [Rosen's Text, Fourth ed., p. 706, Fig. 43-24 or Fifth ed., p. 572, Fig. 45-24]

---

*Elbow dislocations may have associated fractures that may block reduction or render it unstable. Because of this (and the potential for significant neurovascular sequelae) consultation with an orthopedic surgeon should be obtained (if at all possible) in an emergent situation prior to attempted reduction.

d. Radial head subluxation (Nursemaid's elbow)
  (1) Subluxation of the radial head (without associated ulnar fracture) occurs with some regularity in children < 5 years old.
  (2) Mechanism of injury — abrupt longitudinal traction on the hand or forearm with the arm in pronation pulls the annular ligament over the radial head (annulus).
  (3) Clinical presentation — The child presents with his arm dangling at his side, unwilling to move it; the elbow is flexed and the arm is held in passive pronation. There is resistance to and pain with full supination and with direct palpation over the radial head.
  (4) X-rays (if obtained) are usually normal. They are only helpful in excluding other diagnoses and should only be ordered when the history is unclear or reduction is unsuccessful.
  (5) Reduction is accomplished by placing the thumb of one hand on the radial head and using the other hand to supinate the forearm and flex the elbow. A click is often palpated over the radial head as it reduces; (full pronation with elbow flexion has also been described and may be less painful.) Unless the subluxation was prolonged, the child should be asymptomatic and using his arm normally within 5 - 10 minutes post-reduction. Immobilization post-reduction is unnecessary in most cases.

E. Radial and Ulnar Injuries

1. Radial Head fracture
  a. Often results from a fall on the outstretched hand.
  b. Examination — reveals tenderness and swelling over the radial head; pain is increased with forearm supination; also check for distal radio-lunar dissociation (Essex-Lopresti lesion).
  c. Although nondisplaced fractures may not be visible on initial x-ray evaluation, a bulging anterior fat pad sign or a posterior fat pad sign is usually present, suggesting the diagnosis.
  d. Associated injury to the articular surface of the capitellum is common.
  e. Treatment is determined by the type of fracture present.
    (1) Nondisplaced fractures — are treated with sling immobilization followed by early range of motion exercises as tolerated. If the swelling is very painful, the joint may be aspirated through the posterolateral triangle, but this is rarely necessary.
    (2) Comminuted and displaced fractures — are treated with immobilization in a long-arm posterior splint and early (2 - 5 days) orthopedic referral for screw fixation or radial head excision (with or without silastic implant) if one of the following exists:
      (a) Marked comminution of the fracture
      (b) Angulation of the articular surface that is > 30°
      (c) > 2mm offset in a two-part fracture
      (d) Fracture involving more than one-third of the articular surface

2. Galeazzi fracture
   a. This is a fracture of the distal radial shaft associated with a distal radioulnar dislocation (radiographic signs may be subtle).
   b. Mechanisms of injury
      (1) Direct blow to the back of the wrist
      (2) Fall on the outstretched hand in forced pronation
   c. Treatment is open reduction and internal fixation.

3. Nightstick fracture
   a. This is an isolated fracture of the shaft of the ulna.
   b. Mechanism of injury — a direct blow to the subcutaneous border of the ulna that usually occurs when a patient raises his forearm up to protect his face from a blow
   c. Treatment
      (1) Nondisplaced fractures — immobilization in a long arm cast
      (2) Displaced fractures (those with >10° angulation or displacement > 50% of the diameter of the ulna) — orthopedic referral for open reduction and internal fixation

4. Monteggia's fracture
   a. A fracture of the proximal third of the ulna combined with dislocation of the radial head (usually anterior)
   b. Mechanisms of injury
      (1) Direct blow to the posterior aspect of the ulna
      (2) Fall on the outstretched hand with forearm in forced pronation
   c. The ulnar fracture is often apparent on AP and lateral views of the forearm, but the radial head dislocation is missed in as many as 25% of cases. This can be avoided by remembering to assess the alignment of the radial head with the capitellum; if the radial head is in its normal anatomic position, a line drawn through the radial shaft and head should intersect the capitellum in all views.
   d. Associated injury to the radial nerve is common.*
   e. Treatment — open reduction and internal fixation of the ulnar fracture followed by closed reduction of the radial head dislocation is the preferred treatment in adults and is associated with the best functional outcome. Children, however, can usually be treated with closed reduction under general anesthesia.

5. Fractures of both the radius and ulna
   a. Are usually displaced.
   b. Most common mechanism of injury — a direct blow to the forearm
   c. Associated injuries — peripheral nerve deficits (radial, ulnar and median) occur infrequently with closed injuries but can be seen with open fractures.
   d. Development of compartment syndrome should be a major concern.

*Usually resolves spontaneously in 6 - 8 weeks.

e. Treatment
   (1) Nondisplaced fractures (rare) → immobilization in a bivalved long arm cast
   (2) Displaced fractures → generally require open reduction and internal fixation with compression plates in adults. Children, however, can sometimes be treated with closed reduction.
f. Complications → compartment syndromes (both anterior and posterior), malunion and nonunion.

F. Hand and Wrist Injuries/Infections

1. Essential anatomy
   a. The eight carpal bones

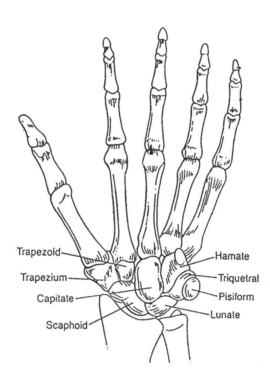

   b. The <u>ulnar nerve</u>
      (1) Runs deep to the flexor carpi ulnaris tendon and through Guyon's canal.
      (2) Innervates the following muscles:
         (a) Hypothenar eminence
         (b) Interosseous muscles
         (c) Lumbrical muscles of the ring and little fingers
         (d) Adductor pollicis brevis
         (e) In the forearm — the flexor carpi ulnaris and ulnar aspect of the flexor digitorum profundus

(3) Provides sensation to palmar and dorsal aspects of the ulnar side of the hand, the little finger and the ulnar half of the ring finger.

(4) Testing

    (a) Motor test of normal function → abduction of fingers against resistance (patient can spread fingers apart).

    (b) Sensation → is best tested over the volar tip of the <u>little</u> finger.

(5) Loss of ulnar nerve function → inability to hold a piece of paper between fingers (early) or claw hand (late).

c. The <u>median nerve</u>

(1) Runs through the carpal tunnel between the flexor carpi radialis and the palmaris longus.

(2) Innervates the following muscles:

    (a) Pronator teres

    (b) Flexor carpi radialis

    (c) Flexor digitorum superficialis and profundus (radial part)

    (d) Flexor pollicis longus

    (e) Pronator quadratus

(3) The thenar motor branch supplies the

    (a) Abductor pollicis brevis

    (b) Opponens pollicis

    (c) Flexor pollicis brevis

(4) The common digital branches — innervate the lumbrical muscles of the index and middle fingers

(5) Provides sensation to the palm on the radial side of the hand and the palmar aspect of the radial three and one-half fingers as well as the dorsal aspect of the tips of the index and middle fingers and the radial half of the ring finger.

(6) Testing

    (a) Motor test of normal function → opposition of the thumb to each finger while watching thenar muscles for contractions.

    (b) Sensation → is best tested over the volar tip of the <u>index</u> finger.

    (c) Loss of median nerve function → carpal tunnel syndrome. With thenar atrophy in the late stages → monkey hand.

d. The <u>radial nerve</u>[*]

(1) Innervates the following muscles:

    (a) Triceps

    (b) Brachioradialis

    (c) Extensor carpi radialis longus

    (d) Extensor carpi radialis brevis

    (e) Supinator

    (f) Extensor digitorum communis

    (g) Extensor digiti minimi

    (h) Extensor carpi ulnaris

    (i) Abductor pollicis longus

    (j) Extensor pollicis brevis

    (k) Extensor pollicis longus

    (l) Extensor indicus proprium

[*]Does not innervate any of the intrinsic muscles of the hand.

(2) Provides sensation to the dorsum of the radial aspect of the hand, the dorsum of the thumb and the dorsal aspect of the index and middle fingers as well as the radial half of the ring finger as far distally as the PIP joints.

(3) Testing

(a) Motor test of normal function → extension of wrist and fingers against resistance

(b) Sensation → is best tested over the dorsal web space between the thumb and index finger.

(4) Primary function → extension of the wrist and metacarpophalangeal (MCP) joints

(5) Loss of radial nerve function → wrist drop; loss of finger extension.

e. The intrinsic muscles of the hand

(1) Thenar

(2) Hypothenar

(3) Abductor pollicis

(4) Lumbricals

(5) Interossei

f. The six groups of extrinsic extensor muscles

(1) Abductor pollicis longus + extensor pollicis brevis

(2) Extensor carpi radialis longus and brevis tendons

(3) Extensor pollicis longus tendon

(4) Extensor indices proprius + extensor digitorum communis

(5) Extensor digiti minimi

(6) Extensor carpi ulnaris

g. The extrinsic flexor muscles

(1) Flexor pollicis longus

(2) Flexor digitorum superficialis

(3) Flexor digitorum profundus

(4) Flexor carpi ulnaris

(5) Flexor carpi radialis

(6) Palmaris longus

2. Regional nerve blocks — can be particularly useful when treating finger and hand injuries.

a. Digital blocks

(1) Local infiltration into the restricted space of the finger is very painful and can impair capillary refill; digital blocks are, therefore, better than local infiltration for most finger injuries.

(2) Sensation to the finger (dorsal and volar surfaces and the interphalangeal joints) is provided by the palmar and dorsal digital nerves which run along the lateral aspects of each phalanx.

(3) Digital blocks are performed by using one of three approaches (each of which has advantages and disadvantages).

(a) Dorsal approach — needle is directed into the dorsum of the hand at the metacarpals.

(b) Palmar approach — needle is directed into the palm over the metacarpal head (very painful).

(c) Web space approach — needle is directed into the interdigital web space.

    b. Nerve blocks (wrist)
       (1) Are useful for extensive hand injuries (particularly the palm, which is very painful to inject into) and MCP joint injuries, but they require more time and training to learn and, therefore, are less commonly used.
       (2) Sensation to the hand is provided by the median, ulnar and radial nerves; therefore, if complete anesthesia of the hand is needed, all three of these nerves must be blocked (which means that multiple injections are required).
       (3) These blocks are performed on the volar aspect of the wrist at the proximal skin crease where the tendons are easily palpated and provide landmarks to guide the injections.

Note: More detailed information regarding the performance of these blocks can be found in Tintinalli's Text, Fifth ed., pp. 260-263 or Sixth ed., pp. 269-270 and in Roberts and Hedges Clinical Procedures in Emergency Medicine, Fourth ed., pp. 574-583.

  3. Infections in the hand
    a. Paronychia
       (1) Infection of the lateral nail fold that sometimes extends to involve the proximal nail fold (eponychium).
       (2) Causative agents are usually *Staph. aureus* or Strep.
       (3) Patients presenting early with cellulitis may respond to oral antibiotics (a penicillinase-resistant oral penicillin or a first-generation cephalosporin) and warm soaks alone.
       (4) If purulent material is present, the nail fold should be incised and drained; this should be followed by daily warm soaks; use antibiotics only if a surrounding cellulitis is present.
       (5) If subungual pus is present, the adjacent portion of the nail should be removed.
    b. Felon
       (1) Infection of the pulp space of the fingertip
       (2) Causative agent is usually *Staph. aureus*
       (3) Treatment — incision and drainage at the point of maximum tenderness and fluctuance:
         (a) Make a central longitudinal incision starting one-half cm. distal to the distal flexion crease (to avoid the flexor tendon sheath) and extending into the pulp space. This approach is preferred due to fewer long-term complications.
         (b) Pack the wound, splint the finger and start the patient on an oral antistaphylococcal antibiotic.
         (c) Remove the packing in 48 - 72 hours and start warm soaks.
       (4) Complications
         (a) Flexor tenosynovitis and osteomyelitis
         (b) Skin instability, loss of sensation and a disrupted pad also may occur but are infrequent when the central longitudinal approach is used.

c. <u>Herpetic Whitlow</u>
   (1) A <u>viral</u> infection of the distal finger
   (2) Caused by the herpes simplex virus (type I or type II)
   (3) Typically occurs in health care providers with exposure to oral secretions and in patients with coexistent herpes infections.
   (4) Presentation — localized burning, itching and pain precede the development of the classic clear herpetic vesicles; typically, only one finger is involved.
   (5) Diagnosis — can usually be made clinically, but if doubt remains or the presentation is atypical, it can be confirmed with Tzanck smear (reveals multinucleated giant cells) or viral culture.
   (6) Treatment
      (a) Splinting, elevation and analgesics for pain relief
      (b) An oral antiviral agent effective against herpes simplex (e.g. acyclovir, famciclovir) if patient is seen early in the course of the infection (or is immunocompromised)
      (c) A dry dressing and instructions to prevent autoinoculation or transmission to others
      (d) Surgical drainage is <u>contraindicated</u>; it can result in secondary infection and delayed healing.
d. <u>Human bite infections involving the MCP joint</u> ("fight bites")
   (1) Can result in severe complications including deep palmar space infections, functional loss and amputation; these wounds must be aggressively treated and associated tendon injuries must be ruled out.
   (2) These injuries commonly result from punching someone in the mouth. (Beware, many patients initially deny this mechanism of injury.)
   (3) A common mistake is to suture a human bite laceration over the metacarpophalangeal (MCP) joint; these lacerations should <u>never</u> be closed primarily but allowed to heal by secondary intention.
   (4) Frequently found pathogens include anaerobes (especially *Eikenella corrodens* and anaerobic Streptococcus), *Staph. aureus* and Neisseria species.*
   (5) Treatment
      (a) Consult with an orthopedic surgeon.
      (b) Obtain x-rays to R/O fractures and retained foreign bodies.
      (c) Obtain aerobic and anaerobic wound cultures.
      (d) Irrigate the joint with normal saline.
      (e) Splint and elevate the hand.
      (f) Hospitalize the patient and start IV antibiotics (ampicillin/sulbactam).
e. <u>Pyogenic flexor tenosynovitis</u>
   (1) Typically results from a puncture wound
   (2) Causative agents are usually *Staph. aureus* or Strep.
   (3) Diagnosis is based on the presence of Kanavel's four cardinal signs of flexor tenosynovitis

*Prophylaxis with amoxicillin/clavulanate may prevent this complication.

        (a) Finger held in slight flexion

        (b) Symmetric swelling of the finger

        (c) Tenderness along the flexor tendon sheath

        (d) Pain with passive extension of the finger

    (4) Treatment

        (a) Hospitalization and emergent orthopedic/hand consultation for surgical drainage

        (b) IV antibiotics

           <u>1</u> If the tenosynovitis was caused by penetrating trauma → penicillinase-resistant antistaphylococcal penicillin or a first-generation cephalosporin.

           <u>2</u> If there is no history (or evidence) of trauma in a sexually active adult, consider disseminated GC and treat empirically with ceftriaxone until culture results are available.

        (c) Elevation and splinting

        (d) Tetanus prophylaxis as needed

  f. <u>Deep palmar space infection</u>

    (1) Is characterized by swelling and tenderness that is localized to the palmar space.

    (2) Treatment is incision and drainage in the operating room and IV antibiotics.

4. High-pressure injection injuries (are true surgical emergencies).

  a. A 1 - 3mm wound caused by a grease or paint gun is the hallmark of a high-pressure injection injury. The fluid frequently travels down the tendon sheath and damages the flexor tendon with tenderness typically present along the course of injection.

  b. The prognosis of these injuries is poor despite the deceptively normal appearance of the hand on initial presentation; up to 70% of these injuries result in some form of amputation and several months of lost work time despite early and aggressive management. Factors affecting prognosis include:

    (1) Location of entry wound and the underlying anatomy affected.

    (2) Physical and chemical qualities of the substance injected (viscosity, corrosiveness); substances that are <u>low</u> in viscosity and corrosive in nature (paint solvents) produce the most damage.

    (3) Velocity of injection; the higher the velocity the greater the penetration.

    (4) Duration of exposure to the injected substance; the greater the duration of exposure, the worse the prognosis.

  c. Treatment

    (1) Obtain an x-ray to determine the degree of spread of material injected; it may be radiopaque. [Harwood-Nuss, 3rd. ed., Fig. 121-1]

    (2) Splint and elevate the extremity.

    (3) Administer a parenteral broad-spectrum antibiotic.

    (4) Update tetanus prophylaxis as indicated.

    (5) Provide oral or parenteral analgesia.
       (Note: Digital blocks are contraindicated → increased tissue pressure → vascular compromise)

    (6) Obtain <u>immediate</u> orthopedic consult for operative debridement.

5. Carpal injuries
   a. Scaphoid (navicular) fracture
      (1) Is the most common carpal fracture.
      (2) Mechanism of injury — fall on the outstretched hand
      (3) Initial AP, lateral and scaphoid x-ray views of the wrist may not demonstrate a fracture in $\geq 10\%$ of cases. Repeat x-rays of the wrist in 2 weeks will often demonstrate the fracture line.
      (4) Clinical findings of a fracture include:
         (a) Tenderness in the region of the anatomic snuff box
         (b) Pain referred to the anatomic snuff box with longitudinal compression of the thumb or with supination of the hand against resistance.
         [If these findings are present, treat as a fracture.]
      (5) Treatment
         (a) Nondisplaced and clinically-suspected fracture — immobilization in a thumb spica cast or splint and referral to an orthopedist.
         (b) Displaced fractures — usually require open reduction and fixation.
      (6) Complications
         (a) Avascular necrosis of the proximal fragment (the more proximal, oblique or displaced the fracture, the greater the risk because the vascular supply enters the distal part of the bone.)
         (b) Delayed union, malunion and nonunion
   b. Triquetrum dorsal chip fracture
      (1) Is the second most common carpal fracture
      (2) Mechanisms of injury
         (a) Fall on the outstretched hand
         (b) Direct blow to the dorsum of the hand
      (3) Clinical finding — tenderness immediately distal to the ulnar styloid on the dorsal aspect of the wrist
      (4) Best visualized on the lateral view of the wrist
      (5) Treatment — immobilization in a volar splint
   c. Lunate fracture
      (1) Is the third most common carpal fracture
      (2) Mechanism of injury — a fall on the outstretched hand
      (3) Clinical findings — pain and tenderness over the middorsum of the wrist that is increased by axial compression of the third metacarpal.
      (4) Plain x-rays of the wrist are often normal; therefore, treatment should be initiated on clinical grounds alone.
      (5) Treatment — immobilization in a thumb spica cast and orthopedic referral.
      (6) Avascular necrosis of the proximal segment (Kienbock's disease) is a serious complication of these fractures; it is seen most often in patients with congenital shortening of the lunate but it also results from inadequate immobilization of a lunate fracture.

    d. Dislocations

       (1) Mechanism of injury — violent hyperextension

       (2) All are referred to an orthopedic surgeon

       (3) <u>Lunate dislocation</u>

         (a) The lunate may dislocate either volarly (most common) or dorsally [<u>Tintinalli's Text,</u> Fifth ed., p. 1778, Fig. 262-7 A and B <u>or</u> Sixth ed., p. 1680 Fig. 269-8 A and B]

         (b) There is pain, swelling and marked loss of flexion with the wrist, hand and arm held in anatomic position. Occasionally, the patient complains of tingling in the three radial digits (acute carpal tunnel syndrome).

         (c) Findings on wrist x-ray [<u>Rosen's Text,</u> Fourth ed., p. 677, Fig. 42-12 A and B <u>or</u> Fifth ed., p. 543, Fig. 44-12 A and B]:

           <u>1</u> The diagnosis may be suggested on the AP view: the lunate is normally squarish in appearance but, when it dislocates, it becomes triangular in shape ("piece of pie" sign). There is also foreshortening of the wrist and loss of the normal space between the capitate and the lunate.

           <u>2</u> The diagnosis is confirmed by a good lateral view which demonstrates displacement of the lunate volarly relative to the capitate and carpus, which remain in their normal alignment ("spilled teacup" sign).

         (d) Associated scaphoid injuries are common.

       (4) <u>Perilunate dislocation</u> (most common wrist dislocation)

         (a) This may be associated with a fracture or dislocation of the scaphoid. The lunate remains in anatomic position relative to the forearm while the capitate is displaced dorsally due to disarticulation of the capitolunate joint. [<u>Tintinalli's Text,</u> Fifth ed., p. 1777 Fig. 262-6 A and B <u>or</u> Sixth ed., p. 1679, Fig. 269-7 A and B]

         (b) As with a lunate dislocation, a perilunate dislocation is best diagnosed by a true lateral film of the wrist. [<u>Rosen's Text,</u> Fourth ed., p. 676, Fig. 42-11 <u>or</u> Fifth ed., p. 542, Fig. 44-11]

       (5) <u>Scapholunate dislocation</u>

         (a) Clinical clues: pain with wrist hyperextension and a snapping sensation when the wrist is deviated in either the radial or ulnar direction.

         (b) Radiologic signs [<u>Rosen's Text,</u> Fourth ed., p. 675, Fig. 42-10 <u>or</u> Fifth ed., p. 541, Fig. 44-10]

           <u>1</u> AP film:

             <u>a</u> The scaphoid is foreshortened and has a dense ring-shaped image around its distal edge ("signet ring" sign).

             <u>b</u> There is a widening > 3mm in the space between the lunate and scaphoid ("Terry Thomas" sign).

           <u>2</u> Lateral film: the angle between the scaphoid and the lunate is increased (> 60 degrees).

         (c) Place the arm in a radial gutter splint or posterior mold for orthopedic referral.

6. Metacarpal injuries
   a. Metacarpal neck fractures
      (1) Result from a punch with a clenched fist.
      (2) Almost all are unstable.
      (3) The <u>proximal</u> fragment angulates in the <u>dorsal</u> direction while the <u>distal</u> fragment angulates in the <u>volar</u> direction.
      (4) The amount of <u>angulation</u> that is acceptable varies directly with the normal mobility of the involved metacarpal; the greater the mobility of the metacarpal, the greater the degree of angulation that can be tolerated.
         (a) Metacarpal neck fractures of the ring and little fingers ("Boxer's fracture"); up to 20 and 40 degrees of angulation, respectively is acceptable.
         (b) Metacarpal neck fracture of the index and long fingers; ≤ 15 degrees of angulation is acceptable.
      (5) Rotational deformities, if present, must be completely corrected; look for malalignment of the plane of the fingernails when the fingers are viewed in the partially flexed position [<u>Tintinalli's Text,</u> Fourth ed., p. 1225, Fig. 224-18; not found in Fifth or Sixth edition.]
   b. MCP joint dislocations
      (1) MCP dislocations of fingers are rare while those of the thumb are relatively common.
      (2) They are usually dorsal and result from hyperextension forces.
      (3) Types of MCP dislocations:
         (a) Simple (= subluxation)
         (b) Complex (= complete dislocation)
      (4) X-rays
         (a) Should be taken both pre-and post-reduction to R/O associated fractures and confirm adequate reduction.
         (b) The lateral view usually demonstrates an obvious dislocation.
      (5) Treatment — is determined by the type of dislocation present:
         (a) Simple dislocations — Following adequate anesthesia,* these dislocations can usually be managed with closed reduction, splinting in flexion and referral to a hand surgeon.
         (b) Complex dislocations — often cannot be reduced by closed reduction because of interposition of the volar plate in the MCP joint or entrapment of the metacarpal head between the lumbrical tendon and a flexor tendon. Irreducible MCP joint dislocations should be splinted and referred to a hand surgeon for open reduction and operative repair.
      (6) Complications of MCP joint injuries include:
         (a) Volar plate injuries
         (b) Bony avulsions
         (c) Thickening and stiffness of the joint
         (d) Bennett's fracture/subluxation → An unstable fracture at the base of the first metacarpal, often caused by punching; it should be suspected when evaluating a "sprained thumb."

*Adequate anesthesia of the MCP joint requires a wrist block of the ulna, median and/or radial nerves, depending on which finger is involved.

7. Gamekeeper's or skier's thumb (torn <u>ulnar</u> collateral ligament)
   a. Mechanism of injury — acute and forceful radial deviation of the thumb; commonly occurs in skiing accidents when the ski pole forcefully abducts the thumb at the MCP joint as the hand hits the ground in a fall.
   b. Examination — reveals tenderness along the ulnar aspect of the thumb, which is most exquisite at the MCP joint. Thumb grasp and pinch are weak.
   c. Obtain x-rays of the thumb to R/O associated fractures (present in up to 30% of cases).
   d. Assess joint stability:
      (1) Apply a lateral stress (abduction) to the MCP joint of the injured thumb (following adequate anesthesia).*
      (2) Stress the normal thumb in the same manner.
      (3) The presence of ≥ 10° - 20° of laxity in the injured thumb when compared to the normal thumb is consistent with a complete tear and requires surgical repair.
   e. Treatment — is based upon the degree of joint stability:
      (1) Incomplete tear (some stability: < 10° laxity) → thumb spica cast or splint (for 3 - 6 weeks) and follow-up with a hand surgeon.
      (2) Complete tear (no stability: ≥ 10° - 20° laxity) → surgical repair

8. Distal forearm fractures
   a. <u>Colles' fracture</u>
      (1) Transverse fracture of the metaphysis of the distal radius with <u>dorsal</u> displacement of the distal fragment.
      (2) Mechanism of injury — a fall on the outstretched hand
      (3) Exam reveals the classic "dinner fork" deformity of the wrist produced by the dorsal displacement of the fracture.
      (4) Associated injuries:
         (a) Ulnar styloid fracture (present in 60% of cases)
         (b) Median nerve injury
      (5) Treatment
         (a) Nondisplaced fractures → immobilize in a long arm cast or coaptation (sugar-tong) splint and refer to an orthopedic surgeon for follow-up.
         (b) Displaced fractures → require prompt reduction, usually accomplished with traction (using Chinese finger traps) and manipulation; it should be followed by a coaptation (sugar-tong) splint or cast immobilization and orthopedic referral. Adequate local anesthesia can be achieved by injecting 5 - 10mL of lidocaine directly into the hematoma of the fracture at the fracture site.
            <u>1</u> Immobilization should ultimately be in slight flexion and ulnar deviation to maintain/restore the normal length and tilt of the radius.
            <u>2</u> If a cast is applied, it should be split (bivalved) prior to the patient being discharged.

*You must learn how to do this; failure to diagnose this injury may result in chronic instability of the thumb and debilitating osteoarthritis.

b. Smith's fracture
   (1) Transverse fracture of the distal radial metaphysis with <u>volar</u> displacement of the distal fragment.
   (2) Mechanisms of injury
       (a) Fall on the outstretched hand with the forearm in supination
       (b) Direct blow to the dorsum of the distal radius or wrist with the hand flexed and the forearm pronated.
   (3) Associated injury of the median nerve should be ruled out.
   (4) Treatment — Following adequate anesthesia (hematoma block), these fractures are reduced with traction (using Chinese finger traps) and manipulation; this is followed by immobilization in a long-arm splint or cast and referral to orthopedics for follow-up.

9. Tendon injuries
   a. General principles of evaluation:
       (1) First, observe the resting posture of the hand; any change in the normal flexion cascade is suspicious for a tendon injury.
       (2) Second, examine the wound with the hand/finger in the position it was in at the time of the injury; this will aid you in determining the location of the tendon injury relative to the skin laceration (if present).
       (3) Finally, evaluate the wound/tendon as the hand/finger is taken through its full range of motion.
   b. <u>Flexor tendon injuries</u> — should be repaired (in the OR) by an orthopedic surgeon. These tendons are most often injured in association with lacerations. Closed traumatic disruption, however, can also occur. A common example is the "jersey finger" in which the flexor digitorum profundus tendon is avulsed when one football player grabs the jersey of another and his finger gets caught. Examination of the flexor tendons is as follows:
       (1) <u>Flexor digitorum profundus tendon</u> — Immobilize the PIP and MCP joints in extension and ask the patient to flex the tip of the finger; inability to flex the DIP joint indicates a profundus tear which is usually associated with a volar plate slip at the PIP joint.
       (2) <u>Flexor digitorum superficialis tendon</u> — Hold the uninjured fingers in extension and ask the patient to flex the injured finger; this blocks the action of the profundus tendon and allows an isolated test of the superficialis tendon.
   <u>Note</u>: It is not adequate merely to test the function of these tendons as patients with 90% full-thickness lacerations will still have normal (although painful) range of motion. These partial tears are detected by evaluating the <u>strength</u> of these tendons against resistance; patients with partial tears will have weakness <u>against resistance</u>. Direct visualization of the tendon <u>through the entire range of motion</u> is crucial. Treatment of partial tendon lacerations is controversial and should be determined in consultation with an orthopedic surgeon. Many are treated with protective splinting alone.

ORTHOPEDIC

c. <u>Extensor tendon injuries</u> — are usually closed. (Be able to identify on pictorial)
  (1) <u>Mallet finger</u>
    (a) Extensor tendon laceration or disruption at the DIP joint (may or may not be associated with avulsion chip fracture).
    (b) The patient is unable to extend the DIP joint actively.
    (c) Mechanism of injury — is usually a blow to the tip of the extended finger producing sudden forced flexion.
    (d) Treatment
      <u>1</u> If there is no associated fracture → splint the DIP in <u>extension to slight hyperextension</u> for 6 - 8 weeks.
      <u>2</u> If there is an associated fracture → the treatment is either splinting as above or surgical pinning of the avulsed fragment using Kirschner wire fixation.
    (e) A delayed complication of an old untreated mallet finger is the "swan neck deformity" in which there is hyperextension of the PIP joint in addition to the mallet flexion deformity of the DIP joint. It is the result of increased extension forces on the PIP joint and is produced by proximal and dorsal migration of the lateral bands.
  (2) <u>Boutonnière deformity</u>
    (a) Rupture of the central slip of the extensor tendon at the PIP.
    (b) The deformity is characterized by flexion of the PIP joint and hyperextension of the DIP joint.
    (c) Mechanism of injury — a direct blow to (or laceration of) the PIP joint or forced flexion of the PIP joint against resistance.
    (d) This deformity is not always present immediately after the injury but, rather, often develops over time (1 - 2 weeks post-injury) because the lateral bands of the extensor tendon slip volar to the axis of the PIP joint and so become paradoxical flexors of this joint.
    (e) Treatment: Splint the PIP in extension and then refer to an orthopedic/hand surgeon for possible operative repair.
d. <u>De Quervain's stenosing tenosynovitis</u>
  (1) This is an inflammation of the extensor tendons of the thumb:
    (a) Abductor pollicis longus
    (b) Extensor pollicis brevis
  (2) Patients present with the complaint of pain along the radial aspect of the wrist that is exacerbated with use of the thumb. Palpation reveals tenderness over the radial styloid.
  (3) Mechanism of injury — overuse of the thumb
  (4) A positive <u>Finkelstein's test</u> (pain on ulnar deviation of the wrist while the thumb is flexed and held in the palm by the other fingers) confirms the diagnosis.

(5) Treatment
    (a) Administer an oral NSAID.
    (b) Splint in position of function.
    (c) Inject the first dorsal compartment with a marcaine and triamcinolone combination; this can be done on the initial evaluation or reserved for those patients who, on follow-up, have failed conservative therapy. [Note: Repeated injections are associated with a risk of subsequent tendon rupture.]

10. Compartment syndrome (Volkmann's ischemia) of the upper extremity
  a. Usually involves the flexor (volar) compartment of the forearm.
  b. Arises from increased pressure in the muscle compartment of the limb (forearm) that compromises the circulation to the muscles and nerves of that compartment.
  c. It can be precipitated by an increase in compartment contents, a decrease in compartment size or externally applied pressure. Causes include:
    (1) Supracondylar fracture of the elbow
    (2) Fracture of the radius and ulna
    (3) Forearm crush injury
    (4) Extravasation of blood into the forearm
    (5) Arterial injection of drugs
    (6) Constrictive dressing or cast
    (7) Burns
  d. Classic signs and symptoms:
    (1) **Pain** that is:
      (a) Out of proportion to the injury
      (b) Increased with passive stretching of the involved muscles
      (c) Increased with active contraction of the involved muscles
      [Note: These are the earliest findings.]
    (2) **Paresthesia** or hypesthesia of the nerves traversing the compartment (early finding)
    (3) **Paralysis** or paresis of the involved muscles
    (4) **Palpable tenseness and tenderness** of the compartment
    (5) **Pallor**, cyanosis or mottling of the skin (late finding)
    (6) **Pulselessness** or reduced distal pulses — rarely present (late finding)
  e. Management of suspected compartment syndrome:
    (1) Remove constrictive dressings or casts (if present).
    (2) Obtain immediate orthopedic consultation and measure intra-compartmental pressure.
    (3) Surgical decompression via fasciotomy is indicated if the pressure is > 30mmHg (normal pressure is < 10mmHg and typically near zero).
    [Note: Do not elevate the limb, as this does not significantly affect venous outflow and may further decrease perfusion.]
  f. If left untreated, compartment syndrome will result in Volkmann's ischemic contracture; affected muscles necrose and are replaced with fibrotic tissue, thus producing a paralyzed and deformed arm.

11. Amputated digits
    a. Preservation of the amputated part
        (1) After irrigating the amputated part with normal saline to remove gross contamination, wrap it in sterile gauze moistened with Ringer's lactate or saline and place it in a sterile, watertight container.
        (2) Store this container in ice water.
    b. Criteria for reimplantation:
        (1) A young, stable patient
        (2) A sharply incised wound with minimal associated damage
        (3) An amputated thumb
        (4) Multiple-digit amputation
        (5) Hand or forearm amputation
        (6) Amputation in a child
    c. Contraindications to reimplantation:
        (1) Absolute
            (a) Unstable patient with other life-threatening injuries
            (b) Severe crush injury
        (2) Relative
            (a) Severely damaged or contaminated part
            (b) Single-digit amputation (other than the thumb)
            (c) Avulsion injury
            (d) Serious underlying systemic illness (e.g. CHF, DM)
            (e) Prolonged warm ischemia ($\geq$ 12 hours)
            (f) Prior injury/surgery to affected part
            (g) Emotionally unstable patient

III. Pelvis and Hip Injuries

A. Essential Anatomy of the Pelvis

1. Pelvic bones: innominate (consists of the ilium, ischium and pubis), sacrum and coccyx.

2. On the AP view of the pelvis, the symphysis pubis is usually $\leq$ 5mm in width and the sacroiliac joint is normally 2 - 4mm in width.

3. The lumbar and sacral nerves run through the pelvis.

4. The ileopectal line divides the upper (false) pelvis and the lower (true) pelvis. Injuries to the true pelvis may be associated with injuries to the following structures:

- Bladder or urethra
- Descending colon
- Sigmoid colon
- Rectum
- Anus
- Nerve roots
- Vasculature

B. Pelvic Fractures

1. Mechanism of injury
   a. Motor vehicle and motorcycle accidents (most common cause of injury in adults)
   b. Falls
   c. Crush injuries
   d. Pedestrian hit by motor vehicle (leading cause of injury in children)

2. Classification — There are several different systems that have developed over the years to classify pelvic fractures. The central focus of most of these systems is the underlying stability of the pelvis. The *Young* system has become the one most favored by emergency physicians because it is valuable in predicting pelvic fracture-related hemorrhage and local vascular injury. This system is based on the mechanism of injury (AP compression or lateral compression) as well as the degree of pelvic instability (ligamentous tear: see Fig. I).

AP Compression (usually caused by an MVA from the <u>front</u>)

- **Type I**   **Disruption of the pubic symphysis < 2.5 cm of the diastasis; no significant posterior pelvic injury.**

- **Type II**   **Disruption of the pubic symphysis > 2.5cm with tearing of the anterior sacroiliac, sacrospinous and sacrotuberous ligaments (see Fig. 2).**

- **Type III** **Complete disruption of the pubic symphysis and posterior ligament complexes (iliolumbars unilaterally or bilaterally) with hemipelvic displacement.**

Lateral Compression (caused by injuries from the <u>side</u>: T-bone MVAs, pedestrians struck from the side, fall from a height.)

- **Type I**   **Posterior compression of the sacroiliac joint without ligament disruption; oblique pubic ramus fracture (Fig. 3).**

- **Type II**   **Rupture of the posterior sacroiliac ligament; pivotal internal rotation of the hemipelvis on the anterior SI joint with a crush injury of the sacrum and an oblique pubic ramus fracture (Fig. 4).**

- **Type III** **Type II findings plus evidence of an AP compression injury to the contralateral hemipelvis (Fig. 5).**

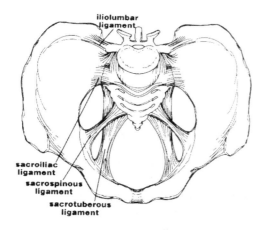

Fig. 1
Ligamentous anatomy of the pelvis

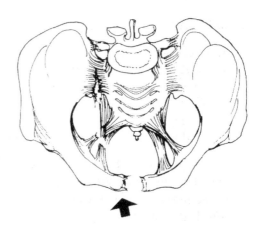

Fig. 2
Anterior Compression

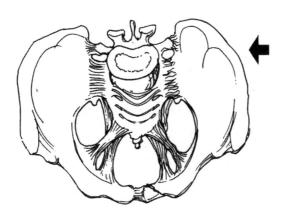

Fig. 3
Lateral Compression Type I

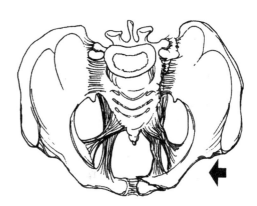

Fig. 4
Lateral Compression Type II

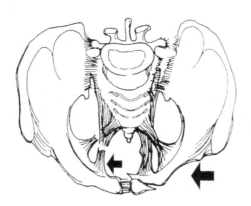

Fig. 5
Lateral Compression Type III

Reproduced with permission. K.Martox, et.al, Trauma 2000. McGraw-Hill, Inc.

3. Signs of pelvic fracture
   a. <u>Destot's sign</u>: a superficial hematoma above the inguinal ligament or on the scrotum
   b. <u>Earle's sign</u>: on rectal exam, a large hematoma or tenderness along the fracture line or palpation of a bony prominence
   c. <u>Roux's sign</u>: the distance measured from the greater trochanter to the pubic spine is diminished on one side as compared to the other (indicates an overlapping fracture of the anterior pelvic ring)

4. Computerized tomography
   a. Is superior to standard x-ray films in evaluating the acetabulum, posterior (femorosacral) arch and the sacroiliac joint.
   b. Often provides information on the degree of pelvic instability and the presence of a retroperitoneal hematoma.

5. Associated injuries
   a. Hemorrhage
      (1) The primary cause of death in patients with pelvic fractures; up to 6 L of blood can be accommodated in the retroperitoneal space.
      (2) Occurs most frequently in patients with Type III and posterior fractures.
      (3) 50% of patients require transfusion.
      (4) May initially be controlled by application of MAST trousers or an antishock pelvic clamp; external fixation and angiographic embolization are also useful in selected patients and may subsequently be required.
   b. Injuries of the urethra and bladder
      (1) Are the most commonly associated pelvic injuries.
      (2) Urethral injuries (particularly posterior urethral tears in men) are more common than bladder injuries.
   c. Vaginal laceration or rupture (relatively uncommon, but may be seen with anterior pelvic fractures)
   d. Nerve damage (most commonly occurs in association with posterior pelvic fractures)
   e. Ruptured diaphragm (not uncommon and is often missed)
   f. Rectal injuries
      (1) Are uncommon.
      (2) They generally occur in association with ischial and urinary tract injuries.
      (3) Prophylactic antibiotics should be administered without delay.
   g. Thoracic aortic rupture (incidence is eight times greater in patients with pelvic fractures than in patients with blunt abdominal trauma)
   <u>Note</u>: Due to the lesser degree of protection provided by the developing pelvis, children have a higher rate of concomitant injuries.

6. Complications of pelvic fractures
   a. Sepsis
   b. Thromboembolic complications (pulmonary and fat emboli)
   c. Malunion or delayed union
   d. Chronic pain

7. Specific pelvic fractures
   a. Pubic rami
      (1) A <u>single</u> pubic ramus fracture is the most common pelvic fracture — a fall on the buttocks....may be missed (or not visible) on plain film; order an MRI if in doubt.
      (2) A "straddle injury" is a fracture of <u>all four</u> pubic rami — a fall on the crotch with the legs apart.
   b. Iliac crest (result from impact collisions)
      (1) Duverney fracture (pelvic wing fracture)
      (2) Ilium fracture → pelvic ring disruption, visceral injuries
   c. The multiple fractured pelvis (Malgaigne fracture)
      (1) Involves the pubic rami bilaterally and the ilium or sacrum
      (2) Results from vertical shear forces (e.g. fall from a height)

C. Hip Dislocations (an orthopedic emergency*)

1. Anterior — 10% of hip dislocations [Be able to identify on pictorial].
   a. Are classified according to the final resting position of the femoral head as either:
      (1) Superior iliac — femoral head is palpable in the area of the superior iliac spine.
      (2) Superior pubic — femoral head rests near the pubis.
      (3) Inferior (obturator) — femoral head lies in the obturator foramen.
   b. Mechanism of injury: extreme abduction causes the femoral head to be pushed out through a tear in the anterior capsule. Causes include:
      (1) Auto accident
      (2) A fall
      (3) A blow to the back while squatting
   c. Limb appearance: (varies with the type of dislocation present)
      (1) With anterior <u>superior</u> dislocations, the limb is slightly <u>abducted</u>, externally rotated and <u>extended</u> [<u>Tintinalli's Text,</u> Fifth ed., p. 1812 Figs. 265-20 A + C <u>or</u> Sixth ed., p. 1723, Figs. 273-22 A + C]
      (2) With anterior <u>inferior</u> dislocations, the limb is abducted, externally rotated and <u>flexed</u> [<u>Tintinalli's Text,</u> Fifth ed., p. 1812, Figs. 265-20 B and D <u>or</u> Sixth ed., p. 1723, Figs. 273-22 B and D]
   d. Associated physical findings
      (1) Diminishing femoral or distal pulses (or progressive swelling of the leg) indicates the need for immediate reduction of the hip.
      (2) If the femoral nerve is involved:
         (a) ↓ quadriceps function
         (b) ↓ DTR at knee
         (c) ↓ sensation on anteromedial thigh

2. Posterior — 80 - 90% of hip dislocations [Be able to identify on x-ray]
   a. Mechanism of injury: the majority of cases result from auto accidents in which a direct force is applied to the flexed knee (hitting the dashboard) that is transmitted to the femoral head, which is pushed out through the posterior capsule.

*...in the absence of a prosthetic femoral head

b. Limb appearance: shortened, adducted, internally rotated and flexed. [Tintinalli's Text, Fifth ed., p. 1813, Figs. 265-21 A and B or Sixth ed., p. 1724, figs. 273-24 A and B]

c. Associated physical findings
   (1) Evidence of acetabular/femoral fractures
   (2) Knee injury
   (3) Sciatic nerve injury
      (a) ↓ muscle function below the knee
      (b) ↓ ability to flex the knee
      (c) ↓ sensation on posterolateral leg and sole of the foot

3. Treatment — Early reduction is required since avascular necrosis of the femoral head increases in direct proportion to delay in reduction. Immediate closed reduction (using IV sedation and analgesia) should be attempted in the ED as soon as appropriate x-rays have been obtained to R/O associated injuries. If this is unsuccessful, closed reduction under general anesthesia is indicated. Neurovascular assessment should be performed prior to and following any reduction attempts.

4. Complications of hip dislocations
   a. Early complications
      (1) Anterior dislocations → femoral artery, vein and nerve injury
      (2) Posterior dislocation → sciatic nerve injury (10% of patients)
   b. Late complications (in addition to osteoarthritis)
      (1) Anterior dislocation → femoral artery/vein thrombosis → pulmonary embolism and avascular necrosis of the femoral head
      (2) Posterior dislocation → avascular necrosis of the femoral head (15 - 30% of patients)

D. Hip Fractures

1. Classification
   a. Hip fractures are classified as:
      (1) Intracapsular (femoral head and neck fractures) or
      (2) Extracapsular (trochanteric, intertrochanteric and subtrochanteric)
   b. This classification system has prognostic value in that intracapsular fractures are far more likely to result in a disrupted vascular supply and subsequent avascular necrosis than extracapsular fractures.

2. **Clinical pictures** of hip fractures
   a. You are examining an elderly patient who complains of hip pain after a fall. The patient limps when he walks or he may be unable to walk. The affected leg is shortened, abducted and in slight external rotation → femoral neck fracture.
   b. You are examining a patient who complains of hip pain after a fall. The leg is shortened and in marked external rotation → intertrochanteric fracture (fracture line between the greater and lesser trochanters).

3. Clinical pearls
   a. The ability to ambulate does <u>not</u> R/O a fracture; some patients with nondisplaced or minimally displaced fractures may be able to bear weight.
   b. Negative plain films do <u>not</u> R/O a fracture; patients with negative plain x-rays who are unable to ambulate require further work-up (tomograms, CT scan, MRI or bone scan).
   c. Femoral neck fractures are common in the elderly and are associated with significant complications, the most frequent of which is avascular necrosis (occurs in 15 - 35% of patients).

E. Clinical Pictures of Pediatric Hip Disorders

1. You are examining an infant with some other condition. Since you routinely perform the Ortolani maneuver in all children < 1 yr. of age, you detect a "click" on the affected side → <u>congenital hip dislocation</u>. This disorder is much more common in females, particularly first borns.

2. You are examining a child < 4 yrs. of age who presents with fever, irritability and a toxic appearance. The parents tell you that he limps and, when he walks, you observe a limp on the affected side. With the child lying supine on the cart, you see that the affected leg is flexed, abducted and externally rotated → septic arthritis of the hip caused by *Staphylococcus aureus*. Ultrasound of the hip reveals an effusion. Arthrocentesis performed by the orthopedic surgeon under fluoroscopic guidance confirms the diagnosis; synovial fluid analysis typically reveals 80,000 - 200,000 WBCs with a predominance (>75%) of PMNs.

3. You are examining a nontoxic-appearing child between the ages of 18 months and 12 years who presents with hip, knee or thigh pain and a limp or inability to bear weight. This child is usually a male and, most typically, five or six years old → <u>transient (toxic) synovitis</u> (nonspecific inflammation of the synovium of the hip, often following a nonspecific viral illness). This is a diagnosis of exclusion. Fluoroscopically-guided aspiration of the hip (performed by an orthopedic consultant) is sometimes needed to distinguish this entity from septic arthritis. Synovial fluid analysis typically reveals 5000 - 15,000 WBCs with fewer than 25% PMNs.

4. You are examining a child (frequently a male) between 4 and 9 years of age who presents with a limp. He may also c/o muscle spasm and groin or hip pain that radiates to the inner aspect of his thigh and knee. The child is afebrile and nontoxic in appearance. Exam of his hip reveals limitation of abduction and internal rotation and spasm. The WBC count and sedimentation rate are normal. X-ray findings vary with the time course of the disease process. Widening of the joint space and smaller size of the ossific nucleus of the femoral head are the initial findings, followed by the development of a subchondral stress fracture line in the femoral head (Caffey's crescent line). Subsequent findings include increased density of the femoral head with later fragmentation and distor-

tion → <u>Legg-Calvé-Perthes Disease</u> (osteochondrosis of the femoral head). A technetium bone scan (shows decreased uptake in the femoral head) or MRI (shows low signal intensity in the femoral head) can be used to confirm the diagnosis if doubt remains.

5. You are examining an adolescent or preadolescent (usually a male) who presents with groin pain after activity. He may also c/o hip stiffness, knee pain and a limp. The build of this youth is classic: he is typically obese with underdeveloped genitalia or tall, thin and rapidly growing. There is often a history of trivial antecedent trauma. The affected leg is <u>externally</u> rotated and <u>ad</u>ducted (and may be shortened). Further evaluation reveals tenderness around the hip and decreased range of motion (<u>internal</u> rotation and <u>ab</u>duction [full flexion] are limited). Radiographs (AP and bilateral frogleg lateral views of the hips) confirm the diagnosis → <u>slipped capital femoral epiphysis (SCFE)</u>; earliest findings (preslippage stage) are irregular widening of the epiphyseal plate, decalcification of the epiphyseal border of the metaphysis and globular swelling of the joint capsule; with slippage, there is posterior and inferior (medial) displacement of the femoral head and loss of Shenton's line (a curved line formed by the top of the obturator foramen and the inner side of the neck of the femur). Bilateral involvement eventually develops in up to 40% of these children.

<u>Note</u>: All of the above-described hip disorders require orthopedic referral.

IV. Knee Injuries

A. *Essential Anatomy*

1. There are five <u>stabilizers</u> (two static and three dynamic) of the <u>lateral aspect</u> of the knee:
   a. Lateral collateral ligament ┐
   b. Joint capsule ┤— static (ligamentous) stabilizers
   c. Iliotibial tract ┐
   d. Popliteus muscle ┤— dynamic (muscular) stabilizers
   e. Biceps femoris muscle ┘

2. There are four <u>stabilizers</u> of the <u>medial aspect</u> of the knee:
   a. Medial collateral ligament ┐
   b. Medial joint capsule ┤— static stabilizer
   c. Semimembranosus muscle ┐
   d. Pes anserinus ┤— dynamic stabilizers

<u>Note</u>: <u>Medial</u> collateral ligament injury is much more common than injury to the lateral collateral ligament.

3. The quadriceps tendon permits extension and is the primary dynamic stabilizer of the knee. It is formed by four muscles:
   a. Rectus femoris
   b. Vastus lateralis
   c. Vastus intermedius
   d. Vastus medialis

4. The cruciate ligaments are two internal bands extending from the tibia to the femur — one anteriorly, the other posteriorly. They control antero-posterior and rotatory stability of the knee and prevent hyperextension. The anterior cruciate ligament (ACL) is the <u>most frequently</u> injured ligament in the knee. It has a rich blood supply which accounts for the high incidence of hemarthrosis when this ligament is injured. The posterior cruciate ligament (PCL) is significantly stronger than the anterior cruciate and collateral ligaments; thus, injury to it is rare and is usually associated with severe knee injuries.

B. Baker's Cyst

1. An inflammation of the semimembranosus or medial gastrocnemius bursa produced by protrusion of the synovial membrane through the posterior aspect of the knee's capsule.

2. In adults, these cysts are usually due to an intra-articular abnormality of the knee such as chronic inflammatory arthritis or a torn meniscus. In children, however, these cysts appear to be a primary lesion.

3. Patients usually relate a history of intermittent swelling behind the knee and may c/o local discomfort.

4. Examination reveals a tense and occasionally painful fluid-filled sac in the <u>medial</u> aspect of the popliteal fossa.

5. Rupture of the cyst with inferior dissection of the synovial fluid causes calf pain and swelling, often simulating thrombophlebitis or a DVT of the calf.

6. Treatment
   a. In adults, management is directed toward correction of the underlying joint pathology.
   b. In children, treatment is generally unnecessary since most of these cysts resolve on their own in 1 - 2 years.

C. Osgood-Schlatter's Disease (traumatic tibial apophysitis)

1. Is due to repetitive microscopic injury that produces inflammation of the apophysis of the tibial tubercle and leads to partial avulsion and separation of the tibial tubercle.

2. It is commonly seen in adolescents (particularly males) who are active in sports and is often bilateral (25% of cases).

3. These youths present with pain and swelling in the region of the tibial tuberosity that is increased with forceful leg extension (climbing stairs, running, jumping).

4. Treatment: ice, nonsteroidals and decreased participation in sports.

D. Rupture of the Quadriceps Mechanism

1. May result from one of the following injuries:
   a. Quadriceps tendon rupture
   b. Patellar tendon rupture
   c. Patellar fracture
   d. Avulsion of the tibial tuberosity

2. With a complete disruption, the patient can stand but he cannot walk or extend his knee and, on physical exam, there is diffuse swelling around the knee and a palpable deficit; with incomplete disruption, active extension is weak and painful.

3. Treatment
   a. Obtain early orthopedic consultation.
   b. Complete ruptures → early surgical repair
   c. Partial tear → immobilization in full extension

E. Chondromalacia Patellae (patellofemoral pain syndrome/patellar malalignment syndrome)

1. Most common cause of knee pain.

2. Usually occurs in young adults (particularly females) and is often bilateral.

3. Causes include patellofemoral malalignment, recurrent patellar subluxation/dislocation and excessive knee strain (athletes).

4. Patients present with the complaint of intermittent peripatellar pain that is exacerbated by prolonged sitting and climbing steps.

5. Examination reveals:
   a. Pain with compression of the patellae into the femoral groove (patellar compression test) and with knee extended and quadriceps tightened.
   b. Quadricep muscle contraction in anticipation of pain when the patella is displaced laterally while the knee is extended and relaxed (patellar apprehension test).
   c. Findings of patellar malalignment (Q angle > 20°) may also be present. The Q angle is formed by the intersection of two lines: one drawn from the anterior superior iliac spine to the center of the patellae and the second drawn from the center of the patellae through the tibial tuberosity (the normal Q angle is 15°).

6. Treatment: rest and NSAIDs, followed by isometric quadricep-strengthening exercises (quadricep contraction with adduction).

F. Mechanisms of Knee Injury

1. <u>Valgus (abduction) stress</u> — most common mechanism of injury
   a. Definition: <u>outward</u> stress on lower leg with angulation of the foot away from the midline.
   b. Injured structure/associated history or complaint:
      (1) Med. collateral lig./ski injury (61%)
      (2) Ant. cruciate lig./patient stumbled, caught himself and now cannot climb steps.
      (3) Medial meniscus/patient complains of knee "locking" in place or clicking (medial meniscus attached to MCL).

2. <u>Varus (adduction) stress</u> — uncommon mechanism of injury
   a. Definition: <u>inward</u> stress on lower leg with angulation of the foot toward the midline
   b. Injured structure/associated history or complaint
      (1) Lat. collateral lig./skier fails to maintain a snow-plow and the tips of his skis cross (significant disruption → peroneal nerve injury)
      (2) Lat. post. capsule/knee buckling or giving way
      (3) Lat. meniscus/knee "locking" or clicking

3. <u>Hyperextension stress</u>
   a. Definition: backward stress with the knee extended
   b. Usually results in injury to the cruciate ligaments.
   c. Injured structure/associated history or complaint
      (1) Ant. cruciate ligament/hyperextension of the knee
      (2) Rupture of the posterior capsule/knee buckling, collapsing or giving away
      (3) Isolated post. cruciate ligament/a blow to the anterior aspect of the tibia with the knee in extension or hyperextension

4. <u>Anterior and posterior forces</u> of the tibia on the femur
   a. Usually occur with the knee in flexion.
   b. Injured structure/associated history or complaint
      (1) Ant. cruciate lig./tibia is forced anteriorly relative to the femur
      (2) Post. cruciate lig./tibia is forced posteriorly relative to the femur

5. <u>Rotational stress</u>
   a. Definition: rotation of the knee (tibia relative to femur) with the foot firmly planted on the ground
   b. Internal rotation → ruptures the anterior cruciate ligament.
   c. External rotation → disrupts the anterior cruciate and/or the medial capsular and medial collateral ligaments.
   d. Associated history: a sudden stop and pivot while running

<u>Note</u>: Partial ligament ruptures are often more painful than complete tears and injuries to cruciate ligaments occur more frequently in women. (2006 LLSA Reading, "Does this Patient have a Torn Meniscus or Ligament of the Knee?")

G. Hemarthrosis in association with a negative x-ray indicates the presence of one of the following:

1. Ligamentous tear
   a. Hemarthrosis usually develops within 2 hours of injury.
   b. Torn anterior cruciate ligament is responsible for 75% of all hemarthroses of the knee.

2. Peripheral meniscus tear
   a. Effusion develops gradually (6 to 24 hours post injury).
   b. Usually occurs in association with <u>rotational</u> force to a <u>weight bearing</u> knee.

3. Osteochondral fracture
   a. Hemarthrosis develops immediately.
   b. Usually occurs in children, particularly adolescent males

<u>Note</u>: When aspiration of a hemarthrosis reveals the presence of fat globules (lipohemarthrosis) a fracture is likely.

H. Physical examination of the knee should include the following tests:

1. <u>Stability tests</u>
   a. Valgus stress in 30° of flexion → instability indicates rupture of the medial collateral ligament.
   b. Valgus stress in extension → instability indicates rupture of the medial collateral ligament as well as potential injury to the cruciate ligaments and posterior capsule.
   c. Varus stress in 30° of flexion → instability indicates rupture of the lateral collateral ligament.
   d. Varus stress in extension → instability indicates rupture of the lateral collateral ligament as well as potential injury to the iliotibial tract, popliteus muscle, lateral capsule and cruciate ligaments.
   e. Anterior and posterior drawer signs (test the ant. + post. cruciate ligs.)
   f. Lachman test (another test of the anterior cruciate ligament; it is more sensitive and accurate than the anterior drawer sign).
   g. McMurray's and Ege's tests (aid in diagnosing meniscal tears)
      (1) <u>McMurray's Test</u> → joint line tenderness
      (2) <u>Ege's Test</u> → pain and/or a click on maximum rotation of the knee with the patient in a squatting position (<u>external</u> rotation → <u>medial</u> meniscus tear; <u>internal</u> rotation → <u>lateral</u> meniscus tear)
2. <u>Patellar compression and apprehension test</u>: Pain is elicited with chondromalacia patellae (an overuse syndrome often seen in young women).

I. Knee Dislocation (a true orthopedic emergency)

1. Results from violent trauma, most commonly from MVAs and vehicle-pedestrian accidents.

2. Knee dislocations are classified according to the direction of the <u>tibial displacement</u> relative to the femur:
   a. There are 5 types: anterior, posterior, medial, lateral and rotary.
   b. Anterior and posterior dislocations are the most common (50 - 60%).

3. Diagnosis is essential since the incidence of associated injuries is high:
    a. Complete disruption of all major ligaments plus meniscal injury
    b. Popliteal artery injury (21 - 32%); particularly common with anterior and posterior dislocations (up to 40%)
    c. Peroneal nerve injury (25 - 35%)
        (1) Clinical diagnosis
            (a) Paresthesia of the dorsal aspect of the foot
            (b) Diminished dorsiflexion of the foot (foot drop)
            (c) Decreased sensitivity between the first and second toes
        (2) Seen most often with medial and posterolateral dislocations
    d. Tibial nerve injury* (less common than peroneal nerve injury)
    e. Proximal tibial fractures

4. Diagnostic caveats
    a. The knee with complete disruption of all major ligaments (and the joint capsule) may exhibit less swelling and pain than the less severely injured knee with a tense hemarthrosis.
    b. The knee may relocate spontaneously and the diagnosis of dislocation may be missed.
    c. Any patient who presents following trauma with a grossly unstable knee (a tear in three of the four major ligaments of the knee) should be assumed to have a spontaneously-reduced dislocation until further evaluation rules this injury out.
    d. Popliteal artery injury may be present even if the pulses are intact or the foot is warm.

5. Clinical management
    a. The dislocated knee should be reduced <u>immediately</u> (in the neutral position)** by longitudinal traction in a sedated patient. Do not wait for x-ray confirmation.
    b. The popliteal, dorsalis pedis and tibialis posterior pulses should be checked <u>before and after</u> reduction.
    c. Following reduction, the knee should be immobilized in a posterior splint in 15° flexion.
    d. An arteriogram must be performed in all cases of knee dislocation, even if pulses return after reduction.***
        (1) An arteriogram in the Radiology Dept. is mandatory if the knee is not going to be surgically explored immediately.
        (2) If immediate surgical intervention is indicated, arteriography should be performed in the OR, since performance in the Radiology Dept. is associated with an additional delay of one to two hours before surgery.
    e. The peroneal and tibial nerves should be tested prior to and following reduction.
    f. Immediate orthopedic (and possibly vascular) surgery consultation is indicated whenever this injury is suspected.

---

*Plantar foot numbness/paresthesias and weakness with plantar flexion
**Extension of the knee stretches the popliteal artery.
***Doppler flowmeter measurement may be considered in "low-energy" type dislocations if distal pulses are strong post-reduction.

g. Immediate surgical intervention is indicated for:
   (1) Popliteal artery injuries (arterial repair should be accomplished within 6 hours to avoid the complications of prolonged ischemia).
   (2) Open dislocations
   (3) Irreducible dislocations

J. *Patellar Subluxation/Dislocation*

1. Generally occurs in adolescent females with chronic patellofemoral anatomic abnormalities such as genu valgum (knock-knees), patellae alta (high-riding patellae), a large Q (quadriceps) angle or generalized joint laxity.

2. Lateral subluxation/dislocation is the most common.

3. Mechanisms of injury:
   a. Sudden flexion and external rotation of the tibia on the femur with concomitant contraction of the quadriceps
   b. Direct blow to the patella with the knee in flexion or extension

4. Clinical management
   a. Obtain AP and lateral x-rays of the knee prior to and following reduction to R/O associated osteochondral fracture of the patellae or lateral femoral condyle.
   b. Reduction — is accomplished by flexing the patient's hip and applying gentle, medially-directed pressure over the lateral aspect of the patellae while extending the knee. [Note: Patellar subluxations often reduce spontaneously.]
   c. Immobilization in full extension
   d. Crutches — patient should be non-weight-bearing
   e. Orthopedic referral for possible surgical intervention
   f. Isometric quadriceps exercise should be initiated as soon as the patient can do them without pain.

K. *Patellar Fracture*

1. One of several possible injuries to the extensor mechanism of the knee.

2. Transverse fractures are the most common (50 - 80% of cases).

3. Mechanisms of injury:
   a. Direct blow (most common), e.g. against the dashboard of a car
   b. Forceful contraction of the quadriceps muscles

4. Patients typically present with tenderness + swelling over the patella and limited, painful knee extension (if the extensor mechanism is intact) or inability to extend the knee (if the extensor mechanism is torn).

5. X-ray evaluation should include AP, lateral and sunrise (skyline) views.

6. Clinical management
   a. If the fracture is nondisplaced or minimally displaced and the extensor mechanism is intact → treatment consists of immobilization in full extension, partial weight-bearing advancing to full weight-bearing as tolerated and orthopedic referral.
   b. If the fracture fragments are widely displaced (> 3mm) or there is loss of extensor function → orthopedic referral for surgical intervention is required. [Note: When fracture fragments are widely separated, associated concomitant knee joint injury is frequently present.]

L. Tibial Plateau Fracture (most common fracture of the knee)

1. The most common mechanism of injury is a strong valgus stress with axial loading.

2. Most condylar fractures (55 - 70%) involve the lateral plateau.

3. Vascular complications are common.
   a. Fracture fragments in the subcondylar area → popliteal artery
   b. Displaced fracture of the lateral condyle → ant. tibial artery

---

V. Lower Leg Injuries

A. The soft tissue surrounding the tibia and fibula is divided into four compartments:

1. Anterior compartment
   a. Dorsiflexor muscles of the ankle and foot (tibialis anterior, extensor digitorum longus, extensor hallucis longus and peroneus tertius)
   b. Anterior tibial artery
      (1) The most frequently injured structure in this compartment
      (2) Injury occurs secondary to fractures of the
         (a) Lateral tibial plateau
         (b) Proximal third of the tibia
   c. Deep peroneal nerve
      (1) Provides sensation to the first dorsal web space of the foot
      (2) May be injured due to fracture of the lateral tibial plateau

2. Lateral (peroneal) compartment
   a. Everter and plantar flexor muscles of the foot (peroneus brevis and longus muscles)
   b. Superficial peroneal nerve
      (1) Provides sensation to the dorsum of the foot
      (2) Is frequently injured due to fracture of the fibular neck or proximal shaft

3. Deep posterior compartment
   a. Tibialis posterior, flexor digitorum longus and flexor hallucis longus muscles
   b. Posterior tibial and peroneal arteries
   c. Posterior tibial nerve (provides sensation to the sole of the foot)

4. Superficial posterior compartment
   a. Gastrocnemius, plantaris and soleus muscles
   b. Sural nerve (provides sensation to the lateral aspect of the foot and the distal calf)

B. Anterior Compartment Syndrome

1. Is more common than the lateral or posterior compartment syndromes and is usually seen with fractures of the proximal tibia.

2. Usually occurs in association with tibial fractures, but can result from prolonged strenuous exercise (particularly in runners) or other causes.

3. Signs and symptoms
   a. Anterior tibial pain that is:
      (1) Out of proportion to the injury ──────┐
      (2) Increased with passive plantar flexion of the foot ──┤ earliest findings
      (3) Increased with active dorsiflexion of the foot ──────┘
   b. Decreased two-point sensory discrimination (most consistent finding)
   c. Paresthesia or hypesthesia in the distribution of the deep peroneal nerve (early finding)
   d. Weak dorsiflexion of the ankle and toes
   e. Palpable tenseness and tenderness of the compartment
   f. Pallor of the skin (late finding)
   g. Pulselessness or reduced distal pulses (a very late—and frequently absent—finding). The presence of peripheral pulses does not R/O increased intracompartmental pressure; pulses often remain intact.

4. Treatment
   a. Remove constrictive dressing or cast (if present).
   b. Obtain immediate orthopedic consultation and measure intracompartmental pressure.
   c. Surgical decompression via fasciotomy is indicated if the intracompartmental pressure is > 30mmHg.

C. Stress Fractures of the Fibula

1. Result from over-training and usually occur at the distal fibula.

2. Patients present with pain exacerbated with ambulation.

3. Initial x-rays are usually negative.

4. Treatment is symptomatic.

VI. Ankle Injuries

A. *Essential Anatomy*

1. Three groups of ligaments unify the bony structures of the ankles:
   a. Medial collateral (deltoid) ligament
      (1) Provides medial support to the ankle
      (2) Originates from the medial malleolus and inserts on the navicular and talus
   b. Anterior talofibular, calcaneofibular and posterior talofibular ligaments → provide lateral support.
   c. Ligaments of syndesmosis → bind the lower portions of the tibia and fibula together.
      (1) Anterior and posterior tibiofibular ligaments
      (2) Transverse tibiofibular ligament
      (3) Interosseous ligament (provides the strongest bond between the tibia and fibula at the ankle joint)
2. Four groups of muscles traverse the ankle joint:
   a. Anteriorly → dorsiflexion of the ankle
      (1) Tibialis anterior
      (2) <u>Extensor</u> digitorum longus
      (3) <u>Extensor</u> hallucis longus
   b. Medially → inversion of the foot
      (1) Tibialis posterior
      (2) <u>Flexor</u> digitorum longus
      (3) <u>Flexor</u> hallucis longus
   c. Posteriorly → plantar flexion
      (1) Gastrocnemius
      (2) Plantaris
      (3) Soleus
   d. Laterally → eversion and plantar flexion
      (1) Peroneus longus
      (2) Peroneus brevis

B. *Sprains (ligamentous injury)*

1. <u>Lateral</u> collateral ligament sprains
   a. Are the most common (85 - 90%).
   b. Result from inversion + internal rotation of the plantar-flexed foot.
   c. Ligamentous injury occurs in sequence, starting anteriorly with the anterior talofibular ligament and progressing posteriorly to the calcaneofibular ligament, followed by the posterior talofibular ligament.
   d. The most frequently injured ligament → anterior talofibular

2. <u>Medial</u> collateral ligament sprains — are uncommon
   a. Result from eversion and external rotation of the foot.
   b. Are often associated with either a fracture of the fibula or a tear of the tibiofibular syndesmosis.

3. Distal tibiofibular syndesmotic ligament sprains — are also uncommon.
   a. Result from dorsiflexion and eversion forces with an axial load.
   b. Have a prolonged recovery period.

4. Classification of sprains — is based upon the clinical presentation and the degree of instability present (as demonstrated by stress testing).
   a. First Degree
      (1) Mild localized tenderness
      (2) Minimal swelling
      (3) No instability or functional loss
      (4) Able to bear weight
      (5) No abnormal motion
   b. Second Degree
      (1) Moderate swelling and tenderness
      (2) Moderate functional loss
      (3) Increased pain with stress testing
   c. Third Degree
      (1) Marked tenderness
      (2) Egg-shaped swelling over the affected ligament(s) within two hours of injury
      (3) Significant functional loss
      (4) Inability to bear weight
      (5) Resistance to motion of the foot
      (6) Positive stress test

5. <u>Stress Tests</u> for ankle stability — are useful in confirming specific ligamentous injury and in distinguishing second from third degree sprains.
   a. Anterior drawer test → abnormal movement indicates a rupture of at least the anterior talofibular ligament.
   b. Inversion stress (or talar tilt) test
      (1) Needs to be done only if the anterior drawer test is positive.
      (2) Abnormal movement indicates rupture of <u>both</u> the anterior talofibular and the calcaneofibular ligaments.
   c. External rotation test → pain at the syndesmosis or a sensation of lateral talar movement indicates injury to the distal tibiofibular syndesmotic ligament.
   <u>Note</u>: Accurate results require the presence of good muscle relaxation obtained with application of ice or infiltration of a local anesthetic.

6. Associated injuries
   a. Maisonneuve fracture
      (1) A proximal fibular fracture that occurs in association with rupture of the deltoid ligament or an avulsion fracture of the medial malleolus at the insertion site of the distal talofibular ligament.
      (2) This diagnosis should be suspected in patients presenting with a history of eversion injury and significant medial malleolar tenderness and swelling.
   b. Osteochondral fracture of the talar dome
   c. Avulsion fracture of the 5th metatarsal — occurs with flexion-inversion injuries of the foot
   d. Peroneal tendon dislocation or subluxation

7. Treatment — is determined by the degree of injury; all sprains should initially be managed with ice, elevation and compression. The management of third degree sprains, however, is controversial (operative vs non-operative) and requires orthopedic consultation.
   a. First (and most second degree) sprains — ice, elevation, immobilization in a protective device (air cast, brace, splint, Unna boot) and crutches as needed. As pain and swelling decrease, this should be followed by graded exercises to increase dorsiflexion and peroneal strength, weight bearing as tolerated and re-evaluation by the PMD.
   b. Severe second degree sprains — ice, elevation, splint immobilization (sugar-tong or posterior mold), crutches and early orthopedic re-evaluation for possible casting.
   c. Third degree sprains — ice, elevation, splint immobilization, crutches and orthopedic evaluation within 24 hours (or while in the department); some of these patients, depending on their level of athletic involvement and other associated injuries, may be considered for primary surgical repair.

C. Ankle Dislocations

1. Are described according to the direction of <u>talar displacement</u> relative to the tibia. There are five types:
   a. Anterior
   b. Posterior ⎤
   c. Medial ⎦— common
   d. Lateral
   e. Superior (diastasis) — uncommon

2. Pure ankle dislocations are uncommon; most occur in association with malleolar fractures.

3. Management
   a. All of these dislocations require <u>immediate</u> neurovascular assessment and <u>emergent</u> orthopedic consultation in the ED.
   b. If there is any evidence of neurovascular compromise or skin tenting, reduction should be accomplished <u>immediately</u> (prior to x-ray evaluation). If, however, these findings are absent, pre-reduction films should be obtained first to R/O the presence of associated fractures.
   c. Following administration of adequate analgesia or conscious sedation, promptly reduce the dislocation with gentle in-line traction.
   d. Once reduction has been accomplished, reassess the patient's neurovascular status, order post-reduction films and place the patient in a posterior splint.

D. Tendon Injuries

1. Achilles tendon rupture
   a. The patient gives a history of sudden excruciating pain at the back of his ankle that lessens instantly and often reports having heard or felt a "pop" or "snap".
   b. Commonly occurs in sedentary, middle-aged males (mean age 35 years) engaging in weekend athletic activities.
   c. Up to 25% of cases are initially misdiagnosed as ankle sprains.
   d. Mechanism of injury:
      (1) Forceful dorsiflexion of the foot with the ankle in a relaxed state
      (2) Direct trauma to a taut tendon
      (3) An extra stretch applied to a taut tendon
   e. Examination reveals:
      (1) Swelling of the distal calf
      (2) A palpable defect in the tendon 2 - 6cms proximal to its calcaneal insertion site
      (3) Weak plantar flexion when compared to the uninjured leg
   f. Diagnosis is made with the Thompson's test (also called Simmonds test) — which is performed with the patient in the prone position.
      (1) Normal function — squeezing the calf produces plantar flexion of the foot.
      (2) With a complete tear, plantar flexion will not occur.
      Note: Ultrasound or MRI can be used to confirm the diagnosis if doubt remains, but this is usually unnecessary.
   g. Treatment:
      (1) Initial management — ice, elevation, analgesia, immobilization in a posterior splint in passive equinus (plantar flexion) along with crutches and orthopedic consultation within 48 - 72 hours.
      (2) Definitive care (casting versus surgical repair) — remains controversial; it is usually determined by the patient's age, his activity level and underlying medical conditions. Surgical repair appears to be associated with a better outcome (increased strength and mobility, and decreased incidence of rerupture) but is typically reserved for young athletic patients.

2. Peroneal tendon subluxation/dislocation
   a. Results from a tear of the superior peroneal retinaculum from its attachment on the fibula. This allows the peroneus brevis and longus tendons to sublux anteriorly over the lateral malleolus.
   b. It is often misdiagnosed as an ankle sprain.
   c. Mechanism of injury: forced dorsiflexion of the ankle with reflex contraction of the peroneal muscles.
   d. The patient typically c/o pain and a clicking or slipping sensation at the back of his ankle.
   e. Diagnosis is made by physical exam.
      (1) There is tenderness, swelling and ecchymosis at the posterior aspect of the lateral malleolus.
      (2) Tensing of the peroneal muscles intensifies the pain.

(3) Eversion is weak.

(4) Anterior subluxation of the tendons with the patient's foot dorsi-flexed and everted against resistance confirms the diagnosis.

 f. Plain x-rays may reveal a small avulsion fracture of the lateral ridge of the distal fibula (pathognomonic for this injury) in 50% of cases.

 g. Treatment: splint in midplantar flexion and refer to orthopedist for possible surgical repair.

E. Ankle Injuries in Children

1. Because ligaments are <u>stronger</u> than bone in children, fractures at the epiphyseal plate are more common than ligamentous injuries.

2. These fractures usually result from indirect forces and are classified according to the Salter-Harris classification system (described on p. 409 of this chapter).

3. Tillaux fracture → A Salter III fracture of the lateral distal tibia commonly seen in adolescents participating in sporting events; consider this diagnosis if the history is suggestive and there is swelling over the anterior ankle.

VII. Foot Injuries

A. Essential Anatomy

1. The foot is divided into three parts:
 a. Hindpart (calcaneus and talus)
 b. Midpart (navicular, cuboid, cuneiforms)
 c. Forepart (metatarsals and phalanges)

2. The hindpart is separated from the midpart by Chopart's joint; the midpart is separated from the forepart by Lisfranc's joint.

3. First metatarsal head bears twice the weight of the other metatarsals.

4. During the push-off phase, the second and third metatarsals bear the most weight; hence, they are prone to stress fractures.

B. Fractures

1. Calcaneus
 a. The calcaneus is the most frequently fractured tarsal bone. (The talus is the second most commonly fractured.)
 b. A calcaneal fracture is usually due to a compression injury (e.g. fall from a height with the patient landing on his feet).

c. Exam reveals swelling, tenderness and ecchymosis of the hindfoot and inability to bear weight on the fracture.

d. 10% are bilateral and another 10% are associated with compression fractures of the dorsolumbar spine.

e. 26% are associated with other injuries to the lower extremities.

f. Whenever a calcaneal body fracture is diagnosed, Bohler's angle should be measured to determine whether or not the fracture is depressed. This is done by measuring the intersection of two lines on the lateral film. One is drawn from the superior margin of the posterior tuberosity of the calcaneus and extended through the superior tip of the posterior facet. The other line is drawn from the superior tip of the anterior process and extended through the superior tip of the posterior facet. This angle normally measures 20° - 40°. If the angle is less than 20°, the fracture is depressed. [Rosen's Text, Fifth ed., p. 724, Fig. 51-22 or Tintinalli's Text, Sixth ed., p.1743, Fig. 277-2]

g. Treatment
   (1) Intra-articular or displaced calcaneal fractures — management remains controversial (non-operative versus immediate surgical reduction); obtain emergent orthopedic consultation in the ED.
   (2) Nondisplaced or minor extra-articular fractures — ice, elevation, immobilization in a posterior splint, crutches, consultation with an orthopedic surgeon and arrangement for early follow-up on an outpatient basis.

2. Lisfranc's (tarsometatarsal) fracture-dislocation
   a. Mechanisms of injury:
      (1) Axial load — a fall on the plantar-flexed foot
      (2) Compressive forces — crush injury
      (3) Rotational forces — twisting of the body around a fixed foot
   b. Exam reveals significant midfoot swelling and pain, decreased range of motion and inability to bear weight. Paresthesias of the midfoot may also be present.
   c. X-ray findings:
      (1) The key to making this diagnosis is to look for the normal alignment along the medial aspect of the middle cuneiform with the medial aspect of the base of the second metatarsal; any disruption of this alignment is indicative of a dislocation.
      (2) The second metatarsal functions as the primary stabilizing force of the joint; thus, a fracture through the base of the second metatarsal (Fleck's sign) is indicative of a disrupted Lisfranc joint.
      (3) Separation between the base of the first and second metatarsals is highly suggestive of subluxation and is the most reliable finding.
   d. Treatment — involves either closed reduction under general anesthesia or open reduction and surgical fixation; thus, early orthopedic consultation in the ED is indicated.

3. <u>Jones fracture</u> (diaphyseal fracture of the fifth metatarsal)
   a. A transverse fracture of the <u>proximal diaphysis</u> of the fifth meta-tarsal. (In children, the proximal physis of the fifth metatarsal may be mistaken for a fracture.)
   b. Mechanism of injury: a forceful load applied to the ball of the foot laterally (such as a pivot).
   c. Unlike avulsion fractures of the base of the fifth metatarsal (Dancer's fracture), these fractures are slow to heal and are associated with a high incidence of delayed union or nonunion.
   d. Treatment — these fractures require emergent consultation in the ED. Nondisplaced fractures are usually managed with immobilization in a non-weight-bearing short-leg cast, while displaced fractures (and fractures in athletes) are typically managed surgically.

VIII. Musculoskeletal Disorders

A. Arthritis — can be produced by many conditions and may be classified in several ways. Classification of arthritides by pattern of joint involvement (polyarticular, monarticular, migratory) is very useful, but there is some overlap.

1. Conditions associated with <u>symmetric polyarticular</u> joint pain:
   a. Rheumatoid arthritis (RA)
      (1) Most commonly affects women; there is a genetic predisposition related to HLA-DR 4 haplotype.
      (2) Most commonly affects the hand (MCP and PIP joints), wrist and elbow in an additive manner.
   b. Systemic lupus erythematosus (SLE)
      (1) Women 15 - 40 years of age are most commonly affected.
      (2) Arthralgias and arthritis are the most common presenting complaints; both small and large joints are affected.
      (3) An erythematous malar ("butterfly") rash is a typical feature of SLE and often accompanies joint involvement.
   c. Rheumatic fever (RF)
      (1) A <u>migratory</u> polyarthritis
      (2) Primarily affects the large joints of the extremities (knees, ankles, elbows and wrists)
   d. Bacterial endocarditis (<u>migratory</u>)
   e. Hepatitis B (<u>migratory</u>)
   f. Rubella
      (1) Occurs with both natural and vaccine-induced rubella.
      (2) Most commonly affects young women.
      (3) Finger, wrist and knee involvement is typical.

2. Conditions associated with <u>asymmetric polyarticular</u> joint pain:
   a. Reiter's syndrome (reactive arthritis)
      (1) Usually affects young males 15 - 35 years of age; the HLA-B27 antigen occurs in up to 75% of these patients.
      (2) Classic clinical triad: urethritis, conjunctivitis and arthritis; however, this syndrome has also been documented to occur following dysentery and cervicitis.
      (3) Oligoarthritis usually develops 1 - 6 weeks following an episode of urethritis (due to chlamydia) or dysentery (due to Salmonella, Shigella, Yersinia or Campylobacter).
      (4) The weight-bearing joints of the lower extremities are most commonly affected (usually four or five).
      (5) Must be differentiated from gonococcal arthritis.
   b. Gonococcal arthritis
      (1) A <u>migratory</u> arthritis that primarily affects young adults, particularly women.
      (2) The wrists, fingers, knees and ankles are most affected.
      (3) An associated rash (erythematous macules or pustules with a necrotic or purpuric center) which is distributed primarily on the extremities, accompanies the arthritis in 2/3 of patients (arthritis/dermatitis syndrome).
   c. Henoch-Schönlein purpura
      (1) Most commonly occurs in young children ages 4 - 11.
      (2) Classic clinical triad: <u>migratory</u> arthritis, palpable purpuric rash on the lower extremities/buttocks and colicky abdominal pain.
      (3) The ankles and knees are most commonly affected.
   d. Lyme disease
      (1) An oligoarthritis that typically affects the large joints (particularly the knees); it can be <u>migratory</u> and usually occurs in those patients not treated with appropriate antibiotics.
      (2) Arthritic symptoms develop in Stage III of the disease (months to years after the initial infection).

3. Conditions associated with <u>monarticular</u> joint pain:
   a. Septic arthritis (a medical emergency)
      (1) *Staph. aureus* is the most common cause.
      (2) In most adults, the knee is the most commonly affected joint. In IV drug abusers, however, the favored sites are the sacroiliac, sternoclavicular and intervertebral joints. In children, the knee and hip are most commonly affected.
      (3) **Clinical picture**: A 58-year-old woman with a long history of rheumatoid arthritis presents with fever and left knee pain for the past 24 hours. On exam, her knee is swollen, warm and tender. Laboratory evaluation reveals a leukocytosis and a markedly elevated ESR. Aside from some soft-tissue swelling, her x-rays are unremarkable. Arthrocentesis reveals purulent fluid (> 100,000 WBCs with a predominance of PMNs), a low glucose and gram-positive cocci in clusters on Gram stain.

b. Gout
   (1) A disease of middle-aged men and elderly adults.
   (2) Caused by deposition of uric acid crystals.
   (3) Usually affects the lower extremities, particularly the great toe ("podagra").
   (4) Evaluation of synovial fluid reveals <u>needle-shaped</u> crystals that exhibit <u>negative</u> birefringence under polarized light.
   (5) **Clinical picture:** An obese 48-year-old man presents with left knee pain. He states that the pain developed over a period of a few hours and is so bad that even the weight of a bedsheet on his knee is too much to bear. The patient denies recent trauma and prior injury to this knee, but does admit to over-indulging in rich food and alcohol the past couple of days. This PMH is remarkable only for hypertension for which he is being treated with a loop diuretic. On exam, his knee is erythematous, swollen, hot and tender. X-ray evaluation reveals only soft-tissue swelling. Synovial fluid analysis demonstrates 20,000 WBCs with a predominance of PMNs, a negative Gram stain and needle-shaped, negatively birefringent crystals.
c. Pseudogout (chondrocalcinosis)
   (1) Primarily affects men and women in their sixties (and older).
   (2) Caused by the deposit of <u>calcium pyrophosphate</u> crystals.
   (3) The most commonly affected joint is the knee, followed by the wrist, ankle and elbow.
   (4) Evaluation of synovial fluid reveals <u>rhomboid-shaped</u> crystals that exhibit weakly <u>positive</u> birefringence under polarized light.
   (5) X-rays of the affected joint may reveal calcification of the cartilage (chondrocalcinosis).
   (6) **Clinical picture:** A 68-year-old woman presents with left knee pain for the past two days. She denies acute trauma and prior injury to this knee. On exam, her knee is erythematous, swollen and tender. X-rays reveal presence of calcium deposits. Arthrocentesis demonstrates 20,000 WBCs with a predominance of PMNs, a negative Gram stain and rhomboid-shaped crystals that are positively birefringent.
d. Osteoarthritis (degenerative joint disease)
e. Trauma
f. Aseptic arthritis
g. Hemarthrosis
<u>Note</u>: Patients with monarticular joint pain should always be considered to have an infectious arthritis until proven otherwise.

4. Conditions associated with <u>migratory</u> arthritis:
   a. Rheumatic fever
   b. Bacterial endocarditis
   c. Hepatitis B
   d. Septicemia (gonococcal, meningococcal, strep, staph)
   e. Henoch-Schönlein purpura
   f. Lyme disease

g. Serum sickness

h. Pulmonary infections (mycoplasmosis, histoplasmosis, coccidio-mycosis)

5. Synovial fluid analysis is the most important diagnostic study in the evaluation of an acute arthritis.

    a. Mnemonic for laboratory analysis: "CAPS"

        C - culture, cell count, crystals

        A - appearance

        P - protein

        S - sugar, stain (gram stain)

        <u>Note</u>: if there is only enough fluid for one test, it should be C&S

    b. Crystals

        (1) <u>Gout</u>: negatively birefringent (urate) and needle-shaped.

        (2) <u>Pseudogout</u>: positively birefringent (calcium pyrophosphate) and rhomboid-shaped.

    c. White blood cell count

        (1) < 200 with < 25% PMNs is normal.

        (2) 200 - 2,000 with < 25% PMNs is noninflammatory (osteoarthritis, traumatic arthritis).

        (3) 2,000 - 50,000 with ≥ 50 - 75% PMNs is inflammatory (rheumatoid arthritis, gout, pseudogout).

        (4) 5,000 - > 50,000 (usually > 40,000) with > 75% PMNs is septic.

    d. Glucose — is significantly decreased (relative to serum glucose) in both septic and rheumatoid arthritis.

    e. Gram stain — usually positive, except for gonococcal infection which is only positive in 25% of cases.

B. Back Pain

1. Differential diagnosis

   • Aortic aneurysm

   • Peptic ulcer

   • Pyelonephritis

   • Pancreatitis

   • Vertebral disc compression/fracture

   • Osteoporosis

   • Carcinoma (primary or metastatic)

   • Ankylosing spondylitis (associated with inflammatory bowel disease)

   • Infection

   • Osteomyelitis

   • Ectopic pregnancy

   • Strain or sprain

   • PID

2. General facts (pearls)

    a. Back pain is the most frequent (and the most costly) cause of workman's compensation payments.

    b. Most back pain (including pain secondary to disc disease) is self-limited; it will resolve in 6 - 7 weeks or less, regardless of treatment.

   c. Most back pain is benign (particularly in healthy, young- and middle-aged adults).

   d. A serious cause of back pain is more likely in patients < 20 yrs old (incidence of 10%) and in patients > 55 yrs. of age (incidence of 20%).

   e. 80% or more of low back pain occurs in the L_4 - S_1 region; L_5 - S_1 is the most frequent location.

   f. When x-rays are indicated (which they are not in the majority of cases) AP and lateral views alone are usually sufficient.

     (1) Most healthy 18 - 55-year-olds with atraumatic, nonspecific, mechanical low back pain can be managed initially <u>without</u> x-ray evaluation.

     (2) Lumbosacral films should be obtained as part of the initial evaluation in the following circumstances:

       (a) Age < 18 or > 55 years (higher incidence of serious causes)

       (b) Trauma

       (c) Persistent, unremitting back pain > 4 - 6 weeks duration

       (d) Prior referral

       (e) Suspicion of serious underlying pathology based on the patient's:
- PMH (cancer, IV drug abuse)
- Vital signs (fever)
- Atypical symptoms (night pain)

3. Lumbar disc syndromes

   a. Impingement of a herniated disc on the anterior nerve root produces pain in a dermatomal pattern:

     * L_1 — groin
     * L_2 — upper thigh
     * L_3 — mid thigh and medial knee
     * L_4 — lower thigh, anterior knee and medial foot
     * L_5 — Lateral lower leg, first interdigital web space and dorsal foot
     * S_1 — posterolateral calf and lateral foot

   b. Physical findings of nerve root involvement:

     (1) ↓ Knee jerk = L_3 + L_4

     (2) ↓ Dorsiflexion of foot = L_5

     (3) ↓ Ankle jerk (↓ plantar flexion) and numbness of lateral foot = S_1

   c. Cauda equina syndrome (neurosurgical emergency)

     (1) A serious complication of lumbar disc disease

     (2) Results from a massive <u>midline</u> lumbar disc herniation which compresses several nerve roots of the cauda equina.

     (3) Patients complain of lower back/leg pain and incontinence (or retention) of bowel and bladder. With progression, the patient will also develop numbness of the feet and trouble walking.

     (4) Exam reveals loss of sensation in the "saddle" distribution and loss of anal tone (S_3, S_4, S_5).

     (5) An MRI or emergency myelogram may be used to confirm the diagnosis + locate the disc level but should not delay treatment.

(6) Treatment: <u>Immediate</u> neurosurgical consultation for operative disc decompression; decompression must be performed quickly (within several hours) if permanent disability is to be avoided.

4. <u>Spondylolisthesis</u>
   a. Definition: the <u>forward</u> displacement of a vertebral body on the one below (most commonly L_5 on S_1).
   b. The amount of forward displacement is graded; the higher the grade, the worse the slippage:
      - Grade I: up to 25%
      - Grade II: 25 to 50%
      - Grade III: 50 to 75%
      - Grade IV: 75 to 100%
   c. Best seen on the lateral view of the lumbar spine series.
   d. This disorder is often asymptomatic (only 25% of patients with this disorder develop back or leg pain); therefore, this finding on x-ray may be incidental and not necessarily the cause of the patient's back/leg pain.

5. Treatment
   a. Outpatient management protocol for patients with low back pain without neurologic findings ("lumbar strain"):
      (1) Bedrest for 1 - 2 days followed by a gradual increase in physical activity, avoiding those activities that exacerbate pain (heavy lifting, twisting).
      (2) Analgesics (including NSAIDs)
      (3) Muscle relaxants
      (4) Follow-up in 7 days
      (5) Instructions to return immediately if problems develop (worsening pain, loss of motor strength, bowel or bladder incontinence)
   b. Inpatient management is indicated for patients with:
      (1) Cauda equina syndrome
      (2) Severe or progressive neurologic deficit
      (3) Multiple nerve root involvement
      (4) Unmanageable pain
      (5) Inadequate support system at home

C. *Charcot's Joint*

1. Most common presentation is a painful, swollen ankle.

2. At the present time, the usual cause is diabetic peripheral neuropathy (not syphilis).

3. X-ray of the ankle reveals the classic "bag of bones" appearance.

Journal References

ACAD EMERG MED, Dominguez, S., et. al., April 2005, 12(4):366, "Prevalence of Traumatic Hip and Pelvic Fractures in Patients with Suspected Hip Fracture and Negative Initial Standard Radiographs: A Study of Emergency Department Patients.

CRITICAL DECISIONS IN EMER MED, September 1997, Reinhardt, R., "Emergency Evaluation and Management of the Nontraumatic Acute Joint."

EMERGENCY MEDICINE AUSTRALASIA, Cooper, J.G., et.al., April 2005, 17(2):132, "Local Anaesthetic Infiltration Increases the Accuracy of Assessment of Ulnar Collateral Ligament Injuries

EMERGENCY MEDICINE NEWS, Davenport, B., March 2001, "Knee Dislocations are Always a Threat for Vascular Injury."

EMERGENCY MEDICINE REPORTS, Stewart, Charles, May 29, 1995, "Traumatic and Inflammatory Disorders of the Shoulder: Assessment Strategies, Complications, and Interventional Techniques."

EMERGENCY MEDICINE REPORTS, Stewart, Charles, Jan. 6, 1997, "Knee Injuries: Diagnosis and Repair."

EMERGENCY MEDICINE REPORTS, Stewart, Charles, Feb. 16, 1998, "Winter Sports-Related Injuries: Current Standards for Diagnosis and Treatment."

EMERGENCY MEDICINE REPORTS, Wiens, D., July 10, 1995, "Acute Low Back Pain: Differential Diagnosis, Targeted Assessment, and Therapeutic Controversies."

J ARTHROSCOPY RELATED SURG, Akseki, D., et.al., November 2004 (9):951, "McMurray's Test and Joint Line Tenderness."

J MUSCULOSKELETAL MEDICINE, Austin, S., Beaty, J., May 1995, "Supracondylar Fractures of the Distal Humerus in Children."

J MUSCULOSKELETAL MEDICINE, Itamura, J., Burkhead, Jr., W., Shankwiler, J., November, 1995, "Decision Making in Shoulder Dislocation."

J MUSCULOSKELETAL MEDICINE, Kaiser, J., Holland, B., July 1995, "Using Imaging Studies in the Diagnosis of Low Back Pain."

J MUSCULOSKELETAL MEDICINE, Keating, J., June 1995, "Evaluating Low Back Pain: A Primary Care Approach."

Specific Text References

Clinical Procedures in Emergency Medicine. 4th ed., Roberts, J.R., Hedges, J.R., (Saunders, Philadelphia, 2004).

Fractures and Dislocations, Closed Management (Volume 2). Connolly, J. F., (Saunders, Philadelphia, 1995).

Handbook of Orthopedic Emergencies. Hart, Rittenberry, Vehara (Lippincott-Raven, Philadelphia, 1999).

<u>Primer on the Rheumatic Diseases</u>. Klippel, J. H., Weyand, C. M., Wortmann, R. L., 11th ed., (Arthritis Foundation, Atlanta, Ga, 1998).

<u>Radial Head Subluxation: Comparing Two Methods of Reduction</u>. McDonald, Whitelaw, Goldsmith (Academic Emergency Medicine, 1999).

<u>Rockwood and Green's Fractures in Adults</u>. 5th ed., Buckholz, R.W., Heckman, J.D., (Lippincott, Williams & Wilkens, Philadelphia, 2001).

General Text References, Acep Clinical Policies and LLSA Reading Lists for all chapters located in the back of both volumes.

NOTES

MAJOR TRAUMA

📖 **Note: Manual Update**

For New ATLS guidelines published after this printing, refer to Written Board Manual/Guideline Update link on our website - www.emeeinc.com.

It is assumed that the written board candidate is ATLS certified. The following chapter covers only the essentials of trauma recognition and management that were felt to be pertinent to this exam. If the reader feels that he/she is weak in this area, a review of the ATLS manual is strongly recommended prior to sitting for the written board exam.

---

1. The smallest amount of blood loss that consistently produces a decrease in the systolic BP in adults is:

    (a) Loss < 15% of blood volume
    (b) Loss 15 - 30% of blood volume
    (c) Loss 30 - 40% of blood volume
    (d) Loss > 40% of blood volume

2. All of the following statements regarding Class I hemorrhage are accurate except:

    (a) It represents a blood loss up to 15% of blood volume.
    (b) It is treated with crystalloids in the trauma victim.
    (c) Capillary refill is delayed with this degree of hemorrhage.
    (d) It is associated with a slight increase in HR (< 100 BPM).

3. The leading cause of death and disability in trauma victims is:

    (a) Head injury
    (b) Back injury
    (c) Abdominal injury
    (d) Thoracic injury

4. Which of the following statements regarding cardiac tamponade is inaccurate?

    (a) It is most commonly caused by blunt chest trauma.
    (b) Clinical findings include hypotension, decreased pulse pressure, JVD, pulsus paradoxus and muffled heart tones.
    (c) Initial therapy is with IV fluids and pericardiocentesis.
    (d) It can manifest as PEA.

5. A patient with chest trauma is hypotensive on presentation and c/o SOB. Exam reveals JVD, tracheal deviation and decreased breath sounds associated with hyperresonance to percussion on one side of his chest. Other than providing O_2, starting IVs and placing the patient on a cardiac monitor, what is the most appropriate initial therapy for this patient?

    (a) Pericardiocentesis
    (b) Tube thoracostomy
    (c) Intubation
    (d) Needle thoracostomy

6. The components of Beck's Triad include all of the following except:

    (a) Muffled heart tones
    (b) Pulsus paradoxus
    (c) Hypotension
    (d) JVD

7. The most common abdominal organ injured in blunt trauma is:
   (a) Spleen
   (b) Liver
   (c) Pancreas
   (d) Kidney

8. All of the following modalities are useful in the treatment of myoglobinuria except:
   (a) Acidifying the urine
   (b) IV mannitol
   (c) Alkalinizing the urine
   (d) Increasing the urine output (by increasing IV fluid resuscitation)

9. All of the following statements regarding drowning are accurate except:
   (a) Freshwater drownings are more common than saltwater drownings.
   (b) 10 - 15% of drownings are "dry" (no water enters the lungs).
   (c) The initial management of the drowning victim is determined by the type of drowning that occurred (wet, dry, saltwater, freshwater).
   (d) Death in these victims is usually due to hypoxia.

10. It is recommended that all trauma patients receive supplemental oxygen. The suggested FIO_2 is:
    (a) >.85
    (b) >.60
    (c) >.50
    (d) >.40

11. All of the following CXR findings are consistent with the diagnosis of traumatic rupture of the aorta except:
    (a) Widening of the superior mediastinum
    (b) Apical pleural cap
    (c) Deviation of the trachea to the right
    (d) Elevation of the left mainstem bronchus

12. Which of the following modalities provides the best assessment of retroperitoneal organs (e.g. pancreas, duodenum)?
    (a) Physical exam
    (b) Diagnostic peritoneal lavage (DPL)
    (c) Computerized tomography (CT)
    (d) All of the above modalities are equally effective.

13. Although all of the following techniques should be used when available, the most reliable method of confirming ET tube position is by:

    (a) Listening over the upper lung fields for equal breath sounds
    (b) Checking the position of the tube on a post-intubation CXR
    (c) Establishing end-tidal CO_2 monitoring
    (d) Seeing the ET tube pass through the vocal cords

14. Neurologic evaluation of a trauma patient reveals a lack of response in the categories of eye opening, verbal response and motor response. What is this patient's Glasgow Coma Score?

    (a) 0
    (b) 3
    (c) 4
    (d) 5

15. All of the following statements regarding epidural hematomas are accurate except:

    (a) Associated parietal or temporal skull fracture is common.
    (b) CT reveals a lens-like, biconvex lesion.
    (c) Signs and symptoms are due to the mass effect of an arterial bleed.
    (d) Pupillary findings typically occur contralateral to the side of the lesion.

16. All of the following statements regarding basilar skull fractures are accurate except:

    (a) Placement of an NG tube and nasotracheal intubation are contraindicated in the presence of these fractures.
    (b) Skull films are more useful than clinical findings in making the diagnosis.
    (c) Clinical findings include CSF rhinorrhea or otorrhea, hemotympanum, raccoon's eyes, Battle's sign and the "ring sign" on filter paper.
    (d) Patients should receive neurosurgical consultation and possible admisson for observation.

17. Listed below are several C-spine injuries and their mechanism of injury. Which is incorrectly matched?

    (a) Jefferson fracture: axial loading mechanism
    (b) Hangman's fracture: flexion injury
    (c) Clay-shoveler's fracture: flexion injury or direct trauma
    (d) Unilateral facet dislocation: flexion-rotation injury

18. The best view for visualizing a Jefferson fracture is:
    (a) Open-mouth odontoid
    (b) Cross-table lateral
    (c) AP
    (d) Oblique

19. All of the following statements regarding pulmonary contusions are accurate except:
    (a) They usually result from blunt chest wall trauma.
    (b) Associated rib fractures may be present.
    (c) CXR findings are typically diffuse and develop in a delayed fashion (24 - 72 hours post-injury).
    (d) Pneumonia is the most common and most significant complication.

20. Cardiac contusions most commonly involve the:
    (a) Left ventricle
    (b) Right ventricle
    (c) Left atrium
    (d) Right atrium

21. The earliest clinical finding in a patient with a compartment syndrome is:
    (a) Pain
    (b) Paralysis
    (c) Palpable tenseness and tenderness of the involved compartment
    (d) Pulselessness

Answers: 1. c, 2. c, 3. a, 4. a, 5. d, 6. b, 7. a, 8. a, 9. c, 10. a, 11. d
12. c, 13. d, 14. b, 15. d, 16. b., 17. b, 18. a, 19. c, 20. b, 21. a

Use the pre-chapter multiple choice question worksheet (p. xxv) to record and determine the percentage of correct answers for this section.

MAJOR TRAUMA

I. General Information

A. Trauma is the leading cause of death between the ages of 1 - 44. Many of the injuries are readily treatable (and death preventable) primarily because these patients are youthful and otherwise healthy.

B. The primary role of the emergency physician is to <u>assess</u>, <u>resuscitate</u> and <u>stabilize</u> the trauma patient on a <u>priority basis</u>; this includes both suspicion and recognition of potentially serious problems. Trauma management, on the other hand, falls in the realm of general surgery and the various surgical specialties.

C. There are three peak times for trauma deaths:

1. First peak time (<u>immediate</u> death)*
   a. Occurs within <u>seconds to minutes</u> of injury; these patients generally die at the scene.
   b. Death is usually due to:
      (1) Massive head injury
      (2) High C-spine injury with high spinal cord disruption
      (3) Cardiac laceration
      (4) Aortic rupture
      (5) Laceration of other great vessels
      (6) Airway obstruction

2. Second peak time (<u>early</u> death)
   a. Occurs within <u>minutes to a few hours</u> of injury, the so-called "golden hour."
   b. Death in these patients is generally secondary to:
      (1) Subdural and epidural hematomas
      (2) Ruptured spleen/lacerated liver
      (3) Multiple injuries associated with hypovolemic shock
      (4) Fracture of the pelvis or multiple long bones
      (5) Hemopneumothorax
      (6) Tension pneumothorax
      (7) Cardiac tamponade
      (8) Massive hemothorax
      (9) Aortic dissection/rupture
   c. Application of ATLS guidelines regarding rapid ABC assessment and stabilization (definitive airway management, fluid resuscitation and blood replacement) reduces the mortality/morbidity rate of these patients.

*Greatest number of fatalities occur in this time frame.

3. Third peak time (<u>delayed</u> death)
   a. Occurs days to weeks following the initial injury.
   b. Death in these patients is usually due to:
      (1) Multisystem organ failure
      (2) Sepsis

II. General Approach to the Trauma Patient

A. Primary Survey: assessment and management of the ABCs

1. Airway and C-spine
   a. Airway control is the single most important prehospital/arrival priority.
   b. Immediately assess the airway for potential compromise; a compromised airway is a non-patent or poorly-protected airway. Check the following:
      • If the patient can speak . . . the airway is patent.
      • If the respirations are noisy . . . partial obstruction is present.
      • If the gag reflex is depressed/absent or if secretions are pooling . . . the airway is poorly protected → potential for aspiration.
   c. Beware of the potential for associated cervical spine injuries; <u>always</u> maintain the cervical spine in neutral position with in-line manual cervical immobilization or appropriate immobilization devices when evaluating and managing the airway. Significant C-spine injury should be suspected in the multiple-injured patient with an altered LOC or evidence of blunt injury above the clavicle.
   d. Methods
      (1) Open the airway using the chin lift or jaw thrust maneuver.
      (2) Remove dentures and foreign bodies if present.
      (3) Consider placement of a nasopharyngeal (conscious patient) or oropharyngeal (<u>un</u>conscious patient) airway.
      (4) Patients who cannot speak, are not handling secretions and have a <u>depressed/absent</u> gag reflex require definitive airway management (nasotracheal/orotracheal intubation or a surgical airway).
      (5) Orotracheal intubation is the procedure of choice (even in the presence of suspected C-spine injury). Hyperventilation prior to rapid sequence induction is not generally recommended due to the risk of aspiration. If intubation is unsuccessful, a surgical airway is indicated.
         (a) <u>Nasotracheal intubation with in-line manual cervical immobilization</u> . . . is usually restricted to patients ≥ 12 years of age who are breathing and should not be performed in kids < 9 years of age. Contraindications include: apnea, midfacial fractures/trauma and basilar skull fracture.

       (b) <u>Orotracheal intubation with in-line cervical immobilization</u> . . . should be performed if the patient is <u>not</u> breathing, has midfacial injuries or a basilar skull fracture.

       (c) <u>Fiberoptic endoscopy</u> . . . may be used to facilitate difficult nasotracheal or orotracheal intubation if the patient's condition permits and the physician is skilled in this technique.

       (d) <u>Surgical cricothyroidotomy</u> . . . is necessary if attempts at intubation are unsuccessful. [<u>Note</u>: Most authors consider a surgical airway the procedure of choice for patients with severe midfacial injuries; however, most clinicians would make a single attempt at orotracheal intubation with in-line manual cervical immobilization before proceeding to a surgical airway.]

         <u>1</u> Consider using a laryngeal mask airway (LMA) or an esophageal-tracheal combitube (ETC) as a bridging device; the ETC is easier to insert than the LMA and also has less risk of aspiration.

         <u>2</u> In children less than 12 years of age, needle crichothyroidotomy followed by transtracheal jet insufflation is the procedure of choice (because the cricothyroid membrane is not yet palpable).

   (6) Following intubation, verify the position of the ET tube by:

       (a) Listening over the upper lung fields (axillae or apices) for equal breath sounds

       (b) Listening over the epigastrium to R/O the presence of borborygmi

       (c) Checking the position of the ET tube on a post-intubation CXR

       (d) Establishing end-tidal CO_2 monitoring[*]

      <u>Note</u>: Although all of the above techniques should be used, the <u>most reliable</u> method of confirming ET tube placement is <u>seeing</u> the tube pass through the vocal cords.

   (7) In pediatric patients, the same guidelines for airway management apply but with two exceptions:

       (a) In children < 9 yrs. of age, orotracheal intubation should be performed with <u>uncuffed</u> tubes and

       (b) In children < 12 yrs. of age, <u>needle</u> cricothyroidotomy is preferred over surgical cricothyroidotomy

2. Breathing

   a. Determine the rate, depth and pattern of respiration; then place the patient on a pulse oximeter to assess the adequacy of ventilation.

   b. Administer supplemental oxygen to <u>all</u> trauma patients; use high-flow oxygen (10 - 12L/min) to deliver an FIO_2 > .85; for intubated or "cric" patients, breathing should generally be assisted.

---

[*]When cardiac arrest confounds attempts to assess placement using end-tidal CO_2, an aspiration device (e.g. esophageal detector device) may be useful.

    c. Look for and correct any injuries to the chest wall that may acutely impair ventilation:
- Perform needle thoracostomy to alleviate <u>tension</u> pneumothorax; follow immediately with thoracostomy tube placement.
- Seal sucking chest wounds -- cover with a sterile occlusive dressing, taped down on three of its four sides.

    d. Ventilator settings in the trauma patient may be different than usual due to changes in hemodynamic status.
- (1) Positive pressure ventilation in a hypovolemic patient may worsen hypotension; low tidal volumes are appropriate (5mL/kg at a rate of 20 - 30 breaths/min).
- (2) Close monitoring of pulse and blood pressure and frequent ABGs will ultimately determine the ventilator settings.

3. Circulation and hemorrhage control
    a. Check pulses for quality, rate and regularity
    b. Evaluate skin color, capillary refill and level of consciousness.
    c. Control external bleeding with direct pressure or the application of a transparent pneumatic splint.
    d. Consider application of MAST/PASG to control bleeding from pelvic or lower extremity fractures.
    e. Use large-bore catheters (at least 16-gauge) and draw blood for lab.
    f. Initiate treatment of shock with a <u>warmed</u> crystalloid solution; rapidly administer 1 - 2 liters of Ringer's lactate (or normal saline).[*] If the patient fails to respond, blood should be administered.
    g. Place the patient on a cardiac monitor and check a rhythm strip.
    h. Treat tamponade with pericardiocentesis.
    i. Consider ED thoracotomy for patients with penetrating thoracic injuries who arrive pulseless but with myocardial activity.
    [<u>Note</u>: ATLS recommends that a surgeon be present.]

4. Disability (neuro exam)
    a. Assess pupil size, reactivity and symmetry.
    b. Determine the patient's level of consciousness; use the AVPU method or the Glasgow Coma Scale:
- (1) The AVPU method — provides a <u>qualitative</u> assessment of the patient's level of consciousness; AVPU is an acronym for:
  - **A**lert
  - Responds to **V**ocal stimuli
  - Responds to **P**ainful stimuli
  - **U**nresponsive
- (2) The Glasgow Coma Scale (GCS) — provides a <u>quantitative</u> assessment of the patient's level of consciousness based upon the patient's <u>best</u> response in three categories (eye opening, verbal response and motor response); scores range from a minimum of 3 (no response) to a maximum of 15 (best response in all categories).

*Fluid bolus in kids is 10mL/kg

c. Patients with severe head injury plus an altered level of consciousness (or a GCS score ≤ 8) usually require intubation. The presence of non-purposeful motor responses also suggests the need for a definitive airway. If either (or both) of these conditions exist, make sure the airway is protected.

5. Exposure/environmental control — completely undress the patient to facilitate a thorough exam, but remember to cover him with warmed blankets to prevent iatrogenic hypothermia.

B. Initial Testing/Continued Treatment

1. Order lab studies, e.g. Type & cross, CBC with platelets, PT(INR)/PTT, BUN/cr, lytes, glucose, amylase, lipase, ETOH, tox screen, B-HCG, UA, ABGs, CK, etc. as appropriate. (Selective ordering is recommended.)

2. Order the following x-rays unless they are clearly not indicated: cross-table lateral C-spine, AP chest and abdomen.

3. Provide continuous ECG, pulse oximetry and blood pressure monitoring.

4. Place NG (or orogastric) tube and Foley catheter — after having first evaluated the patient for the presence of contraindications (cribriform plate fracture, blood at the urethral meatus, scrotal hematoma or a high-riding prostate on rectal exam).

5. Determine if there is a need to transfer the patient to a hospital that can provide a higher level of care. If such a need exists, administrative personnel should initiate the transfer process while the secondary survey is completed and the patient is stabilized.

C. Secondary Survey/Final Case Management

1. Obtain an "AMPLE" medical history and inquire about the mechanism of injury.

2. Perform a complete physical exam — a "finger or tube" in every orifice. Be sure to complete the rectal exam, checking for sphincter tone, blood, high-riding prostate and bowel wall integrity.

3. Order additional diagnostic studies as indicated, e.g. x-rays of thoracolumbar spine and/or extremities, DPL, CT, ultrasound, etc.

4. Assess and reassess lab data, response to fluids, vital signs and overall stability of the patient.

5. Don't forget tetanus booster and antibiotics when indicated.

D. Pediatric Pearls

1. Airway Management
    a. Use of sedating agents prior to intubation is based on the presence or absence of hemorrhagic shock.
        (1) Hypovolemic kids → etomidate (0.3 mg/kg)
        (2) Normovolemic kids → etomidate (same dose) and midazolam (same dose)
    b. Uncuffed ET tubes are used in kids ≤ 9 yrs. old; nasotracheal intubation should not be performed in children < 9 yrs old.
    c. Surgical crichothyroidotomy can be performed when the crichothyroid membrane is palpable (~12 yrs. old).

2. Shock evaluation
    a. The decrease in circulating blood volume required to produce minimal signs of shock is 30%.
    b. The lower limit of normal systolic BP is 70mmHg plus twice the age in years.

3. Evaluation of abdominal trauma
    a. Helical CT scanning (with or without trauma) can be used in the hemodynamically stable child.
    b. DPL is used to detect intra-abdominal bleeding in the hypotensive child or when ultrasonography/FAST is not readily available.

4. Younger children (< 11 yrs. old) with cervical spine injuries are most commonly injured in the upper C-spine.

III. Hemorrhagic Shock

A. Hemorrhage - induced hypovolemia is the most common cause of shock in the trauma patient.

B. The earliest signs of hemorrhagic shock are tachycardia and cutaneous vasoconstriction.

C. Once shock is identified, the initial treatment is volume resuscitation with a warmed crystalloid solution; continued management is determined by the patient's response to initial therapy.

D. The amount of blood loss present can be estimated based on the patient's initial clinical presentation as follows:
1. Class I hemorrhage: blood volume loss 0 - 15% (0 - 750mL)
    a. Minimal clinical signs and symptoms; the patient is normotensive with slightly ↑ HR (< 100)
    b. Although the healthy adult can easily compensate for this small volume loss via compensatory mechanisms, the trauma patient should be treated with crystalloids; blood products are not required.

2. Class II hemorrhage: blood volume loss 15 - 30% (750 - 1500mL)
   a. Clinical signs and symptoms: tachypnea, tachycardia > 100, <u>narrow</u> pulse pressure, delayed capillary refill, mild anxiety, slight decrease in urine output.
   b. Blood products may or may not be required; treat first with crystalloids and monitor response.

3. Class III hemorrhage: blood volume loss 30 - 40% (1500 - 2000mL)
   a. Clinical signs and symptoms: tachypnea, tachycardia (HR $\geq$ 120), decrease in systolic BP, delayed capillary refill, decreased urine output, change in mental status.
   b. Blood products and crystalloids should be used; if possible, wait for at least type-specific blood.

4. Class IV hemorrhage: blood volume loss > 40% (> 2 liters)
   a. Clinical signs and symptoms: obvious shock, tachycardia (HR $\geq$ 140), decreased systolic BP, extremely <u>narrow</u> pulse pressure, scant urine output, delayed capillary refill, confusion, lethargy.
   b. Death is imminent without aggressive treatment: use blood warmers and administer an initial bolus of 2 liters of crystalloid; transfuse Type O blood (Rh neg for premenopausal females,[*] Rh neg or pos for males). Immediate surgery is often required.
   <u>Note</u>: The crystalloid to blood replacement ratio is 3:1; the patient should receive 3mL of crystalloid for each 1mL of blood lost. Remember that aggressive and continuous volume resuscitation is not a substitute for manual or operative control of hemorrhage.

IV. Common Injuries By Anatomical Location

A. Head Injuries

1. Head injury is the leading cause of death + disability in trauma cases.

2. The most frequent cause of death in patients sustaining severe head injury is uncontrolled intracranial hypertension.

3. Assume a cervical spine injury exists in head-injured patients; if your clinical assessment or the mechanism of injury <u>suggests</u> the possibility of neck injury, immobilize the C-spine and order films.

4. An altered level of consciousness is the hallmark of brain injury.

5. With the exception of patients with minor head injuries, almost all head-injured patients require CT scanning and most require neurosurgical consultation. Medical personnel must accompany the head-injured patient outside the ED (radiology suite) to monitor the stability of the patient.

---

[*]Rh neg not needed after pregnancy is not an issue.

6. A head injury must be ruled out in any patient who is not fully alert. This includes intoxicated patients who have a higher incidence of head and other serious injuries than do non-intoxicated people; they should receive a CT scan <u>or</u>, at the very least, be observed until improved.

7. Alert patients who complain of headache and/or sensory changes should be scanned or observed as should those with a history of unconsciousness (unless very brief), persistent amnesia or a skull fracture.

8. Patients with a decreased level of consciousness, lateralized extremity weakness and abnormal pupillary function (especially a dilated, unreactive pupil) often have a mass lesion and may need emergent surgery.

9. Patients with head trauma resulting from <u>non</u>vehicular accidents (e.g. falls) are <u>more likely</u> to need surgical intervention than those with a head injury resulting from vehicular accidents, particularly if they are comatose and/or have lateralizing motor deficits.

10. The Glasgow Coma Scale (GCS) provides a <u>quantitative</u> assessment of the patient's level of consciousness and can be used to categorize the severity of head injury as mild (GCS 14 - 15), moderate (GCS 9 - 13) or severe (GCS 3 - 8); all patients with a GCS < 8 (and most patients with a GCS of 8) are comatose.

11. Never assume that brain injury is the cause of hypotension; except as a terminal event, hypotension is seldom the result of isolated head injury.

12. Avoid secondary brain injury by preventing/treating hypoxia, ischemia, hypercarbia, increased ICP and hyperpyrexia.

13. The <u>Cushing response</u> to elevated ICP consists of <u>hypertension</u>, <u>bradycardia</u> and a <u>decreased respiratory rate</u>; the hypertension represents the brain's effort to maintain cerebral perfusion pressure (CPP). Maintaining the CPP (mean arterial pressure minus ICP) at 60 - 70mmHg is recommended as a means of improving cerebral blood flow.

14. Specific types of head injuries are categorized as: diffuse brain injuries (concussions, diffuse axonal injuries), focal brain injuries (contusions, hemorrhages, hematomas) or skull fractures. <u>Diffuse</u> brain injuries do <u>not</u> have mass lesions necessitating emergency surgery whereas <u>focal</u> brain injuries, because of their mass effect, may require emergency surgery. The management of skull fractures is determined by the type of fracture and the presence of associated brain injuries.
    a. <u>Cerebral concussion</u>
       (1) Classic clinical scenario; head injury → <u>brief</u> loss of neurologic function. These patients are often amnestic and, therefore, will frequently ask the same questions over and over again. Headache with or without vomiting is generally present, but there are <u>no</u> <u>focal findings</u>.
       (2) Clinical features
           • <u>Brief</u> loss of neurologic function (confusion, amnesia, and/or loss of consciousness)
           • Vomiting (±)
           • Rapid clinical improvement is the rule.

(3) Loss of consciousness results from impairment of the reticular activating system.

(4) CT scan is negative.

(5) Admission depends on severity of symptoms, other associated injuries and the home situation.

b. <u>Diffuse axonal injury (DAI)</u>

    (1) Clinical features
- Prolonged coma (often lasting days to weeks) ± posturing
- (±) Autonomic dysfunction (high fever, HTN, sweating)

    (2) Results in widely scattered <u>microscopic</u> neuronal damage throughout the brain.

    (3) CT scan → no mass lesion

    (4) Patients require admission and neurosurgical consultation; overall mortality is 33%.

c. <u>Cerebral contusion</u>

    (1) Clinical features — are similar to those of a concussion <u>except</u>:
- Neurologic dysfunction is more profound and prolonged; patients often demonstrate mental confusion, obtundation or coma.
- Focal deficits may be present if contusions occur in the sensorimotor strip.

    (2) These lesions generally occur in the frontal and temporal lobes and are visible on CT scan. They may be produced at the site of impact (coup contusions) or at the opposite pole of the brain (contrecoup contusions).

    (3) Admit these patients for observation and obtain neurosurgical consultation. No further therapy is indicated unless complications develop.

    (4) Potential delayed complications (hours or days) include development of cerebral edema or an intracerebral hematoma at the site of the contusion → mass effect; hematomas are best detected by repeating the CT 12 - 24 hours after the initial scan.

d. <u>Epidural hematoma</u>

    (1) Classic clinical scenario: head injury → LOC → lucid interval (≤ 30%) → coma → a fixed and dilated pupil <u>on the side of the lesion</u> and contralateral hemiparesis. The mechanism is a transtentorial herniation which compresses the III nerve and the corticospinal tract. This scenario, however, is not always present; patients do not always lose consciousness, pupillary dilation can occur on the side opposite the lesion and hemiparesis may occur on the same side of the lesion.

    (2) Signs and symptoms are usually caused by the mass effect of an <u>arterial bleed</u> (usually the middle meningeal artery). They may become evident within an hour of the injury or take 4 - 6 hours (or more) to develop.

    (3) CT scan demonstrates the classic <u>lens-like</u>, <u>biconvex</u> lesion (be able to recognize on CT). Associated parietal or temporal skull fracture is common with this injury (80%).

(4) Treatment
   (a) Obtain stat neurosurgical consultation; immediate surgical decompression is required to assure optimal outcome.
   (b) Elevate head of bed.
   (c) To decrease ICP, intubate and ventilate to maintain a $PaCO_2$ of 35 - 40mmHg. If acute neurologic deterioration occurs despite these and other measures, <u>brief</u> periods of hyperventilation to a $PaCO_2$ of 25 - 30mmHg are acceptable. Cerebral perfusion pressure = MAP (mean arterial pressure) minus ICP; cerebral ischemia may result if the $PaCO_2$ falls below 30mmHg.
   (d) Use of mannitol to decrease ICP should be discussed with the neurosurgeon before employed.
   (e) Mortality = 0 - 20% (depending on neuro status: normal neuro exam → 0%; coma → 20% without rapid detection and evacuation)

e. <u>Subdural hematoma</u>
   (1) These lesions are more common than epidural hematomas and more often associated with significant primary, intrinsic brain damage (usually covering the entire surface of the hemisphere).
   (2) Patients with brain atrophy (alcoholics, the elderly) are especially susceptible to these lesions; brain atrophy → bridging veins spanning a greater distance and being more easily torn.
   (3) Symptoms are caused by "mass effect" of a <u>venous</u> bleed; they range from a mild headache and confusion to lethargy and coma (with or without localizing signs). They develop within 24 hours of injury in patients with <u>acute</u> subdurals but are delayed up to two weeks or more, respectively, in patients with <u>subacute</u> and <u>chronic</u> subdurals.
   (4) CT demonstrates the classic <u>crescent-shaped</u> lesion (be able to recognize on CT).
   (5) Stabilization is the same as for an epidural hematoma.
   (6) Immediate neurosurgical intervention is required (except perhaps for chronic subdurals).
   (7) Mortality rate for <u>acute</u> subdurals = 30% (with early evacuation) → 60% (with later evacuation).
      (a) There is a higher mortality in patients who are unconscious from the time of injury.
      (b) Those with a history of a lucid interval (50 - 70%) have a better prognosis.

f. <u>Skull fractures</u>
   (1) Skull fractures are important in that they identify patients at high risk for having or developing an intracranial hematoma.
   (2) <u>Most</u> patients with skull fractures require neurosurgical consultation and admission for observation.
   (3) Types
      (a) Linear, non-depressed skull fractures → no specific treatment
      (b) Depressed skull fractures → may require operative elevation of the bony fragment
      (c) Open skull fractures → require early operative intervention

(d) "Egg shell" skull fractures require evaluation for child abuse

(e) Basilar skull fracture → clinical findings are more useful than skull x-rays[*] in making the diagnosis but may require several hours to develop:
- CSF rhinorrhea or otorrhea
- "Ring sign" on filter paper
- Battle's sign
- Raccoon's eyes
- Hemotympanum

15. Posttraumatic Epilepsy
  a. A high incidence is associated with:
    (1) An intracranial hematoma
    (2) A depressed skull fracture
    (3) Seizures occurring within the first week of head injury
  b. Anticonvulsant therapy
    (1) Phenytoin, fosphenytoin or phenobarbital are currently the agents of choice in the acute phase.
    (2) There is evidence that phenytoin reduces the incidence of seizures within the first week of injury, but not thereafter.
    (3) For patients with prolonged seizures, diazepam or lorazepam are used (in addition to phenytoin) until the seizure stops.

B. Facial Injuries

1. The Le Forte classification should be reviewed. Schematics and sample films can be found in Tintinalli's Text. However, texts do not provide an adequate review of facial films demonstrating the wide variations of Le Forte fractures. Your best source is a university hospital teaching file or written board course with a radiology review session. In clinical practice, CT scanning with 3-D reconstruction is typically required for preoperative diagnosis.

2. Extensive facial injuries may necessitate a surgical airway.

3. Orbital "blowout" fractures — most commonly occur through the floor of the orbit, but may also occur medially in the region of the lamina papyracea of the ethmoid bone.
  a. Orbital <u>floor</u> fractures
    (1) Signs and symptoms
      (a) Pain and diplopia on upward gaze
      (b) Enophthalmos
      (c) Hypesthesia in the distribution of the infraorbital nerve (ipsilateral cheek and lip)
      (d) Limitation of <u>upward</u> gaze due to entrapment of the inferior rectus and inferior oblique muscles
      (e) Subcutaneous orbital emphysema
    (2) X-ray findings (best seen on modified Waters view)
      (a) Air-fluid (blood) level in maxillary sinus
      (b) Prolapse of orbital tissue into the maxillary antrum ("teardrop" sign)

---

[*]CT and MRI (if available) may better delineate the extent of a basilar skull fracture.

(c) Bony disruption of the orbital floor

(d) Clouding of the maxillary sinus

(e) Orbital emphysema

   b. <u>Medial wall</u> fractures

      (1) Signs and symptoms

         (a) Epistaxis

         (b) Emphysema of the lids or conjunctiva

         (c) Limitation of <u>lateral</u> gaze due to entrapment of the medial rectus muscle (uncommon)

      (2) X-ray findings

         (a) Unilateral clouding of the ethmoid sinus

         (b) Orbital emphysema

   c. Treatment

      (1) R/O associated ocular injuries (e.g. rupture of the globe, hyphema); they occur in up to 30% of patients with these fractures; CT scanning may be helpful.

      (2) Prescribe decongestants and consider prophylactic antibiotics.

      (3) Advise patients to avoid Valsalva maneuvers such as blowing their nose, which can worsen orbital emphysema.

      (4) Refer patients to an ophthalmologist for follow-up; symptoms usually resolve on their own, but surgical correction is sometimes needed.

      <u>Note</u>: Further discussion of these fractures can be found in the ENT chapter on p. 218 and in the Eye chapter on pp. 1089 - 1090.

4. Dental injuries generally require antibiotics, analgesics and referral.

C. Neck and Back Injuries

1. A cervical spine injury should be suspected in any patient with:
   a. An injury above the clavicle
   b. A high-speed vehicular injury
   c. A fall > 10 feet
   d. An electrical injury
   e. An altered level of consciousness
   f. A diving accident
   g. A football injury sustained while tackling

2. Thoracic and lumbar injuries should be suspected in patients sustaining multiple trauma, particularly if the trauma was to the trunk and the patient c/o pain at these sites or has neuro findings/complaints. In patients undergoing chest and/or abdominal helical CT scanning, screening for thoracic or lumbar spine fractures can be performed on reformatted CT data, obviating the need for plain x-ray screening.

   a. <u>Chance</u> fractures
     (1) Tranverse fractures through the vertebral body caused by flexion about an axis <u>anterior</u> to the vertebral column (most frequently seen following MVAs in which the patient was restrained only by a lap belt).
     (2) May be associated with retroperitoneal and abdominal visceral injuries.
   b. Fracture-dislocations
     (1) Caused by extreme flexion or severe blunt trauma to the spine → disruption of the posterior elements (pedicles, facets, laminae) of the vertebra.
     (2) Since the thoracic spinal canal is narrow in relation to the spinal cord, fracture-subluxations of the thoracic spine commonly result in complete neurologic deficits.
[Note: Chance fractures and fracture-dislocations are extremely un-stable and usually require internal fixation.]

3. Protect the spinal cord (which ends at L_2) until stability of the entire spine has been assured, i.e. absent or improving neurologic complaints, a normal neuro exam and negative x-rays or CT.
   a. Obtain x-rays while the patient is immobilized.
     (1) Patients with neurologic complaints or findings should have C-spine films even in the absence of bone pain or tenderness in these areas. [Note: in the future, x-rays may become obsolete (in favor of CT) but we are not there yet.]
     (2) When evaluating the cross-table lateral C-spine film, be sure to visualize <u>all</u> 7 cervical vertebrae (COUNT THEM) <u>and</u> the C_7-T_1 interspace; if they are not visualized on the initial cross-table lateral film, repeat it while applying traction to the arms or obtain a swimmer's view.
     (3) Do <u>not</u> rely on the cross-table lateral alone to R/O cervical frac-tures; open-mouth odontoid and AP views must also be obtained.*
     (4) Detection of a C-spine injury necessitates x-ray evaluation of the entire spinal column.
   b. A CT scan should be ordered if plain films are not clearly negative or the patient has neurologic complaints/findings associated with "normal" films; for suspicious areas, axial CT scans should be ob-tained at 3mm intervals.
   c. Further evaluation with MRI and/or dynamic flexion views is indi-cated if the patient ....
     (1) Is obtunded (neuro exam not possible) <u>or</u>
     (2) Has neuro complaints/findings with normal plain films or CT.
       (a) MRI can detect the following injuries:
         <u>1</u> Spinal epidural hematoma
         <u>2</u> Herniated disc
         <u>3</u> Spinal cord contusion/disruption
         <u>4</u> Paraspinal ligamentous/soft tissue injury
       (b) When MRI is not available (or appropriate), CT myelography may exclude the presence of acute spinal cord compression caused by a traumatic herniated disc or epidural hematoma.

*The combination of lateral C-spine + swimmer's view is ~ 85% sensitive for fracture.

4. Common bony injuries
    a. Jefferson Fracture (C_1 ring blowout) — an axial loading injury. It is best seen on the open-mouth odontoid view. Associated C_2 fractures occur in ~40% of these patients.
    b. Odontoid fracture — Look for swelling anterior to C_2 on the cross-table lateral view and for abnormalities on the open mouth odontoid view; additional views including tomograms and CT are occasionally needed. There are three types of odontoid fractures:
        (1) Type I ... is rare (involves tip of the dens)
        (2) Type II ... traverses the dens at the junction of the body of C_2*
        (3) Type III ... involves the vertebral body of C_2
    c. Hangman's fracture (unstable bipeduncular fracture of C_2) — is an extension injury
    d. Facet dislocations — may be either unilateral or bilateral. Unilateral dislocations result from flexion-rotation injuries while bilateral dislocations are produced by flexion injuries. The lateral view reveals $\geq 25\%$ (unilateral) to $\geq 50\%$ (bilateral) anterior displacement of the superior vertebral body relative to the adjoining inferior vertebral body.
    e. Clay-shoveler's fracture — an avulsion fracture of the spinous process of C_6 - T_3 (C_7 most common). It results from a flexion injury or a direct blow to the spinous process.

5. Immediate neurosurgical consultation is required for patients with positive x-rays as well as those with neurologic complaints or findings, i.e. sensory or motor.

6. Administer high-dose methylprednisolone (a 30mg/kg IV bolus followed by a 5.4 mg/kg/hr. infusion) after neurosurgical consultation to patients with evidence of a nonpenetrating spinal cord injury who presented within eight hours of injury.**

D. Thoracic Trauma

1. Statistics
    a. Thoracic injuries are responsible for 25% of all trauma deaths.
    b. Between 10 - 30% of thoracic injuries require surgical correction.

2. Pulmonary injuries
    a. <u>Pneumothoraces</u>
        (1) Tension pneumothorax
            (a) This diagnosis should be made <u>clinically</u> (rather than by x-ray) since it can be rapidly fatal due to severe ventilatory and circulatory compromise.

---

*Worst prognosis
**The National Acute Spinal Cord Injury Study (NASCIS) showed that administration of steroids <u>after</u> eight hours of injury resulted in a poor outcome.

    (b) Clinical features
      <u>1</u> Respiratory distress (late sign = cyanosis)
      <u>2</u> Hypotension
      <u>3</u> Tachycardia (late sign = PEA)
      <u>4</u> Tracheal deviation (<u>away</u> from the side of the pneumo)
      <u>5</u> Distended neck veins
      <u>6</u> Ipsilateral absent breath sounds
      <u>7</u> Ipsilateral hyperresonance on percussion
    (c) Treatment: immediate needle thoracostomy of the affected hemithorax followed by tube thoracostomy.

(2) Simple pneumothorax
    (a) Primary clinical findings are decreased breath sounds and hyperresonance to percussion on the affected side; there may be some dyspnea.
    (b) Diagnosis is most easily made on an <u>expiratory</u> view of the chest.
    (c) Treatment: tube thoracostomy.

(3) Open pneumothorax ("sucking chest wound")
    (a) If the opening in the chest wall is approximately two-thirds of the diameter of the trachea or more, air moves preferentially through the chest wall defect → ineffective ventilation → hypoxia.
    (b) Treatment
      <u>1</u> Cover the defect with a sterile occlusive dressing (petrolatum gauze, plastic wrap); tape it down on <u>three</u> of its four edges.
      <u>2</u> Place a chest tube in an area distant from the wound site.

b. <u>Pulmonary contusion</u> (most common <u>potentially</u> lethal chest injury)
    (1) Mechanism of injury: usually results from direct chest wall trauma (e.g. MVA with rapid deceleration).
    (2) Clinical manifestations include dyspnea, tachypnea, tachycardia and chest wall tenderness/ecchymosis at the site of injury. Associated rib fractures may also be present.
    (3) ABG reveals hypoxemia and a widening alveolar-arterial oxygen gradient.
    (4) CXR findings are <u>localized</u> to the site of injury and range from a patchy, irregular alveolar infiltrate to frank consolidation. They are usually <u>present on arrival</u> and always develop within 6 hours of injury; after that time, they tend to "blossom" on x-ray. [<u>Note</u>: the x-ray findings in ARDS, by comparison, are <u>diffuse</u> and <u>delayed</u> (usually developing 24 - 72 hours post-injury). These points are helpful in distinguishing these two pulmonary processes.]
    (5) The goal of therapy in management of pulmonary contusions is adequate ventilation and perfusion to promote healing and prevent complications (e.g. pneumonia, pneumothorax).
    (a) Mild to moderate contusions (< 18% total lung volume or about one lobe) are treated with supplemental oxygen, pulmonary hygiene (nasotracheal suctioning, chest physiotherapy) and pain control (intercostal nerve blocks) which allow the patient to take deep breaths regularly and cough adequately.

(b) Severe contusions (> 28% total lung volume or > one lobe) associated with significant hypoxemia ($pO_2 <$ 65mmHg) require early intubation and mechanical ventilation.

   <u>1</u> Use of intermittent mandatory ventilation (IMV) with lower tidal volumes* (5 -7mL/kg) and PEEP to prevent alveolar collapse usually provide much better ventilation - perfusion matching than standard controlled ventilation.

   <u>2</u> When only <u>one</u> lung has been severely contused and significant hypoxemia persists despite the use of IMV + PEEP, mechanical ventilation may improve if each lung is ventilated <u>separately</u> with a double-lumen endobronchial catheter; this technique helps prevent hyperexpansion of the normal lung and gradual collapse of the injured, poorly compliant lung.

      <u>a</u> Place the normal lung "down" by turning the patient to the decubitus position (helps improve ventilation/perfusion matching of the contused lung).

      <u>b</u> Administration of nitric oxide gas (although experimental at this time) has proven to be a superb adjunct in many patients since the gas only reaches ventilated alveoli where it exerts its vasodilatory effects, thus improving perfusion as well as ventilation.

(6) Pneumonia is the most common and most significant complication; it significantly worsens the prognosis.

c. <u>Hemothorax</u>

(1) Primary x-ray finding (requires at least 200mL of fluid to be seen) is blunting of the costophrenic angles on an upright CXR; effusions can easily be missed on a supine film.

(2) Twenty-five percent of cases have concomitant pneumothoraces; seventy-three percent have associated extrathoracic injuries.

(3) Clinical findings include diminished breath sounds, dullness to percussion and decreased tactile fremitus.

(4) Treatment

   (a) Most hemothoraces are self-limited and need only tube thoracostomy.

   (b) Consider autotransfusion in patients with massive hemothoraces.

   (c) Thoracotomy is indicated if: blood loss is $\geq$ 1500mL in the initial chest tube drainage, there is persistent bleeding requiring continuous blood transfusion, the patient remains hypotensive or decompensates, blood loss is > 200mL/hr for 2 - 4 hours or there is a 50% hemothorax.

3. <u>Blunt cardiac injuries</u> .... usually result from high-speed vehicular accidents in which the chest wall strikes the steering wheel; they are all associated with potentially fatal complications, although they should be viewed clinically as a continuous spectrum of myocardial damage:

- Concussion (no permanent cell damage)
- Contusion (permanent cell injury)

*Reduce the risk of barotrauma

- Infarction (cell death)
- Tamponade (bleeding into the pericardium)
- Rupture (exsanguination)

a. Myocardial concussion

   (1) Mechanism of injury: a sharp, direct blow to the mid-anterior chest wall "stuns" the myocardium and results in a dysrhythmia, hypotension or loss of consciousness.

   (2) If the episode resolves (spontaneously or with treatment) there are no histopathologic changes. However, prolonged cellular dysfunction may lead to a non-perfusing rhythm (V-Fib, asystole) and irreversible cardiac arrest.

b. Myocardial contusion

   (1) Mechanism of injury: high-speed deceleration → heart moves forward and forcibly strikes the sternum.[*]

   (2) Site of injury: the right ventricle (most commonly).

   (3) *Suspecting* this diagnosis is more important than *making* it since it is often elusive:

   (a) What was the mechanism of injury? Is it compatible with a myocardial contusion?

   (b) How severely damaged is the vehicle (including the dashboard and steering wheel)?

   (c) What was the estimated speed of the vehicle before impact?

   (d) What was the position of the victim when found? Was he belted? Were the airbags inflated?

   (e) What were the initial vital signs and level of consciousness? Are they changing?

   (f) Any cardiac dysrhythmia at the scene, en route or in the ED?

   (g) Is there evidence of chest wall trauma?

   (4) Diagnostic studies are utilized primarily to identify the low-risk patients who can be safely sent home; in general, the higher the index of suspicion (based on accurate prehospital and emergency dept. assessments) the more sophisticated the testing.[**]

   (a) ECG findings

   <u>1</u> Although ECG is neither sensitive nor specific, presence of abnormalities on the <u>initial</u> ECG is correlated with the risk of developing subsequent cardiac complications.

   <u>2</u> Findings are variable and may include:
   - Sinus tachycardia (most sensitive, least specific)
   - Multiple PVCs
   - Atrial fibrillation
   - Bundle branch block (most often RBBB)
   - ST - T wave changes

   (b) 2-D echocardiographic findings include:

   <u>1</u> Impaired regional systolic function (particularly right ventricular free wall dyskinesis)

   <u>2</u> Increased echo brightness

   <u>3</u> Increased end-diastolic wall thickness

[*]Injuries that occur during early systole or late diastole (when the ventricles are blood-filled) are the most damaging.

[**]Cardiac enzymes have, at most, a very limited role in the evaluation of blunt trauma

(5) Management strategy
   (a) Patients with conduction abnormalities (or other significant injuries) should be admitted to a critical care unit.
   (b) Asymptomatic patients with normal vital signs, a low-risk profile and normal ECG may be released after a short period of observation.
   (c) Symptomatic patients with a low-risk profile and normal serial ECGs can probably be sent home after a period of observation (6 - 12 hrs); if there is some concern after this time, consider ordering 2-D echocardiography.
   (d) Symptomatic patients with a moderate-risk profile and normal serial ECGs should have echocardiography performed; they may be sent home after a 12-hour observation period if the echo is clearly normal.
   (e) High risk patients (or those with questionable findings on diagnostic studies) should be admitted for observation and cardiac monitoring, since these patients are at risk for the development of dysrhythmias and cardiac dysfunction.

c. <u>Traumatic myocardial infarction</u>
   (1) Although rare, a blunt injury may cause coronary artery occlusion by arterial spasm, an intimal tear, thrombosis or compression from adjacent hemorrhage and edema (which may occur with capillary bleeding in a contused heart).
   (2) What is important is that a traumatic MI can be a part of the continuous spectrum of injury in that cardiac damage does not have to be confined just to the myocardium but may extend to involve the coronary arteries as well.
   (3) Obviously, patients with pre-existing CAD are at greatest risk. If there are any ischemic findings on the ECG, obtain old cardiograms for comparison and order serial ECGs and enzymes to R/O evolving changes.
   (4) If there is any doubt, the patient needs to be admitted and treated as an MI. However, **thrombolytic agents are contraindicated in this setting** since the myocardium is presumably contused and actively bleeding to some degree.

d. <u>Pericardial tamponade</u>
   (1) Penetrating trauma is the most frequent cause but tamponade can also occur with blunt trauma and iatrogenic trauma (CVP placement, pacemaker insertion); the most common site of perforation from catheter placement is the right atrium.
   (2) Mechanism of injury in tamponade caused by blunt injury: rapid deceleration with cardiac compression during early systole or late diastole → blood-filled ventricles → rigid myocardial wall → rents/tears/lacerations → impending myocardial rupture.

(3) Clinical diagnosis
  (a) Beck's triad: hypotension, JVD and muffled heart tones; however, JVD may <u>not</u> present if there is marked hypovolemia.
  (b) Decreased pulse pressure
  (c) Rising CVP (earliest response)
  (d) Kussmaul's sign (distention of neck veins with inspiration)
  (e) A CVP > 15cmH$_2$O in association with hypotension and tachycardia (most reliable sign).
  (f) Electrical alternans (pathognomonic for tamponade but is rarely present in the <u>acute</u> scenario).
  (g) PEA (pulseless electrical activity) can be a manifestation of cardiac tamponade but also occurs with tension pneumothorax and hypovolemia.
  (h) The presence of pericardial fluid on ultrasound is highly suggestive of active bleeding in the pericardium.
(4) Treatment: IV fluids followed by pericardiocentesis; definitive treatment is open thoracotomy by a qualified surgeon.
e. <u>Myocardial rupture</u>*
  (1) Mechanism of injury: compression of a blood-filled chamber (usually a ventricle but may be an atrium, especially the right)
  (2) The patient is protected from immediate exsanguination if the pericardium is intact.
  (3) The clinical picture is usually one of pericardial tamponade in a patient with other known or suspected thoracic injuries (e.g. hemothorax, pneumothorax, aortic dissection/rupture).
  (4) The management strategy begins with IV fluids and CVP catheter insertion. Then order the following studies:
    (a) <u>Chest x-ray</u>: shows position of the CVP line and presence of other intrathoracic injuries.
    (b) <u>Cardiac ultrasound</u> (if time permits): confirms the presence of acute pericardial tamponade.
  (5) Immediate decompression of cardiac tamponade and control of hemorrhage are the mainstays of ED treatment.
    (a) Pericardiocentesis is only a temporizing measure until surgical correction can be undertaken.
    (b) If the patient's clinical status deteriorates in the ED, emergency thoracotomy and pericardiotomy may be required prior to definitive repair in the OR.
4. <u>Traumatic aortic rupture</u>
  a. Mechanism of injury: sudden deceleration ($\geq$ 45 mph MVA impact, damaged steering wheel or 20 - 30 foot fall)
  b. Site of injury: most ruptures occur at the <u>ligamentum arteriosum</u> (the point of greatest aortic fixation) just distal to the left subclavian artery and progress from the intima outward toward the adventitia.
  c. 80 - 90% of patients die at the scene and as many as 50% of remaining survivors will die within 24 hours if they are not diagnosed and treated expeditiously.

---

*Most common cause of death in non-penetrating cardiac injuries

    d. Diagnosis — is usually suspected from the history of a deceleration injury plus findings on CXR and is confirmed by angiography, dynamic contrast-enhanced CT or transesophageal echocardiography (TEE).

        (1) CXR findings (any, all or none may be present):

            (a) Widening of the superior mediastinum (> 8cm) on an upright PA CXR taken at a distance of 6 feet (most common finding)

            (b) Obliterated or indistinct aortic knob

            (c) Deviation of the trachea and/or esophagus (NG tube) to the right

            (d) Depression of the left mainstem bronchus > 40 degrees below horizontal

            (e) Obliteration of the space between the pulmonary artery and the aorta

            (f) Left apical pleural cap (obliteration of the medial aspect of the left upper lobe apex)

            (g) Multiple rib fractures

            (h) Widening and/or displacement of the paratracheal stripe to the right

            (i) Widening of the left or right paraspinous stripe

            (j) Left hemothorax

            (k) Fractures of the first or second ribs or the scapula

        (2) Signs and symptoms can include:

            (a) Retrosternal or interscapular pain (25%) — most common

            (b) Dyspnea

            (c) Harsh systolic murmur over the precordium or in the interscapular area

            (d) Upper extremity HTN in association with decreased or absent femoral pulses (pseudocoarctation syndrome)

            (e) Pulse deficits

            (f) Voice change or hoarseness (in the absence of laryngeal injury)

            (g) Ischemic pain of the extremities

            (h) Paraplegia

        (3) Definitive diagnosis

            (a) Contrast-enhanced dynamic CT (using state-of-the-art spiral CT) — is extremely accurate for demonstration or exclusion of direct aortic injury.

                1 Axial CT images can be supplemented by 2-D multiplanar reformations (MPR) or 3-D surface contour views that can simulate thoracic aortography → better delineates extent of injury and its relationship to branch vessels.

                2 Spiral CT is very useful because it permits reconstruction of axial images that allows production of better 2-D (MPR) and 3-D images.

                3 If CT demonstrates traumatic aortic injury (or is not clearly negative), aortography should be performed.

            (b) Transesophageal echocardiography — is a diagnostic alternative if both CT and angiographic findings are equivocal; however, results are highly operator-dependent and patient cooperation is required.

(4) Treatment is prompt surgical repair. While awaiting surgery, the patient's BP should be carefully controlled so as to minimize the shearing effect on the intact adventitia of the aorta; intravenous beta-blockers (e.g. esmolol*) in combination with nitroprusside should be used as needed to maintain the systolic BP between 100 and 120mmHg.

E. Abdominal Injuries

1. Clinical caveats
   a. <u>All</u> patients involved in high-speed or bicycle accidents should be evaluated for abdominal injury.
   b. Benign initial exam — occurs in 20% of patients with abdominal injury; <u>serial</u> exams are important.
   c. Your goal is to identify the presence of a surgical abdomen; prolonged evaluation to determine the specific injury is unnecessary and can be detrimental.

2. Ultrasonography (US)/FAST exam
   a. Is the initial (and sometimes only) diagnostic modality of choice for evaluating both hemodynamically stable and unstable patients with blunt thoracoabdominal trauma.
   b. Should be used in combination with other diagnostic modalities (such as IVP for blunt renal trauma) and clinical assessment:
      (1) Unstable patient + positive US → laparotomy
      (2) Stable patient + positive US → CT (to R/O the need for operative intervention)
      (3) Unstable patient + negative US → repeat US or perform DPL
      (4) Stable patient + negative US → observation
      <u>Note</u>: A negative or equivocal US does NOT rule out the need for further testing.
   c. Advantages
      (1) Noninvasive
      (2) Detects the presence of intra-abdominal, pericardial or pleural fluid
      (3) Rapid, safe and portable (can be performed in the controlled environment of the trauma suite) and may be repeated prn based on protocol or change in the patient's condition
      (4) Can be performed without interfering with resuscitative efforts
      (5) Does <u>not</u> require administration of contrast agents
      (6) Has a sensitivity of 60 - 95% and a specificity of 100% (when <u>six</u> "windows" are used, which is not usually done in the ED)
   d. Disadvantages
      (1) Can miss bowel and retroperitoneal injuries
      (2) Cannot differentiate fluids, e.g. ascites vs blood
      (3) Imaging is impaired in patients who are markedly obese, those with subcutaneous air/emphysema or excessive bowel gas.
      (4) Evaluations are operator-dependent, i.e. determined by skill level.
   <u>Note</u>: Studies evaluating the efficacy of US for penetrating trauma are limited and inconclusive at this time.

---

*Much easier to titrate than propranolol.

Diagnostic Study	DPL	Ultrasound (FAST)	CT Scan
Indication	Document bleeding if the blood pressure is low; (Unstable patient)	Document fluid if the blood pressure is low; (Unstable or stable pt.)	Document organ injury if normal blood pressure; (Stable patient)
Advantages	Early diagnosis; very sensitive and detects bowel injury (98% accurate)	Early diagnosis; noninvasive, easily repeatable; 86 - 97% accurate; performed rapidly	Most specific for injury (92% - 98% accurate)
Disadvantages	Invasive; misses injuries to diaphragm and retroperitoneum; is less specific than US or CT; may overdiagnose injuries	Operator dependent; misses diaphragm,bowel and some pancreatic injuries; bowel gas and subcut. air distortion	Cost and time; misses diaphragm, bowel and some pancreatic injuries; transport out of ED required

3. Computerized tomography
   a. Is the diagnostic study of choice for evaluating <u>hemodynamically stable</u> patients with blunt thoracoabdominal and genitourinary trauma and is often used in concert with the FAST exam (i.e. initial evaluation with the FAST exam followed by CT).
      (1) Normal vital signs + normal US → CT may be deferrred
      (2) Normal vital signs + positive US → CT may delineate extent of the injuries
   b. It can also be used to complement DPL when:
      (1) DPL results are equivocal
      (2) Retroperitoneal injury is suspected
      (3) Technical difficulties arise in performing DPL
   c. Advantages
      (1) Noninvasive
      (2) Provides information on specific organ injury*
      (3) Can diagnose retroperitoneal and pelvic organ injuries
   d. Disadvantages
      (1) May necessitate the administration of oral and IV contrast
      (2) Takes more time than DPL to perform
      (3) Requires an expert to interpret it
      (4) Has a rather high false-negative rate (2 - 25%) -- misses certain injuries, e.g. diaphragm, pancreas, bladder and bowel
   <u>Note</u>: The value of CT in assessing those patients with penetrating abdominal trauma is limited but growing.

4. Diagnostic peritoneal lavage
   a. Is used to identify intra-abdominal bleeding (or bowel injury) that requires immediate laparotomy in the <u>unstable</u> patient if a FAST exam is not available or is inconclusive; it is rapidly performed, readily available and has a sensitivity of 98%.

*When liver or spleen injury is suspected, CT <u>may</u> reliably exclude injuries that require emergent operative intervention (ACEP Clinical Policy).

b. Indications
  (1) In blunt abdominal trauma this includes:
    (a) Suspected or known blunt abdominal trauma in a patient with an unreliable or equivocal exam (due to intoxication with drugs or alcohol, distracting injuries, spinal cord lesion, etc.) or injury to adjacent structures (lower ribs, pelvis or lumbar spine).
    (b) Lap belt sign with suspicion of bowel injury
    (c) Unexplained hypo/hypertension
    (d) Lack of availability of patient for serial examinations (i.e. requires anesthesia for treatment of other injuries).
  (2) In penetrating trauma, this includes:
    (a) Stab wounds (SWs) with known or suspected peritoneal violation
    (b) Gunshot wounds (GSWs) when peritoneal violation is unclear.
c. Contraindications
  (1) The only absolute contraindication to DPL is an indication for laparotomy (i.e. free air under the diaphragm, intraperitoneal bladder rupture).
  (2) Relative contraindications include:
    (a) Previous abdominal surgery
    (b) Morbid obesity
    (c) Advanced cirrhosis (ascites)
    (d) Severe coagulopathy
    (e) Gravid uterus
d. The major pitfalls of DPL are that it can miss significant retroperitoneal bleeding and isolated hollow viscus perforation.
e. Procedure
  (1) DPL can be performed using either a closed, semi-open or open technique; if performed during pregnancy, the open technique (or mini-lap) should be done using a supra-umbilical approach when the gravid uterus is palpable above the uterus.
  (2) Prior to lavage, the stomach and bladder are decompressed (NG tube and Foley catheter).
  (3) A peritoneal lavage catheter is then placed and aspiration of free intraperitoneal blood is attempted. If blood is aspirated, DPL is considered positive and is terminated.
  (4) If no blood is obtained, 1 liter (or 10mL/kg in children) warmed NS or LR is instilled into the peritoneal cavity and allowed to drain back out. This effluent is then sent to the lab for analysis.
f. RBC criteria for a positive lavage:
  (1) $\geq 100,000$ RBCs/mm^3 for blunt trauma and anterior abdominal stab wounds.
  (2) > 5000 RBCs/mm^3 for SWs of the lower chest and abdominal GSWs.
  Note: The RBC count is the most accurate parameter for evaluating lavage fluid. Other criteria (WBC count, amylase, bile) are less reliable and only rise after a delay of several hours.

F. Pelvic and Extremity Injuries

1. Since pelvic injuries are frequently encountered in major blunt trauma cases, an AP pelvis film is a <u>standard</u> trauma order.

2. During primary survey, extremity evaluation is limited to identifying (and treating) exsanguinating hemorrhage as well as assessing perfusion. It is only during the secondary survey that a more detailed evaluation of the extremities is performed.

3. Once all life-threatening problems have been identified and treated, known and suspected fractures should be immobilized with splints and/or traction, as appropriate, to control pain and bleeding as well as prevent further injury.

4. Following appropriate x-ray evaluation, dislocations should be rapidly reduced.

5. Distal neurovascular function should be assessed promptly and reassessed before and after all extremity manipulations (e.g. joint reduction, application of splints and/or traction).

6. If open wounds/fractures are identified, the patient's tetanus immune status must be assessed and updated as appropriate.

7. Systemic antibiotics should be administered to patients with open fractures and contaminated wounds.

8. Fractured bones bleed extensively — Count on at least 2 units of blood for a femoral fracture, 6 units for pelvic fractures.

9. Compartment syndromes can occur later, especially in the lower leg and forearm.
    a. Classic signs of a compartment syndrome (the "6Ps"):
        (1) Pain —out of proportion to the injury + increased with passive stretching and active contraction of the involved muscles
        (2) Paresthesias
        (3) Paralysis
        (4) Pallor
        (5) Palpable tenseness and tenderness of the compartment
        (6) Pulselessness (a very late finding)
    b. Pain is the <u>earliest</u> finding and is followed by the development of paresthesias; all the others are late findings.
    <u>Note</u>: Specific bony injuries and further discussion of compartment syndrome can be found in the orthopedic section.

V. Special Problems

A. *Drowning*

1. 10 - 15% of drownings are "dry" (no aspiration occurs, there is laryngo-spasm with glottis closure); the remaining 85 - 90% of drownings are "wet" (aspiration occurs).

2. Postural drainage has no proven efficacy and is not recommended.

3. Assess these patients for co-morbidity: hypothermia (use a rectal thermometer that is calibrated to record low temperatures), hypotension and C-spine injuries.

4. Death in these individuals is usually due to hypoxia → cardiac arrest

5. The CXR may be normal or it may reveal a pattern of either generalized pulmonary edema or perihilar pulmonary edema.

6. The most common cause of dysrhythmias is hypoxemia.

7. The most reliable prognostic indicators are the duration of submersion and resuscitation.

Note: A more detailed discussion of this topic can be found in the Pulmonary chapter on pp. 384 - 389.

B. *Electrical Shock*

1. There are three major insults that result from electrical shock:
   a. Conduction system changes secondary to damage of the body's electrical system:
      (1) Cardiac conduction (asystole, V. fibrillation or other cardiac dysrhythmias); V. fibrillation is the most common cause of death in the acute phase of electrical injuries.
      (2) CNS conduction (respiratory problems, apnea, seizures, etc.) — occurs because the body's electrical system is the preferential path for current conduction since it has the least resistance.
   b. Thermal tissue damage
      (1) The passage of current generates heat → cutaneous burns and muscle injury
      (2) Muscle injury → rhabdomyolysis → acute myoglobinuric renal failure (if untreated)
   c. Blunt trauma
      (1) An electric shock can throw the victim down or into the air → fractures (particularly long-bone fractures and spinal compression fractures) and dislocations.
      (2) An electric shock delivered at a frequency of 40 - 110cps → tetanic contractions → scapular fractures and shoulder dislocations.

2. Management
   a. IV-O_2-cardiac monitor
   b. Place a Foley catheter to monitor urine output.
      (1) Mannitol diuresis increases renal tubular flow and may be required to maintain an output >1mL/kg/hour.
      (2) With significant electrical injury, consider alkalinization of the urine with bicarb to decrease precipitation of hemochromogens in the renal tubules.
   c. With severe electrical injuries (increased risk of adynamic ileus), an NG tube should also be placed.
   d. Initiate fluid resuscitation with NS or LR:
      (1) If there are signs of shock (hypotension/tachycardia, diaphoresis, altered LOC), a fluid bolus (20mL/kg) is indicated.
      (2) The subsequent rate should be adjusted as needed to maintain a urine output of at least 0.5 - 1mL/kg/hr.
      (3) If there is evidence of myoglobinuria, the rate should be increased until the urine output is 1.5 - 2.0mL/kg/hr.
   e. Order CK and urine for myoglobin as well as serum potassium and calcium levels (to R/O hyperkalemia and hypocalcemia).
   f. Obtain an ECG on all patients.
   g. Check carefully for entrance + exit wounds; most common entrance sites are the hand and skull; the most common exit site is the heel.
   h. Evaluate patients for evidence of blunt trauma.
   i. Cleanse cutaneous burns and apply a topical antibiotic dressing (e.g. silver sulfadiazine, mafenide acetate).
   j. Administer tetanus prophylaxis as needed.
   k. Check for compartment syndromes.
   l. Never debride soft tissue injuries involving the hands, digits or face in the ED.
   m. Evaluate patients who sustain electrical injuries of the head and neck for cataracts and refer them to an ophthalmologist for follow-up; cataracts may develop shortly after injury or they may be delayed months to years.
   n. Lip burns require close observation and referral to a plastic or oral surgeon; delayed hemorrhage (3 - 14 days post-injury) occurs in 10 - 15% of these patients.

3. Disposition
   a. Hospitalization is indicated for all patients with high-voltage burns (> 1000 V) and for those patients with low-voltage burns (< 1000 V) who are symptomatic (e.g. dysrhythmias, chest pain, cutaneous findings, abnormal urine)
   b. Asymptomatic patients with low-voltage injuries may be discharged to home following a period of observation and cardiac monitoring in the ED if their ECG and physical exam are normal and if they have no evidence of cutaneous involvement or urinary heme pigment.

4. Important differences between electrical injuries and thermal burns:
   a. Electrical injuries cause extensive muscle damage → myoglobin release (so they are more like a crush injury than a thermal burn).

b. In electrical injuries, the extent of cutaneous injury in no way correlates with the amount of underlying tissue damage (neurovascular and musculoskeletal); it is often just the tip of the iceberg.

Note: Further discussion of electrical injuries can be found in the chapter on environmental injuries.

C. Rhabdomyolysis

1. Clinical pathophysiology: injury to muscle → release of myoglobin → damage to kidneys → acute renal failure (90% of patients recover).

2. Commonly associated electrolyte abnormalities are hypocalcemia (63%) and hyperkalemia (40%).

3. Myoglobin is difficult to assay in serum and is only transiently found in urine so serial CKs are done to monitor the patient's progress.

4. Treatment
   a. The most important aspect of treatment is aggressive IV fluid (NS or LR) hydration; administer fluids at a rate that is sufficient to maintain the urine output at 1.5 - 2.0mL/kg/hr.
   b. If this does not clear the pigment, administer mannitol; give 25gms IV initially and then add 12.5gms to each subsequent liter of fluid and titrate to maintain urine output > 50mL/hour until the myoglobin is cleared. Furosemide (2mg/kg IV) may also be administered to promote diuresis.
   c. Alkalinization of the urine with sodium bicarbonate is also helpful; it increases the solubility of myoglobin and facilitates its excretion; 44mEq of $NaHCO_3$ may be added to each liter of IV fluid.

D. Thermal Burns

As with all traumatized patients, start with the ABCs. Airway patency and fluid resuscitation are of prime importance:

1. Inhalation injury should be considered in patients with facial burns, singed facial and nasal hair, evidence of oropharyngeal inflammation, carbon deposits in the oropharynx, carbonaceous sputum and/or a history of fire exposure in a confined space; treat with humidified oxygen and early intubation.

2. Early intubation is indicated in patients with:
   a. Circumferential burns of the neck
   b. Suspected airway injury

3. Early burn resuscitation requires fluid replacement based on the percent of body burned.
   a. Estimate the percent of body surface area (BSA) burned using one of the following:
      (1) "Rule of Nines" (head 9% — each arm 9% — chest, back and each leg 18% — perineum 1%)

    (2) "Rule of Palms" (The surface area of the <u>victim's palm</u> is approximately 1% of his BSA).

    (3) Lund and Browder charts (are more precise than the other two methods, particularly in children)

  b. There are many fluid replacement formulas; a general rule is to administer a crystalloid solution (LR) in an amount equal to 2 - 4mL/kg/%BSA burned/24 hrs. In infants and small children, daily maintenance fluids should also be administered.

    (1) Give the first half of these fluids over the initial 8 hours (from time of burn).

    (2) Give the second half of these fluids over the next 16 hours.

    (3) Adjust fluid administration as needed based on the patient's urine output, heart rate and mentation.

<u>Note</u>: A more detailed discussion of burns and their management is found in the chapter on Environmental Emergencies pp. 992 - 1002.

E. *Pregnant Patients...* are fundamentally <u>two</u> patients

 1. Introduction

  a. Trauma is the most common cause of nonobstetric <u>maternal</u> death during pregnancy.

  b. Because fetal survival depends entirely on maternal integrity, initial management should be directed at resuscitation and stabilization of the mother; prevention of maternal hypoxia and hypotension ensures the best outcome for both mother and fetus.

  c. Early obstetrical, pediatric and trauma service consultations should be obtained.

 2. Airway and Breathing

  a. Use continuous pulse oximetry.

  b. Administer supplemental 100% oxygen by mask; because fetal blood functions in a lower portion of a left-shifted oxygen-hemoglobin dissociation curve, an increase in oxygen tension produces a significant increase in fetal saturation.

  c. If intubation is required in the breathing patient, rapid sequence induction (with thiopental, ketamine, or etomidate) utilizing the Sellick maneuver and neuromuscular blockage (with succinylcholine* or vecuronium) is recommended.

  d. Thoracostomy tube placement (when indicated) should be at the 3rd or 4th ICS to avoid diaphragmatic injury.

 3. Circulatory Status: hemodynamic parameters are misleading.

  a. An increased HR and decreased BP (classic signs of shock) may reflect the normal physiologic changes that occur in association with pregnancy or supine positioning.

---

*Consider using a low-end dose because pseudocholineserase levels fall in pregnancy.

    b. Total blood volume increases by 30 - 50% during normal pregnancy.
       (1) As a result of this, a pregnant woman may lose 30 - 35% of her blood volume (up to 1.5 liters) before displaying clinical signs of hypovolemia.
       (2) Maternal blood loss of this volume results in decreased uterine blood flow and fetal hypoxia. Thus the fetus may be in shock despite the presence of normal maternal vital signs.
    c. Positioning of the pregnant patient on her back → the <u>supine hypotension syndrome</u>, wherein the uterus compresses the <u>IVC</u> → decreased preload and cardiac output. To prevent this, patients > 20 wks. gestation should be positioned on the <u>left</u> side. If a spinal injury is suspected, the backboard should be tilted 15° to the left.
    d. Classic signs of shock (tachycardia, hypotension) can represent normal physiologic changes associated with pregnancy.
    e. Lactated Ringer's solution should be used for initial resuscitation; normal saline may cause hyperchloremic acidosis.
    f. If clinical signs of shock do not resolve after 2 liters of a crystalloid solution has been administered, blood products should be transfused.

4. Obstetric evaluation is conducted during the secondary survey and it should include:
    a. Fundal height and tenderness
    b. Uterine contractions
    c. Fetal movement
    d. Fetal heart rate (FHR < 120 or > 160 indicates fetal distress*)
    e. Inspection of the vulva and outer vaginal vault for blood and secretions (ferning and blue discoloration of nitrazine paper may aid in distinguishing alkaline amniotic fluid from urine).
    f. Pelvic (and rectal) exams should be performed.
       (1) Perform a careful sterile speculum exam: inspect the cervix for dilation, effacement and cloudy white or green fluid coming from the os (suggests prolapse of the umbilical cord--an obstetric emergency requiring immediate C-section).
       (2) Perform a bimanual exam (unless you suspect premature rupture of membranes) to determine fetal station, presence of contractions or evidence of injury.

5. Patients with gestations > 20 weeks should undergo continuous cardiotocographic monitoring. The fetus may be in jeopardy, even with minor maternal injury. Uterine irritability, ruptured membranes, vaginal bleeding, abnormal fetal heart tones/rate (repetitive decelerations, absence of accelerations, beat-to-beat variability) or significant maternal injuries require immediate obstetric consultation and admission to the hospital.

6. A gestational age > 24 wks is considered to be viable (uterine fundus > 3 - 4cm / 2 - 3 fingerbreadths above the umbilicus). Estimate gestational age by fundal height or by ultrasonography (femur length or biparietal diameter).

---

*May be the first sign of maternal hemodynamic compromise.

7. Traumatic uterine rupture may present as maternal shock or there may only be minimal signs and symptoms. Ultrasound is very sensitive in detecting uterine rupture and is the diagnostic modality of choice if the equipment and expertise are immediately available. Abdominal x-ray findings include:
   a. Free intraperitoneal air
   b. Extended fetal extremities
   c. Abnormal fetal position

8. Placental abruption (abruptio placenta) is the most common cause of fetal death following blunt trauma.*
   a. Signs and symptoms include:
      (1) External vaginal bleeding (absent in up to 30% of cases)
      (2) Abdominal cramps/pain
      (3) Uterine tenderness/rigidity
      (4) Expanding fundal height
      (5) Maternal shock
      (6) Fetal distress
   b. Diagnosis is confirmed by:
      (1) Cardiotocographic monitoring (most sensitive modality)
      (2) Uterine ultrasonography
   c. Since abruption may cause DIC, clotting studies should be performed.

9. Abdominal trauma during pregnancy can result in fetomaternal hemorrhage (FMH). In an Rh-negative woman carrying an Rh-positive fetus, this can result in isoimmunization if it is not detected and treated. Thus, all Rh-negative women who sustain abdominal trauma during pregnancy should be given RhoGAM. In women who are < 12 weeks pregnant, a "mini-dose" of MICRhoGAM (50mcg) is appropriate; for women > 12 weeks pregnant, the standard dose (300mcg) should be administered. The Kleihauer-Betke test, which detects fetal cells in the maternal circulation, is most useful in the setting of significant blunt abdominal trauma (especially to the uterus) in which a large fetal transfusion may occur.

10. Prevention: use of seat belts significantly decreases the risk of serious and fatal maternal injuries; properly worn, three-point restraints (lap and shoulder) are the safest.

F. Mast Suit

1. Use of the Pneumatic Antishock Garment (PSAG) or Military Antishock Trousers (MAST) is somewhat controversial; these suits work by increasing peripheral vascular resistance and myocardial afterload, and by tamponading venous and small arterial bleeding in the areas covered by the suit.

2. Indications include:
   a. Immobilization of unstable pelvic fractures with continuing bleeding and hemodynamic compromise.
   b. Intra-abdominal trauma associated with significant hypovolemia in patients who are being transferred to the OR or another facility.

*Late in pregnancy, abruption can occur following relatively minor injuries.

3. Contraindications
   a. Pulmonary edema
   b. Known ruptured diaphragm
   c. Uncontrolled bleeding outside the confines of the suit
   d. Pregnancy (relative contraindication to inflation of the abdominal compartment)

G. Penetrating Trauma

1. Most penetrating injuries result from gunshot and stab wounds (rather than impalements); all penetrating wounds require surgical evaluation.

2. Gunshot wounds (GSWs)
   a. Bullets and other missiles (shot) can ricochet and cause much more extensive damage than is visible externally.
   b. GSWs to the lower thorax may involve the abdomen as well. The intraperitoneal cavity extends from the 4th ICS anteriorly to the 6 - 7th ICS posteriorly and laterally.
   c. GSWs of the abdomen are associated with a high incidence of peritoneal cavity penetration and intraperitoneal injuries; most require mandatory laparotomy.

3. Stab wounds (SWs)
   a. Injuries produced by stab wounds are confined to the path of the instrument.
   b. SWs of the abdomen have a relatively low incidence of intraperitoneal injuries (when compared with GSWs) and hence can be managed selectively; in a patient with stable vital signs, local wound exploration is followed by diagnostic laparoscopy.
   c. SWs to the neck that penetrate the platysma muscle should be extensively evaluated, either surgically in the OR or with further diagnostic studies; admission for observation is also indicated.

H. Additional Pearls

- The spleen is the most common abdominal organ injured in blunt trauma, followed by the liver.

- The liver is the most common abdominal organ injured in penetrating trauma, followed by the small bowel.

- The most common cause of sudden death following an MVA or fall from a great height is traumatic aortic rupture.

- A sternal fracture or chest wall contusion may be associated with a potentially more serious injury, i.e. myocardial contusion.

- Pelvic fractures are associated with bladder injury; check for hematuria and do a urethrogram/cystogram.

- Posterior knee dislocations may be associated with injury to the popliteal artery and/or nerve; arteriography is indicated (after surgical consultation) even if pulses are present; if you are skilled in joint reduction, you may attempt <u>one</u> gentle reduction maneuver.

- Solitary lap belts are associated with jejunal injuries and mesenteric lacerations.

- Up to 20% of patients with severe renal trauma do not have hematuria; if there is a high index of suspicion, order an IVP/cystogram or CT scan with infusion.

- The most common injury likely to present <u>late</u> is a contused bowel; initial CT may be normal.

- <u>Continuous reevaluation</u> of the trauma patient is a must.

VI. Pediatric Spine and Spinal Cord Injuries

A. Epidemiology

1. The pediatric age group accounts for 5% of all spinal cord injuries.

2. Etiology of C-spine fractures/dislocations: MVA (~ 40%), diving/falling accidents (~ 35%) and sport injuries (~ 25%).

3. Children < 8 years old have a high incidence of <u>upper</u> cervical spine and craniovertebral junction injuries. Factors which favor this injury pattern are: flat (horizontally oriented) facet joints, ligament laxity, disproportionately large head and relatively weak neck muscles.

4. Children > 12 yrs. old have <u>low</u> cervical spine injuries (similar to adults).

5. Neurologic deficits due to manipulation during resuscitation develop in ~10% of children who were neurologically intact initially.

B. Prehospital Management

1. Pediatric long-spine board; in kids < 8 yrs. old, padding should be placed underneath the <u>shoulders</u> to maintain neutral alignment of the spine.

2. Hard cervical collar

3. Securing straps

4. Soft spacing devices (e.g. blanket rolls) should be placed between head and securing straps to prevent lateral movement.

C. Developmental Anatomy

1. C_1 (atlas)
   a. Three ossification centers
   b. Neural arches ossify in utero
   c. Body ossifies (now visible on x-ray) at 1 year of age
   d. Neurocentral synchondroses fuse at age 7 years.

2. C_2 (axis)
   a. Four ossification centers — all visible at birth
   b. Secondary center at apex of odontoid appears between the ages of 3 and 6 years. Summit ossification center fuses at puberty.
   c. Between the ages of 3 and 6 years, the neurocentral synchondroses (between body and neural arches) and the odontoid-body synchondrosis fuse.
   d. The odontoid — C_2 body fusion line disappears in approximately 66% of the population near age 11. A fused or unfused synchondroses may mimic a fracture line.

3. C_3 - C_7
   a. At puberty, secondary ossification sites appear at the spinous processes and at the superior and inferior aspects of the main body.
   b. These centers fuse by age 25 and may be confused with fractures.

D. Radiologic Variables

1. Absent lordosis (~ 15% of patients) on lateral radiograph

2. Pseudosubluxation*
   a. Most pronounced at C_2 - C_3 level; 40% of kids < 7 yrs. old and 20% of kids up to 16 years of age exhibit anterior displacement of C_2 on C_3.
   b. May also be seen at the C_3 - C_4 level.

3. Predens space
   a. About 20% of children < 8 years old have a gap exceeding 3mm.
   b. Consider all distances greater than 5mm as abnormal.

4. Prevertebral soft tissues
   a. Suggested normal values are < 7mm anterior to C_2 or less than 3/4 of the adjacent vertebral body's width.
   b. Crying and forced expiration increase the distance.

5. Anterior wedging of cervical bodies (especially C_3 and C_4)

6. SCIWORA (**S**pinal **C**ord **I**njury **W**ithout **R**adiographic **A**bnormality)
   a. Incidence: accounts for up to two-thirds of pediatric cervical cord injuries; children ≤ 8 years of age are most commonly affected.
   b. Pathophysiology: microvascular blood supply insult or direct injury to the spinal tracts from extreme subluxations and distortion of the spinal ligaments.
   c. May see delayed onset of neurological deficits (up to 4 days).
   d. With a Hx of transient paresthesias, assume a potential injury.
   e. SCIWORA is a diagnosis of exclusion — bony, ligamentous and disc injuries must be ruled out.

*Subluxation up to 3mm can be considered normal

Journal References

ANN THOR SURG, Downing, S. W., et. al., 2001, "Experience with Spiral Computed Tomography as the Sole Diagnostic Method for Traumatic Aortic Rupture."

AUDIO-DIGEST: EMER. MED., Betts, James M., November 6, 1995, "The Burned Child," (side A), Carter, C. Tom, "ED Care of the Burned Adult," (side B).

BR MED J, Newlands, C., August 21, 1999, 319:516, " Orbital Trauma."

EMER MED CLINICS OF NORTH AMERICA, Shah, A.J. and Kilcline, B.A., 2003, 21: (615-629): "Trauma in Pregnancy."

EMER MED CLINICS OF NORTH AMERICA, Eckstein, M. and Chan, D., February 1998, "Contemporary Issues in Trauma."

EMERGENCY MEDICINE REPORTS, Coluccielo, Stephen A., September 1995, "The Challenge of Trauma in Pregnancy: Guidelines for Targeted Assessment, Fetal Monitoring and Definitive Management."

J TRAUMA, Tyburski, J.G., May 1, 1999, 45(5):833-8, "Pulmonary Contusions: Quantifying the Lesions on Chest X-ray films and the Factors Affecting Prognosis."

TRAUMA REPORTS, Corpron, C., Jan/Feb 2004, Vol. 5, No. 1, "Delayed or Missed Diagnoses: Avoiding these Pitfalls in the Trauma Patient."

TRAUMA REPORTS, Jones, R., September 2000, Vol. 1, No. 2, "Clinical Use of Ultrasound in Thoracoabdominal Trauma."

TRAUMA REPORTS, Hanlon, D., May/June 2001, Vol. 2, No. 3, "Current Concepts in the Management of the Pregnant Trauma Patient."

TRAUMA REPORTS, Woods, W., July/August 2003, Vol 4, No. 4, "Pediatric Cervical Spine Injuries: Avoiding Potential Disaster."

WORLD J SURG, Nagy, K. K., Krosner, S. M., Roberts, R. R., et. al., 2001, "Determining Which Patients Require Evaluation for Blunt Cardiac Injury Following Blunt Chest Trauma."

Specific Text References

Advanced Trauma Life Support for Doctors - Instructor (and Student) Course Manual. American College of Surgeons, 7th ed., (Chicago, 2004).

Sabiston's Textbook of Surgery - The Biological Basis of Modern Surgical Practice, Townsend, Beauchamp, Evers and Mattox, 16th ed., (W.B. Saunders Co., Philadelphia, 2001).

Trauma. Martox, K. L., Feliciano, D. V., Moore, E. E., 4th ed., (McGraw-Hill, New York, 2000).

Trauma Management: An Emergency Medicine Approach. Ferrera, P. C., Colucciello, S. A., Marx, J. A., Verdile, V.P., Gibbs, M. A. (Ed), (Mosby, St. Louis, 2001).

Web and Other Sources

ANNALS OF EMER MED, February, 2004, 43:2, "Clinical Policy: Critical Issues in the Evaluation of Adult Patients Presenting to the Emergency Department with Acute Blunt Abdominal Trauma."

CRITICAL DECISIONS IN EMER MED, Euerle, B., Butler, K., January 2004, Vol. 18, No. 1, "Diagnostic Ultrasonography in Emergency Medicine."

General Text References, Acep Clinical Policies and LLSA Reading Lists for all chapters located in the back of both volumes.

UROGENITAL EMERGENCIES

📖 Note: CDC Update

For New STD guidelines published after this printing, refer to the Written Board Manual/Guideline Update link on our website - www.emeeinc.com.

In this chapter, you will see a certain amount of overlap (repetition) of content. The STDs are best reviewed as a "unit" for exam purposes so they are presented as a separate section. Only those STDs that belong under Gynecologic Disorders reappear in that section and then, only from a clinical (not academic) perspective.

UROGENITAL EMERGENCIES

Additional Note

There are many antibiotics and dosing regimens in this chapter. You are not expected to memorize them but you should be familiar with them so that you will recognize specific antibiotics and corresponding doses when they appear on your exam.

---

1. Which of the following statements regarding syphilis, chancroid, lympho-granuloma venereum and genital herpes simplex is most accurate?

   (a) Treatment of these STDs should be withheld until lab confirmation has been obtained.
   (b) Doxycycline is the recommended drug of choice for each of these STDs.
   (c) Patients with these STDs commonly complain of a vaginal or penile discharge.
   (d) These STDs are characterized by genital ulcers and/or inguinal lymphadenopathy.

2. A female patient presents with the complaint of an itchy, malodorous vaginal discharge which is yellow-gray in color. On exam, her vaginal mucosa has a stippled appearance and the vaginal pH is 6.0. Wet mount reveals motile pear-shaped organisms with flagella at one end. The patient tells you she is 5 weeks pregnant. How would you treat her for this condition?

   (a) Prescribe metronidazole 2gms PO in one dose.
   (b) Recommend vaginal douching Q HS with yogurt × 7 days.
   (c) Prescribe clotrimazole vaginal suppositories, two Q HS × 7 days.
   (d) Recommend vinegar douches Q HS × 7 days.

3. A pregnant patient presents in her first trimester with a foul-smelling vaginal discharge. Exam reveals diffuse vaginal erythema, foamy grayish-yellow-green discharge; wet mount reveals many PMNs and flagellated, motile, tear-drop-shaped organisms. The most appropriate therapy for this patient is:

   (a) Metronidazole
   (b) Doxycycline
   (c) Clotrimazole cream or suppositories
   (d) Clindamycin

4. Which of the following is not considered a risk factor for PID?

   (a) Use of an IUD
   (b) Use of BCPs
   (c) Multiple sexual partners
   (d) Adolescence

5. The most common cause of PID in college students is:

   (a) *Chlamydia*
   (b) *N. Gonorrhea*
   (c) Anaerobic bacteria
   (d) Genital tract mycoplasmas

6. All of the following are considered safe for administration during pregnancy except:

   (a) Tetanus toxoid
   (b) Penicillins/cephalosporins
   (c) Erythromycin (except for estolate)
   (d) Measles vaccine

7. All of the following statements regarding thromboembolic disease in pregnancy are accurate except:

   (a) The risk of thromboembolism is 5 - 6 times greater in pregnant women (and in the immediate postpartum period) than in nonpregnant women.
   (b) The initial diagnostic study of choice for ruling out a pulmonary embolus is an angiogram.
   (c) The initial diagnostic study of choice for ruling out a DVT is a venogram.
   (d) Treatment is with heparin.

8. All of the following statements regarding vulvovaginal candidiasis are accurate except:

   (a) Candida albicans is part of the normal vaginal flora in up to 20% of women.
   (b) Causes of colonization or overgrowth include diabetes mellitus, pregnancy, menstruation and BCPs.
   (c) Diagnosis is with a KOH prep which reveals "clue cells."
   (d) Treatment of partners is generally unnecessary as this is not a sexually transmitted disease.

9. A young, sexually active woman presents with a history of RLQ pain for the past several hours. Her LMP was 6 weeks ago but she says that is not unusual for her. Her vital signs are stable but she looks visibly uncomfortable. On abdominal exam, you note tenderness confined to the RLQ and pelvic exam reveals right adnexal tenderness and fullness. Which of the following possible diagnoses is least likely?

   (a) Ectopic pregnancy
   (b) PID
   (c) Hemorrhagic corpus luteum cyst
   (d) Adnexal torsion

10. Referring to the patient discussed in question 9, which of the following lab tests would be least likely to help you in narrowing the differential and establishing a definitive diagnosis?

    (a) CBC
    (b) Culdocentesis
    (c) B-HCG
    (d) Pelvic ultrasound

11. The incidence of transmission of Rubella from an infected mother to her fetus is greatest when maternal infection occurs:

    (a) In the first month of pregnancy
    (b) In the second month of pregnancy
    (c) In the third month of pregnancy
    (d) Is the same in the first 3 months of pregnancy

12. The drugs considered to be safest for administration during pregnancy are those classified by the FDA as:

    (a) Category X drugs
    (b) Category D drugs
    (c) Category C drugs
    (d) Category A drugs

13. All of the following statements regarding the diagnosis of intrahepatic cholestasis of pregnancy are accurate except:

    (a) Patients usually present in their third trimester with pruritus and mild jaundice.
    (b) Associated lab findings include a 7 - 10 fold increase in the alkaline phosphatase level and markedly elevated serum transaminases.
    (c) Symptoms are treated with cholestyramine.
    (d) It is associated with an increased risk of premature delivery and fetal compromise.

14. Which of the following is not considered to be a risk factor for abruptio placenta?

    (a) HTN
    (b) Abdominal trauma
    (c) Primiparity
    (d) Smoking

15. A patient is brought in by ambulance for evaluation. The paramedics state that she had been out shopping with a friend and had a grand mal seizure. A chem strip done in the field showed a glucose of 120. There is no known history of a prior seizure disorder. On evaluation, your patient looks to be about 17 yrs. old and at least eight months pregnant. She is lethargic and hyperreflexic (+3/4) and has a BP of 170/100. The most appropriate initial medication for this patient is:

    (a) Hydralazine
    (b) Valium
    (c) Lasix
    (d) Magnesium sulfate

16. Signs of magnesium toxicity include all of the following except:
    (a) Loss of DTRs
    (b) Respiratory depression
    (c) Flushing
    (d) Bradydysrhythmias

17. Appropriate initial evaluation of a woman with vaginal bleeding in the third trimester includes all of the following except:
    (a) Evaluation of the fetal heart tones
    (b) Pelvic exam
    (c) CBC, type and Rh, DIC profile
    (d) Ultrasound

18. A woman who is 34 weeks pregnant presents with RUQ pain of several hours duration. On exam, she has a temperature of 100.4° F and diffuse RUQ tenderness. CBC reveals a white count of 17,000; her alkaline phosphatase and LFTs are normal; her U/A reveals pyuria without bacteria. The most likely diagnosis is:
    (a) Pyelonephritis
    (b) Salpingitis
    (c) Appendicitis
    (d) Cholecystitis

19. A woman who is four days postpartum presents with vaginal bleeding. Exam reveals a temperature of 101° F, a purulent discharge and uterine tenderness. The most likely cause of her postpartum bleeding is:
    (a) Retained placental tissue
    (b) Endometritis
    (c) Uterine atony
    (d) Genital tract trauma sustained during delivery

20. All of the following statements regarding the Kleihauer-Betke test are accurate except:
    (a) It can be used to detect and quantify fetomaternal hemorrhage (FMH).
    (b) It is useful in determining the amount of RhoGAM administered to an Rh-negative woman who has sustained FMH.
    (c) Its use is generally limited to women who are at least 12 weeks pregnant.
    (d) A negative test means that no FMH has occurred.

21. A patient presents with acute renal failure. Urinalysis reveals a specific gravity of 1.025 and occasional hyaline casts but is otherwise normal. The urine sodium is < 20, the fractional excretion of sodium (FE_{Na}) is < 1% and the renal failure index (RFI) is < 1%. What type of renal failure does this patient have?

    (a) Prerenal azotemia
    (b) Renal azotemia
    (c) Postrenal azotemia
    (d) Cannot be determined from the information provided

22. The most common cause of acute renal azotemia is:

    (a) Glomerulonephritis
    (b) Malignant hypertension
    (c) Acute tubular necrosis (ATN)
    (d) Vasculitis

23. Complications of acute renal failure include all of the following except:

    (a) Hyperkalemia
    (b) Volume overload
    (c) Hypocalcemia
    (d) Hypomagnesemia

24. The most sensitive test for detecting rhabdomyolysis is:

    (a) Urine myoglobin
    (b) Serum myoglobin
    (c) Serum creatinine kinase
    (d) All of the above are equally sensitive

25. What is the most common cause of life-threatening infection in renal transplant patients?

    (a) Hepatitis B
    (b) Toxoplasmosis
    (c) Cytomegalovirus
    (d) *Strep. pneumoniae*

26. All of the following kidney stones are radiopaque except:

    (a) Cystine
    (b) Uric acid
    (c) Magnesium ammonium phosphate
    (d) Calcium oxalate

27. All of the following infections may be associated with the development of penile ulcers except:

    (a) Herpes simplex
    (b) Chancroid
    (c) Gonorrhea
    (d) Syphilis

28. A healthy 24-year-old female presents with a 2-day history of frequency, urgency and dysuria. She is afebrile and exam reveals only mild suprapubic tenderness. U/A reveals pyuria and bacteriuria. The most appropriate antibiotic for this patient is:

(a) Augmentin
(b) Ciprofloxacin
(c) Amoxicillin
(d) TMP-SMX

29. A healthy 28-year-old male presents with rectal itching and a discharge. When specifically asked, he states that his sexual preference is male and that he practices anal receptive intercourse. Exam reveals a purulent discharge and inflammation. The most appropriate initial therapy for this patient is:

(a) Ceftriaxone 250mg IM
(b) Doxycycline 100mg PO bid × 10 days
(c) Ceftriaxone 125mg IM <u>plus</u> doxycycline 100mg PO bid × 7 days
(d) Erythromycin base 500mg PO qid × 7 days

30. All of the following drug classes are typically associated with urinary retention except:

(a) Sympatholytics
(b) Alpha-adrenergic stimulants
(c) Cyclic antidepressants
(d) Antihistamines

31. An elderly gentleman from a nursing home (NH) is sent to the ED for evaluation of abdominal distention and discomfort. Exam reveals a markedly distended bladder. A Foley catheter is passed and returns 2000mL initially and 900mL/hr over the next 3 hours. The most appropriate management of this patient is:

(a) Discharge to the NH with the catheter in place
(b) Removal of the catheter and discharge to the NH
(c) Admission to the hospital for IV fluid resuscitation and correction of electrolyte imbalance
(d) None of the above

Answers: 1. d, 2. a, 3. a, 4. b, 5. a, 6. d, 7. c, 8. c, 9. b, 10. a, 11. a, 12. d, 13. b, 14. c, 15. d, 16. c, 17. b, 18. c, 19. b, 20. d, 21. a, 22. c, 23. d, 24. c, 25. c, 26. b, 27. c, 28. d, 29. c, 30. a, 31. c

Use the pre-chapter multiple choice question worksheet (p. xxv) to record and determine the percentage of correct answers for this section.

SEXUALLY TRANSMITTED DISEASES

I. Gonorrhea

A. Clinical Presentations (may be asymptomatic)

1. In males, the usual complaint is a purulent urethral discharge that is frequently associated with dysuria. Rectal gonorrhea (venereal proctitis) should be suspected in the presence of a rectal discharge in men who have sex with men.

2. In females, the disease may be misdiagnosed in the early stages as non-specific vaginitis, cervicitis or UTI since the presenting complaint is frequently dysuria, a vaginal discharge or both. Abdominal pain does not occur until the infection has spread to the uterus and fallopian tubes (PID).

3. Pharyngeal or anal infection may occur in either sex. Although generally asymptomatic, patients with anal infection may c/o discharge, rectal pain, tenesmus and/or constipation. Patients with pharyngeal infection are rarely symptomatic.

4. Gonococcal conjunctivitis occurs in both sexes, and is usually the result of inoculation of the eye by a contaminated finger. A copious purulent discharge, marked conjunctival injection and unilateral involvement are characteristic.

5. Hematogenous dissemination also occurs in both sexes and may produce any of the follow complications:
   a. Joint disease
      (1) Most common cause of septic arthritis in patients under fifty, especially teenagers and young adults.
      (2) Diagnosis should be considered in any young patient with joint pain. A classic (but not necessarily common) presentation is a fever, rash and multiple joint pain that includes a tenosynovitis.
   b. Endocarditis
   c. Sepsis
   d. Meningitis

   [A rash may be associated with any of these complications, but is most frequently seen if fever is present. The skin lesions of gonococcemia are typically erythematous macules or pustules with a necrotic or purpuric center. Petechiae are also seen.]

B. Diagnosis

1. Gram-negative intracellular diplococci should be seen on gram stain smears from skin lesions in both sexes, urethral discharge in males or cervical discharge in females; this provides a tentative diagnosis of GC.

2. *Neisseria Gonorrhea* should be identified on culture of suspected lesions or discharges or by nucleic acid amplification tests (PCR/LCR of DNA).

3. Failure to obtain a positive smear or culture is common. Repeated cultures should be done if clinical suspicion remains.

C. Treatment

1. Should be started as soon as the diagnosis is suspected clinically or there is a history of exposure. Do not wait for culture results, as this may result in the development of more advanced disease and continued transmission of the infection.

2. Due to the prevalence of concurrent chlamydial infection (up to 45% of patients with gonorrhea have a coexisting chlamydial infection), all patients should receive simultaneous antibiotic coverage for both gonorrhea and chlamydia.

3. Given the increasing incidence of penicillinase-producing *N. gonorrhea* and tetracycline-resistant *N. gonorrhea*, ceftriaxone is currently the drug of choice for the treatment of gonorrhea.

4. Drug regimen of choice for uncomplicated infections (no hematogenous dissemination):
   a. Ceftriaxone 125mg IM (may be used in the pregnant patient) plus
   b. Doxycycline 100mg PO bid × 7 days or Azithromycin 1gm PO.
      (1) Effective in treating concurrent chlamydial infection as well as incubating syphilis:
         (a) If a GC culture is negative, *Chlamydia trachomatis* is the most likely offending organism (since it is the most common STD).
         (b) Untreated chlamydial PID can lead to tubal injury with subsequent infertility problems.
         (c) Epididymitis in males < 35 yrs. of age without a urethral discharge is most commonly a chlamydial infection and is considered to be the most common STD in males.
      (2) Doxycycline (a form of tetracycline) is contraindicated in pregnancy and should probably not be used in children < 8 years old. In these patients, erythromycin base 500mg PO qid × 7 days may be substituted for doxycycline.

5. Alternative drug therapy for uncomplicated infections for patients who cannot take ceftriaxone:
   a. Cefixime 400mg PO (single dose) plus doxycycline 100mg PO bid × 7 days or

    b. Quinolones
       (1) Should not be given to patients who acquired the infection in Cleveland, Seattle, California, Hawaii, Asia or the Pacific islands since the incidence of quinolone-resistant *N. Gonorrhea* is significant in these areas. In these cases, cefixime or ceftriaxone should be used. [CDC Guidelines 2002]
       (2) Due to increasing antimicrobial resistance, the CDC currently recommends that fluoroquinolones no longer be used as treatment for gonorrhea in MSM (men who have sex with men).
       (3) The quinolones (and doxycycline) are both contraindicated in children and during pregnancy; use alternative therapy in these patients (spectinomycin or erythromycin).
       (4) Specific agents
          (a) Ciprofloxacin 500mg PO (single dose) <u>or</u> ┐ plus doxycycline
          (b) Ofloxacin 400mg PO (single dose) <u>or</u> ┤ 100mg PO bid
          (c) Levofloxacin 250mg PO (single dose) ┘ x 7 days

6. Alternative drug therapy for uncomplicated infections in patients who cannot take cephalosporins and quinolones: Spectinomycin 2gms IM (may be used in the pregnant patient).

7. Patients with gonococcal conjunctivitis should be hospitalized and also receive timely ophthalmologic consultation.

8. Patients with disseminated gonorrhea should be hospitalized for initial therapy.

9. Advise treatment of sexual contacts (even if signs and symptoms of active disease are absent).

10. Recommend abstinence until sexual partners have been evaluated, treated and antibiotic therapy has been completed.

11. Obtain a serologic test for syphilis (RPR or VDRL) in all patients evaluated and treated for gonorrhea.

12. Recommend a follow-up culture, one week after the completion of therapy, for patients who have symptoms that persist after treatment.

II. Syphilis

A. Etiology

1. A common STD (especially in MSM) caused by a spirochete (*Treponema pallidum*) found in infected skin lesions, mucous membranes, saliva, semen and blood.

2. Transmission occurs primarily by direct contact with an infected lesion (usually genital). Syphilis may also be acquired congenitally and by a blood transfusion (if the donor was in a very early stage of the disease).

B. Clinical Phases and Diagnostic Tests

1. Primary Syphilis
   a. A small papule develops at the site of inoculation (usually genital) which becomes a painless, indurated ulcer — the classic chancre. Chancres develop after an incubation period of 10 - 90 days, are present for 3 - 6 weeks and resolve spontaneously.
      (1) Scrapings obtained from the chancre, and examined under dark-field microscopy, reveal moving corkscrew-like treponemes.
      (2) Serologic tests (VDRL or RPR) are often negative.
   b. Inguinal lymphadenopathy (buboes) may be present; nodes are enlarged, non-tender, firm and rubbery; they develop approximately 4 weeks after the initial exposure.
      (1) Material obtained from the nodes is dark-field positive.
      (2) Serologic tests are usually positive.

2. Secondary Syphilis
   a. Is characterized by constitutional signs/symptoms and a rash.
   b. Rash and lymphadenopathy are the most common symptoms.
   c. The rash of secondary syphilis emerges 4 - 8 weeks after the initial appearance of the chancre and lasts for several months. It may be difficult to distinguish from the rash of RMSF (Rocky Mountain Spotted Fever) since both occur on the palms and soles. Definitive differentiation is with serologic testing (VDRL, RPR or FTA-ABS).
      (1) Erythematous (red) macules, papules or plaques (condylomata lata) suggest syphilis; the classic rash is maculopapular, non-pruritic, symmetric and commonly involves the palms and soles.
      (2) A fine pink (not red) rash interspersed with macules suggests RMSF.

3. Tertiary Syphilis — Onset occurs after a latent (dormant) period of several years and is characterized by development of cardiovascular and/or neurologic disorders such as thoracic aneurysm, dementia and tabes dorsalis. Serology tests are positive. [Note: Consider neurosyphilis in your differential diagnosis of HIV+ patients with neurologic disease.]

C. Treatment

1. Exposed patients should be evaluated clinically and serologically, then treated on a presumptive basis. (Note: all patients who have syphilis should be tested for HIV infection).

2. Sexual partners should be notified and treated.

3. Penicillin G is the treatment of choice for syphilis, regardless of stage; doxycycline is the alternative choice for the PCN-allergic patient.

4. Primary, secondary and early latent (< 1 year duration) syphilis
   a. Benzathine PCN G 2.4 million units IM or
   b. Doxycycline 100mg PO bid × 14 days or ⎤ nonpregnant
   c. Tetracycline 500mg PO qid × 14 days or ⎦ patients*
   d. Ceftriaxone 1gm IM/IV qd × 8 - 10 days

*Pregnant patients who are allergic to penicillin should be desensitized and treated with penicillin.

5. Tertiary syphilis
   a. Cardiovascular syphilis and/or late latent syphilis (> 1 year duration)
      (1) Benzathine PCN G 2.4 million units IM weekly for three wks. <u>or</u>
      (2) Doxycycline 100mg PO bid × four weeks <u>or</u> ⎤ <u>non</u>pregnant
      (3) Tetracycline 500mg PO qid × four weeks ⎦ patients[*]
   b. Neurosyphilis
      (1) Aqueous crystalline PCN G 3 - 4 million units IV Q4 hrs. × 10 - 14 days <u>or</u>
      (2) If compliance assured → Procaine PCN G 2.4 million units IM qd <u>plus</u> probenecid 500mg PO qid, both for 10 - 14 days.
      <u>Note</u>: PCN-allergic patients require desensitization followed by one of the above regimens or Ceftriaxone 2gm IM/IV qd × 10 - 14 days (for patients without a prior anaphylactic reaction to penicillin).

6. Follow-up serologic testing (VDRL or RPR) should be recommended as treatment failure may occur with any drug regimen.

7. Treatment may result in the development of the Jarisch-Herxheimer reaction, an acute febrile reaction accompanied by headache, myalgias and rash intensification. This self-limited reaction usually occurs 1 - 2 hours after antibiotic therapy is started (certainly within the first 24 hours) and is treated with antipyretics and bedrest.

III. Chancroid

A. *Etiology*

1. Although chancroid is the least reported STD, the incidence is rising.

2. The infecting organism, *Hemophilus ducreyi*, is acquired through sexual contact from discharges of ulcerations or suppurating lymphatic tissue; the incubation period is 2 - 10 days.

B. *Clinical Presentation*

The initial sign is a small pustule or papule that quickly breaks down into one or more painful chancres. Most patients present with a *"pain triad"*:

- <u>painful</u> <u>necrotic</u> chancre (dirty ulcer, ragged)
- <u>painful</u> urination on contact with the chancre
- <u>painful</u> inguinal lymphadenopathy that is suppurative and frequently associated with extensive tissue destruction; bubo formation (50% of cases) with spontaneous rupture is common.

---

[*]Pregnant patients who are allergic to penicillin should be desensitized and treated with penicillin.

C. Diagnosis

1. If your lab has experience with this organism, obtain an aspirate from the inguinal bubo and send it to the lab for gram stain and culture.
   a. Gram stain reveals short, gram-negative bacilli in a linear or parallel formation ("school of fish").
   b. A positive culture confirms the diagnosis, but a negative culture does not rule it out.

2. If your lab does not have the capability to isolate this organism, diagnosis should be based on clinical presentation. [Note: HIV testing should be done if chancroid is suspected; there is a high rate of co-infection.]

D. Treatment

1. Azithromycin 1gm PO in a single dose <u>or</u>

2. Ceftriaxone 250mg IM in a single dose <u>or</u>

3. Ciprofloxacin 500mg PO bid × 3 days. [<u>Note</u>: Quinolones are contraindicated in pregnancy and in children < 17 yrs. old] <u>or</u>

4. Erythromycin base 500mg PO qid × 7 days or until lesions are healed. [All four regimens are effective for the treatment of chancroid in HIV-infected patients.]

5. Advise treatment of sexual contacts, even if they are asymptomatic.

6. Recommend abstinence until sexual partners have been treated and antibiotic therapy has been completed.

IV. Lymphogranuloma Venereum

A. Etiology

This is an uncommon STD caused by *Chlamydia trachomatis*. It usually occurs in young men, 20 - 40 years old, and is characterized by tender inguinal and/or femoral lymphadenopathy that is usually unilateral.

B. Clinical Presentation

A small, shallow, <u>painless</u> vesicle or ulcer appears 3 - 21 days after exposure. It usually goes unnoticed by the patient. Two to twenty-four weeks after the exposure, localized, tender inguinal lymphadenopathy develops. When the nodes enlarge, coalesce and ulcerate, constitutional symptoms may occur. The *"groove sign"* may appear and is characterized by the proliferation of inguinal lymphadenopathy above and below the inguinal ligament.

C. Diagnosis

1. The LGV complement fixation test (which has replaced the Frei skin test) is diagnostic, but is not available in many hospital laboratories.

2. Culture is also diagnostic, but many labs do not have this capability.

3. The diagnosis is usually made by identification of leukocytes with intracellular inclusion bodies from aspirates of infected tissue.

D. Treatment

1. Should be initiated as soon as the diagnosis is suspected, without waiting for lab confirmation.

2. Doxycycline 100mg PO bid × 3 weeks is the treatment of choice but should be avoided in pregnancy, while nursing, and in children < 8 yrs. old. Pregnant women should be treated with erythromycin* 500mg PO qid × 3 weeks.

3. Treatment of sexual partners should be recommended.

V. Trichomoniasis

A. Etiology

1. A common, although minor, STD caused by the flagellated protozoan *Trichomonas vaginalis* that is transmitted by contact (usually genital) with infected secretions of the genital and urinary tracts.

2. The incubation period is usually a week with symptoms occurring in women, but not men.

B. Clinical Presentation

Patients complain of a malodorous, itchy, vaginal discharge that is typically frothy or foamy. On exam, the discharge may be yellow or have a gray-green appearance; the vaginal mucosa and cervix may have a stippled or punctate "strawberry" appearance. The vaginal pH is usually ≥ 5.5

C. Diagnosis — is by wet mount and direct visualization of the motile trichomonads, which are pear-shaped and have several flagella at one end.

D. Treatment

1. Metronidazole (Flagyl): a single dose of 2gm or 500mg bid × 7 days are equally effective.
   a. Use the 7-day regimen if single dose therapy fails.
   b. For repeated failures, use 2gms qd × 3 - 5 days.

*Not the estolate formulary

2. Sexual partners should be treated.

3. Advise patients to avoid ingestion of alcoholic beverages during treatment with metronidazole and for at least 24 hours thereafter as ingestion may precipitate an "Antabuse" reaction (flushing, headache, nausea, vomiting, palpitations and abdominal discomfort).

VI. Granuloma Inguinale (Donovanosis)

A. Etiology — a rare STD caused by *Calymmatobacterium granulomatis* that has an incubation period of 1 - 12 weeks.

B. Clinical Presentation — depends on the stage of the disease

1. A painless papule, vesicle or nodular lesion of the genitalia.

2. Beefy-red, velvety ulcers with a rolled border on the genital and/or anal regions; they bleed easily on contact.

3. Subcutaneous granulomas (pseudobuboes) in the inguinal nodes may develop over the next few months.

4. Extensive tissue destruction which may lead to subsequent squamous cell carcinoma.

C. Diagnosis

1. Is usually made by biopsy.

2. Donovan bodies (monocytes engulfing clusters of organisms that resemble microscopic safety pins) confirm the diagnosis, but few laboratory personnel have experience in identifying this organism.

D. Treatment

1. Trimethoprim-sulfamethoxazole one DS tab PO bid <u>or</u>

2. Doxycycline 100mg PO bid

   [Both drugs should be taken for at least 3 weeks and neither drug should be given to pregnant patients.]

3. Alternative drug regimens
   a. Ciprofloxacin 750mg PO bid <u>or</u>
   b. Erythromycin 500mg PO qid

   [Both drugs should be taken for at least 3 weeks; pregnant and lactating women should be treated with erythromycin (<u>not</u> Cipro).]

VII. Acquired Immunodeficiency Syndrome (AIDS)

A. AIDS is a disease complex resulting from an incompetent immune system. It begins when a patient becomes infected with a lymphotropic retrovirus called the human immunodeficiency virus (HIV). This virus causes a reduction in the number of normally immunocompetent cells (especially T helper lymphocytes). This leads to the development of either Kaposi's sarcoma or one of several opportunistic infections (most commonly *Pneumocystis carinii* pneumonia [PCP], cryptococcal meningitis or toxoplasma brain abscess).

B. High-Risk Populations

1. Homosexuals, bisexuals and heterosexuals exposed to a partner at risk; presence of other STDs (e.g. chancroid) increases the risk of transmission.

2. IV drug users

3. Prostitutes

4. Patients who underwent tattooing or acupuncture

5. Patients who received blood transfusions between 1978 and 1985

6. Infants born to an HIV-infected mother

C. Most Frequent Modes of HIV Virus Transmission

1. Sexual intercourse

2. Parenteral (blood is probably the most infectious; risk to health care worker is 0.3 - 0.4% per exposure)

3. Perinatal maternal-fetal inoculation

4. Breast milk

D. **Clinical Presentation** – is usually one of the complicating conditions. Respiratory symptoms such as dyspnea and cough are particularly frequent. Other common complaints include: fever, fatigue, weight loss, diarrhea and lymphadenopathy. The primary infection is often asymptomatic but a mononucleosis-type illness (acute retroviral syndrome) may occur 2 - 6 wks. post-exposure. HIV antibody testing should be done as soon as the diagnosis is suspected:

1. ELISA — Currently the best available screening test

2. Western blot assay — a confirmatory test for positive ELISA results

E. Recognizing AIDS-Related Diseases

1. *Pneumocystis carinii* pneumonia (most common opportunistic infection in HIV patients)
   a. **Clinical picture**: high fever, nonproductive cough and dyspnea; there are little (if any) findings on chest exam.
   b. Diagnostic tests
      (1) ABGs
         (a) Early — mild hypoxemia (pO_2 70 - 90 torr)
         (b) Later — progressive hypoxemia with respiratory alkalosis
      (2) Check x-ray
         (a) Early — little or no findings
         (b) Later — progressive bilateral interstitial infiltrates (not always symmetric, not always bilateral)
      (3) Sputum Gram stain — may yield a diagnosis in 60% of cases. (An acid-fast stain to rule out TB should also be done)
      (4) Bronchoscopy — with bronchoalveolar lavage has a diagnostic yield of 90%.
      (5) Gallium lung scan — is helpful in demonstrating diffuse parenchymal disease, but is nonspecific.
   c. Treatment (40 - 60% of AIDS patients will develop this infection and it is rapidly fatal if untreated)
      (1) Supplemental O_2 and volume repletion as needed
      (2) Trimethoprim-sulfamethoxazole or Pentamidine
      (3) Corticosteroids (if pO_2 is < 70 torr or A-a gradiant is > 35)

2. Cryptococcal meningitis (most common cause of meningitis in HIV patients)
   a. **Clinical picture**: fever (at times low grade), headache (with or without nuchal rigidity) and photophobia; seizures and cranial nerve palsies may also occur.
   b. Specific diagnostic tests
      (1) Do a CT scan first to R/O an intracranial mass lesion.
      (2) If CT is negative, do an LP and send the spinal fluid for the usual studies plus:
         (a) India ink prep (75% sensitive) and/or fungal culture
         (b) Cryptococcal antigen titer (95% sensitive)
         [Note: The serum cryptococcal antigen titer has the highest sensitivity (98%)]
   c. Treatment
      (1) Amphotcricin B (with or without Flucytosine)
      (2) Immediate infectious disease consult

3. CNS Toxoplasmosis (most common cause of focal encephalitis and the leading cause of intracranial mass lesions in AIDS patients)
   a. **Clinical picture**: fever, headache, focal neurological signs and symptoms, altered mental status or seizures.
   b. Specific diagnostic tests
      (1) CT scanning with contrast — often shows ring-enhancing lesion(s) (the "signet ring" sign).
      (2) MRI — lesions in the basal ganglia are suggestive
      (3) Brain biopsy if CT and MRI are negative
   c. Treatment: Pyrimethamine and Sulfadiazine with folinic acid (to reduce the incidence of hematologic toxicity)

4. Kaposi's sarcoma (is seen in 43% of AIDS patients, primarily in male homosexuals; second most common opportunistic infection and most common cancer in AIDS patients)
   a. **Clinical picture**: reddish-brown or bluish-red subcutaneous nodules most commonly found on the face (including the oral cavity), genitalia and feet. These painless, nonpruritic lesions have a spongy texture, and range from several millimeters to several centimeters in diameter. They are most frequently seen on the skin of the distal extremities.
   b. Immediate oncology consult is indicated.

5. Oral candidiasis (Thrush) often antedates the development of AIDS.
   a. **Clinical picture**: although sometimes asymptomatic, patients usually complain of a sore or dry mouth and examination reveals raised white lacy plaques on the tongue and buccal mucosa.
   b. Specific test: KOH prep
   c. Treatment is usually clotrimazole troches or a nystatin suspension.

   Note: The complaint of painful swallowing is suggestive of candidal esophagitis, which, if present, confirms the diagnosis of AIDS. Endoscopic verification should be obtained.

6. Herpes Zoster (Shingles) can be a severe and recurrent problem at any stage of HIV infection. Acyclovir orally (in large doses) or parenterally is the treatment of choice.

7. Cytomegalovirus (CMV) retinitis is the most common ocular complication of AIDS and, if untreated, leads to blindness. Parenteral treatment with foscarnet or ganciclovir is indicated.

8. There are a host of other AIDS-related diseases that can affect one or more organ systems, but these are less commonly seen (except for tuberculosis which is covered at length in the Pulmonary Emergencies chapter, pp. 344 - 351). The treatment of AIDS and the opportunistic infections with which it is associated is rapidly evolving; early consultation with an infectious disease specialist regarding therapeutic options for these infections is highly recommended.

VIII. Herpes Progenitalis (Herpes Simplex Virus Type II, Herpesvirus Hominis)

A. Etiology

1. A common STD caused most often by Type II Herpes Simplex Virus, and occasionally by Type I.

2. Transmission is generally by sexual contact with an infected individual; it may occur in the absence of visible lesions if viral shedding is present.

3. Incubation period ranges from 8 to 16 days.

B. Clinical Manifestations

1. Recurring, painful, genital lesions that appear as clusters of vesicles on an erythematous base and subsequently denude forming ulcers.

2. The lesions may be found at any site, but the most commonly affected areas are:
   a. The cervix and vulva in females (swelling of the vulva may be so severe that the patient may not be able to void urine)
   b. The glans and prepuce in males

3. Attacks are often heralded by a prodrome of pain, hyperesthesia, burning or paraesthesia at the skin site.

4. Headache, fever, arthralgias and regional adenopathy may also be present, particularly with the first clinical episode.

5. Newborns who acquire the virus at birth may develop devastating complications.

C. Diagnosis

1. The clinical findings are usually sufficient evidence of the diagnosis.

2. If there is some question, the diagnosis can be confirmed by one of the following:
   a. Direct immunofluorescent testing
   b. Identification of multinucleated giant cells on Tzanck smear
   c. Viral culture

D. Treatment Recommendations

1. Acyclovir (PO or IV) remains the antiviral agent of choice; it accelerates healing, shortens the duration of viral shedding and provides partial control of symptoms. Use of <u>topical</u> acyclovir is not recommended. Famciclovir and Valacyclovir are acceptable alternatives. Foscarnet is often effective for treatment of acyclovir-resistant genital herpes. (Neither acyclovir nor any other treatment regimen has succeeded in preventing the recurrence of lesions.)

2. Indications for treatment with oral acyclovir:
   a. Patients with primary lesions
   b. Patients with associated herpes cervicitis, urethritis, proctitis, stomatitis or pharyngitis
   c. Patients with recurrent genital herpes
   d. Episodic infections in HIV+ patients

3. Indications for hospital admission and treatment with IV acyclovir:
   a. Patients with severe genital infections
   b. Immunocompromised patients with severe infections/disseminated disease.
   c. Patients who cannot tolerate or do not respond to oral medication
   d. Neonatal herpes

4. Prescribe analgesics as needed.

5. If an associated cellulitis is present, prescribe anti-staphylococcal antibiotics.

6. Advise patients to avoid sexual contact when lesions are present.

GYNECOLOGIC DISORDERS

I. **Vulvovaginitis (inflammation of vagina and external genitalia)**

A. ***Trichomonas Vaginitis (a sexually transmitted disease).***

   1. Is caused by *Trichomonas vaginalis*, a flagellated protozoan.

   2. Clinical presentation: patients present with vulvovaginal itching and a foul-smelling discharge. Associated dysuria and lower abdominal pain may also be present. Symptoms usually develop after an incubation period of 4 - 28 days.

   3. Diagnosis
      a. Profuse, occasionally foamy, yellow-green discharge associated with diffuse vaginal erythema and a "strawberry cervix and vagina" (punctate hemorrhages).
      b. Wet mount demonstrates a flagellated, motile, tear-drop-shaped organism and many PMNs.
      c. Vaginal pH $\geq$ 5.5

   4. Treatment (partner must also be treated)
      a. Recommended regimen (includes pregnant patients): metronidazole 2gms PO in one dose---should not be used for male partners.
      b. Alternative regimen: metronidazole 500mg PO BID $\times$ 7 days.
      Note: Metronidazole can produce a disulfiram-like (Antabuse-like) reaction if taken in conjunction with alcohol. Therefore, patients must be advised to avoid ingesting alcohol while taking metronidazole and for at least 24 hours following the completion of therapy.

   5. Clinical importance
      a. It can produce inflammatory changes on the Pap smear.
      b. 90% of males with this infection are <u>asymptomatic</u>; therefore, sexual partners must be treated if reinfection is to be prevented.
      c. It has been associated with an increased risk of premature rupture of membranes, preterm delivery and postpartum endometritis.

B. ***Vulvovaginal Candidiasis***

   1. Pathophysiology
      a. Normal vaginal flora in up to 20% of healthy women.
      b. Colonization or overgrowth of the organism (*Candida albicans*) can be caused by:
         (1) Diabetes mellitus
         (2) Pregnancy and post-menopause
         (3) Drugs (oral contraceptives, antibiotics, steroids)
         (4) Menstruation

---

2. Clinical presentation: extreme itching with a thin watery to thick white discharge sometimes associated with dysuria or dyspareunia.

3. Diagnosis
   a. Physical exam: thick, white "cottage cheese" discharge; vulvovaginal erythema and edema; satellite lesions on perineum (sometimes).
   b. Pseudohyphae and spores may be seen on 10% KOH prep.
   c. pH of vaginal secretions is normal (≤ 4.5)

4. Classification of vulvovaginal candidiasis (VVC)
   a. Uncomplicated VVC
      (1) Sporadic/Infrequent VVC
      (2) Mild-to-moderate VVC
      (3) Likely to be *C. albicans*
      (4) Nonimmunocompromised patient
   b. Complicated VVC
      (1) Recurrent or severe VVC
      (2) Non-albicans candidiasis
      (3) Pregnancy
      (4) Debilitated, diabetic or immunocompromised patient

5. Treatment
   a. Uncomplicated VVC -- Fluconazole 150mg PO in one dose or <u>one</u> of the following vaginal preparations Q HS × 3 days:
      (1) Butoconazole 2% cream
      (2) Clotrimazole 2 (100mg) vaginal tablets
      (3) Miconazole 200mg vaginal suppository
      (4) Terconazole 80mg suppository or 0.8% cream
   b. Complicated VVC -- use one of the following vaginal preparations Q HS × 7 days:
      (1) Butoconazole 2% cream
      (2) Clotrimazole 100mg vaginal tablet
      (3) Miconazole 100mg vaginal suppository
      (4) Terconazole 0.4% cream

C. *Bacterial Vaginosis* *(most common cause of vulvovaginitis)*

1. Pathophysiology
   a. Previously thought to be caused by a single organism, it is now evident that multiple anaerobes are implicated in the pathogenesis of this vaginal infection.
   b. It is believed to result from changes in the vaginal microflora that foster the synergistic activity of the normal mixed flora and anaerobes which ultimately results in the predominance of the anaerobic organisms.

2. Clinical presentation: patients present with complaints of a fishy smelling discharge and mild itching.

3. Diagnosis—three of the following four criteria must be present:
   a. Homogeneous, grey-white, noninflammatory discharge that coats the vaginal <u>wall</u> rather than pooling on the vaginal floor.
   b. Positive amine odor test (fishy odor when KOH is added to a sample of the vaginal secretions)
   c. pH of vaginal secretions > 4.5
   d. "Clue cells" (vaginal epithelial cells covered with bacteria) on wet mount

4. Treatment:
   a. Metronidazole 500mg PO bid × 7 days
   b. Alternative regimens:
      (1) Clindamycin cream 2% intravaginally* Q HS × 7 days <u>or</u>
      (2) Metronidazole gel 0.75% intravaginally qd × 5 days <u>or</u>
      (3) Clindamycin 300mg PO bid × 7 days

5. Clinical importance — in pregnant patients, bacterial vaginosis is associated with an increased incidence of premature rupture of membranes, preterm labor, preterm birth and post-caesarean endometritis.

D. <u>**Genital Herpes Simplex**</u> **(a sexually transmitted disease)**

1. Is caused by the herpes simplex virus (HSV), a DNA virus; most ($\geq 80\%$) genital infections are caused by HSV-2; however, up to 20% of infections are caused by HSV-1.

2. Clinical presentation: patients with primary infection present with painful lesions, abdominal pain, fever, arthralgia, H/A and malaise. Dysuria is often present and can be severe enough to produce urinary retention. The symptoms begin 2 to 20 days following exposure and last up to 3 weeks in patients with a primary infection. Hepatitis, aseptic meningitis and autonomic dysfunction (bladder/bowel incontinence, loss of sensation in the sacral nerve distribution)...can also occur. Recurrent episodes are common but less severe; systemic symptoms are generally absent and the episodes are shorter in duration.

3. Diagnosis
   a. Physical exam
      (1) Characteristic lesions (grouped, fluid filled vesicles or ulcers on an erythematous base)
      (2) Tender inguinal lymphadenopathy
   b. Lab studies
      (1) Tzanck smear (scraping of an ulcer stained with Wright or Giemsa stain) reveals multinucleated giant cells; immunofluorescent staining for HSV is another option.
      (2) Positive culture
      (3) Positive ELISA
      (4) Positive direct immunofluorescent assay

*Oral metronidazole or clindamycin is the preferred treatment for pregnant women with bacterial vaginosis.

4. Treatment
   a. Acyclovir
      (1) Primary infections — are treated with 200mg 5 × per day × 7 - 10 days or until clinical resolution occurs. Acyclovir decreases viral shedding, accelerates healing and shortens the duration of symptoms, but does not affect the frequency or severity of recurrence.
      (2) Patients with frequent (> 6 per year) recurrences — benefit from daily suppressive therapy. The dose is 400mg PO bid. This regimen decreases the recurrence rate by 75%.
      (3) Patients with severe disease or those with complications requiring hospitalization are treated with IV acyclovir. The dose is 5 - 10mg/kg IV Q 8 hrs. for 2 -7 days or until clinical resolution occurs, then PO therapy to complete at least 10 days.
         [Note: IV acyclovir is recommended for pregnant women with severe herpes infection.]
      (4) Famciclovir or Valacyclovir are acceptable alternative antiviral medications.
   b. Analgesics, (topical viscous lidocaine and/or oral agents) as needed.
   c. Local soaks with Domeboro's solution.

5. Clinical importance
   a. HSV has been epidemiologically associated with both cervical cancer and cancer of the vulva.
   b. Genital herpes has been associated with an increased risk of acquiring HIV infections.
   c. C-section is indicated in term-pregnant patients with active genital herpes because of the high neonatal mortality rate (50 - 80%) and morbidity associated with contraction of neonatal herpes during vaginal delivery.

   Note: Further discussion of this topic can be found in the chapter on Dermatologic Emergencies in the section on herpes infections, pp. 1212 - 1214.

II. Cervicitis

A. Primary Pathogens: chlamydia, gonorrhea and/or trichomonas.

B. Usual Clinical Presentation: vaginal discharge and dysuria; may be asymptomatic.

C. Diagnosis

1. Vulvovaginal area is normal but the cervix is friable and inflamed with a purulent endocervical discharge.

2. Culture for GC and send a chlamydia prep.

3. On wet mount and gram stain, look for WBCs, trichomonads and GC; if only WBCs are seen, assume chlamydia.

D. Treatment

1. Trichomonal cervicitis is treated with metronidazole 2gms PO as a single dose <u>or</u> 500mg PO bid × 7days.

2. Gonococcal cervicitis is treated with:
   a. Ceftriaxone 125mg IM in a single dose <u>or</u>
   b. Cefixime 400mg PO in a single dose <u>or</u>
   c. Ciprofloxacin 500mg PO in a single dose <u>or</u>
   d. Ofloxacin 400mg PO in a single dose <u>or</u>
   e. Levofloxacin 500mg PO × 7days.
   <u>Note</u>: Because concurrent infection with Chlamydia trachomatis is common in these patients, a regimen effective against chlamydia (described below) should also be prescribed.

3. Chlamydial cervicitis should be suspected if the Gram stain reveals PMNs but no organisms. It is treated with:
   a. Azithromycin 1gm PO in a single dose (the preferred treatment) <u>or</u>
   b. Doxycycline 100mg PO bid × 7 days
   c. Alternative regimens include:
      (1) Ofloxacin 300mg PO bid × 7 days <u>or</u>
      (2) Erythromycin base 500mg PO qid × 7 days or amoxicillin 500mg PO tid × 7 days (recommended for pregnant women) <u>or</u>
      (3) Erythromycin ethylsuccinate 800mg PO qid × 7 days <u>or</u>
      (4) Levofloxacin 500mg PO × 7days.
   <u>Note</u>: Some of the above drugs are contraindicated in pregnant or lactating women and in children/adolescents:
      • Ciprofloxacin and Ofloxacin — are contraindicated during pregnancy and in patients ≤ 17 years old.
      • Doxycycline — is contraindicated in pregnant/lactating women and in children < 8 years old.
      • Erythromycin estolate — is contraindicated in pregnancy.

III. Miscellaneous Vulvovaginal Conditions

A. Contact Vulvovaginitis

1. Signs and symptoms: itching and irritation with erythema and edema but no discharge.

2. Work-up for an infectious etiology is negative.

3. Treatment
   a. Determine the cause (cosmetics, toiletries, laundry detergent) and eliminate it.
   b. Cool sitz baths and wet compresses of Domeboro's solution will suffice in mild-moderate cases; topical steroids are indicated for severe cases.

B. Vaginal Foreign Body

1. Children may insert any object; adults may forget tampons, pessaries, diaphragms or condoms.

2. Signs and symptoms: a foul-smelling and sometimes bloody discharge.

3. Remove the object, prescribe Betadine douche and arrange for follow-up.

4. Consider the possibility of sexual abuse when vaginal foreign bodies are found in prepubertal girls.

C. Bartholin's Abscess

1. A Bartholin's gland or duct cyst can become infected with various organisms (*E. coli, N. gonorrhea, chlamydia* or mixed anaerobes) → painful unilateral swelling of the posterior-lateral aspect of the vaginal opening. Pain is increased with sitting and walking; associated swelling and erythema of the labia majora is common.

2. Treatment
   a. Incision + drainage (on the mucosal aspect of the vestibule) followed by sitz baths
   b. Antibiotics if cellulitis is also present
   c. Word catheter placement for 1 - 2 weeks (to facilitate healing and re-epithelialization)
   d. Elective marsupialization

IV. Pelvic Inflammatory Disease (usually an STD)

A. Pathophysiology/Etiology

1. The most common cause is ascension from asymptomatic cervicitis.

2. Risk factors
   a. Multiple sexual partners
   b. Previous PID
   c. Adolescence
   d. IUD use (especially during the first few months of use)
   e. Instrumentation of the cervix or uterine cavity
   f. Recent menses
   g. Douching
   h. Cigarette smoking

3. Normal host barriers (uterotubal cervical mucus, lysozymes and local immunoglobulin IGA as well as the cervix itself) are usually very competent in preventing infection; menstruation is the most common cause of breakdown of these barriers. During pregnancy, fusion of the chorion and decidua forms another natural barrier; it obliterates the cavity between the cervix and the fallopian tubes, making PID during pregnancy an uncommon event.

4. Pathogenic organisms — *N. gonorrhea* and *chlamydia* are the major pathogens; together they account for approximately 80% of cases.
   a. Chlamydia (25% - 50% of cases)
      (1) The most common cause of PID in college students.
      (2) Is an obligate intracellular parasite that penetrates the submucosa and muscularis layers producing a more indolent infection than GC.
      (3) These infections may occur at any time in the menstrual cycle and have the greatest propensity for causing permanent tubal obstruction and infertility.
   b. *N. gonorrhea* (25% - 50% of cases)
      (1) The most common cause of PID in urban areas.
      (2) Is a gram-negative intracellular diplococcus.
      (3) Virulence is related to its ability to attach to tubal epithelial cells and infection is usually limited to the mucosal surface.
      (4) These infections generally develop shortly after the menses.
   c. Other pathogens include:
      (1) Anaerobic bacteria
      (2) Aerobic bacteria
      (3) Genital tract mycoplasmas

B. Classic Clinical Picture (only one-third of cases)

The patient is a sexually active young woman who complains of bilateral lower abdominal pain for several days (often following menses) associated with an abnormal vaginal discharge. Constitutional symptoms, i.e. fever > 100.4°, chills and general malaise are frequently present. Gastrointestinal complaints such as nausea and vomiting may also be present but are less common. On physical exam, there is lower abdominal tenderness, cervical motion tenderness and bilateral adnexal tenderness.

C. Clinical Caveats: unilateral lower abdominal and adnexal tenderness is probably not PID; bilateral lower abdominal and adnexal tenderness may be PID...or something else. Rule out the following in either case:

1. Ectopic pregnancy
2. Tubo-ovarian abscess
3. Adnexal torsion
4. Appendicitis

A beta-HCG and ultrasonography can help sort this out but direct visualization with laparoscopy is even better

D. Diagnostic Studies

1. Routine labs (CBC, sed rate) may be supportive but are nonspecific.
   a. Leukocytosis > 10,500/mm^3 supports the diagnosis but may not be present.
   b. The sed rate is elevated in most cases (>15mm/hr.)

2. Endocervical specimens should be obtained for:
   a. Gram stain (98% specific but only 67% sensitive for gram negative intracellular diplococci)
   b. GC culture
   c. Chlamydia prep

3. Measurement of beta-HCG — is useful in ruling out an ectopic.

4. Laparoscopy — is the most accurate way to diagnose PID. Although neither practical nor necessary for all cases, it should be considered for equivocal or refractory cases. It allows:
   a. Direct visualization and culture of the involved organs
   b. Exclusion of other diagnoses (appendicitis, diverticular disease)

5. Culdocentesis — is no longer a common procedure in the ED due to the widespread availability of ultrasonography. If performed, note the following:
   a. A dry tap is nondiagnostic; other diagnostic modalities must be used.
   b. The differential diagnosis at this point includes:
      (1) Ectopic pregnancy
      (2) Adnexal torsion
      (3) Appendicitis (Remember, this is RLQ, not adnexa)
      (4) PID
      (5) Ruptured ovarian cyst
   c. If a specimen of fluid is obtained, send it to the lab for a white count and bacterial determination.

E. Criteria for Diagnosing Acute PID

1. Minimal clinical criteria (all 3 must be present):
   a. Lower abdominal tenderness
   b. Adnexal tenderness (usually bilateral)
   c. Cervical motion tenderness

2. Additional criteria helpful in increasing the specificity of the diagnosis:
   a. Routine criteria:
      (1) Oral temperature > 101° (> 38.3°C)
      (2) Abnormal vaginal or cervical discharge
      (3) Elevated ESR or C-reactive protein
      (4) Lab evidence of cervical infection with GC or chlamydia
      (5) Leukocytosis > 10,500/mm^3
   b. Definitive criteria:
      (1) Confirmation of fluid-filled tubes (with or without free pelvic fluid) or a tubo-ovarian abscess on sonography

(2) Histopathologic confirmation of endometritis on endometrial biopsy

(3) Findings consistent with PID on laparoscopic exam

F.   Treatment (all regimens should cover GC, chlamydia, anaerobes, gram-negative rods and streptococci).

1.   Outpatient

a.   Ceftriaxone (Rocephin) 250mg IM or another parenteral third generation cephalosporin or Cefoxitin* 2gm IM with probenecid 1gm PO plus doxycycline 100mg PO bid × 14 days is the traditional therapy; single-dose therapy with azithromycin 1gm PO or levofloxacin 500mg PO is also acceptable.

b.   Another alternative regimen is ofloxacin 400mg PO bid × 14 days plus metronidazole 500mg PO bid × 14 days. This regimen provides better anaerobic coverage but does not cover incubating syphilis . . . and it's more expensive.

2.   Inpatient

a.   Indications for admission:

(1) Patient is toxic

(2) Presence of nausea and vomiting

(3) Failure to respond to outpatient therapy within 72 hours

(4) Suspicion of a tubo-ovarian or pelvic abscess (which may require surgery)

(5) Concurrent pregnancy

(6) Concurrent HIV infection

(7) Uncertain diagnosis (another surgical emergency cannot be ruled out)

(8) Young age (potential for future fertility issues)

(9) Timely clinical follow-up (within 72 hours of starting antibiotics) cannot be arranged.

b.   Drug therapy

(1) Cefoxitin 2gm IV Q 6hrs. or cefotetan 2gm IV Q 12hrs. plus doxycycline 100mg IV or PO bid. Patients are continued on this regimen for at least 24 hrs. after they show clinical improvement; following discharge, patients are continued on doxycycline 100mg PO bid for a total of 14 days.

(2) An alternative drug regimen is clindamycin 900mg IV Q 8 hrs. plus gentamicin — loading dose 2mg/kg IV followed by a maintenance dose of 1.5mg/kg IV Q 8 hrs. This regimen is continued for at least 24 hours after the patient shows signs of improvement. Following discharge, the patient should be continued on doxycycline 100mg PO bid or clindamycin 450mg PO qid for a total course of 14 days.

---

*Theoretical limitations in Cefoxitin's coverage of anaerobes may require the addition of metronidazole to the treatment regimen.

3. Newer outpatient/inpatient treatment regimens utilizing azithromycin and amoxacillin/clavulanic acid plus doxycycline are currently being evaluated for the treatment of PID. The 2002 STD guidelines reported by the CDC state the data are insufficient to recommend azithromycin or an oral regimen of amox/clav + doxy. However, IV therapy with amox/clav+ doxy is acceptable alternative therapy of inpatients. [Check guideline/manual link on website for updated guidelines in 2006]

G. Clinical Importance

1. PID is a significant cause of ectopic pregnancy, infertility and chronic pelvic pain.

2. Complications include:
    a. Formation of tubo-ovarian abscess
    b. Fitz-Hugh-Curtis syndrome (perihepatitis)
    c. Obstetrical complications
        (1) Intrauterine growth retardation
        (2) Septic abortion
        (3) Premature rupture of membranes/preterm delivery

3. Sexual partners should be evaluated and treated empirically to prevent reinfection (if they had sexual contact within 60 days of symptom onset).

V. Adnexal Torsion

A. Pathogenesis

1. An abnormal ovary or fallopian tube twists around its vascular pedicle → blood supply is compromised → painful anoxic degeneration of the ovary or fallopian tube occurs with eventual gangrenous necrosis.

2. Ovarian torsion usually occurs in association with an ovary that is en-larged due to a cyst or tumor or is overstimulated (ovarian hyperstimu-lation syndrome) by the use of fertility drugs; fallopian tube torsion usually occurs in association with hydrosalpinx, neoplasm, adhesions, trauma or previous ligation.

3. May occur at any age (although most are in the mid-twenties) and at any time during the menstrual cycle.

B. Clinical Differentiation from Pelvic Infections (PID, TOA)

1. <u>Vital signs</u>: absence of fever <u>or</u> tachycardia out of proportion to the fever.

2. <u>History</u>
   a. The onset of pain is usually sudden (frequently during or immediately after sexual intercourse); the patient may even remember the exact moment. Pelvic infections have a more gradual onset.
   b. The pain is usually unilateral (more commonly on the right), becomes increasingly severe but may subside and, if so, the patient may not appear to be acutely ill when you see her (not so with pelvic infections).
   c. Often there is a history of similar episodes in the past that resolved spontaneously.

3. <u>Pelvic exam</u>
   a. While cervical motion tenderness is present, unilateral adnexal tenderness is the rule (although bilateral adnexal tenderness does occur in some patients).
   b. A significant finding is a small discrete tender adnexal mass. (Inflammatory masses tend to be larger and less well-defined).

C. Diagnostic Studies

1. Routine labs are usually normal.

2. Culdocentesis: may yield a serosanguineous fluid (from hemorrhagic necrosis).

3. Ultrasound: may reveal the adnexal mass when the physical exam does not.

4. Laparoscopy: the definitive diagnostic procedure.

<u>Note</u>: Pregnancy testing should be done to R/O ectopic or concomitant intra-uterine pregnancy.

D. Treatment: surgical correction or resection is the definitive therapy of choice; however, laparoscopy alone is being used with increasing frequency since "untwisting" may be possible if torsion is diagnosed early or is caused by the ovarian hyperstimulation syndrome.

E. Consequences of a Missed or Late Diagnosis

1. Scarred tube → ↓ fertility and ↑ risk of tubal pregnancy

2. Ovarian necrosis → peritonitis and shock

VI. Abnormal Vaginal Bleeding (nonpregnancy-related)

A. *There are Multiple Etiologies:*

1. Alterations in the endocrine system secondary to:
   a. Ovarian tumors
   b. Corpus luteum cyst
   c. Menarche or menopause
   d. Excessive exercise
   e. Poor diet

2. Drugs
   a. The most common drugs implicated in "breakthrough" bleeding (that which occurs between periods) are:
      (1) Anticonvulsants (phenytoin, phenobarbital, carbamazepine, etc.)
      (2) Some antibiotics (penicillins, tetracyclines and TMP-SMX)
   b. Other pharmaceutical causes of abnormal bleeding are:
      (1) Anticoagulants
      (2) Exogenous estrogen or progesterone
      (3) Oral contraceptives (→ breakthrough <u>and</u> withdrawal bleeding)

3. Pelvic infections
   a. Vulvovaginitis
   b. Cervicitis
   c. Endometritis
   d. PID

4. Neoplasms (of both external and internal genitalia)
   a. Cervical polyps or carcinoma (bleeding often provoked by coitus)
   b. Leiomyomas (fibroids)
   c. Endometrial polyps or carcinoma
   d. Ovarian tumors

5. Postoperative (generally occurs when absorbable sutures dissolve)

6. Trauma
   a. Foreign bodies
   b. "Straddle" injury

7. IUDs

8. Medical problems
   a. Coagulopathies (especially von Willebrand's disease -- the most common hereditary disorder associated with menorrhagia)
   b. Thrombocytopenia
   c. Hypothyroidism
   d. Cirrhosis

9. Dysfunctional uterine bleeding

B. Responsibilities of the Emergency Physician:

1. R/O life-threatening hemorrhage by evaluating hemodynamic stability (orthostatic vital signs, Hb/Hct).

2. Stabilize patients with life-threatening bleeding (the minority) with IV fluids and blood products as needed.

3. Identify treatable causes through a careful H&P; important points are:
   a. Assume that any woman of childbearing age with abnormal vaginal bleeding is pregnant (intrauterine or ectopic) until proven otherwise; check a pregnancy test.
   b. Estimate the blood loss by determining the duration and amount of bleeding as well as the presence of clots (a history of heavy bleeding associated with clotting > 7 days indicates substantial blood loss).
   c. In addition to a pelvic exam, check other potential sites of bleeding which might be confused with vaginal bleeding (perineum and rectum); also, check for bladder tenderness and order a U/A if there is any question as to the source of the bleeding.

4. Order other appropriate lab work as indicated.

   Note: Iron-deficiency anemia suggests prior excessive bleeding in the absence of severe bleeding on physical exam; assessment of the hemoglobin level (plus microscopic examination of a peripheral smear) or a serum iron (ferritin) concentration is a clinically useful means of uncovering iron-deficiency anemia.

5. Management of cervical bleeding
   a. Mild - moderate → Monsel's solution or silver nitrate
   b. Severe (post-op or trauma-induced) → appropriate suturing

6. Refer to a gynecologist for a complete investigation (including an endometrial biopsy if the patient is > 35 years of age).

VII. Hemorrhagic Corpus Luteum Cyst

A. Etiology:

1. Corpus luteum of pregnancy persists up to eight weeks into the pregnancy.

2. Persistent corpus luteum in a nonconception cycle occurs for unknown reasons and causes amenorrhea until it degenerates; this is followed by heavy menstrual bleeding.

B. The Clinical Picture may be indistinguishable from a ruptured ectopic pregnancy. Sudden onset of lower abdominal pain in an amenorrheic patient or one in early pregnancy may be the only clue. The diagnosis is easier to make in the pregnant patient because the serum pregnancy test will be positive

and ultrasound will show intrauterine pregnancy. (The likelihood of a co-existing normal and ectopic pregnancy is exceedingly rare.) In the nonpregnant patient, a negative B-HCG and an adnexal mass coupled with a missed period or two can be easily interpreted as an ectopic; ultrasound will help sort this out. Laparoscopy is necessary for definitive diagnosis as well as to establish if cystic bleeding has stopped.

C. _Treatment_ is surgical (unless cystic bleeding has stopped and the patient is stable) and usually requires ovarian cystectomy.

VIII. Mittelschmerz

A. _Etiology_ — mittelschmerz is the pain that occurs in association with rupture of a follicular cyst and extrusion of an ovum from the ovary. The pain is believed to be due to follicular fluid irritation of the parovarian visceral peritoneum.

B. _It occurs_ at <u>midcycle</u> (on days 12 to 16 in women with 28 to 30-day cycles) after a normal menses.

C. _The pain_ is unilateral, varies in intensity, lasts from a few hours to a day and may be associated with slight vaginal spotting.

D. _Treatment_ is supportive with analgesics.

IX. Sexual Assault

A. _General Approach_

1. The purpose of this evaluation is to diagnose and treat the victim's physical and emotional injuries as well as to collect legal evidence.

2. Since the patient was a victim of a violent crime, she may feel fearful, helpless and guilty. For this reason, the interview and examination should be performed patiently in a quiet, private area and by the same doctor-nurse-counselor team from start to finish; offer to call the crisis counselor immediately to be with the patient during the interview and exam as well as arrange for follow-up care at a rape crisis center.

3. Explain all procedures and obtain consent for the physical exam, evidence collection, photographs and treatment.

4. Divide the history-taking into two segments: a standard medical history (to determine the need for medical evaluation and treatment) and a history of the assault (to correlate with the physical findings).

Document your findings carefully and completely. Diagnoses such as "rape" or "sexual assault" are considered legal conclusions rather than medical definitions; instead, use one of the following: "Reported Rape," "Rape by History," "History and Exam Consistent with Chief Complaint of Rape" or "Alleged Sexual Assault."

B. History of the Event

1. Where and when did the assault occur?

2. What happened during the assault? Use the patient's own words and then ask about the following:
   a. Number of assailants
   b. Use of force, weapons, objects or restraints
   c. Orifices penetrated and an impression of whether or not ejaculation occurred
   d. Use of alcohol or drugs

3. What happened after the assault?
   a. Did the patient bathe, void, defecate, brush teeth or change clothes?
   b. Does she complain of pain or have any other symptoms?

4. Has the patient had sexual intercourse in the last 72 hours? (If so, it may confuse the lab analysis of sperm and acid phosphatase).

5. Determine pregnancy risk
   a. When was the last menstrual period? (midcycle is high risk)
   b. Is the patient using any birth control method?

C. Physical Examination

1. Note the general appearance of the patient as well as her clothing.

2. Perform a general physical exam, noting especially any signs of trauma.

3. Perform a pelvic exam, looking for evidence of trauma or infection.

D. Laboratory and Evidence Collection

1. The following tests are medically indicated:
   a. Culture for GC
   b. Chlamydia prep
   c. Serology (VDRL or RPR)
   d. B-HCG (to R/O pre-existing pregnancy)
   e. X-rays as indicated
   f. Consider HIV and hepatitis B testing for all patients.
   g. Wet mount of the cervix and vagina to determine whether sperm or acid phosphatase are present and to look for evidence of *Trichomonas vaginalis* and bacterial vaginosis.

2. Evidence:
   a. Know what the police want before you examine the patient or use a standard kit that contains supplies for the collection of any or all of the following:
      (1) Debris from skin
      (2) Dried secretions on skin
      (3) Combed and plucked head and pubic hairs
      (4) Fingernail scrapings and clipped fingernails
      (5) Saliva sample
      (6) Oral, anal and vaginal smears (for sperm and acid phosphatase)
      (7) Blood sample
      (8) Nasal mucus sample
   b. Any of the above may be duplicated and sent to the hospital lab as your protocol dictates although the results will probably not be admissible as evidence.
   c. The emergency physician should personally collect and examine a wet mount for motile sperm. Sperm motility is a good sign of recent intercourse. If you wait for the pathologist to examine the specimen, sperm motility may be lost. Remember, however, that penetration (not ejaculation) is the hallmark of rape.
   d. Maintain an unbroken chain of evidence.
      (1) Specimens must always be in view or under lock and key.
      (2) Sign the outside of each sealed container when transferring custody.

E. Treatment

1. Traumatic injuries: standard care.

2. Infection prevention:
   a. Offer prophylactic antimicrobial therapy for syphilis, GC, chlamydia, trichomonas and bacterial vaginosis.
   b. Offer prophylactic therapy for Hepatitis B and HIV (Combivid 1 tab bid or Viracept 3 tabs tid; treat for one month)
   c. Schedule follow-up visits for repeat serology and cultures.

3. Pregnancy prevention: offer postcoital contraception (2 Ovral tablets PO stat and in 12 hrs.); refer for repeat pregnancy test prn.

4. Counseling: The initial contact should be made while the patient is in the ED by an individual experienced in rape counseling; if this is not possible, early referral is essential.

OBSTETRIC EMERGENCIES

I. Diagnosis of Pregnancy

ANY WOMAN OF CHILDBEARING AGE WHO PRESENTS TO THE ED IS PREGNANT UNTIL PROVEN OTHERWISE.

A. *Signs and symptoms*

1. Menstrual period: missed, light or late

2. Breast swelling and tenderness at 4 weeks

3. Fatigue, nausea and urinary frequency at 5 - 6 weeks

4. Cervical softening (tip at 4 weeks, isthmus at 6 - 8 weeks)

5. Chadwick's sign: (bluish discoloration of cervix at 6 - 8 weeks)

6. Uterus enlarged and soft at 6 - 8 weeks

B. *Pregnancy Tests*

1. All available tests detect human chorionic gonadotropin (HCG) with varying sensitivities and specificities. Production of HCG begins at the time of implantation (8 - 9 days post-conception). Levels of HCG double every 2 days during the initial weeks of a normal pregnancy, peak at 8 weeks and remain detectable up to 60 days postpartum or postabortion. With the newer assays, pregnancy can be detected as early as 23 - 25 days following the LMP. Pregnancy tests which measure the B-HCG subunit have the greatest specificity. Enzyme-linked immunoabsorbent assay (ELISA) is the standard assay. You need to be aware of the sensitivity and specificity of the pregnancy assay being used in your lab and the reference standard being employed (first, second or third international reference preparation) in order to be able to correctly interpret the test result you obtain.

2. Causes of false negatives
   a. Too early in pregnancy
   b. Dilute or old urine
   c. Ectopic pregnancy
   d. Incomplete abortion

3. Causes of false positives
   a. Urine tests only: gross hematuria or proteinuria
   b. Serum tests only
      (1) Tubo-ovarian abscess
      (2) Thyrotoxicosis
      (3) Molar pregnancy

(4) Drugs
    (a) Marijuana
    (b) ASA
    (c) Methadone
    (d) Methyldopa
    (e) Phenothiazines
    (f) Anticonvulsants
    (g) Antidepressants
    (h) Antiparkinsonian drugs

[Note: Urine ELISA testing (rather than serum testing) reduces the incidence of false positive and negative results since this assay is not affected by drugs or physiologic abnormalities.]

C. Physiologic Changes of Pregnancy

1. Cardiovascular changes
   a. Heart rate — increases by 15 to 20 beats/min. above baseline (to an average of 80 to 90 beats/min.) by the third trimester.
   b. Blood pressure
      (1) Systolic and diastolic blood pressure decrease by 10 to 15mmHg in the second trimester (to an average of 102/55) and then gradually return to prepregnant levels in the third trimester.
      (2) Following the 20th week of gestation, uterine compression of the inferior vena cava in the supine position can decrease venous return by as much as 30% and produce hypotension. This can be relieved by either placing the patient in the left lateral decubitus position, inserting a wedge under the right hip or manually displacing the uterus.
   c. Cardiac output — increases by ~30% during the first trimester, increases further (~50%) in the second trimester and is maintained at this level for the remainder of the pregnancy.

2. Respiratory changes
   a. Respiratory rate — increases slightly (or not at all)
   b. Tidal volume — increases by 40%
   c. Functional residual volume — decreases by 25% (due to elevation of the diaphragm)
   d. pCO_2 — decreases to 30 - 33mmHg

3. Hematologic changes
   a. Blood volume — increases up to 50% at term.
   b. Hct. — decreases to the low 30% range by the 30th week.
   c. WBC count — increases (due to an increase in PMNs); counts up to 18,000 are normal in the second and third trimesters while counts up to 25,000 may be seen during labor.
   d. ESR — is increased to 70 - 80mm/hr.
   e. Fibrinogen level is increased (average level is 400 to 450mg/dL).
   f. PT(INR)/PTT — are normal despite elevations in factors VII, VIII, IX, X and XII.

II. Drugs and Radiation Exposure in Pregnancy

A. Drugs

1. In an attorney's eyes, all drugs are harmful and, since we do not know about the adverse maternal/fetal effects of many of them, they should be used only when absolutely indicated for maternal or fetal health.

2. The teratogenic risk associated with drugs is greatest in the first trimester and is usually dose-related.

3. The FDA classification of drugs in pregnancy classifies drugs into five categories (A,B,C,D,X) according to their safety:
   a. Drugs in category A have been studied in humans and are considered safe for use in pregnancy.
   b. Drugs in category B have been studied in animals and are generally considered safe.
   c. Drugs in category C should be used with caution.
   d. Drugs in categories D and X should be avoided (if possible); studies have demonstrated use in pregnancy associated with risk to the fetus.

4. Drugs that are generally recognized as safe:
   a. Penicillins
   b. Cephalosporins
   c. Erythromycin (except the estolate)
   d. Azithromycin
   e. Aztreonam
   f. Spectinomycin
   g. Acetaminophen
   h. Narcotics (morphine, meperidine)
   i. Heparin
   j. Asthma drugs
      (1) Inhaled beta-adrenergic agents (especially terbutaline)
      (2) Steroids
      (3) Theophylline (a category C drug)
      (4) Inhaled anticholinergic agents
      (5) Cromolyn
   k. Antiemetics if dehydration or poor maternal nutrition is a threat; Reglan (metoclopramide) is the drug of choice (category B)* followed by trimethobenzamide, promethazine and prochlorperazine which are category C drugs.

5. Immunizations:
   a. Those derived from <u>killed</u> viruses (tetanus, diphtheria, hepatitis B, rabies) can be <u>safely</u> administered in pregnancy.
   b. Those derived from <u>live attenuated viruses</u> (measles, mumps, rubella, smallpox) are <u>contraindicated</u> in pregnancy.

---

*The newer class of antiemetics (5-HT$_3$ receptor antagonists) are still being evaluated for hyperemesis gravidarum. Benefits are: no sedation or extrapyramidal side effects; they can even be used effectively if the patient is on chemotherapy. Their general efficacy, however, is controversial. Zofran (ondansetron) is the prototype.

B. *Radiation Exposure*

1. The risk of birth defects from a 1-rad exposure (1000 mrads) is thousands of times smaller than the <u>spontaneous</u> risks of congenital malformations or genetic disease. If exposure to the fetus is < 5 - 10 rads, there is no significant increase in birth defects; also, coned radiographic beams aimed >10 cm away from the fetus are not harmful.
   a. The initial trauma series (plain films of C-spine, chest and pelvis) all deliver < 1 rad.
   b. CT scanning exposes the fetus to a higher level of radiation which can be reduced by shielding the uterus for part of the study. With shielding, fetal exposure from ....
      (1) Head and chest scans → < 1 rad
      (2) Abdominal scan (above the uterus) → < 3 rad
      (3) Pelvic scans (centered over the fetus) → < 3 - 9 rads
      Spiral scanning can reduce the dosage even further (up to 30%).
   c. MRI scanners do not use radiation, produce no birth defects, but are often not available on a 24 - hour basis.

2. Clinical guidelines
   a. Do not withhold necessary radiographic studies; shield the uterus and limit the scope of the exam when possible.
   b. If the patient is not sterilized (or is not using another reliable contraceptive method) postpone <u>elective</u> x-rays until a negative serum pregnancy test is obtained or until after the first ten days following a normal period.

III. Medical Complications of Pregnancy

A. *Nausea and Vomiting*

1. 50 - 70% of women are affected, usually in the first trimester (probably due to ↑HCG levels);[*] persistence of symptoms past 14 weeks or presence of abdominal pain suggests the possibility of another cause.

2. Treatment
   a. Frequent small meals (dry crackers before rising, toast and cereal when symptomatic) and supplemental Vitamin B_6 may be helpful.
   b. IV hydration (D_5LR or D_5NS) and antiemetics (second line treatment only) are indicated if hyperemesis gravidarum develops (starvation, dehydration, acidosis).
   c. Hospitalization is indicated if emesis cannot be controlled with the above measures.

---

[*]Some recent literature suggests that *H. Pylori* is a potential cause, since patients treated with erythromycin got better. However, erythromycin is a promotility agent ... so who knows? Also, some studies suggest a Vitamin B_6 deficiency as the cause and recommend supplemental B_6.

B. UTI and Pyelonephritis

1. Pregnant women are more prone to these infections (and their associated complications) than nonpregnant women. The increased susceptibility is related to the following physiologic changes which are induced by the gravid state:
   a. Increased mechanical pressure on the ureters and bladder by the uterus
   b. Poor emptying of the bladder with voiding
   c. Inhibition of ureteral peristalsis and dilatation by progesterone-induced smooth muscle relaxation

2. Both symptomatic and asymptomatic bacteriuria should be treated; untreated bacteriuria in pregnancy is associated with a 20 - 40% risk of progression to pyelonephritis.

3. Treatment
   a. Send urine for culture and place patients on a 7-day course of an antibiotic active against *E. coli*, *Proteus* and *Klebsiella*. Resistance rates have increased. The following commonly used antibiotics do eradicate bacteriuria in 70 - 80% of patients:
      (1) Cephalosporins
      (2) Nitrofurantoin (not effective against proteus)
      (3) Amoxicillin (drug of choice in third trimester) or amoxicillin-clavulanate
      (4) Sulfas (use should be restricted to the first + second trimesters)[*]
   b. Consider chlamydial vaginitis as the cause of the urinary tract symptoms if the bacteriuria proves to be culture negative; a single 1-gram dose of azithromycin is safe and effective.
   c. Admit pregnant patients with pyelonephritis to the hospital for IV antibiotics (a cephalosporin with or without an aminoglycoside) and hydration. These patients are at increased risk of developing pre-term labor and septic shock. Urine cultures should be sent and obstetric consultation should be obtained.

C. Thromboembolism

1. Pregnancy is a hypercoagulable state:
   a. The synthesis of coagulation factors VII, VIII, IX, X and XII is increased.
   b. Venous distensibility is increased.
   c. Compression of the inferior vena cava by the enlarging uterus promotes venous stasis.

2. The risk of thromboembolism is 5 - 6 times greater in pregnant women than nonpregnant women and is highest in the immediate postpartum period as well as those delivered by C-section.

---

[*]Sulfas given in the last few weeks of pregnancy may contribute to hyperbilirubinemia and kernicterus in the newborn.

3. Initial diagnostic studies of choice are:
    a. Doppler ultrasonography or impedance plethysmography — to R/O DVT (abnormal results should be confirmed with the patient on her left side)
    b. CXR (with shielding) — to R/O other pulmonary diseases when considering the diagnosis of PE*
    c. ABG — an alveolar-arterial (A-a) oxygen gradient >20 to 25mmHg is abnormal and suggestive of PE*
    d. Ventilation/perfusion scan — to R/O PE
    e. Spiral CT to R/O PE is safe in the 2nd and 3rd trimesters.

4. Treatment is with heparin (or LMWH) which do not cross the placenta.

D. Rubella Syndrome (cataracts, deafness, patent ductus arteriosus)

1. Order a pregnancy test in all women of childbearing age with rubella:

Time of maternal infection	Fetal infection
First month	50%
Second month	25%
Third month	10%

2. If the pregnancy test is positive, the patient should be referred for genetic counseling.

E. Intrahepatic Cholestasis of Pregnancy (Idiopathic Jaundice of Pregnancy, Pruritus Gravidarum)

1. Presents as mild jaundice (bilirubin < 5mg%) and pruritus in the third trimester.

2. Alkaline phosphatase is elevated 7 - 10 times normal and serum transaminase levels are normal or slightly elevated.

3. It is associated with an increased risk of premature delivery and fetal compromise.

4. Treatment
    a. Is on an outpatient basis if the diagnosis is clear.
    b. Pruritus is treated with cholestyramine resin (Questran) 10 - 12 grams/day.
    c. It resolves spontaneously with delivery.

5. Recurrence with subsequent pregnancies is not uncommon.

---

*When interpreting these studies, recall that: (1) the diaphragms are symmetrically elevated in late pregnancy; and (2) respiratory alkalosis with a slight increase in the A-a gradient is normal in pregnancy and due to progesterone-induced stimulation of the minute ventilation.

F. Herpes Simplex Infection*

1. Women with primary mucus membrane infections in the third trimester have an increased risk of dissemination...which may be life-threatening.

2. Neonatal infection can be contracted via passage through an infected birth canal and is associated with significant mortality (50%) and morbidity (particularly neurologic sequelae).

3. Active infection at the time of delivery carries a 30 - 40% risk of infecting the infant.

4. The presence of active lesions in a patient who is in labor is an indication for C-section.

G. Chronic Hypertension

1. BP is ≥ 140/90mmHg; it was identified prior to conception or prior to the 20th week of gestation and persists for > 6 weeks postpartum.

2. It can be exacerbated by pregnancy.

3. Treatment
   a. Bed rest
   b. Methyldopa
   c. Cardioselective beta blockers (atenolol, metoprolol)
   d. Labetalol
   e. Hydralazine
   Start with the simplest treatment first (a); if that doesn't work, try drug therapy (b), (c), (d) and (e) in that order.

4. Clinical importance — hypertension in pregnancy is associated with increased risk of superimposed pre-eclampsia, abruptio placentae, prematurity, intrauterine growth retardation and stillbirth.

H. Pre-eclampsia

1. Definition: elevation of the systolic or diastolic blood pressure that occurs after the 20th to 24th week of pregnancy in a previously normotensive or hypertensive woman; patients with a history of chronic hypertension are more prone to develop pre-eclampsia and eclampsia.

*Most (if not all) of the complications associated with lesions during pregnancy can be avoided by taking antiviral meds in the third trimester. Famciclovir and Valacyclovir are pregnancy category B.

2. Diagnosis	Mild	Severe
Elevated Blood Pressure	Systolic ≥ 140 or ≥ 20 above baseline; diastolic ≥ 90 or ≥ 10 above baseline	≥ 160/110
Proteinuria	0.3gm/24hrs.	> 5gms/24 hrs.
Edema (generalized)	Often but not always present	Present
Oliguria	Absent	Present
Associated Symptoms • Headache • Visual disturbances • Abdominal pain • Pulmonary edema or cyanosis	Absent	Present
Associated Lab Findings • Thrombocytopenia • ↑ Liver enzymes • ↑ Bilirubinemia • ↑ Serum creatinine	Absent	Present
• ↑ Uric acid	Usually Present	Present
Intrauterine Growth Retardation	Absent	Present

3. Predisposing factors
   a. Primiparity: > 60% of cases occur during the first pregnancy.
   b. Age: primigravidas at the extremes of age (< 17 or > 35 yrs. old) are at increased risk.
   c. Pregnancies associated with a large placenta (multiple pregnancies, hydatidiform mole, diabetes mellitus)
   d. History of chronic HTN or renal disease
   e. Family history of pre-eclampsia (mother, sister) or pregnancy-induced HTN

4. HELLP syndrome
   a. A very severe form of pre-eclampsia characterized by:
      (1) **H**emolysis
      (2) **EL**evated liver enzymes and
      (3) **L**ow **P**latelets (< 100,000/mm^3)
   b. It is associated with increased maternal mortality.
   c. Symptoms — may include any of those associated with simple pre-eclampsia; however, RUQ pain with nausea and vomiting are the most common.
   d. Signs — commonly include generalized edema, RUQ tenderness, jaundice, GI bleeding and hematuria.

5. Treatment
  a. If hypertension is the only finding:
    (1) Order a 24-hour urine for protein.
    (2) Encourage the patient to decrease her activity level and recommend home BP monitoring.
    (3) Refer the patient to an obstetrician for close follow-up in 2 to 3 days.
  b. If other findings are also present (especially proteinuria), hospitalization is indicated.
    (1) Order absolute bed rest with the patient lying on her left side.
    (2) Obtain a quantitative 24-hour urine for protein as well as renal function studies.
    (3) Observe for progression.
  c. Antihypertensive therapy is not required unless the systolic BP is > 170 or the diastolic BP is > 105; target pressure is 130 - 150 systolic and 90 - 100 diastolic.
    (1) Hydralazine is the drug most commonly used but others work well, too (diazoxide[*], labetalol, nifedipine and nitroprusside).
    (2) ACE inhibitors (all the "prils": captopril, enalapril, etc.) are contraindicated because of the possibility of fetal renal damage.
    (3) Prophylactic treatment with magnesium is also recommended to prevent seizures in the pre-eclamptic patient (loading dose of 4 - 6gms over thirty minutes followed by a 2 gm/hr. drip to maintain a serum level of 4 - 7 mEq/L).

I. Eclampsia (pre-eclampsia + grand mal seizures or coma)

1. Important facts
  a. Eclampsia may occur without prior proteinuria.
  b. Eclampsia can occur up to 10 days postpartum.
  c. Intracranial hemorrhage is the major cause of maternal death.

2. Warning signs of impending seizure
  a. Headache
  b. Visual disturbances
  c. Hyperreflexia
  d. Abdominal pain (epigastric or RUQ)

3. Definitive treatment is DELIVERY (obtain stat OB/GYN consult). Until that can be accomplished, give drug therapy. (Do not do a pelvic exam or transport the patient prior to drug therapy.)
  a. Magnesium sulfate
    (1) Has both antiepileptic and antihypertensive properties which usually controls seizure activity but may not be adequate for BP control; Valium and/or hydralazine may also be needed.
    (2) Loading dose is 4 - 6gm IV over 5 - 15 minutes; then continuous IV infusion at 1 - 3gm/hr; patient should be placed on a cardiac monitor and have a Foley in place.
    (3) Excretion is 100% renal so maintain the urine output at a rate > 25mL/hr.

[*]most commonly used

(4) Follow DTRs — Stop maintenance infusion if DTRs disappear.

(5) Watch for signs of magnesium toxicity:

    (a) Respiratory depression

    (b) Bradydysrhythmias

    (c) Loss of DTRs

(6) Antidote: calcium gluconate (1gm slow IVP)

b. Phenytoin (10mg/kg IV over 1 min.) or diazepam (5mg/min. IV Q 5 minutes prn up to 20 - 30mg) may be given for seizures resistant to magnesium therapy. If phenytoin is used, the potential for toxicity is reduced by giving this lower-than-normal loading dose since serum phenytoin levels tend to be higher in pregnant patients (due to hypo-albuminemia); diazepam can produce both maternal and fetal depression but is a good choice for prolonged seizures (or status epilepticus) resistant to magnesium therapy.

c. Hydralazine (Apresoline) — is indicated for the treatment of HTN associated with eclampsia that does <u>not</u> improve with administration of magnesium sulfate. Its use is generally restricted to patients who continue to have a diastolic BP > 110mmHg. Dose is 5 - 10mg IV slowly Q 20 minutes as needed to keep the diastolic BP between 90 and 100mmHg.

d. Labetalol — is also safe and effective in controlling HTN in eclamptic patients. It should be used when hydralazine is ineffective or unavailable. The initial dose is 20mg IV. . . and can be doubled every 10 minutes until BP control is achieved or 300mg has been given.

J. Rh Immunoprophylaxis

1. <u>Rh-negative mothers</u> who are carrying Rh positive babies and are exposed to any of the clinical events described below are at risk for developing Rh isoimmunization. This can negatively affect the outcome of both their current and subsequent pregnancies producing fetal anemia, fetal hydrops and fetal loss.

2. Events imposing a risk:

    a. Miscarriages

    b. Ectopics

    c. Term deliveries

    d. Trauma

    e. Placenta Previa

    f. Abruptio Placenta

    g. Vaginal bleeding of unknown etiology

3. To prevent this, check the type and Rh of all pregnant women with any risk factors and administer Rh immune Globulin (Rho-GAM) to those women who are <u>Rh-negative</u> and have not been sensitized in the past.

4. Dosing of MICRhoGAM

    (1) A mini-dose of 50mcg IM should be given for spontaneous abortions < 12 wks. gestation; > 12 wks. requires a standard dose of 300mcg IM, possibly more (see the Kleihauer-Betke test on p. 570).

    (2) It should be administered within 72 hours of the event.

K. Premature Rupture of Membranes (PROM) -- the leading cause of endometritis and puerperal sepsis

1. Definition: rupture of fetal membranes prior to onset of labor.

2. Diagnosis
    a. History of watery vaginal discharge in small or large amounts.
    b. Perform a careful <u>sterile</u> speculum exam without using a lubricant (which can give a false positive) and obtain sterile swabs of the posterior vaginal vault for:
        (1) A Nitrazine test — amniotic fluid is alkaline (blood and semen give false positives) and turns the yellow paper to blue-green.
        (2) Microscopic exam of a dried slide — amniotic fluid should show ferning (blood and inflammation give false negatives).
    c. Obtain cervical cultures for GC, chlamydia, Group B Strep, aerobes and anaerobes for patients with preterm (occurring before 37 weeks gestation) ROM. A digital exam should <u>not</u> be done in suspected or confirmed cases.

3. Treatment is hospitalization.
    a. If gestational age is > 37 weeks → delivery within 12 - 24 hours.
    b. If gestational age < 37 weeks → time of delivery depends on fetal lung maturity and development of infection (chorioamnionitis)

4. Clinical importance — these patients are subject to the development of chorioamnionitis.

L. Postpartum (Puerperal) Fever

1. Look for all usual causes of fever first:
    a. Wound infection (caesarean or episiotomy)
    b. UTI (especially if there is a Hx of catheterization or forceps delivery)
    c. Pneumonia
    d. Phlebitis

2. Endometritis
    a. Swollen tender uterus with foul lochia 1 - 3 days postpartum.
    b. Hospitalize for IV broad-spectrum antibiotics.
    c. Cultures demonstrate normal flora.

3. Pelvic thrombophlebitis
    a. May mimic endometritis so suspect this diagnosis if the patient does not respond quickly to antibiotics.
    b. Can cause pulmonary embolus.

M. Mastitis

1. Etiology
   a. Usually caused by *Staphylococcus aureus* (acquired from a contaminated nursery)
   b. Usually occurs as a complication of breast-feeding (but can occur antepartum and in non-breast-feeding postpartum women).
   c. The usual mode of transmission is inoculation of breast milk from the infant's nasopharyngeal secretions; cracked nipples can also be a route of entry for organisms.

2. Signs and symptoms
   a. Cellulitis involving one segment of a breast (initial infection)
   b. Abscess formation (may result if the initial infection is untreated)

3. Diagnostic criteria:
   • Painful swollen breast
   • Fever (often high)
   • No pus expressed from the nipple (unless there is an abscess close to it)
   • Gram stain of expressed milk often reveals Staph. aureus

4. Treatment
   a. Simple mastitis
      (1) Warm compresses and analgesics for symptomatic relief
      (2) Breast-feeding should be continued (as long as the bacteria is not antibiotic-resistant) because this assures continued drainage; the infant will not be harmed because he is already colonized.
      (3) Oral antibiotics (penicillinase resistant, i.e. dicloxacillin or a cephalosporin)
   b. Mastitis with abscess formation
      (1) Incision and drainage may be performed in the ED only if the abscess is small and superficial—Use a circumareolar incision or one following a line radiating out from the nipple and pack open; refer larger ones to a surgeon for drainage in the OR.
      (2) Continued drainage with a breast pump is indicated since higher concentrations of bacteria may be harmful to the infant; some authors recommend discontinuation of breast feeding until the infection has cleared.

IV. Surgical Complications of Pregnancy

A. Ectopic Pregnancy (EP)

1. Is the leading cause of maternal death in the first trimester and the second leading cause (overall) of maternal mortality.

2. Usually presents 5 to 8 weeks after the last normal menses.

3. Risk factors (~50% of EPs have no associated risk factors)
   a. High risk
      (1) Previous ectopic, tubal surgery or sterilization procedure
      (2) Documented tubal scarring/pathology
      (3) Diethylstilbestrol exposure in utero
      (4) Presence of IUD*
   b. Moderate risk
      (1) History of PID
      (2) Infertility (in-vitro)
      (3) Multiple sex partners
   c. Low risk
      (1) Previous pelvic/abdominal surgery
      (2) Cigarette smoking
      (3) Vaginal douching
      (4) Age of first intercourse < 18 yrs.

4. Clinical characteristics
   a. Patients classically present with a history of amenorrhea followed by abdominal pain and abnormal vaginal bleeding. However, this classic triad is present in only 15% of patients and is neither sensitive nor specific. The menstrual history may, in fact, be "normal" but pay attention to any subtle deviations from normal; the onset, character, location and intensity of the pain is quite variable and not particularly helpful; however, a clinical clue (if present) is shoulder pain referred from an irritated diaphragm (Kehr's sign).
   b. Pelvic exam findings
      (1) Vaginal bleeding (may be absent)
      (2) Unilateral adnexal tenderness ± a palpable mass
      (3) Uterus may be normal in size or slightly enlarged
      (4) Fullness of the cul-de-sac

*An IUD prevents only intrauterine (not extra-uterine) pregnancies

The following tables may help you remember (and rank) the signs and symptoms of an ectopic pregnancy:

Symptoms	% of women with symptoms
Abdominal Pain	80 - 100%
Amenorrhea	75 - 95%
Vaginal Bleeding	50 - 80%
Dizziness	20 - 35%
Pregnancy Symptoms	10 - 25%
Urge to Defecate	5 - 15%
Passing Tissue	5 - 10%

Signs	% of women with signs
Adnexal Tenderness	75 - 95%
Abdominal Tenderness	80 - 95%
Adnexal Mass	50%
Uterine Enlargement	20 - 30%
Orthostatic Changes	10 - 15%
Fever	5 - 10%

5. Differential diagnosis
    a. PID
    b. Appendicitis
    c. Adnexal torsion
    d. Dysfunctional uterine bleeding
    e. Corpus luteum cyst
    f. Spontaneous abortion (complete or incomplete)
    g. Mittelschmerz

6. Diagnostic studies
    a. Pregnancy tests: trust only the most sensitive (B-HCG radio-immuno-assay) to R/O this diagnosis; the value of progesterone levels has yet to be clarified.

b. Pelvic ultrasound
  (1) Is most useful in establishing a diagnosis in patients who present ≥ 5 weeks following their LMP; a gestation sac is <u>not</u> visible prior to this time.
  (2) Transabdominal sonography (TAS) is most useful in ruling out the presence of an intrauterine pregnancy (IUP). Visualization of a yolk sac (within the gestational sac) or a "double ring" sign is one of the earliest findings confirming an IUP.
  (3) Transvaginal sonography is an extremely sensitive technique; it can identify landmarks consistent with a normal IUP at 5 wks. of gestation and may <u>occasionally</u> identify the actual ectopic.

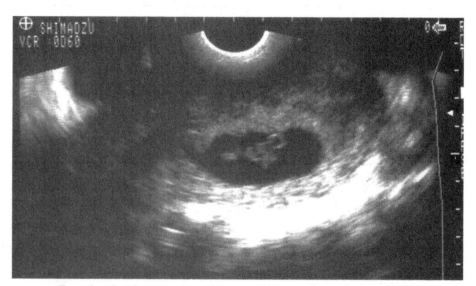

(Reproduced with permission of Dr. Chris DiOrio, Asst. Professor. Dept. of EM, University of South Carolina, Palmetto Health Alliance, Columbia, SC)

c. Serial quantitative HCGs — In patients with an empty uterus on US and a positive qualitative HCG, quantitative HCG levels can be useful in clarifying the diagnosis and determining management.
  (1) A quantitative HCG > 6000-6500mIU/ml + an empty uterus on transabdominal ultrasound <u>or</u> a quantitative HCG >1200 - 1500 mIU/ml + an empty uterus on transvaginal ultrasound = ectopic pregnancy → laparoscopy
  (2) Stable patients with a quantitative HCG < 6000 - 6500mIU/ml + empty uterus on transabdominal ultrasound <u>or</u> a quantitative HCG < 1500mIU/ml + an empty uterus on transvaginal ultrasound can be followed with serial quantitative HCGs every two days as outpatients to see if the HCG levels increase in a normal fashion; it should double every two days with a normal IUP. This type of management should be undertaken in consultation with an OB/GYN consultant and should be restricted to patients who are stable and reliable. If HCG levels fall → D&C → if no villi are found → pregnancy is assumed to be ectopic → laparoscopy.

    d. Culdocentesis
       (1) Should be considered for the unstable patient and in situations where ultrasonography is not available in a timely fashion.
       (2) Aspiration of nonclotting blood (a "positive" culdocentesis) is an indication for surgery.
       (3) A dry tap does NOT rule out the diagnosis.

  7. Treatment
    a. Establish an IV and provide fluid resuscitation prn.
    b. Draw blood for lab work (CBC, Rh typing as well as type + screen/ crossmatch) early on in suspected cases.
    c. Administer Rh immune globulin (MICRhoGAM) to women who are Rh-negative.
    d. Definitive therapy
       (1) Stable patients with unruptured EPs measuring < 4cm by ultrasound are eligible for methotrexate therapy.
       (2) Stable patients with unruptured (or minimally ruptured) EPs measuring > 4cm by US → laparoscopic salpingectomy.
       (3) Unstable patients (or those in whom a laparoscopic approach is difficult) → laparotomy.

B. *Vaginal bleeding in pregnancy*

  1. First trimester bleeding
    a. Prior to 12 weeks, vaginal bleeding is due to one of the following:
       (1) Nonpregnancy-related conditions
          (a) Infections
          (b) Trauma
          (c) Neoplasms
       (2) Ectopic pregnancy
       (3) Abortion
       (4) Molar pregnancy
    b. <u>Threatened abortion</u>…is the most common cause of bleeding in a primigravida.
       (1) Definition: any amount of bleeding without passage of products of conception or cervical dilatation.
       (2) Incidence: 30 - 40% of clinically pregnant women have first trimester bleeding; 50% of these women ultimately miscarry.
       (3) Treatment
          (a) Bedrest for 24 hours
          (b) No douching, tampons or intercourse until bleeding resolves
          (c) Rh immune globulin (MICRhoGAM) for Rh-negative women
          (d) Follow-up with obstetrician in 2 to 3 days
    c. <u>Inevitable abortion</u>
       (1) Definition: the cervical os is open and vaginal bleeding is present.
       (2) Treatment: D&C; MICRhoGAM for Rh-negative women.

d. Incomplete abortion
  (1) Definition: the cervical os is open, vaginal bleeding is present and products of conception are present at the cervical os or in the vaginal canal.
  (2) Treatment:
    (a) Visible products of conception should be removed with a ring forceps to control bleeding.
    (b) D&C; MICRhoGAM for Rh-negative women.
e. Complete abortion
  (1) Definition: all products of conception have been passed, the cervix is closed, the uterus is firm and nontender and the bleeding has almost stopped.
  (2) Treatment: D&C (unless the patient has brought in all material she has passed which, upon inspection, appears to be all products of conception or complete expulsion has been confirmed by US); MICRhoGAM for Rh-negative women.
f. Missed abortion
  (1) Definition: failure to pass products of conception beyond two months after fetal death; pregnancy test converts from positive to negative.
  (2) Treatment: D&C; MICRhoGAM for Rh-negative women.

2. Late first trimester or second trimester bleeding → Molar Pregnancy
  a. Signs and symptoms
    (1) Abdominal pain with severe nausea and vomiting (HCG levels higher than normal)
    (2) Pre-eclampsia before 24 weeks
    (3) Vaginal passage of characteristic grape-like clusters of vesicles
    (4) Uterus large for dates
    (5) Anemia
  b. Diagnosis: ultrasound (findings are typically described as a "snow-storm" appearance) or discovery of molar tissue.
  c. Treatment: D&C plus careful follow-up of HCG titers to R/O chorionic carcinoma; MICRhoGAM for Rh-negative women.

3. Second trimester bleeding
  a. Vaginal bleeding in the second trimester is due to:
    (1) Nonpregnancy related conditions (infection, trauma, neoplasm) or
    (2) Abortion
  b. If abortion was the cause of bleeding, treatment depends on the type of abortion:
    (1) A threatened AB is treated the same as in the first trimester.
    (2) If an inevitable, incomplete or missed abortion occurs, evacuation of the uterus is usually done by oxytocin-induced labor in the hospital.
    (3) Following a complete abortion, the treatment is D&C unless the patient has brought in all products of conception.
    (4) MICRhoGAM should be administered to those women who are Rh-negative.

4. Third trimester bleeding (after 28 weeks gestation)
   a. <u>Placenta previa</u> is responsible for 20% of cases of third trimester bleeding.
      (1) Definition: implantation of the placenta in the lower uterine segment such that it covers all or part of the cervical os.
      (2) Clinical presentation: <u>painless bright red vaginal bleeding</u> that is sometimes intermittent and progressively severe over a period of 1 - 2 weeks; on abdominal exam, the uterus is usually soft and nontender.
      (3) Risk factors:
         (a) Prior C-section
         (b) Grand multiparity
         (c) Previous placenta previa
         (d) Multiple gestations
         (e) Multiple induced abortions
         (f) Maternal age > 40
      (4) Management guidelines
         (a) Establish IV access, draw blood for type and crossmatch and preop labs; establish cardiac and fetal monitoring.
         (b) Call OB/GYN consultant immediately if patient is unstable and order ultrasound for placental location.
         (c) Pelvic exam (digital and speculum)
            <u>1</u> Should <u>not</u> be done unless ultrasound rules out placenta previa — A diagnostic ultrasound is followed by C-section.
            <u>2</u> Should be done in OR by the obstetrician under "double setup" conditions in patients who are bleeding rapidly, in labor or are hemodynamically unstable. In this manner, an immediate C-section can be rapidly performed if uncontrolled bleeding results.
         (d) Administer MICRhoGAM to Rh-negative women.
   b. <u>Abruptio placenta</u> — 30% of cases of third trimester bleeding.
      (1) Definition: premature separation of a normally implanted placenta from the uterine wall causing visible or hidden bleeding. Significant unseen blood loss can occur before or without vaginal bleeding.
      (2) Clinical characteristics
         (a) <u>Painful uterine bleeding</u>
            <u>1</u> Bleeding is typically light (but may be heavy) and is usually dark or clotted.
            <u>2</u> At times, only pain is present and this can vary from mild to severe.
         (b) Uterine findings vary from soft and nontender to slightly tender to rock hard.
      (3) Severity of placental separation
         (a) <u>Grade 0 or 1</u> (up to 40% cases): slight bleeding, little or no uterine irritability; no fetal distress or coagulation factor consumption.

        (b) <u>Grade II</u> (45% of cases): moderate vaginal bleeding or hidden maternal blood loss, increased uterine irritability, fetal distress and coagulation changes.

        (c) <u>Grade III</u> (~15% of cases): uterine tetanic contractions, hypotension, coagulopathy and increased possibility of fetal death.

    (4) Risk factors

        (a) HTN (most common)

        (b) Smoking, chronic alcohol consumption

        (c) Cocaine use

        (d) Multiparity

        (e) Increased maternal age

        (f) Previous abruptio placentae

        (g) Abdominal trauma

    (5) Treatment

        (a) Establish IV access, draw blood for type and crossmatch, preop labs and a DIC profile; establish cardiac and fetal monitoring.

        (b) Fluid resuscitation and blood replacement as needed.

        (c) Obtain immediate OB/GYN consultation and perform ultrasound to R/O placenta previa (ultrasound is <u>not</u> useful in diagnosing abruptio placenta).

        (d) Stable patients may be observed in the hospital with close surveillance if a surgical team is available.

        (e) If the patient is unstable → immediate delivery by C-section (unless patient is in advanced labor); place the patient in the left lateral decubitus position to relieve inferior vena caval compression (can increase cardiac output by 30 - 40%).

        (f) Administer MICRhoGAM to Rh-negative mothers.

  c. <u>Uterine rupture</u>

    (1) Causes in an unscarred uterus:

        (a) Oxytocin stimulation

        (b) Cephalopelvic disproportion

        (c) Grand multiparity

        (d) Placenta percreta (abnormal adherence of the placenta to the uterine wall with invasion of the myometrium all the way to its peritoneal covering)

        (e) Blunt abdominal trauma

    (2) Causes in a scarred uterus:

        (a) Previous hysterotomy, myomectomy, C-section or curettage

        (b) Manual removal of placenta

5. Postpartum hemorrhage

  a. Immediate postpartum hemorrhage

    (1) Definition: blood loss > 250mL immediately after delivery or > 500mL within the first 24 hours after delivery.

    (2) Causes include:

        (a) Uterine atony (most common cause)

        (b) Retained placental tissue

        (c) Genital tract trauma (lacerations, uterine rupture, inversion)

    (3) Pelvic exam

        (a) Palpate for a large, soft, atonic uterus.

        (b) Manually locate and remove placenta if it does not pass.

        (c) Look for and treat lacerations (pack or repair) and inversion.

    (4) Treatment for uterine atony

        (a) Bimanual massage (one hand on abdomen, one in vagina). If uterine contractions are not induced, suspect uterine rupture.

        (b) IV oxytocin (Pitocin); add 10 - 40 units to a liter of IV fluid; run at a rate sufficient to control uterine atony (~10mL/min.)

        (c) Methylprostaglandin F_2 alpha 0.25mg IM (or methylergonovine 0.2mg IM) if bleeding persists despite above measures.

  b. Delayed postpartum hemorrhage

    (1) Definition: hemorrhage occurring <u>more</u> than 24 hours after delivery (most often 1 - 2 wks. postpartum).

    (2) Causes include:

        (a) Retained placental tissue (confirm with ultrasound)

        (b) Endometritis

    (3) Treatment

        (a) Control bleeding with oxytocin or methylergonovine.

        (b) Start antibiotics on patients with evidence of endometritis (fever, purulent discharge and/or uterine tenderness)

C. Appendicitis in Pregnancy

1. This is the most frequent surgical emergency of pregnancy.

2. Incidence of appendicitis is not higher in pregnancy but the development of complications (especially rupture) occurs more frequently in the pregnant patient because of delay in diagnosis.

3. After the first trimester, the diagnosis can be elusive because the normal leukocytosis of pregnancy frequently does not elevate further and the pain location changes (may gradually move up to the right flank or RUQ).

4. In the third trimester, appendicitis is most frequently misdiagnosed as pyelonephritis because the appendix occupies a position in close proximity to the right kidney at this point in pregnancy, and can thereby produce right flank pain and pyuria (without bacteriuria).

  a. <u>High fever</u>, chills, <u>bacteriuria</u> and pyuria must all be present before the diagnosis of pyelonephritis is certain.

  b. If "pyelonephritis" has not improved with IV antibiotics in 24 hours and the patient is not afebrile in 48 hours, reconsider the diagnosis ...it may be appendicitis.

5. While ultrasonography can be helpful in ruling out other diagnoses, laparoscopy or laparotomy is the preferred diagnostic procedure.

D. Abdominal Trauma in Pregnancy

1. Important point to consider: you have <u>two</u> patients and maternal circulation will be maintained at the expense of the fetus; trauma-induced maternal shock carries with it a fetal mortality rate of almost 80%; during the initial evaluation, concentrate on the clinical status of the mother because fetal survival depends wholly on maternal integrity.

2. The patient should be kept on her left side at all times (except during the abdominal exam) to avoid a supine hypotensive syndrome caused by pressure of the gravid uterus on the inferior vena cava which reduces venous return; cardiac output can be augmented 30 - 40% by placing the patient in the left lateral decubitus position.

3. Ringer's lactate should be used for fluid resuscitation.

4. Factors contributing to the difficulty of evaluation:
   a. Due to the physiologic anemia of pregnancy (↑in plasma vol. > ↑in RBC vol.), the normal hematocrit in late pregnancy is 31 - 35%.
   b. Due to the increased plasma volume associated with pregnancy (40 - 50% increase compared with the nonpregnant state), a pregnant patient can lose 30 - 35% of her blood volume before demonstrating the usual signs of hypovolemic shock.
   c. The BP is decreased in the second trimester (usually < 125/75); however, a systolic BP < 80 is always abnormal.
   d. The WBC is elevated in the second and third trimesters (as high as 18,000).
   e. Abdominal findings are altered by the presence of an enlarged uterus.

5. All pregnant women (> 20 weeks gestation) who sustain abdominal trauma should undergo a minimum of 4 hours of cardiotocographic monitoring once their vital signs have been stabilized. Signs of fetal distress include:
   a. Fetal bradycardia or tachycardia
   b. Late decelerations (bradycardia following a contraction)
   c. Loss of fetal beat-to-beat variability

6. Abdominal trauma during pregnancy results in fetomaternal hemorrhage in up to 30% of patients. In an Rh-negative woman carrying an Rh-positive fetus, this can result in isoimmunization if it is undetected and untreated. Thus, all Rh-negative women who sustain abdominal trauma during pregnancy should receive MICRhoGAM. Although the standard dose of 300mcg is sufficient in most cases of gestation > 12 weeks, the Kleihauer-Betke test can be helpful in quantifying the exact dose of MICRhoGAM to be given.

7. The Kleihauer-Betke test
   a. Should be used in pregnant women who have sustained abdominal trauma to detect and quantify the amount of fetomaternal hemorrhage (FMH) that has occurred. This information is useful in determining the amount of MICRhoGAM to administer since FMH > 30mL requires more than the standard dose.

     b. It is only used in women who are at least 12 weeks pregnant since the fetal volume of blood up until this point is < 30mL and, therefore, is covered by the standard dose of MICRhoGAM.

     c. It is only useful when it is positive; a negative test does not R/O a small FMH capable of sensitizing an Rh-negative mother.

8. Abruptio placenta is the number one cause of fetal death following blunt trauma.

9. In the evaluation of abdominal trauma in the pregnant patient, <u>culdocentesis can be substituted for peritoneal lavage</u>. (This is an important point because pregnancy is a relative contraindication for peritoneal lavage.)

10. Admission criteria include any of the following:
     a. Significant blunt abdominal trauma in a stable patient carrying a fetus > 20 weeks gestation
     b. Vaginal bleeding
     c. Uterine irritability
     d. Persistent abdominal pain, cramping or tenderness
     e. Evidence of maternal hypovolemia
     f. Fetal heart tones < 120 or >160
     g. Presence of late decelerations
     h. Amniotic fluid leak
     i. Abnormal uterine sonogram, i.e. evidence of fetal injury or a suspicious retroplacental structure (? hematoma)

11. Postmortem C-section and fetal survival — a reasonably good chance if gestational age is > 28 weeks (fetal wt. 1000 gms.) and the interval between maternal death and delivery is < 15 minutes.

V. Complicated Deliveries

A. Dystocia (difficult labor)

1. Types of dystocia
     a. Pelvic: abnormalities of the bony pelvis which affect the presenting fetal part.
     b. Uterine
       (1) Ineffective contractions (hypertonic)
       (2) Maternal inability to assist expulsion
     c. Fetal
       (1) Malpresentation (most common cause of fetal dystocia)
       (2) Multiple gestations
       (3) Large fetal size (secondary to gestational diabetes)
       (4) Congenital anomalies

2. Treatment
   a. Pelvic dystocia → C-section
   b. Uterine dystocia → Tx is based on the nature of the contractions:
      (1) Hypotonic → oxytocin drip
      (2) Hypertonic → Tocolysis
   c. Fetal dystocia → fetal manipulation

   — Maneuvers for shoulder dystocia (head is already delivered) —
   • Flex the mothers legs over her abdomen → rotates the pubic symphysis upward → allows greater exposure of posterior shoulder (McRobert's maneuver) <u>or</u>
   • Rotate fetus into an oblique position + apply suprapubic pressure <u>or</u>
   • Apply suprapubic pressure + gentle downward pressure on the fetal head <u>or</u>
   • Reach into the vaginal canal and gently extract the posterior arm and shoulder -- do not force this!

B. Prolapsed Cord

1. Types of umbilical cord prolapse
   a. Overt: cord lies below the presenting part and can be visualized or palpated
   b. Occult: cord lies adjacent to the presenting part and can be detected by fetal monitoring (FHR changes with intermittent cord compression).

2. Causes of umbilical cord prolapse
   a. Abnormal presentations (especially transverse)
   b. Cephalopelvic disproportion
   c. Multiple gestations
   d. Placenta previa
   e. Prematurity
   f. PROM

3. Management
   a. O_2 administration
   b. Reposition the mother
      (1) Overt cord prolapse → knee to chest position (apply continuous upward pressure on the presenting part to relieve pressure on the cord until the fetus is delivered by C-section)
      (2) Occult cord prolapse → lateral (or Trendelenburg) position:
         (a) If FHR returns to normal with cord compression → vaginal delivery
         (b) Persistence of FHR changes with cord compression → C-section

C. Uterine Inversion

1. Traction on the umbilical cord during delivery can result in partial or complete uterine inversion.

2. Physical exam findings
   a. Partial inversion → crater-like depression over the suprapubic area + descended uterine fundus and cervix on vaginal exam.
   b. Complete inversion → uterus is outside the body and is associated with immediate life-threatening hemorrhage.

3. Management
   a. Immediate anesthesiology (and OB) consult
   b. Two large-bore IV lines with Ringer's lactate run wide-open
   c. Type + crossmatch for 6 - 8 units of blood
   d. Tocolytic drugs (Terbutaline, Ritrodine, $MgSO_4$) to relax the uterus so that manual reimplantation can be achieved
   e. Try to reimplant the uterus <u>without removing the placenta</u> (↑risk of hemorrhage). If this fails, do not proceed further until:
      (1) IVs are secured and running well
      (2) Blood is available
      (3) Anesthesia is being administered to the patient
   f. Gently separate the placenta from the uterus. Then place your hand on top of the fundus with fingers extended (so they touch the border of the cervix) and apply pressure to the fundus (along the axis of the vagina) to push the fundus back through the cervix [remember, the uterus is "inside-out:" it inverted through the cervix and can only be reimplanted by pushing it back again through the cervix]. If manual reimplantation fails, emergency laparotomy is indicated.
   g. Upon completion of successful reimplantation:
      (1) D/C tocolytic therapy
      (2) Initiate oxytocin therapy (while manually maintaining the uterus in position so it does not "re-invert")
      (3) Administer broad-spectrum antibiotics

D. Multiple Births

1. Be suspicious of multiple gestations if the mother...
   a. Used "fertility drugs" prior to pregnancy <u>or</u>
   b. Gained more weight than she expected <u>or</u>
   c. Noticed more fetal movement recently

2. If the uterus is larger than normal for dates (and the history is suspicious) order an ultrasound to confirm the diagnosis.

3. Anticipate potential complications
   a. Spontaneous abortion
   b. Premature... rupture of membranes, labor, infant
   c. Placenta previa
   d. Abnormal presentation
   e. Postpartum uterine atony
   f. Resuscitation of multiple babies

E. Still Birth

1. Maternal risk factors (e.g. excessive obesity, advanced age, illness, drug abuse) have been associated with stillbirth.

2. Causes include:
   a. Congenital anomalies/polyhydramnios
   b. Placenta previa/abruptio
   c. Multiple gestations/breech presentations

F. Emergency Perimortem C-section and Fetal Survival

1. If the fetus is delivered within 5 minutes of maternal cardiac arrest (unassociated with prolonged hypoxia prior to arrest) and gestational age is > 28 weeks → fetal survival is excellent.

2. If the fetus is delivered > 15 minutes after maternal cardiac arrest → fetal survival is poor.

UROLOGIC EMERGENCIES

I. **Acute Renal Failure (ARF)**

A. *Pathophysiology and Causes of ARF According to the Type of Azotemia*

1. Prerenal azotemia
    a. Occurs when normal kidneys are <u>hypo</u>perfused.
        (1) These patients are oliguric (urine volume < 400mL/m²/day).
        (2) In response to volume depletion, the kidney avidly reabsorbs water and salt, producing a concentrated urine (SG 1.020 to 1.030) and a low urine sodium concentration (< 20mEq/L).
        (3) Since renal parenchymal damage is absent, microscopic urinalysis is usually normal with only occasional hyaline casts.
    b. Causes
        (1) Hypovolemia (most common cause)
            (a) Vomiting and diarrhea
            (b) Blood loss of any kind
            (c) Diuretics
            (d) Skin losses (burns)
        (2) Decreased effective blood volume
            (a) Sepsis
            (b) Anaphylaxis
            (c) Third space sequestration (pancreatitis, peritonitis, ischemic bowel)
            (d) Hypo-albuminemic states (cirrhosis, nephrosis)
            (e) Prostaglandin-inhibiting drugs (NSAIDs)
            (f) ACE (angiotensin-converting enzyme) inhibitors
            (g) Decreased cardiac output
                <u>1</u> CHF/pulmonary edema
                <u>2</u> MI
                <u>3</u> Dysrhythmias
                <u>4</u> Tamponade

2. Postrenal azotemia
    a. Occurs when there is obstruction of urine flow at any point from the renal collecting system to the urethra.
        (1) Urine flow rate varies from anuria (with complete obstruction) to normal urine output (with partial obstruction).
        (2) To produce acute renal failure, ureteral obstruction must be bilateral or occur in a patient who has only one functioning kidney.
        (3) Since the renal parenchyma is <u>not</u> affected, microscopic urinalysis may be normal.

---

b. Causes
   (1) Ureteral obstruction
      (a) Stones
      (b) Blood clots
      (c) Sloughed papillae
      (d) Malignancies (intrinsic or extrinsic)
      (e) Iatrogenic (e.g., ligation of ureter during surgery)
   (2) Bladder obstruction
      (a) Enlarged prostate (benign prostatic hypertrophy or malignancy) -- most frequent cause
      (b) Carcinoma of the bladder
      (c) Clot retention
      (d) Neurogenic bladder due to drugs, diabetes or spinal cord injury -- another common cause
   (3) Urethral obstruction
      (a) Strictures
      (b) Phimosis ⎤
                   ⎬ uncommon causes of azotemia
      (c) Meatal stenosis ⎦
      (d) Posterior urethral valves (a common cause in kids)

3. Renal azotemia
   a. Occurs when there is pathology of the kidney or renal tubule
      (1) Signs and symptoms (including urine flow) depend on the site and nature of the disorder.
      (2) In these patients, the renal tubules lose their ability to concentrate and reabsorb sodium; therefore, their urine is dilute (SG 1.010) and the urine sodium concentration is elevated (> 40mEq/L).
      (3) Since the kidney itself is affected, the urine sediment will be abnormal, and the exact findings will vary with the underlying cause of the renal failure:
         (a) Acute tubular necrosis (ATN): renal tubular casts + muddy brown granular casts.
         (b) Acute interstitial nephritis (AIN): eosinophilia, granular and white cell casts.
         (c) Acute glomerulonephritis: RBCs, RBC casts and proteinuria.
   b. Causes of renal azotemia
      (1) Acute tubular necrosis (ATN) is responsible for 90% of cases.
         (a) Ischemia (most common cause of ATN)
            1 Prolonged hypoperfusion
            2 Hemorrhage
         (b) Nephrotoxins
            1 Aminoglycosides
            2 Heavy metals
            3 Contrast
         (c) Pigments
            1 Hemoglobin
            2 Myoglobin

(2) Vascular disease
  (a) Vasoconstrictive disease (malignant HTN, TTP)
  (b) Vasculitis
(3) Thrombosis (renal artery/vein)
(4) Acute interstitial nephritis
  (a) Drug-related (PCN, cephalosporins, sulfonamides, NSAIDs, diuretics, allopurinol, cimetidine); methicillin is the most commonly implicated drug.
  (b) Infection-related (bacterial, protozoan, fungal)
  (c) Immune-related (lupus, leukemia, lymphoma, sarcoidosis)
(5) Glomerular disease
  (a) Postinfectious
  (b) Noninfectious

B. Diagnosis of Renal Failure According to Type of Azotemia

1. The history and physical exam should suggest the type of azotemia you are dealing with:
   a. Signs and symptoms of hypoperfusion → prerenal azotemia
   b. Signs and symptoms of obstruction → postrenal azotemia
   c. History of a primary disorder that can cause renal disease or a Hx of exposure to a contrast material, drug or heavy metal → renal azotemia.

2. Lab studies, procedures and other diagnostic measures that help to identify the cause and site of obstruction in patients with postrenal azotemia:
   a. Postvoid residual urine measurement (by catheter or US)
   b. Urinalysis
   c. Renal ultrasound (98% sensitivity in identifying upper-tract obstruction)
   d. Retrograde pyelography (or antegrade pyelography after placement of percutaneous nephrostomy)[*]

3. Helpful labs in defining specific abnormalities related to renal azotemia include the following:
   a. Microscopic urinalysis (eosinophilia suggests a drug-related cause)
   b. Urine for myoglobin
   c. Urine and serum sodium and creatinine
   d. Urine osmolality (measures concentrating ability)

4. In those cases where you are not sure of the type of azotemia (prerenal, postrenal or renal) learn to calculate the renal indices.
   a. You will need to order the following tests:
      (1) Urine and serum sodium
      (2) Urine and serum creatinine
      (3) Urine osmolality
      [These tests will not be useful in patients with <u>chronic</u> renal failure, those on diuretics or those with a history of obstruction; also, there can be an overlap between categories which just emphasizes the importance of a good H&P in determining the type of azotemia.]

---

[*]IVP and other contrast - related procedures are contraindicated in renal failure

b. Calculating the indices
   ▲ FE_{Na} = fractional excretion of sodium
   ▲ FE_{Na} (%) = $\dfrac{\text{urine sodium/serum sodium}}{\text{urine creatinine/serum creatinine}} \times 100$

   ▲ RFI = Renal Failure Index
   ▲ RFI (%) = $\dfrac{\text{urine sodium}}{\text{urine creatinine/serum creatinine}} \times 100$

c. Interpreting the indices

Test	Prerenal	Postrenal	Renal
Urine osmolality	> 500	< 400	< 300
Urine sodium	< 20	> 40	> 40
$FE_{Na(\%)}$	< 1	> 2	> 2
RFI(%)	< 1	> 2	> 2

C. Treatment

1. <u>Prerenal azotemia</u>: Correct hypoperfusion and its cause.

2. <u>Postrenal azotemia</u>: Relieve the obstruction temporarily by using a catheter first, then refer the patient for definitive management (which may require other upper tract-related instrumentation, e.g. ureteral stent or percutaneous nephrostomy).

3. <u>Renal azotemia</u>:
   a. Remove the offending agent; treat any specific underlying cause.
   b. Attempt to increase urine flow in oliguric patients (UO < 400 to 500mL/day) and convert them to nonoliguric ARF which is easier to manage in terms of fluid and electrolyte status.
      (1) This can be accomplished by administering mannitol, furosemide and/or low-dose dopamine and will be successful in one-third to one-half of patients. The doses are:
         (a) Mannitol 12.5 to 25gms IV
         (b) Furosemide 2 to 6mg/kg IV (max dose of 400mg)[*]
         (c) Dopamine 1 to 3mcg/kg/min IV
      (2) Whether these interventions actually have a favorable effect on mortality has not, as yet, been conclusively demonstrated.
   c. Support with dialysis if necessary.

D. Complications of ARF

1. Hyperkalemia (most immediate life-threatening complication)
   a. Used to be the most common metabolic cause of death in these patients; therefore, a serum potassium and ECG are probably two of the most important labs to obtain in patients with ARF.

---

[*]The use of furosemide has been shown to decrease the need for dialysis and problems associated with fluid overload. However, the ototoxicity of furosemide is proportional to the rate and dose at which it is given and is high in the doses used in the treatment of ARF.

   b. Hyperkalemia primarily manifests as cardiotoxicity (cardiac dysrhythmias and sudden death).

   c. Treatment is determined by the K$^+$ level and the ECG findings and can involve a combination of the following modalities: IV calcium, IV glucose and insulin, IV sodium bicarb, IV sodium chloride (3%), inhaled beta-adrenergic agents, IV diuretics, cation exchange resin (PO or PR) and dialysis. [See section on hyperkalemia in chapter on Fluid and Lyte Emergencies, pp. 854 - 856 for further information.]

2. Hypocalcemia
   a. Is common in ARF, but is usually asymptomatic.
   b. Symptomatic patients are treated with IV calcium gluconate or calcium chloride.

3. Hypermagnesemia — is common but rarely significant; magnesium-containing antacids and laxatives should be avoided in these patients.

4. High anion gap metabolic acidosis — is almost always present but is generally mild and rarely requires correction.

5. Volume overload
   a. Is common in oliguric patients and can lead to CHF and pulmonary edema.
   b. IV diuretics and nitroglycerine can be used as temporizing measures while arrangements for dialysis are being made.

E. Antibiotics to Avoid in the Presence of Renal Failure:

1. Tetracycline
2. Nitrofurantoin
3. Methenamine
4. Penicillin (most common offender)
5. Nalidixic acid
6. Bacitracin (uncommonly used)

F. Indications for Dialysis in ARF

1. Hyperkalemia (ECG or clinical manifestations are resistant to therapy)
2. Fluid overload
3. Significant acidosis
4. Presence of certain toxins (ethylene glycol, methanol)
5. Uremic symptoms (pericarditis, encephalopathy, bleeding complications)
6. BUN > 100mg/dL, creatinine > 10mg/dL (relative indication)

G. Myoglobinuric Renal Failure

1. Pathologic evolution: trauma (especially crush injuries, burns, seizures, prolonged strenuous muscle contraction) → rhabdomyolysis (destruction of skeletal muscle cells) → release of myoglobin into the serum which passes through the kidneys and has a direct toxic effect on the renal tubules → acute tubular necrosis → renal failure (↑ serum creatinine).

2. Diagnosis
   a. Suspect in the following clinical settings:
      (1) Major trauma
      (2) Major burns
      (3) Seizures
      (4) Electrical injuries
      (5) Intoxicated patients (especially alcohol and PCP)
         (a) In the alcoholic, rhabdomyolysis is due to the direct toxic effect of ethanol on the skeletal muscle cell membrane in addition to pressure necrosis of muscle as a result of prolonged immobilization.
         (b) In the PCP OD, rhabdomyolysis is due to the excessive muscle activity and agitation which this drug induces.
   b. Urinary findings
      (1) Color may be smoky (reddish-brown) due to the presence of myoglobin (but do not wait for a color change before pursuing the diagnosis).
      (2) Positive for blood on dipstick exam but no RBCs are seen on microscopic exam (indicates myoglobinuria).
      (3) Renal tubular casts and muddy brown granular casts may be present on microscopic exam.
      (4) Myoglobinuria — may be present; however, it is not a reliable marker for rhabdomyolysis because it is rapidly cleared from the urine and can be absent despite the presence of significant rhabdomyolysis.
   c. Serum myoglobin — may be positive but, like urine myoglobin, is rapidly cleared and is, therefore, not a reliable indicator of rhabdomyolysis.
   d. Serum creatinine kinase (CK)
      (1) Is the most sensitive test for detecting rhabdomyolysis.
      (2) It is released immediately following muscle injury and its clearance from the serum is slow.
   e. Hypocalcemia (63%) and hyperkalemia (< 40%) are the most common electrolyte abnormalities occurring in association with rhabdomyolysis and may be significant enough to require treatment.

3. Management guidelines
   a. Avoid using potentially nephrotoxic drugs
      (1) Nonsteroidal anti-inflammatory agents
      (2) Antibiotics (listed on previous page under E)
   b. Aggressively hydrate with IV fluids (NS or LR) at a rate sufficient to maintain a urine output > 2mL/kg/hr. (This is the most important aspect of therapy in these patients).

c. Administer mannitol: 25gms IV initially, then add 12.5gms to each subsequent liter of fluid to promote diuresis if fluid hydration alone fails to promote an adequate urine output and clear the pigment. Furosemide (2mg/kg IV) may also be used, but this is a controversial issue since it may cause acidification of the urine.

d. Alkalinize the urine with sodium bicarbonate (add 44mEq to each liter of IV fluid) if hydration alone fails to raise the urine pH to > 6.5 (a low urine pH increases the toxicity of myoglobin).

e. Dialysis may be required to support kidney function until recovery takes place in those who do not respond to the above measures.

II. Nephrolithiasis

A. *Pathogenesis of Stone Formation*

1. Stones are formed when the urine is supersaturated with a particular mineral (calcium, phosphate, oxalate, urate, etc.)

2. Most patients with stones (90%) have a specific underlying metabolic derangement such as hypercalcuria, hyperparathyroidism, hyperuricosuria or renal tubular acidosis.

B. *Stone Composition and Etiology*

1. Most kidney stones (≥ 75%) contain calcium (oxalate or phosphate) and are radiopaque; they are sometimes caused by chronic hypercalcemic states such as:
   a. Hyperthyroidism
   b. Hyperparathyroidism
   c. Neoplasm
   d. Sarcoidosis
   e. Multiple myeloma
   f. Distal renal tubular acidosis

2. Struvite stones (magnesium-ammonium-phosphate) are radiopaque and account for an additional 15% and are caused by a chronic UTI associated with urea-splitting organisms (usually Proteus).

3. Uric acid stones (6 - 10%) are radiolucent and are seen in patients with:
   a. Gout
   b. Myeloproliferative disease or leukemia
   c. High protein diet

4. Cystine stones (1-3%) are radiopaque + associated with a familial trait.

5. Xanthine stones are rare and their cause is obscure (?methylxanthine preparations, e.g. theophylline?); they are radiopaque.

C. Epidemiology

1. Highest incidence is in the southeastern U.S. during the summer and fall when the intake of oxalate-rich fresh vegetables is greater and dehydration is more common.

2. Patients are typically between the ages of 20 and 50 years old.

3. Males, particularly sedentary white males, are affected more than females (ratio ~ 3:1).

4. There is a familial and hereditary predisposition.

5. Ninety percent of stones < 5mm in diameter pass on their own.

6. Recurrence of calculus formation is common; about 50% will have a recurrence with the risk increasing with each additional stone episode.

D. Clinical Presentation: unilateral colicky pain in the flank, back or lower quadrant with radiation to the groin, labia or testicles; the pain is usually severe and often accompanied by dysuria, frequency and hematuria; nausea and vomiting occur as the pain increases in severity; if the stone passes into the bladder, the severity of pain diminishes markedly but may persist as a dull ache due to ureteral spasm.

E. Diagnosis

1. Ureteral obstruction is usually due to actual concretions (stones) but it may also be due to crystal aggregates, blood clots, necrotic papillae or even tumors.
   a. 90% of "stones" are radiopaque and may be seen on KUB:
      (1) Calcium oxalate
      (2) Calcium phosphate
      (3) Magnesium-ammonium-phosphate (struvite)
      (4) Cystine (moderately radiopaque)
         [Be able to recognize a radiopaque stone on KUB or IVP — they usually lie over the transverse processes of the lumbar vertebrae]*
   b. Radiolucent "stones" can be detected as filling defects on IVP:
      (1) Uric acid
      (2) Blood clots
      (3) Sloughed papillae
      (4) Tumors
      (5) Xanthine (is about as common as hens teeth)
   c. Definitive diagnosis of the type of stone requires stone analysis and is indicated for recurrent stone - forming patients — a 24-hour urine collection and analysis can provide definitive recommendatios for prevention of stones; studies include: urine volume & pH as well as stone identification (calcium, oxalate, citrate or magnesium).
   d. At some point in time, <u>every</u> patient with a stone should have a serum calcium performed to R/O primary hyperparathyroidism.

*They may be obscured in the mid-third of the ureter where they lie over the sacrum and, occasionally when they lie over a transverse process.

2. Laboratory and Radiographic Studies
   a. CBC (> 15,000 WBCs suggests active infection).
   b. U/A
      (1) Hematuria is typical of urolithiasis but its absence does not exclude the diagnosis; 20% of patients will not have microscopic hematuria. Also, there does not appear to be any correlation between the degree of obstruction and the absence of hematuria.
      (2) If the urinary pH is > 7.6, suspect the presence of urea-splitting organisms (Proteus); a pH < 7.4 suggests the presence of uric acid calculi and also rules out renal tubular acidosis as the cause.
   c. Urine culture if infection suspected
   d. BUN/creatinine (prior to IVP, especially if there is a history of renal disease, DM or HTN)
   e. Serum calcium, phosphorus and uric acid levels
   f. CT scanning — is now the diagnostic study of choice.
      (1) Spiral or helical CTs have largely replaced the IVP because they are faster, have greater sensitivity (98%) and do not use contrast material.
      (2) Both lucent and opaque calculi can be demonstrated as well as hydronephrosis.
      (3) Other anatomical pathology (e.g. abdominal aortic aneurysm) can be identified but scanning does not provide functional info.
   g. IVP (intravenous pyelography)
      (1) This study is generally reserved for situations where a functional or anatomic study is required; it should not replace the non-contrast CT for initial stone workup.
      (2) Findings consistent with the presence of a calculus include:
         (a) A delayed nephrogram (delay in appearance of contrast material on the five-minute film) on the affected side.
         (b) Hydronephrosis/hydroureter
         (c) Columnization (visualization of the entire ureter on a single film)
         (d) Extravasation of contrast (uncommon)
      (3) Is occasionally therapeutic; hyperosmolar contrast load → ↑urine output → passage of stone.
   h. Ultrasonography — is the initial study of choice in pregnant and pediatric patients in the attempt to limit exposure to ionizing radiation.

F. *Treatment*

1. IV hydration with normal saline at a rate sufficient to produce a urine output > 2mL/kg/hr.

2. Pain relief has traditionally been achieved with narcotics (for severe pain) and ketorolac (for mild to moderate pain). However, it now seems clear that ketorolac and narcotics act synergistically with one another. In addition, when used together, the narcotic dosage needed is less than when it is used alone (which also reduces side effects). Start with a low dose of an IV narcotic followed by 30mg of IV ketorolac, then slowly titrate additional doses of IV narcotic until desired pain relief is reached.

3. Patients who are discharged should:
   a. Be encouraged to drink 2 glasses of water every two hours
   b. Strain their urine to collect the stone for analysis
   c. Be referred to a urologist for follow-up
   d. Be advised to return if problems develop (persistent vomiting, fever, chills, unremitting pain)

4. Indications for admission:
   a. Presence of an associated UTI (pyuria, bacteriuria, leukocytosis, fever)
   b. Uncontrolled pain requiring parenteral narcotics
   c. Intractable nausea and vomiting
   d. Hypercalcemic crisis
   e. Renal insufficiency
   f. Solitary kidney (relative)
   g. Intrinsic renal disease (relative)
   h. High-grade obstruction (relative)
   i. Stone > 5mm (relative)

III. Chronic Renal Failure

A. Pathophysiology/Clinical Features

1. First stage (↓renal function = < 50% GFR)
   a. Renal <u>reserve</u> is lost but one half of the renal function (glomerulofiltration rate) can be gone before the serum creatinine rises.
   b. Excretory and regulatory functions are intact.

2. Second stage (renal insufficiency = 20 - 50% GFR)
   a. Mild azotemia with some loss of concentrating ability
   b. Mild anemia
   c. Sudden fluid loss/gain can precipitate acidosis + severe azotemia

3. Third stage (renal failure = 5 - 20% GFR)
   a. Frank azotemia with loss of concentrating ability
   b. Severe anemia
   c. Hypocalcemia, hyperphosphatemia and hypermagnesemia
   d. Hyperkalemia (common cause of cardiac arrest in this stage)

4. Fourth stage: (uremia = < 5% GFR → effects on organ systems)
   a. Cardiovascular
      (1) Hypertension
      (2) CVA
      (3) MI
      (4) CHF
      (5) Dysrhythmias
      (6) Pericarditis (uremic and dialysis-induced)

b. Hematologic
(1) Splenomegaly
(2) Anemia with lymphopenia and granulocyte dysfunction
(3) Prolonged bleeding time (normal INR, Platelet count)
c. Metabolic
(1) Hyperparathyroidism
(2) Hyperlipidemia
(3) Osteomalacia
(4) Goiter
(5) Gonadal dysfunction
(6) Glucose intolerance
d. Neurologic
(1) Subdural hematoma
(2) Peripheral neuropathy
(3) Uremic encephalopathy
(a) Impaired sensorium
(b) Seizures
(c) Gait disturbances
(d) Slurred speech
(e) Asterixis
(4) Wernicke's encephalopathy
(5) "Dialysis dementia" (is progressive and fatal)
e. Immunologic: Patients are more susceptible to bacterial, viral and fungal infections (including TB).
f. Gastrointestinal
(1) Bleeding
(2) Hepatitis
(3) Pancreatitis
(4) Ascites
g. Pulmonary
(1) Pleural effusions
(2) Pulmonary edema

B. Treatment

1. Dialysis
a. Peritoneal dialysis
(1) Access site (abdominal catheter) is at risk for infection and may lead to peritonitis.
(2) Used primarily for treatment of chronic renal failure.
b. Hemodialysis
(1) Access sites (shunts and fistulas) are at risk for infection, clotting and hemorrhage.
(2) Used as a temporary measure for acute renal failure and also for definitive treatment of chronic renal failure.

2. Renal transplantation

IV. Hemodialysis-Related Problems

A. Complications Associated with Vascular Access

1. Hemorrhage
   a. Minor bleeding associated with dialysis puncture or mild trauma:
      (1) Apply nonocclusive pressure to the site. If this is unsuccessful, apply topical thrombin or neutralize excessive anticoagulation with vitamin K or protamine sulfate.
      (2) Recheck access for presence of a thrill.
      (3) Evaluate extent of blood loss.
      (4) Observe in ED for rebleeding.

   b. Extensive bleeding from an aneurysm or pseudoaneurysm — requires prompt evaluation by a vascular surgeon.
      (1) Control bleeding with direct pressure.
      (2) Stabilize patient with IV fluids (NS or LR), O_2 and cardiac monitoring.
      (3) Draw blood work (CBC, INR, type and crossmatch).
      (4) Obtain stat vascular surgery consultation.

2. Thrombosis (signaled by loss of a thrill in the access)
   a. Obtain immediate vascular surgery consultation to determine whether to remove the clot surgically or use a thrombolytic agent.
   b. Do <u>NOT</u> attempt to irrigate the access device as this can result in clot embolization.

3. Infection (usually due to Staph)
   a. More common in artificial than native grafts
   b. Can produce recurrent bacteremia and loss of access site
   c. Local signs (redness, warmth, tenderness and induration of access site) may be absent; some patients present only with a fever or recurrent episodes of bacteremia.
   d. Treatment consists of obtaining blood cultures and administering IV antibiotics (usually vancomycin).

B. Disequilibrium Syndrome

1. Occurs during or immediately after dialysis (most frequently during a patient's first dialysis treatment) especially if a large volume of fluid has been removed.

2. Pathophysiology: Dialysis → production of organic acids by the brain → cerebral intracellular acidosis → ↓pH → neurologic dysfunction.

3. Symptoms range from headache, nausea, vomiting and muscle cramps to altered mental status, grand mal seizures and coma.

4. Symptomatic treatment (rest, analgesics, antiemetics) is all that is needed for most patients; however, other causes of neurologic dysfunction (hypoglycemia, hypocalcemia, intracranial hemorrhage, etc.) should be considered and ruled out, particularly in patients whose symptoms persist or worsen over a period of observation.

V. Complications Associated with Renal Transplantation

A. *Graft Rejection*

1. Types of rejection
    a. Hyperacute rejection (rarest) — occurs within a few minutes to a few hours following surgery and results in irreversible allograft destruction.
    b. Acute rejection (most common) — generally occurs within 1 to 12 weeks following surgery; 90% may be successfully reversed if recognized and treated promptly.
    c. Chronic rejection — is indolent and difficult to arrest.

2. Findings
    a. Tenderness over the allograft (located in the iliac fossa)
    b. Decreased urine output
    c. Fever (low-grade)
    d. Generalized discomfort
    e. Worsening HTN
    f. Precipitous weight gain
    g. Peripheral edema
    h. Increase in serum creatinine[*]

3. Evaluation — should be directed toward ruling out other causes of decreased renal function that occur in renal transplant patients (e.g. volume contraction, drug-induced nephrotoxicity, infection, etc.) and should include:
    a. UA
    b. Serum BUN/creatinine
    c. Renal ultrasonography (and bladder scan for residual urine)
    d. Trough level of cyclosporine

4. Treatment
    a. High-dose steroids (IV or PO) for 3 to 4 days followed by ...
    b. Allograft biopsy (to document the presence of ongoing rejection) in those patients who show little or no improvement and ...
    c. Administration of an antibody preparation directed toward lymphocytes (such as OKT3) to those patients with documented unremitting allograft rejection.

B. *Infections*

1. Due to ongoing immunosuppression, infections (particularly opportunistic ones) are common in these patients and may present with a paucity of findings (fever + typical physical findings may be absent).

---

[*]Acute rejection can be very subtle, presenting with only an increase in the serum creatinine.

2. In an attempt to prevent these infections, patients are given multiple vaccines and prophylactic medications. The regimen generally includes the following:
   a. Pneumococcal vaccine
   b. Hepatitis B vaccine
   c. Nystatin
   d. TMP-SMX (for prevention of pneumocystis carinii pneumonia).
   e. High-dose acyclovir

3. The most common life-threatening infection in these patients (as well as recipients of other solid organ transplants and bone marrow recipients) is cytomegalovirus (CMV) infection.
   a. It generally occurs 1 - 6 months post-transplantation surgery.
   b. Manifestations range from daily fever and malaise to leukopenia, lymphadenopathy, ↑ LFTs, epigastric pain, diarrhea and pneumonia.
   c. Work-up should include a CBC, liver function tests and CXR.
   d. Treatment includes:
      (1) Reducing immunosuppressive therapy and ...
      (2) Administering IV ganciclovir (with or without immune globulin) if lung, GI or liver involvement is present.

4. UTIs develop in 20% of patients in the first four months following renal transplantation.

VI. Urinary Tract Infections (UTIs)

A. Definition: significant bacteriuria in a symptomatic patient.

B. Incidence

1. Females have a steadily increasing incidence with age; peaks occur in infancy, preschool and childbearing years.

2. Males have approximately the same incidence as females during infancy, but then this rapidly declines and remains low until middle age when prostatism occurs.

C. Bacteriology

1. Uncomplicated UTIs ... represent most UTIs
   a. Occur in normal hosts in whom no anatomical defect in the urinary system can be found.
   b. Usually caused by gram-negative aerobic bacilli from the gut; E. coli is the predominant pathogen.
   c. In women, a small percentage of these UTIs are caused by *chlamydia* and *Staph. saprophyticus*.

2. Complicated UTIs
    a. Occur in patients with underlying structural, neurologic or immuno-logic disease.
    b. May be caused by unusual organisms (*Pseudomonas*, *Serratia marces-cens*, etc.); however, typical pathogens predominate.

D. *Normal Host Defense Mechanisms*

1. <u>Acidity</u>: pH < 5.5 discourages bacterial growth.

2. <u>Bladder defense</u>: bladder mucosa destroys the bacteria in the urine remaining on the walls but this defense mechanism is ineffective if bladder emptying is incomplete.

3. <u>Renal defense</u>: local antibodies, leukocytes and phagocytes remove bacteria.

4. <u>Urinary hemodynamics</u>: a large urinary flow dilutes bacteria and elim-inates them from the system.

E. *Clinical Presentations*

1. Infants: poor feeding, irritability, vomiting.

2. Preschoolers: irritability, malaise, dysuria.

3. School age: fever (more often in males), dysuria, frequency.

4. Adults
    a. Dysuria, frequency, urgency and lower abdominal discomfort.
        <u>Note</u>: Patients with upper tract infection may present with lower tract symptoms.
    b. Low-grade fever, chills and malaise may be present; a high temp. is more suggestive of pyelonephritis.
    c. Flank pain and CVA tenderness can be associated with a simple UTI due to referred pain from the bladder. However, if these findings are present, it is safer to assume that the patient has pyelonephritis...A clue to this diagnosis, if present, is a history of <u>shaking</u> chills.
    d. Diabetic women who appear ill, presenting with lower abdominal pain ± a recent Hx of a UTI, may have emphysematous pyelonephritis. This is a life-threatening bacterial infection that can be quickly diagnosed by bedside US (fluid + gas) surrounding the kidney.

F. *Diagnosis*

1. Urinalysis
    a. A good specimen (no epithelial cells) can be obtained with one of the following methods:
        (1) Midstream clean catch
        (2) Catheterization
        (3) Suprapubic aspiration (newborns and infants)

b. Microscopic findings
   (1) Significant pyuria
      (a) Traditionally, significant pyuria was considered to be > 10 WBCs/HPF in women; however, in light of recent research, low-level pyuria of 2 - 5 WBCs/HPF is currently considered to be significant by most authors.
      (b) 1 - 2 WBCs/HPF in men if bacteria are also present.
   (2) Significant bacteriuria
      (a) Any on unspun urine Gram stain under oil
      (b) > 15/HPF (high dry) on spun sediment
c. Diagnosis of a UTI based on a U/A is presumptive.
   (1) False positives occur secondary to contamination with bacteria from the skin or from other causes of pyuria.
   (2) False negatives occur secondary to diuresis or an infection that is due to a more virulent bacterium (in which case, few organisms are required to cause infection) and they may not be seen in significant numbers on microscopic exam.

2. Definitive diagnosis is made by urine culture.
   a. Traditionally, the presence of a colony count > 10^5/mL was considered consistent with the presence of a UTI. Currently, however, a colony count > 10^2/mL is considered significant in the symptomatic patient.
   b. Cultures should be ordered on:
      (1) Infants, children and the elderly
      (2) Adult males
      (3) Pregnant females
      (4) Patients with any of the following:
         (a) Pyelonephritis
         (b) Prolonged symptoms (> 6 days)
         (c) Underlying medical disease/ immunocompromised (DM, sickle cell anemia, CA) or history of kidney stone(s)
         (d) Urologic abnormalities (structural or neurologic)
         (e) History of recent urologic instrumentation
         (f) Those who relapse, require hospitalization or have a chronic indwelling catheter.

G. Treatment

1. In females, look for and rule out cervicitis, PID and vulvovaginitis.

2. In males, look for and rule out urethritis.

3. Outpatient antibiotic therapy for UTIs:
   a. Patients with uncomplicated UTIs should be treated with an agent effective against *E. coli* in your community.
      (1) Trimethoprim-sulfamethoxazole (TMP-SMX) or augmentin*
      (2) Nitrofurantoin
      (3) A fluoroquinolone is indicated ...
         (a) If local resistance to *E. coli* is > 10% <u>or</u>
         (b) If the patient is male with non-STD urethritis (3-day therapy) or cystitis (7 - 10 day regimen)

*First-line drugs only if local resistance patterns to E. coli are < 10%

b. Despite increasing resistance rates to ampicillin, amoxicillin and cephalosporins, these antibiotics remain first-line agents in pregnant patients.
   (1) A 3 - 7 day course is recommended since a single-dose regimen of these drugs may be ineffective in eradicating the vaginal reservoir of *E. coli*.
   2) Nitrofurantoin is becoming a first-line agent because it is efficacious, inexpensive and well-tolerated; due to its short half-life, it must be taken for at least 7 days and should not be given to patients with G6PD deficiency.
c. If chlamydia is the suspected pathogen (history of new sexual partner or the presence of pyuria without bacteriuria) culture for chlamydia and initiate therapy with doxycycline, TMP-SMX or a quinolone* (levofloxacin or ofloxacin).
d. In patients with complicated, resistant or recurrent infections, (but no pyelonephritis) initiate therapy with a quinolone (e.g. Cipro 5 - 7 days) and adjust therapy as needed based upon culture and sensitivity.
e. A 3-day course of antibiotics is optimal if there are no complicating factors; this regimen is low in cost and is associated with good compliance, fewer adverse effects than a traditional 10 - 14 day regimen and cure rates similar to 7-day therapy.
f. Single-dose therapy is not appropriate for the typical ED patients, many of whom have subclinical pyelonephritis and no identified medical doctor.
   (1) Single-dose therapy has not been uniformly accepted in spite of reported cure rates (80 - 100%) with TMP-SMX.
   (2) It should be reserved for the reliable patient with an uncomplicated UTI and an identified personal physician who can reassess the patient within one week.
   (3) Single-dose therapy should be avoided in infants and adult males.
      (a) Children must be protected from upper tract scarring.
      (b) Adult males usually have an associated anatomical defect, e.g. prostatism, kidney stone, tumor.
g. The standard 10 - 14 day course is indicated...
   (1) For pregnant patients
   (2) When symptoms have been prolonged (as subclinical pyelonephritis may be present)
   (3) In the presence of underlying disease
   (4) When chlamydial infection is suspected
h. Consider offering a 2-day course of a bladder analgesic such as Pyridium to patients experiencing painful urination and encourage frequent voiding.

4. Outpatient antibiotic therapy for patients with mild to moderate uncomplicated pyelonephritis who tolerate oral intake:
   a. Consider "sequential" treatment with a parenteral dose of gentamycin, ceftriaxone or a fluoroquinolone before the initiation of oral therapy.
   b. Discharge on a fluoroquinolone for 7 - 14 days with instructions for follow-up in one week.

*Cipro does not have activity against chlamydia

5. Indications for admission in patients with pyelonephritis:
    a. Severely ill / uroseptic
    b. The very young or elderly; adult males > 60 yrs. old
    c. Diagnostic uncertainty
    d. Underlying anatomical urinary tract abnormality or medical problems (including renal failure)
    e. History of obstruction, stones or instrumentation
    f. Progression of uncomplicated UTI / failed outpatient management
    g. Persistent vomiting or inability to tolerate oral antibiotics
    h. Immunocompromised host (diabetes, cancer, sickle cell disease, transplant recipient)
    i. Poor social situation / inadequate access to follow-up

6. Indications for urologic referral to search for an underlying anatomic abnormality:
    a. All children and adult males with UTIs
    b. Any adult with multiple recurrences of infection (> 3/yr.)

7. Patients with obstruction <u>and</u> a UTI (stones are the most common cause) have a potentially life-threatening condition; a GU consultation should be obtained immediately.

VII. Male Genital Problems

A. Anatomy

1. Penis [See <u>Tintinalli's Text</u>, Sixth ed., p.613, Fig. 95-1]
    a. Primarily consists of three cylindrical bodies:
        (1) Two corpora cavernosa
            (a) Form the bulk of the penis and are the major erectile bodies;
            (b) Are encased in a thick layer of connective tissue (tunica albuginea).
        (2) The corpus spongiosum surrounds the urethra.
        (3) All three cylinders are covered by Buck's fascia.
    b. Blood supply: internal pudendal artery → deep and superficial penile arteries.
    c. Lymphatic drainage: inguinal nodes.

2. Scrotum
    a. Thin skin with inner lining of smooth muscle (dartos).
    b. Blood supply: branches of the femoral and internal pudendal arteries.
    c. Lymphatic drainage: femoral and inguinal nodes.

3. Testes
    a. Average size is 4 - 5cm × 3cm; normal position is upright.
    b. Each testis is encased within a tunica albuginea surrounded by a tunica vaginalis and there is a small amount of fluid between the two layers; if the fluid increases, a hydrocele results which can be diagnosed by transillumination.

    c. The testes are anchored to the scrotum at two points — the tunica vaginalis and scrotal ligament; if the tunica vaginalis is capacious and envelopes the entire testicle, the testis will not be properly fixated and will usually lie in a horizontal position (rather than upright) which makes it more prone to torsion.

    d. Blood supply: spermatic and deferential arteries.

    e. Lymphatic drainage: iliacs (external, common) and periaortic nodes.

    f. May have an appendix (which is painful with torsion).

4. Epididymis
    a. A single long duct coiled at the superior pole of the testis on the posterior side; within this structure, sperm mature and gain the ability to move.
    b. May have an appendix (which is painful with torsion).

5. Vas deferens — a muscular tube that extends from the epididymis to the prostate.

6. Prostate
    a. This gland surrounds the urethra at a point between the bladder neck and urogenital diaphragm.
    b. Only the most posterior portion is palpable on rectal exam.

B. Physical Examination

1. Penis and scrotum
    a. Inspect the skin for lesions.
    b. "Milk" the penis to express any discharge to R/O urethritis (which may be asymptomatic).
    c. Palpate the scrotum for excess fluid (hydrocele) and any abnormalities of the testes and epididymis. Make sure the examining room is warm because, in a cold environment, the testes draw up making examination difficult.
       (1) Examine the position of the testes with the patient standing up; palpate for abnormalities with the patient lying down.
       (2) If a hydrocele is present, refer the patient to a urologist for further evaluation to R/O the presence of an underlying testicular tumor.
       (3) A noninflamed epididymis feels like an earlobe on palpation.

2. Prostate
    a. On rectal exam, one palpates a heart-shaped contour and a "ridge" (median raphe) that distinguishes the two lateral lobes.
    b. A normal prostate feels like the tip of a nose; prostatic carcinoma feels like the tip of a chin.

3. Check for inguinal hernia — In an adult, a direct inguinal hernia is usually acquired.

C. Urinalysis — the "Two-Cup Specimen" Technique

1. Patient voids 10-15mL into the first cup (represents urine from the urethra).

2. A midstream specimen is also obtained — represents urine from the bladder, kidneys and prostate.

3. These specimens are then examined for the presence of leukocytes.
   a. The presence of significant pyuria in the first cup and fewer WBCs in the midstream cup suggests urethritis.
   b. The presence of equal numbers of leukocytes in both specimens suggests infection of the bladder, kidneys or prostate.

D. Common Disorders of the Genitalia

1. Urethritis
   a. Etiology
      (1) Gonorrhea (GC)
      (2) Chlamydia (most common cause of non-gonococcal urethritis)
      (3) *Ureaplasma urealyticum* (causes 20 - 40% of non-gonococcal cases of urethritis)
      (4) *Trichomonas vaginalis* (responsible for 2 - 5% of non-gonococcal cases of urethritis)
      Note: Simultaneous infection (which may be asymptomatic) with both gonorrhea and chlamydia occurs in 30 - 50% of cases; antibiotic therapy should target both of these organisms.
   b. **Clinical picture**
      The patient usually complains of dysuria and a urethral discharge but he may be asymptomatic. Gram stain of the discharge reveals $\geq$ 5 WBCs/HPF (oil) and may demonstrate gram negative intracellular diplococci with GC; obtain a culture for GC as well as immunologic preps for chlamydia.
   c. Treatment*
      (1) Recommended regimens for gonorrhea include single-dose therapy with one of the following:
      (a) Ceftriaxone 125mg IM
      (b) Cefixime 400mg PO
      (c) Ciprofloxacin 500mg PO
      (d) Alternative regimens include a single dose of one of the following:
         1 Spectinomycin 2gm IM
         2 Ceftizoxime 500mg IM
         3 Cefotaxime 500mg IM
         4 Cefotetan 1gm IM
         5 Cefoxitin 2gm IM
         6 Enoxacin 400mg PO
         7 Lomefloxacin 400mg PO
         8 Norfloxacin 800mg PO

*If an associated epididymitis is suspected, 7 - 10 days of therapy are required.

(2) A regimen that is effective against chlamydia must also be prescribed. Recommended regimens include:
(a) Doxycycline 100mg PO bid × 7 days <u>or</u>
(b) Azithromycin 1gm PO in a single dose
(c) Alternative regimens include:
<u>1</u>   Erythromycin base 500mg PO qid × 7 days <u>or</u>
<u>2</u>   Erythromycin ethylsuccinate 800mg PO qid × 7 days <u>or</u>
<u>3</u>   Ofloxacin 300mg PO bid × 7 days
<u>Note</u>: These chlamydial regimens are also effective against ureaplasma urealyticum in most instances.
(3) Infection with *trichomonas vaginalis*, if present, should be treated with metronidazole 2gms PO <u>or</u> azithromycin 1gm PO as a single dose. Trichomonal infection should be considered in those patients who present with persistent symptoms (in the absence of non-compliance and re-exposure) despite adequate treatment for gonorrhea and chlamydia.

2. <u>Orchitis</u> (inflammation of the testicle)
   a. <u>Isolated</u> orchitis is rare.
   b. Most cases of orchitis are the result of direct extension of an epididymal infection and occur as a complication of a systemic illness, either bacterial or viral.
   c. Viral orchitis is most often caused by mumps.
   d. The patient presents with testicular pain and swelling (urinary and urethral symptoms are usually absent). In the case of mumps orchitis, symptoms usually evolve several days after the onset of parotitis, whereas bacterial orchitis can have a more acute presentation.
   e. An immediate urologic consult should be obtained to confirm the diagnosis since orchitis is extremely uncommon; testicular torsion and tumor are far more common.

3. <u>Acute Bacterial Prostatitis</u>
   a. Etiology
      (1) Usually bacterial, primarily gram-negative organisms (80% are *E. coli*; 20% Klebsiella, Enterobacter, Proteus or Pseudomonas)
      (2) Mixed bacterial infections are uncommon.
      (3) Tuberculosis is a possibility when renal TB is present.
   b. Diagnosis
      (1) The patient presents with dysuria, frequency, urgency and occasionally urinary retention accompanied by pain in the perineum, pelvis and low back; systemic signs of infection may also occur (chills, fever, myalgias, malaise).
      (2) Exam reveals a tender, swollen prostate that is warm and firm to the touch.
      (3) Prostatic massage should <u>not</u> be done in patients with <u>acute</u> infection because it can precipitate bacteremia; urine culture is sufficient for diagnosis because cystitis is also present in most cases.

c. Treatment
   (1) Antibiotics
      (a) Outpatient:
         <u>1</u> Ofloxacin 300mg PO bid × 30 days <u>or</u>
         <u>2</u> Levofloxacin 500mg PO QD × 30 days
      (b) Inpatient (sepsis, urinary retention): Gentamicin 3 - 5mg/kg/day <u>or</u> Tobramycin 3mg/kg/day <u>plus</u> Ampicillin 2gms Q 6hrs.
   (2) Prompt urologic consultation is indicated for patients who present with acute urinary retention.
   (3) Supportive measures:
      (a) Hydration
      (b) Bedrest
      (c) Analgesics (NSAIDs or narcotics prn)
      (d) Stool softeners/laxatives (especially if narcotics are prescribed)

4. <u>Venereal Proctitis</u>
   a. Etiology — the most common sexually transmitted pathogens:
      (1) *Neisseria gonorrhea*
      (2) *Chlamydia trachomatis*
      (3) *Treponema pallidum*
      (4) Herpes simplex virus (usually type II)
   b. Clinical presentation: symptoms range from none (most rectal GC carriers are completely asymptomatic) to severe and include rectal itching, burning, pain and/or fullness, tenesmus and a discharge; gonorrheal and chlamydial infections are often asymptomatic, but the anal chancre of syphilis and the herpetic lesions of HSV are usually quite painful; there is a history of anal intercourse; rectal exam may be normal but usually reveals inflammation and a purulent discharge; grouped vesicles on an erythematous base or aphthous ulcers may be seen in patients with HSV, while a chancre (primary syphilis) or condyloma lata (secondary syphilis) may be seen in patients with syphilis.
   c. Diagnosis
      (1) Perform anoscopy and a Gram stain to confirm the presence of acute proctitis.
      (2) Rule out HSV infection:
         (a) Immunofluorescent staining <u>or</u>
         (b) Tzanck smear (multinucleated giant cells)
      (3) Perform bacterial and viral cultures.
      (4) Send blood to check for syphilis (VDRL).
   d. Treatment
      (1) Ceftriaxone 125mg IM once <u>plus</u> doxycycline 100mg PO bid × 7 days is the treatment of choice.
      (2) Alternatives to the above regimen are the same as those listed for gonococcal urethritis.
      (3) If herpetic or syphilitic lesions are present, appropriate therapy for these infections should <u>also</u> be given (described below in the section on penile lesions).
      (4) Refer all patients for appropriate follow-up.

5. <u>Penile ulcers</u>
    a. Etiology
        (1) Herpes simplex (types I and II) ⎤ most common causes
        (2) Syphilis ⎬ in young, sexually-
        (3) Chancroid (*H. ducreyi*) ⎦ active patients
        (4) Granuloma inguinale (*Calymmatobacterium granulomatous*)
        (5) Lymphogranuloma venereum (*C.trachomatis*)
        (6) Behçet's syndrome
            (a) Vasculitis of uncertain etiology but thought to be an auto-immune disorder.
            (b) Clinical triad:
                <u>1</u> Chronic oral ulcerations
                <u>2</u> Relapsing iridocyclitis
                <u>3</u> Genital ulcers
            (c) Can be complicated by polyarthritis and erythema nodosum.
            (d) Lasts for many years with relapses and remissions but the condition can be suppressed by corticosteroids.
    b. Diagnosis
        (1) Serologic testing for syphilis — a VDRL or RPR* (nontreponemal tests) should be done initially and, if positive, should be confirmed with an FTA-ABS (a treponemal test). A VDRL should also be repeated at 3, 6 and 12 months following treatment to monitor the patient's response; with successful treatment, VDRL titers should gradually decrease.
        (2) Bacterial and viral cultures of lesions
        (3) Examination of material from base of ulcer:
            (a) Tzanck smear (done with Wright or Giemsa stain) → multi-nucleated giant cells or immunofluorescent staining (herpes)
            (b) Darkfield examination → spirochetes (syphilis)
            (c) Gram stain
                <u>1</u> Gram-negative rods in a linear or parallel arrangement (chancroid)
                <u>2</u> "Donovan bodies" (granuloma inguinale)
            (d) LGV complement fixation test is positive (Lymphogranuloma venereum)
    c. Treatment
        (1) Herpes
            (a) Acyclovir
                <u>1</u> Primary infections — are treated with 200mg PO 5 × per day (or 400mg TID) × 7 - 10 days or until clinical resolution occurs. For proctitis, the dose should be doubled and continued for a minimum of 10 days.
                <u>2</u> Patients with recurrent episodes — may benefit from acyclovir if therapy is initiated within 24 hours of the appearance of lesions. The dosage regimens are:
                    • 200mg PO 5 × per day × 5 days <u>or</u>
                    • 400mg PO tid × 5 days <u>or</u>
                    • 800mg PO bid × 5 days

*Rapid plasma reagent

   <u>3</u> Daily suppressive therapy — is useful for patients with > 6 recurrences per year. The dose is 400mg PO bid.

   <u>4</u> Patients with severe disease or complications requiring hospitalization — are treated with IV acyclovir. The dose is 5 - 10mg/kg IV Q 8 hours for 5 - 7 days or until clinical resolution occurs.

  (b) Other regimens that are equally efficacious:

   <u>1</u> Famciclovir 250mg TID × 7 - 10 days <u>or</u>

   <u>2</u> Valacyclovir 1gm BID × 7 - 10 days

  (c) Symptomatic measures

  <u>Note</u>: Further discussion of this topic can be found in this chapter in the section on genital herpes simplex pp. 536 - 537 and in the chapter on Dermatologic Emergencies, in the section on herpes infections pp. 1212 - 1214.

 (2) Syphilis

  (a) Primary, secondary and early latent (< 1 year duration)

   <u>1</u> Benzathine PCN G 2.4 million units IM (single dose) <u>or</u>

   <u>2</u> Doxycycline 100 mg PO bid × 2 weeks <u>or</u>

   <u>3</u> Tetracycline or Erythromycin 500mg PO qid × 2 wks.

  (b) Late latent (> 1 year duration) and late syphilis (except neurosyphilis)

   <u>1</u> Benzathine PCN G 2.4 million units IM weekly for 3 doses <u>or</u>

   <u>2</u> Doxycycline 100mg PO bid × 4 weeks <u>or</u>

   <u>3</u> Tetracycline 500mg PO qid × 4 weeks

  (c) Neurosyphilis

   <u>1</u> Aqueous crystalline PCN G 2 - 4 million units IV Q 4 hours × 10 - 14 days <u>or</u>

   <u>2</u> Procaine PCN G 2.4 million units IM Q daily PLUS Probenecid 500mg PO qid for 10 - 14 days

   <u>3</u> PCN-allergic patients require desensitization followed by one of the above regimens.

  <u>Note</u>: Pregnant patients allergic to penicillin should be desensitized and treated with the appropriate PCN regimen; all patients with syphilis should be tested for HIV.

 (3) Chancroid (high rate of HIV co-infection)

  (a) Azithromycin 1 gm PO in a single dose <u>or</u>

  (b) Ceftriaxone 250mg IM in a single dose <u>or</u>

  (c) Erythromycin base 500mg PO qid × 7 days or until lesions are healed <u>or</u>

  (d) Ciprofloxacin 500mg PO bid × 3 days

 (4) Granuloma inguinale (all meds must be given at least 3 weeks)

  (a) TMP-SMX DS (one PO) bid <u>or</u>

  (b) Doxycycline 100mg PO bid

  (c) Alternative regimens:

   <u>1</u> Ciprofloxacin 750mg PO bid or

   <u>2</u> Erythromycin base 500mg PO qid

 (5) Lymphogranuloma venereum

  (a) Doxycycline 100mg PO bid × 21 days <u>or</u>

  (b) Erythromycin 500mg PO qid × 21 days

6. <u>Fournier's gangrene</u> (idiopathic scrotal gangrene)
   a. **Clinical picture**
      This patient presents with a painful, erythematous or necrotic scrotum, penis or perineum. He is febrile and appears toxic. The onset of pain and swelling was acute; he denies urinary tract symptoms. The patient is usually older and immunocompromised in some way (diabetes, chronic steroids, chronic alcoholism).
   b. **This is a potentially life-threatening disease.**
   c. Etiology
      (1) Usually due to infection originating from the perianal area.
      (2) Several organisms, both anaerobic and aerobic, are generally involved. *Bacteroides fragilis* is the predominant anaerobe and *E. coli* is usually the predominant aerobe. Other agents include *hemolytic strep*, *Staph.* and *Clostridia* species.
   d. Management
      (1) General supportive measures
      (2) Cultures
      (3) Broad-spectrum parenteral antibiotics against anaerobes and gram-negative enteric organisms
      (4) Prompt urology consultation for surgical debridement
      (5) Hyperbaric oxygen... has been used, but its efficacy is unknown and it is rarely necesssary.

7. <u>Perianal abscess</u>
   a. Clinical evolution: urethral trauma or stricture → extravasation of urine into the scrotum → infection of the scrotum.
   b. Signs and symptoms are similar to Fournier's gangrene but <u>urinary tract symptoms</u> (retention, overflow incontinence) <u>are prominent</u>.
   c. Management: same as above for Fournier's gangrene. If continuity with the urethra is established, a suprapubic catheter is often placed.

8. <u>Balanoposthitis</u>
   a. Is an inflammation of the glans penis (balanitis) and the foreskin (posthitis).
   b. If recurrent, it suggests diabetes as the underlying disorder.
   c. Exam: retraction of the foreskin reveals foul, purulent material and the glans is red, swollen and tender to palpation.
   d. Treatment
      (1) Good hygiene
      (2) Topical antifungal cream
      (3) Consider circumcision
      (4) Broad-spectrum antibiotics (if secondary infection present)[*]
      (5) Work-up for diabetes (if infection recurrent)

9. <u>Phimosis</u>
   a. Definition: inability to retract the foreskin behind the glans; is usually secondary to chronic infection of the foreskin associated with progressive scarring.

---

[*]Strep infection may be indistinguishable from nonspecific balanitis; cultures or empiric therapy should be considered.

      b. Emergency treatment with a dorsal slit of the foreskin is occasionally required in severe cases.

      c. Definitive therapy is circumcision (after the infection has been controlled with broad-spectrum antibiotics)

10. <u>Paraphimosis</u>

      a. Definition: inability to pull retracted foreskin back over the glans.

      b. Emergency treatment is indicated; vascular compromise can occur.

      c. Treatment

         (1) Apply continuous, firm pressure to the glans penis for 5 - 10 mins. to reduce the edema and then pull the foreskin over the glans.

         (2) If manual reduction is unsuccessful, infiltrate the constricting ring with a local anesthetic and make a superficial vertical incision dorsally in the midline (dorsal slit).

         (3) Definitive treatment is circumcision (after inflammation subsides).

11. <u>Constriction injuries to the penis</u> must be treated immediately. Rings, rubber bands, wire, hair and other objects can transect the urethra and cause neurovascular compromise.

12. <u>Fracture of the penis</u>

      a. Acute tear of the tunica albuginea (usually during erection) causes a swollen (or bent) painful penis.

      b. Do a retrograde urethrogram to R/O associated urethral injury and obtain immediate urologic consultation.

      c. Treatment is surgical repair.

13. <u>Peyronie's Disease</u>

      a. Patients present with a history of dorsal penile curvature with painful erections (and may be associated with Dupuytren's contracture of the hand).

      b. Exam reveals a thickened plaque involving the tunica albuginea of the corporal bodies.

      c. This is <u>not</u> an emergency; if the patient is bothered by it, urologic referral is in order.

14. <u>Carcinoma</u> (an aggressive tumor that requires immediate referral)

      a. A nontender or warty growth is usually found on the glans of uncircumcised males > 50 - 60 years old.

      b. On physical exam, always retract the foreskin to look for this.

15. <u>Priapism</u>

      a. This is a sustained erection unrelated to sexual stimulation. There are <u>two forms</u>:

         (1) <u>Low</u>-flow (<u>ischemic</u>) priapism ... is painful

           (a) Pathophysiology: ↓ venous outflow → venous stasis and ischemia that involves the corpus cavernosae but spares the glans and corpus spongiosum → <u>rigid, painful</u> penile shaft and <u>soft</u> glans.*

           (b) A surgical emergency — irreversible damage occurs between 24 - 48 hours.

---

*Because the spongiosum is spared, the patient should be able to void.

(c) Causes

    1 Reversible (may respond to medical therapy)

       a Sickle cell disease or trait (most common cause in children)

       b Intracavernosal injections of papaverine, phentolamine, alprostadil and prostaglandin E1 for erectile dysfunction (most common cause in adults)

       c Leukemic infiltration

    2 Irreversible (generally unresponsive to medical therapy)

       a Medications (antihypertensives, anticoagulants and antidepressents)

       b Illegal substances (alcohol, marijuana, cocaine)

       c Idiopathic

(2) High-flow (non-ischemic) priapism ... is rare and usually painless

    (a) Not a true emergent condition — long-term sequelae are rare.

    (b) Pathophysiology: ↑ arterial blood flow to the corpus cavernosae → ↑ venous blood flow → partially rigid, painless penile shaft and hard glans.

    (c) Causes

       1 Groin or straddle injury → arterial-cavernosal shunt formation (most common cause)

       2 High spinal cord injury/lesion

b. Treatment

  (1) Obtain immediate urologic consultation.

  (2) Manage ischemic priapism in a step-wise fashion to achieve resolution as quickly as possible: dry aspiration → aspiration with irrigation → intracavernous injections of phenylephrine (dilute with NS to a concentration of 100 - 500mcg/mL)

    (a) Repeated injections (1mL Q 3 - 5 mins. prn up to 1 hour) should be performed before deciding that this treatment is unsuccessful and a surgical shunt is required.

    (b) Monitor for adverse effects during and after intracavernous injection(s):

       1 Abnormal vital signs (HTN, tachycardia/bradycardia)

       2 Cardiac dysrhythmias

       3 Headache, palpitations

    (c) In patients with an underlying disorder (sickle cell disease, hematologic malignancy), systemic treatment of the disorder should be administered concurrently with the intracavernous injection(s).

  (3) Initial management of nonischemic priapism should be observation. Corporal aspiration should only be performed if the diagnosis is in question. Selective arterial embolization is recommended for patients who request treatment.

16. Testicular torsion

  a. Incidence may occur at any age but has bimodal peaks: the first few days of life and between ages 12 and 18.

b. **Clinical picture**

Acute onset of severe unilateral testicular pain or lower abdominal pain is typical; there may be a recent history of strenuous physical activity or a past history of testicular pain with spontaneous relief; swelling occurs within hours; examination - - (conducted with the patient in the standing position) reveals a swollen, firm, "high-riding" testicle with a transverse lie; the contralateral testicle may also have a transverse lie since the underlying anatomic abnormality ("bell-clapper deformity"), predisposing the patient to torsion, may be bilateral; an associated reactive hydrocele may be present; loss of the cremasteric reflex is an associated finding with high specificity, but it is not diagnostic and is not always present; urinary symptoms, pyuria, leukocytosis and fever are typically absent; the most common misdiagnosis is "epididymitis" because there is tenderness posteriorly where the epididymis is normally located — but what you are actually feeling is a tender testicle because when the testicle is "torsed" (twisted around) the epididymis is then located anteriorly.

c. Diagnosis

(1) NEVER RULE OUT THE DIAGNOSIS OF TESTICULAR TORSION BASED ON A SINGLE ELEMENT OF HISTORY OR PHYSICAL EXAM FINDING.

    (a) A prior history of torsion and orchiopexy does not R/O the diagnosis (especially if absorbable sutures were used).

    (b) Up to 80% of patients report anorexia, nausea and vomiting.

    (c) Of all the exam findings, presence of the cremasteric reflex is the most helpful in excluding the diagnosis of torsion.

(2) Ultrasound exam and technetium testicular scanning detect the amount of blood flow to the testicle (with the normal side serving as control); flow is decreased or absent on the affected side with torsion; color Doppler ultrasound is more accurate than the traditional Doppler exam and is now the test of choice in most hospitals.* Do NOT delay urologic consultation in order to wait for a scan.

(3) Emergency surgical exploration of the scrotum is the definitive diagnostic test and is indicated if testicular torsion cannot be ruled out with certainty.

d. Management

(1) Obtain immediate urologic consultation.

(2) Order a CBC and U/A (usually normal in torsion) and prepare patient for surgery.

(3) Radionuclide scanning or Doppler exam may be performed if either is immediately available and desired by the urologic consultant, but they should not delay definitive treatment.

(4) Surgery is indicated as soon as the diagnosis is made because testicular viability decreases rapidly; salvage rate is 80 - 100% up to 6 hours of ischemia, 20% after 10 hours and approaches zero after 24 hours.

(5) Symptomatic therapy for patients awaiting surgery is most appropriate.

*Sensitivity ranges from 83 - 100%; however, sensitivity is decreased in younger age groups (especially neonates).

17. <u>Torsion of appendices epididymis and testis</u>
These appendages are small pedunculated structures (without any known function) attached to the epididymis and testis that can torse and produce pain. Early on, pain is localized and <u>a tender nodule is palpated</u> (the "blue dot sign" on transillumination of the testis is pathognomonic). If seen late, pain is diffuse and swelling is present, so the diagnosis is more difficult to make. If the diagnosis is certain, surgery is not required since these structures calcify; but if the diagnosis is uncertain, surgery is indicated to R/O testicular torsion.

18. <u>Epididymitis</u>
   a. Clinical evolution: Inflammation of the epididymis is usually caused by bacterial infection and is more common in young adults than pre-adolescent boys or older men; there is a <u>gradual</u> onset of unilateral pain and swelling (sudden onset is more common with torsion); associated fever and dysuria are common; on exam, you find tenderness and swelling of the epididymis (which is located in its normal posterior position) and elevation of the testicle is associated with relief of pain (Prehn's sign) but this sign is unreliable; it ca<u>nnot</u> be used to distinguish epididymitis from torsion.
   b. Etiology — is age dependent
      (1) *Chlamydia* (usually sexually-transmitted) is the most common pathogen (followed by gonorrhea) in patients < 35 yrs. old.
      (2) *E. coli* and *Pseudomonas* (not sexually transmitted) are the most common pathogens in patients > 35 yrs. old.
   c. Lab studies
      (1) U/A: a few WBCs is common (but may also be seen with torsion).
      (2) Urine culture
      (3) CBC: a leukocytosis of 10,000 to 30,000/mm^3 is common.
      (4) Urethral gram stain
      (5) Urethral culture for GC and chlamydia
   d. Treatment
      (1) Supportive measures:
         (a) Bedrest initially followed by scrotal support
         (b) Ice packs
         (c) Analgesics
         (d) Stool softeners
      (2) Start antibiotics — antibiotic selection should be based upon the patient's age and presumed pathogens:
         (a) Homosexual or sexually-active males (coliforms)
            <u>1</u> Ciprofloxacin 500mg PO bid <u>or</u> ofloxacin 200mg PO bid × 10 - 14 days is the usual regimen.
            <u>2</u> If < 17 yrs. of age → amoxicillin-clavulanate or TMP-SMX PO.
         (b) Heterosexual males < 35 yrs. old (GC, chlamydia and possibly coliforms)
            <u>1</u> Ceftriaxone 250mg [IM] + doxycycline 100mg PO bid × 10 days <u>or</u> ofloxacin 300mg PO bid × 10 days

    <u>2</u> Cautionary advice:

       <u>a</u> Cipro will not work for chlamydia.

       <u>b</u> Single-dose therapy (while appropriate for simple urethritis) is inadequate for simple epididymitis.

  (c) Heterosexual males > 35 yrs. old or bisexual males (usually coliforms, but GC and chlamydia may contribute) → Levaquin 500mg PO bid <u>or</u> ofloxacin 300mg PO bid × 10 days.

(3) Refer to urologist for follow-up in 5 to 7 days.

(4) Admission for IV antibiotics is indicated for:

  (a) Toxic-appearing patients (particularly those who are older and those in whom you suspect a scrotal abscess)

  (b) Immunosuppressed patients

  (c) Patients with severe bilateral epididymitis

19. <u>Urethral stricture</u>

  a. Etiology: trauma, urethral instrumentation or a complication of chlamydial or gonorrheal infection.

  b. Diagnosis

    (1) History of partial or complete retention.

    (2) If unable to pass a catheter, a retrograde urethrogram can determine the extent and location of the stricture.

  c. Treatment is catheterization. If unable to pass a regular or Coudé catheter after 2 - 3 careful attempts, obtain a urologic consult for catheterization utilizing filiforms.

20. <u>Urethral foreign bodies</u>

  a. Occur at any age.

  b. Present with hematuria or signs and symptoms of obstruction or infection.

  c. Diagnosis is made by palpation and confirmed on plain film, retrograde urethrogram or cystoscopy.

  d. Obtain urologic consult for removal.

21. <u>Urinary retention</u>

  a. Etiology

    (1) Benign prostatic hypertrophy with bladder neck obstruction (most common cause in men > 50 yrs. old).

    (2) Strictures (history of an STD or pelvic trauma)

    (3) Drugs

      (a) Antihistamines

      (b) Anticholinergic agents

      (c) Antispasmodic agents

      (d) Cyclic antidepressants

      (e) Alpha-adrenergic stimulants

      (f) Antipsychotic agents

    (4) Meatal stenosis

    (5) Bladder neck contracture

    (6) Bladder CA

    (7) CA of the prostate

    (8) Neurogenic

b. **Clinical picture**
The patient is in distress (unless he has a neurogenic bladder) and he c/o hesitancy or poor stream followed by low abdominal pain and inability to void for 6 - 8 hours. On physical exam, the bladder is often visibly distended and easily palpable.

c. Lab studies
(1) U/A — to R/O co-infection
(2) BUN/creatinine — to assess renal function

d. Management
(1) Pass a Foley catheter; this is both diagnostic and therapeutic.
(2) Observe patients with <u>chronic</u> urinary retention for 2 - 4 hours following the relief of urinary retention for the development of <u>post-obstructive diuresis</u>, a syndrome of massive urine output that can produce volume depletion, electrolyte imbalance and hypotension. These patients require hospitalization and additional lab studies (serum and urine electrolytes).
(3) Most other patients can be discharged to home with the catheter in place and referred to a urologist for work-up.
(4) Antibiotics (trimethoprim or trimethoprim-sulfamethoxazole) should be prescribed if a concomitant UTI is present.
(5) Belladonna and opium (B&O) suppositories should not be prescribed for these patients. Continued use will prevent a successful voiding trial when the catheter is removed.

Journal References

ACAD EMERG MED, Thanassi, M., August 1997, "Utility of Urine and Blood Cultures in Pyelonephritis."

AUDIO-DIGEST EMERGENCY MEDICINE, Birnbaumer, Diane, M., November 1, 1998, "New Drugs and Diagnostic Techniques for Sexually Transmitted Diseases."

AUDIO-DIGEST EMERGENCY MEDICINE, Kilpatrick, S., January 1999, "When the Emergency Physician is the Obstetrician."

AM J EMERG MED, Larkin, G. L., et. al., January 1999, "Efficacy of Ketorolac Tromethamine Versus Meperidine in the ED Treatment of Acute Renal Colic."

AM J EMERG MED, McMurray, B. R., et. al., March 1997, "Usefulness of Blood Cultures in Pyelonephritis."

AM J OBSTET GYNECOL, Sullivan, C. A., et. al., 1996, "A Pilot Study of Intravenous Ondansetron for Hyperemesis Gravidarum."

AM J PERINAT, Younis, C. M., et. al., 1998, "Rapid Marked Response of Severe Hyperemesis Gravidarum to Oral Erythromycin El."

ANN EMER MED, Cordell, W. H., et. al., August 1996, "Comparison of Intravenous Ketorolac, Meperidine and Both (Balance Analgesia) or Renal Colic."

CAN J EMERG MED, Wood, V. M., et. al., April 2000, "The NARC (Nonsteroidal Antiinflammatory in Renal Colic) Trial: Single-Dose Intravenous Ketorolac Versus Titrated Intravenous Meperidine in Acute Renal Colic."

CENTER FOR DISEASE CONTROL AND PREVENTION, MMWR, 1998; 47 (No. RR-1) "1998 Guidelines for Treatment of Sexually Transmitted Diseases."

CLIN INFECT DIS, Gupta, K., et. al., July 2001, "Antimicrobial Resistance Among Uropathogens that Cause Community Acquired Urinary Tract Infections in Women: A Nationwide Analysis."

EMERG MED CLIN NORTH AM, Gallant, Joel E., February 1995, "Infectious Complications of HIV Disease."

EMERG MED CLIN NORTH AM, Coppola, Marco, Della-Giustina, David, August 2003, "Obstetric and Gynecologic Emergencies."

EMERGENCY MEDICINE PRACTICE, Freeman, L., Nov. 2000, Vol. 2, No. 11, "Male Genitourinary Emergencies: Preserving Fertility and Providing Relief."

EMERGENCY MEDICINE REPORTS, Alter, Harrison and Snoey, Eric, January 1997, "Obstructive Uropathy: A Clinical Update."

EMERGENCY MEDICINE REPORTS, Butler, K. H., Reed, K. C., Bosker, G., March 2001, "Urinary Tract Infection (UTI): New Diagnostic Modalities, Alterations in Drug Resistance Patterns and Current Antimicrobial Guidelines."

EMERGENCY MEDICINE REPORTS, Gallagher, S. A., February 15, 1999, "Diagnosis and Management of Urinary Tract Infections: A Disease Stratification Model. Part I: Epidemiology, Detection and Evaluation."

EMERGENCY MEDICINE REPORTS, Gallagher, S. A., February 15, 1999, "Diagnosis and Management of Urinary Tract Infections: A Disease Stratification Model. Part II: Targeted Management and Syndrome Specific Antibiotic Therapy."

EMERGENCY MEDICINE REPORTS, Hals, G., Crump, T., March 2000, "The Pregnant Patient: Guidelines for Management of Common Life-Threatening Medical Disorders in the Emergency Department."

EMERGENCY MEDICINE REPORTS, Hals, G., Tolbert, A., June 19, 2000, "Vaginal Bleeding During the First 20 Weeks of Pregnancy: Guidelines for ED Evaluation and Management. Part I: Clinical Overview and Diagnostic Modalities for Detection of Ectopic Pregnancy."

EMERGENCY MEDICINE REPORTS, Hals, G., Tolbert, A., July 3, 2000, "Vaginal Bleeding During the First 20 Weeks of Pregnancy: Guidelines for ED Evaluation and Management. Part II: Differential Diagnosis and Management of Ectopic Pregnancy and Spontaneous Miscarriage."

EMERGENCY MEDICINE REPORTS, Hals, G., July 17, 2000, "Vaginal Bleeding During the Second 20 Weeks of Pregnancy: Emergency Department Evaluation and Management Strategies for Maximizing Fetal and Maternal Outcomes."

EMERGENCY MEDICINE REPORTS, Haughey, M., Calderón, July 31, 2000, "Trauma in Pregnancy: Optimizing Maternal and Fetal Outcomes. A Systematic Approach to Assessment and Management of the Injured Pregnant Patient."

EMERGENCY MEDICINE REPORTS, Schwab, Robert, November 25, 1996, "Preeclampsia/ Eclampsia: Establishing the Diagnosis and Providing Prompt, Effective Treatment."

EMERGENCY MEDICINE REPORTS, Seamens, C. and Slovis, C.M., October 28, 1996, "Abnormal Vaginal Bleeding in the Nonpregnant Patient."

EMERGENCY MEDICINE REPORTS, Stewart, C. and Bosker, G., January 9, 1995, "The Diverse and Challenging Spectrum of Sexually Transmitted Diseases (STDs): Current Diagnostic Modalities and Treatment Recommendations. Part II: STDs with Skin Manifestations; Herpes, Syphilis, Lymphogranuloma Venereum, Chancroid and Human Papillomavirus."

EMERGENCY MEDICINE REPORTS, Stewart, C. and Bosker, G., August 2, 1999, "Pelvic Inflammatory Disease (PID): Diagnosis, Disposition and Current Antimicrobial Guidelines."

EMERGENCY MEDICINE REPORTS, Stewart, C. and Bosker, G., August 16, 1999, "Common Sexually Transmissible Diseases (STDs): Diagnosis and Treatment of Uncomplicated Gonococcal and Chlamydial Infections."

EMERGENCY MEDICINE REPORTS, Tilden, Jr., F. F. and Robert D. Powers, September 30, 1996, "Ectopic Pregnancy: Avoiding Missed Diagnosis and Reducing Morbidity."

EUR RAD, Kravchich, S., et. al., 2001, "Color Doppler Sonography: Its Real Role in the Evaluation of Children with Highly Suspected Testicular Torsion."

HUMAN REPROD, Mol, B. W., et. al., 1998, "The Accuracy of a Single Serum Progesterone Measurement in the Diagnosis of Ectopic Pregnancy: A Meta Analysis."

INT J FERTIL WOMENS MED, Baker, D. A., Sept./Oct. 1998, "Antiviral Therapy for Genital Herpes in Nonpregnant and Pregnant Women."

J CLIN ANESTH, Goodman, E. J., et. al., December, 2001, "Cephalosporins Can Be Given To Penicillin-Allergic Patients Who do not Exhibit an Anaphylactic Response."

J EMERG MED, Chen, M. Y. M., et. al., 1999, "Can Noncontrast Helical Computed Tomography Replace Intravenous Urography for Evaluation of Patients with Acute Urinary Tract Colic?"

J EMERG MED, Ha, M., et.al., 2004, "Nephrolithiasis."

J EMERG MED, Stone, S. C., et. al., April 2005, 28(3):315, "Emphysematous Pyelonephritis: Clues to Rapid Diagnosis in the Emergency Department."

J TRAUMA, Meunch, M.V., et. al., November 2004, "Kleihauer-Betke Testing is Important in All Cases of Maternal Trauma."

J UROL, Bove, P., et. al., September 1999, "Re-examining the Value of Hematuria Testing in Patients with Acute Flank Pain."

OBSTET GYN, Gracia, C. R., et. al., March 2001, "Diagnosing Ectopic Pregnancy: Decision Analysis Comparing Six Strategies."

OBSTET GYNECOL CLIN NORTH AM, Lavery, J. P., et. al., 1995, "Management of Moderate to Severe Trauma in Pregnancy."

PHARMACOTHERAPY, Longstreth, K.L., Robbins, S.D., Smavatkul, C., Doe, N.S., June 2004 24(6): 808-11, "Cephalexin-Induced Acute Tubular Necrosis".

RADIOLOGY, Preminger, G. M., et. al., May 1998, "Urolithiasis: Detection and Management with Unenhanced Spiral CT - A Urologic Perspective."

SEX TRANSM INFECT, Desmond, N. M., et. al., 1998, "Should Preventive Antiretroviral Treatment be Offered Following Sexual Exposure to HIV? The Case for."

UROLOGY, Miller, O. F., et. al., 1998, "Prospective Comparison of Unenhanced Spiral Computed Tomography and Intravenous Urogram in the Evaluation of Acute Flank Pain."

UROLOGY, Nisbet, A.A., Thompson, I.M., Nov. 2002: 60(5): 775-9, "Impact of Diabetes Mellitus on the Presentation and Outcomes of Fournier's Gangrene".

Specific Text Chapter References

Marco, C. A., "HIV Infection and AIDS." In Tintinalli, J. E., Ruiz, E., Krome, R. L. (eds.) Emergency Medicine: A Comprehensive Study Guide, 4th ed., (McGraw-Hill, New York, 1996)

Marco, C. A., Kelen, G. D., "Human Immunodeficiency Virus Infection and Related Disorders." In Harwood-Nuss, A. L., Linden, C. H., Luten, R. C. (eds.) The Clinical Practice of Emergency Medicine, 2nd ed., (Lippencott-Raven: Philadelphia, 1996)

Specific Text References

Campbell's Urology. Walsh P.C., Retik, A., Vaughan, E.D., Wein, A., eds. 8th ed. (Saunders, Philadelphia, PA, 2002).

Obstetrics & Gynecology. Beckmann, C. R. B., et. al., 2nd ed., (Williams & Wilkins, Baltimore, 1995).

Smith's General Urology. Tanagho, E. A., McAninch, J. W., 14th ed., (Appleton & Lange, Connecticut, 1995).

The Kidney. Brenner, B. M., 5th ed., (Saunders Co, Philadelphia, 1996).

The Sanford Guide to Antimicrobial Therapy. Gilbert, D. N., et. al., (Antimicrobial Therapy Inc., 2002).

Web and Other Sources

1998 SCIENTIFIC ASSEMBLY, Moran, Gregory, J., October 13, 1998, "STD's: What's New? Course #TU-166."

AMERICAN UROLOGICAL ASSOCIATION, 1999, "Priapism: Guideline on the Management of Priapism".

CDC, Center for Disease Control and Prevention, 2003, "Trends in Reportable Sexually Transmitted Diseases in the United States".

PHARMACIST'S LETTER/PRESCRIBER'S LETTER, Steadman, M. S., Allen, J., Detail Document #180603, June 2002, Vol. 18, "Summary Chart of 2002 CDC Treatment Guidelines for STDs."

PRESCRIBER'S LETTER, Vol. 9, No. 828, August 28, 2002, "Sexually Transmitted Diseases."

General Text References, Acep Clinical Policies and LLSA Reading Lists *for all chapters located in the back of both volumes.*

NOTES

NOTES

General Text References

Advanced Trauma Life Support for Doctors - Instructor Course Manual. American College of Surgeons (Chicago, 1997).

Atlas of Emergency Medicine. Knoop, K., Stack, L., Storrow, A., (McGraw-Hill Health Profession Division, New York, 1997).

Atlas of Emergency Medicine. Knoop, K., Stack, L., Storrow, A., 2nd. ed., (McGraw-Hill, New York, 2002).

Cecil Textbook of Medicine. Bennett & Plum, 22nd ed., (W. B. Saunders, Philadelphia, 2004).

Clinical Procedures in Emergency Medicine. Roberts and Hedges, 4th ed., (Saunders, Philadelphia, 2004).

Clinical Toxicology. Ford, Delaney, Ling and Erickson (Saunders, Philadelphia, 2001).

Color Textbook of Pediatric Dermatology. Weston, W., Lane, A. T., Morelli, J. G., 2nd ed., (Mosby-Year Book, St. Louis, 1996).

Comprehensive Textbook of Psychiatry/VI. Kaplan, H. and Sadock, B., 6th ed., (Williams & Wilkins, New York, 1996).

Comprehensive Textbook of Psychiatry/Volume II. Kaplan, H. and Sadock, B., 7th ed., (Lippincott, Williams & Wilkins, Philadelphia, 2000).

Conn's Current Therapy. Rakel, R. E., Bope, E. T., (Saunders, Philadelphia, 2005).

DeGowin's Diagnostic Examination. DeGowin, R. L., and Brown, D. D., 7th ed., (McGraw-Hill, New York, 2000).

Diagnostic Radiology in Emergency Medicine. Rosen, Doris, Barkin, Markovich and Barkin (Mosby-Year Book Inc., St. Louis, 1992).

Emergency Medicine, Howell, et. al., 1st ed., (W.B. Saunders, Philadelphia, 1998).

Emergency Medicine: A Comprehensive Study Guide. Tintinalli, Kelen and Stapczynski, 6th ed., (McGraw-Hill, New York, 2004).

Emergency Medicine: Concepts and Clinical Practice. Rosen, P. and Barkin, R., 5th ed., (Mosby-Year Book Inc., St. Louis, 2002).

Emergency Medicine: The Core Curriculum. Aghababian, R. V., et. al., (Lippincott-Raven, Philadelphia, 1998).

Emergency Medicine Clinics of North America: Bioterrorism. Darling, R. G., Mothershead, J. K., Waeckerle, J. F., Eitzen, E. M., (Saunders, Philadelphia, 2002).

Emergency Medicine Clinics of North America: Emergency Management of Cardiac Arrhythmias. Thakur, R. K., Reisdorf, E. J., (Saunders, Philadelphia, 1998).

Emergency Medicine Clinics of North America: Emergency Psychiatry. Allen, M. H., (Saunders, Philadelphia, 1999).

Emergency Medicine Clinics of North America: Pearls, Pitfalls, and Updates. Moore G. P., Wolfe, R. E., (Saunders, Philadelphia, 1997).

Emergency Medicine Clinics of North America: Pediatric Emergency Medicine: Current Concepts and Controversies. Cantor, R. M., Callahan, J. M., (Saunders, Philadelphia, 2002).

Emergency Medicine Clinics of North America: Pharmacologic Advances in Emergency Medicine. Pollack, C. V., (Saunders, Philadelphia, 2000).

Emergency Medicine Clinics of North America: Psychiatric Emergencies. Richards, C. F., Gurr, D. E., "Psychosis" and Williams, E. R., Shepherd, S. M., "Medical Clearance of Psychiatric Patients." (Saunders, Philadelphia, 2000).

Emergency Pediatrics: A Guide to Ambulatory Care. Barkin, R. M., Rosen, P., 6th. ed., (Mosby, St. Louis, 2003).

Ferri's Clinical Advisor. Ferri, F. F., (Mosby, St. Louis, 2003, 2004, 2005).

Fitzaptrick's Dermatology in General Medicine. Fitzpatrick, T. B., et. al., 5th. ed., (McGraw-Hill, New York, 1999).

Fractures and Dislocations: Closed Management. Connolly, J. F., Vol. 2, (W. B. Saunders, Philadelphia, 1995).

Guidelines 2000 for Cardiopulmonary Resuscitation and Emergency Cardiovascular Care. American Heart Association in collaboration with the International Liaison Committee on Resuscitation (ILCOR), Volume 102, No. 8., August 2000.

Goodman & Gilman's: The Pharmacological Basis of Therapeutics. Hardman, Goodman and Limbird, 9th ed., (McGraw-Hill, New York, 1996).

Handbook of Orthopaedic Emergencies. Hart, Rittenberry and Uehara, (Lippincott-Raven, Philadelphia, 1999).

Harrison's Principles of Internal Medicine. Fauci, Braunwald, et. al., 12th ed., (McGraw-Hill, New York, 1992).

Harrison's Principles of Internal Medicine. Fauci, Braunwald, et. al., 14th ed., (McGraw-Hill, New York, 1998).

Harrison's Principles of Internal Medicine. Fauci, Braunwald, et. al., 15th ed., (McGraw-Hill, New York, 2001).

Harrison's Principles of Internal Medicine. Fauci, Braunwald, et. al., 16th ed., (McGraw-Hill, New York, 2005).

Infectious Disease in Emergency Medicine. Brillman and Quenzer, 2nd ed., (Lippencott-Raven, Philadelphia, 1998).

Intensive Care Medicine. Bippe, Irwin and Alpert, 2nd ed., (Little-Brown, Boston, 1991).

Internal Medicine. Stein, et. al., 5th ed., (Mosby, St. Louis, 1998).

Medicine for the Practicing Physician. Hurst (Butterworths, Boston, 1988).

Pathologic Basis of Disease. Cotran, Kumar, Robbins and Schoen, 5th ed., (W. B. Saunders Co., Philadelphia, 1994).

Pocket Book of Infectious Disease Therapy. Bartlett, (Williams & Wilkins, Baltimore, 1998).

Pocket Book of Infectious Disease Therapy. Bartlett, J. G., (Lippincott Williams & Wilkins, Philadelphia, 2004).

Practical Approach to Emergency Medicine. Stine and Chudnofsky (Little-Brown, Boston, 1994).

Principles and Practice of Emergency Medicine. Schwartz, Hanke, Mayer, et. al., 4th ed., (Williams & Wilkins, Baltimore, 1999).

Principles and Practice of Infectious Diseases. Mandell, G. L., Bennett, J. E. and Dolin, R., 6th ed., (Churchill Livingstone, New York, 2005).

Principles of Surgery. Schwartz, Shires, Spencer, 6th ed., (McGraw-Hill, Inc., New York, 1994).

Providing Emergency Care Under Federal Law: EMTALA. Bitterman, R. A., (ACEP, Dallas, 2001).

Review of Gross Anatomy. Pansky, 5th ed., (Macmillan Publishing Co., New York, 1984).

Robert's Practical Guide to Common Medical Emergencies. Roberts, J. R., (Lippencott-Raven, Philadelphia, 1996).

Rosen's Emergency Medicine: Concepts and Clinical Practice. Marx, Hockberger and Walls, 5th ed., (Mosby, St. Louis, 2002).

Sabiston Textbook of Surgery: The Biological Basis of Modern Surgical Practice. Townsend, C. M., Beauchamp, R. D., Evers, B. M., Mattox, K. L., 16th ed., (W. B. Saunders, Philadelphia, 2001).

Saunders Manual of Medical Practice. Rakel, R. E., 2nd. ed., (Saunders, Philadelphia, 2000).

Scientific American Medicine. (1996-2005).

Textbook of Pediatric Emergency Medicine. Fleisher, Ludwig, et. al., 4th. ed., (Lippencott Williams & Wilkins, Philadelphia, 2000).

Textbook of Pediatric Infectious Diseases. Feigin, R. D., and Cherry, H. D., 4th. ed., (Saunders, Philadelphia, 1998).

The 2002 Tarascon Pocket Pharmacopoeia, Green, S. M., 2nd ed., (Tarascon Publishing, 2002).

The Clinical Practice of Emergency Medicine. Harwood-Nuss, et. al., (Lippencott-Raven, Philadelphia, 1996).

The Clinical Practice of Emergency Medicine. Harwood-Nuss, A., Wolfson, A. B., et. al., 3rd ed., (Lippincott Williams & Wilkins, Philadelphia, 2001).

The Merck Manual of Diagnosis and Therapy. Beers, M. and Berkow, R., 17th ed., (Merck & Co., Pennsylvania, 1999).

The Sanford Guide to Antimicrobial Therapy. Gilbert, D. N., et. al., (Antimicrobial Therapy Inc., 2005).

The Sanford Guide to Antimicrobial Therapy. Gilbert, D. N., et. al., (Antimicrobial Therapy Inc., 2002).

The Year Book of Emergency Medicine. Burdick, Cone, Cydulka, et. al., (Mosby, St. Louis, 2000, 2001, 2002, 2003, 2004 + 2005).

Trauma. Martox, K. L., Feliciano, D. V., Moore, E. E., 5th. ed., (McGraw-Hill, New York, 2004).

Williams Textbook of Endocrinology. Wilson, J. D., Foster, D. W., Kronenberg, H. M., Larsen, P. R., 9th. ed., (W. B. Saunders, Philadelphia, 1998).

Wounds and Lacerations. Trott, A. T., 2nd ed., (Mosby, St. Louis, 1997).

ACEP Clinical Policies

#1 Clinical Policy for the Initial Approach to Patients Presenting with Acute Toxic Ingestion or Dermal or Inhalation Exposure

#2 Practice Parameter: Neuroimaging in the Emergency Patient Presenting With Seizure.

#3 Clinical Policy for the Initial Approach to Patients Presenting with a Chief Complaint of Seizure Who Are Not in Status Epilepticus

#4 Clinical Policy for the Initial Approach to Patients presenting with Altered Mental Status

#5 Clinical Policy: Critical Issues in the Evaluation and Management of Adult Patients Presenting With Suspected Acute Myocardial Infarction or Unstable Angina.

#6 Clinical Policy: Critical Issues for the Initial Evaluation and Management of Patients Presenting with a Chief Complaint of Nontraumatic Acute Abdominal Pain

#7 Clinical Policy: For the Management and Risk Stratification of Community-Acquired Pneumonia in Adults in the Emergency Department

#8 Critical Issues in the Evaluation and Management of Patients Presenting to the Emergency Department with Acute Headache

#9 Clinical Policy: Neuroimaging and Decision making in Adult Mild Traumatic Brain Injury in the Acute Setting.

#10 Critical Issues in the Initial Evaluation and Management of Patients Presenting to the Emergency Department in Early Pregnancy

#11 Clinical Policy: Critical Issues in the Evaluation and Management if Adult Patients Presenting With Suspected Pulmonary Embolism

#12 Clinical Policy: Critical Issues in the Evaluation and Management of Adult Patients Presenting with Suspected Lower-Extremity Deep Venous Thrombosis

#13 Clinical Policy for Children Younger Than Three Years Presenting to the Emergency Department with Fever

#14 Clinical Policy: Critical Issues in the Evaluation of Adult Patients Presenting to the Emergency Department with Acute Blunt Abdominal Trauma.

2004 Lifelong Learning and Self Assessment Reading List

#1 "Immune Thrombocytopenic Purpura", Clines, D.B., Blanchette, V.S., N ENGL J MED, March 2002, 345: 995-1008

#2 "Update on Emerging Infections: News from the Centers for Disease Control and Prevention", Schriger, D.L., Mikulich, V.J. ANN EMERG MED, March 2002, 39: 319-328

#3 "Low Back Pain", Deyo, R.A., Weinstein, J.N., N ENGL J MED, February 2001, 344: 363-370

#4 "Orthopedic Pitfalls in the ED: Pediatric Growth Place Injuries", Perron, S.D., Miller, M.D., Brady, W.J. AM J EMERG MED, January 2002, 30: 50-54

#5 "State of the Art: Therapeutic Controversies in Severe Acute Asthma", Gibbs, M.A., Camargo Jr., C.A., Rowe, B.H., et. al. ACAD EMERG MED, July 2000, 7: 800-815

#6 "Management of Tuberculosis in the United States", Small, P.M., Fujiwara, P.I., N ENGL J MED, July 2001, 345: 189-200

#7 "New Diagnostic Tests for Pulmonary Embolism", Kline J.A., Johns, K.L., Colucciello, S.A. et. al., ANN EMERG MED, February 2000, 35: 168-180

#8 American College of Emergency Physicians. Clinical Policy for the Management and Risk Stratification of Community-Acquired Pneumonia in Adults in the Emergency Department. ANN EMERG MED, July 2001, 38: 107-113

#9 "Difficult Airway Management in the Emergency Department", Orebaugh, S.L. J EMERG MED, January 2002, 22: 31-48

#10 "Causes and Outcomes of the Acute Chest Syndrome in Sickle Cell Disease", Vichinsky, E.P., Neumayr, L.D., Earles, A.N., et.al. N ENGL J MED, June 2000, 342: 1855-1865

#11 "Cocaine-Associated Chest Pain: How Common is Myocardial Infarction?" Weber, J.M., Chudnofsky, C.R., Boczar M., et.al., ACAD EMERG MED, August 2000, 7: 873-877

#12 "Oral Agents for the Treatment of Type 2 Diabetes Mellitus: Pharmacology, Toxicity and Treatment", Harrigan, R.A., Nathan, M.S., Beattie, P. ANN EMERG MED, July 2001, 38: 68-78

#13 "Heat Stroke", Bouchama, A., Knochel, J.P. N ENGL J MED, June 2002, 346: 1978-1988

#14 "High-Altitude Illness", Hackett, P.H., Roach, R.C. N ENGL J MED, July 2001, 345: 107-114

#15 "Illness After International Travel", Ryan, E.T., Wilson, M.E., Kain, K.C. N ENGL J MED, August 2002, 347: 505-516

#16 "The Role of Activated Charcoal and Gastric Emptying in Gastrointestinal Decontamination: A State-Of-The-Art Review", Bond, G.R. ANN EMERG MED, March 2002, 39: 273-288

#17 "Major Radiation Exposure - What to Expect and How to Respond", Mettler, F.A. Jr., Voelz, G.L. N ENGL J MED, May 2002, 346: 1554-1561

#18 "Validity of a Set of Clinical Criteria to Rule Out Injury to the Cervical Spine in Patients with blunt Trauma", Hoffman, J.R., Mower, W. R., Wolfson, A.B. et.al. M ENGL J MED, July 2000, 343: 94-99

#19 Does This Patient Have a Torn Meniscus or Ligament of the Knee?", Solomon, D.H., Simel, D.L., Bates, D.W., et.al. JAMA, October 2001, 286: 1610-1620

#20 "Promoting Patient Safety and Preventing Medical Error in Emergency Departments", Schenkel S. ACAD EMERG MED, November 2000, 7: 1204-1222

2005 Lifelong Learning and Self Assessment Reading List

#1 "Dexamethasone in Adults with Bacterial Meningitis.", deGans, J. Van de Beek, D., N ENGL J MED, November 2002, 347:1549-1556

#2 "Computed Tomography of the Head Before Lumbar Puncture in Adults with Suspected Menigitis." Hasbun, R., Abtahams, J., Jekel, J., et.al., December 2001, 345: 1727-1733

#3 "Treatment of Acute Ischemic Stroke.", Lewandowski, C., Barsan, W., ANN EMERG MED, February 2001, 37: 202-216

#4 "Pediatric Minor Head Trauma.", Schutzman, S.A., Greenes, D.S., ANN EMERG MED, January 2001: 37: 65-74

#5 "Evaluation and Management of Febrile Seizures in the Out-of Hospital and Emergency Department Settings.", Warden, C.R., Zibulewsky, J., Mace, S., et.al., February 2003, 41: 215-222

#6 "Pharmacology of Emergency Department Pain Management and Conscious Sedation.", Blackburn, P., Vissers, R., EMERG MED CLIN N AM, November 2000, 18: 803-826

#7 "Fomepizole for the Treatment of Methanol Poisoning.", Brent, J., McMartin, K., Phillips, S., et.al., N ENGL J MED, February 2001, 244: 424-429

#8 "Management of Drug and Alcohol Withdrawal.", Kosten, T.R., O'Connor, P.G., N ENGL J MED, May 2003, 348: 1786-1794

#9 "Gamma Hydroxybutyric acid (GHB) Intoxication.", Mason, P.E., Kerns, W.P. II, ACAD EMERG MED, July 2002, 9: 730-739

#10 "Ingestion of Toxic Substances by Children.", Shannon, M., January 2000, 342: 186-191.

#11 "Vertigo and Dizziness.", Goldman, B., Tintinalli, J.E., et.al. (eds), EMERGENCY MEDICINE, A COMPREHENSIVE STUDY GUIDE, ed 5, 2000, pp 1452-1463

#12 "Syncope.". Kapoor, W.N., N ENGL J MED, December 2000, 343: 1856-1862

#13 "A Comparison of Coronary Angioplasty with Fibrinolytic Therapy in Acute Myocardial Infarction.", Andersen, H.R., Nielsen, T.T., Rasmussem, K., et.al., August 2003, 349: 733-742

#14 "Intravenous Nesiritide vs Nitroglycerin for Treatment of decompensated Congestive Heart Failure: A Randomized Controlled Trial.", Young, J.B., Publication Committee for the VMAC Investigators, JAMA, March 2002: 287: 1531-1540

#15 "Use of the Electrocardiogram in Acute Myocardial Infarction.", Zimetbaum, PJ., Josephson, M.E., N ENGL J MED, March 2003, 348: 933-940

#16 "West Nile Virus.", Petersen, L.R., Marfin, A.A., Gubler, D.J., JAMA, July 2003, 290: 524-528

#17 "Community-Acquired Pneumonia in Children.", Mettler, F.A. Jr., Voelz, G.L., N ENGL J MED, February 2002, 346: 429-436

#18 "Validation of the Ottawa Knee Rule in Children: A Multicenter Study.", Bulloch, B., Neto, G., Plint, A., et.al., ANN EMERG MED, July 2003, 42: 48-55

#19 "Laceration Management.", Hollander, J.E., Singer, A.J., ANN EMERG MED, September 1999, 3: 356-367

#20 "Principles of Emergency Department Sonography.", Melanson, S.W., Heller, M.B., Tintinalli, J.E., et.al. (eds), EMERGENCY MEDICINE, A COMPREHENSIVE STUDY GUIDE, ed. 5, 2000, pp 1972-1982

2006 Lifelong Learning and Self Assessment Reading List

#1 "Herpes Zoster.", Gnann Jr., J.W., Whitley R.J., N ENGL J MED, August 2002, 347(5): 340-346

#2 "Cellulitis." Swartz, M.N., N ENGL J MED, February 2004, 350(9): 904-912

#3 "A Decision Rule for Identifying Children at Low Risk for Brain Injuries After Blunt Head Trauma.", Palchak, M.J., Holmes, J.F., Vance, C.W., et. al., ANN EMERG MED, October 2003; 42(4): 492-506

#4 "Trauma in Pregnancy.", Shah, A.J., Kilcline, B.A., EMERG MED CLIN N AM, August 2003: 21(3): 615-629

#5 "ACEP Clinical Policy Committee, Clinical Policies Subcommittee on Acute Blunt Abdominal Trauma. Clinical Policy: Critical Issues in the Evaluation of Adult Patients Presenting to the Emergency Department with Acute Blunt Abdominal Trauma.", Shah, February 2004, 43(2): 278-290

#6 "Do Mammalian Bites Require Antibiotic Prophylaxis?", Turner T.W.S., ANN EMERG MED, September 2004, 44(3): 274-276

#7 "CRASH Trial Collaborators. Effect of intravenous corticosteroids on death within 14 days in 10008 adults with clinically significant head injury (MRC crash trial): randomized placebo-controlled trial. ", LANCET, October 2004, 364: 1321-1328

#8 "Thermal Burns", Schwartz, L.R., Balakrishnan C., Emergency Medicine, A Comprehensive Study Guide, 2004, 6th edition, pp. 1220-1226

#9 "Management of Common Dislocations", Ufberg, J. McNamara, R., Clinical Procedures in Emergency Medicine, 2004 4th edition, pp. 946-963

#10 "Acute Infectious Diarrhea.", Thielman, N.M., Guerrant R.., N ENGL J MED, January 2004, 350(1): 38-46.

#11 "A Risk Score to Predict Arrhythmias in Patients with Unexplained Syncope.", Sarasin, F.P., Hanusa, B.H., Perneger, T., Louis-Simonet M., Rajeswaram A., Kapoor, W.N., ACAD EMERG MED, December, 2003, 10 (12): 1312-1317

#12 "Women's Early Warning Symptoms of Acute Myocardial Infarction." McSweeney, J.C., Cody, M., O'Sullivan, P., Elberson, K., Moser, D.K., CIRCULATION, November 2003, 108: 2619-2623

#13 "Prognostic Value of a Normal or Nonspecific Initial Electrocardiogram in Acute Myocardial Infarction", Welch, R.D., Zalenski, R.J., Frederick P.D., et.al., JAMA, October 2001, 286(16): 1977-1984

#14 "Treatment of Deep-Vein Thrombosis", Bates, S.M., Ginsberg, J.S., N ENGL J MED, July 2004: 351(3): 268-277

#15 "Clinical Policy: Neuroimaging and Decisionmaking in Adult Mild Traumatic Brain Injury in the Acute Setting.", Jagoda, A.S., Cantrill, S.V., Wears, R.L., et.al., ANN EMERG MED, August, 2002, 40(2): 231-249

#16 "Comparison of MRI and CT for Detection of Acute Intracerebral Hemorrhage.", Kidwell, C.S., Chalela, J.A., Saver, J.L. et.al., JAMA, October 2004, 292(15): 1823-1830

#17 "Evaluation of Vaginal Complaints.", Anderson, M.R., Klink, K., Cohrssen, A., JAMA, March 2004, 291(11): 1368-1379

#18 "A Randomized Trial of a Single Dose of Oral Dexamethasone for Mild Croup.", Bjornson, C.L., Klassen, T.P., Williamson, J. et.al., N ENGL J MED, September 2004, 351(13): 1306-1313

#19 "Sterile Versus Nonsterile Gloves for Repair of Uncomplicated Lacerations in the Emergency Department: A Randomized Controlled Trial.", Perelman, V.S., Francis, G.J, Rutledge, T., Foote, J., Martino F., Dranitsaris, G., ANN EMERG MED, March 2004, 43(3): 362-370

#20 "Doctors and Drug Companies.", Blumenthal D., N ENGL J MED, October, 2004, 351(18): 1885-1890

INDEX

X

Y

Z